The Complete Guide
to Aromatherapy

The
Complete Guide
to
Aromatherapy

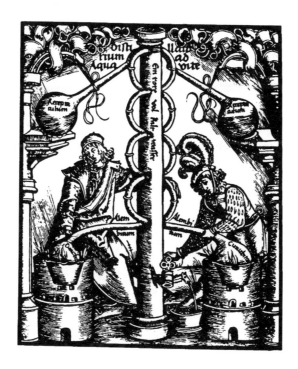

Salvatore Battaglia

Published by

The Perfect Potion (Aust) Pty Ltd

First published in Australia 1995 by

The Perfect Potion
1/15 Virginia Street
Virginia Q. 4014

Second print: 1997

ISBN 0 646 20670 2

Typeset by Page People Pty Ltd, Noosa, Queensland, Australia.

Printed in Australia by Watson Ferguson and Co., Brisbane

About the Author

Salvatore Battaglia is widely recognised as a leading specialist in the field of aromatherapy. He is a qualified acupuncturist and aromatherapist, trained under the world-renowned Madame Micheline Arcier in London, and is responsible for the development of the products at The Perfect Potion.

He conducts both practitioner training and introductory training on aromatherapy, is often called upon to lecture special interest groups and has been a guest speaker on various radio programs. He is a member of the International Federation of Aromatherapists.

Salvatore is the author of *The Enchanting Art of Aromatherapy* and co-editor of the *Aromatherapy Today Journal*.

PLEASE NOTE

This book is concerned with the use of essential oils and natural remedies for a wide range of health issues. Many health issues can have unpredictable effects and it is the author's advice that the best possible expertise should always be consulted.

The author and the publisher, therefore, cannot accept any responsibility for any mishap resulting from the use of any remedy or therapeutic method described in this book.

CONTENTS IN BRIEF

Acknowledgements xvi
Foreword xvii
How to use this book xix

UNIT I BACKGROUND   1
Chapter 1 Introduction to Aromatherapy 3
Chapter 2 History of Aromatherapy 13
Chapter 3 What Are Essential Oils? 23
Chapter 4 Methods of Essential Oil Extraction 29
Chapter 5 Quality Control and Assurance 41

UNIT II ESSENTIAL ISSUES   59
Chapter 6 Research 61
Chapter 7 Essential Oil Chemistry 69
Chapter 8 Pharmacology of Essential Oils 87
Chapter 9 The Biology and Psychology of Essential Oils 99
Chapter 10 Pharmacokinetics 109
Chapter 11 Essential Oil Safety 121

UNIT III THE REMEDIES   137
Chapter 12 The Essential Oils 139
Chapter 13 Carrier Oils 209
Chapter 14 Hazardous Essential Oils 231

UNIT IV PRACTICAL MATTERS   245
Chapter 15 Requirements for Professional Practice 247
Chapter 16 The Consultation 253
Chapter 17 Guidelines to Prescribing 261
Chapter 18 Methods of Administration 271
Chapter 19 The Aromatherapy Massage 277

UNIT V CLINICAL INDEX   289
Chapter 20 Circulatory System 291
Chapter 21 Respiratory System 301
Chapter 22 Musculoskeletal System 313
Chapter 23 Reproductive System 327
Chapter 24 Integumentary System 345
Chapter 25 Nervous System 355
Chapter 26 Lymphatic System 373
Chapter 27 Immune System 383
Chapter 28 Digestive System 403
Chapter 29 Aromatherapy Skin Care 415

APPENDICES AND OTHER INFORMATION
Appendix 1 Glossary 427
Appendix 2 List of Properties 429
Appendix 3 Therapeutic Cross Reference 431
Appendix 4 List of Essential Oils 433
Appendix 5 Acupressure 437
Appendix 6 Useful Addresses 438
References, Bibliography and Indexes: 440

CONTENTS IN DETAIL

UNIT I BACKGROUND 1

1. Introduction to Aromatherapy . . . 3

Defining aromatherapy 4
Holistic aromatherapy 4
The popularity of aromatherapy 5
Aromatherapy as a healing art 7
    The pharmacology of the essential oils 7
    The massage 8
    The therapist/client relationship 8
    The complexity of illness and ill health 9
    Olfaction 9
Medical aromatherapy 10
Aromatherapy and herbalism 10
Conclusion 11

2. History of Aromatherapy 13

Introduction 14
Ancient civilizations 14
    Egypt 14
    Greece 14
    China and India 15
    The Middle East 15
The Middle Ages 17
The scientific revolution 20

3. What Are Essential Oils? 23

Introduction 24
Origin of essential oils 25
    Photosynthesis 25
Biological activity of the essential oils . . . 26
Factors affecting the essential oils 26
    Ecological variables 27
    Harvesting time 27
    Genetics 27
    Chemotype 28
    Overview 28

4. Methods of Essential Oil Extraction 29

Introduction 30
Expression processes 30
    The sponge process 30
    The écuelle à piquer process 31
    Machine abrasion 31
Distillation processes 32
    Principles of distillation 32
    Water distillation 32
    Steam distillation 33
    Water and steam distillation 34
    Fractional distillation 34
    Hydro-Diffusion 35
Solvent extraction processes 35
    Solvent extraction 36
    Enfleurage 37
    Hypercritical carbon dioxide extraction 38

5. Quality Control and Assurance . 41

Introduction 42
The botanical name 42
    Chamomile 42
    Juniper and cedarwood 43
    Lavender 44
    Marjoram 45
    Pine 46
    Sage 46
    Sandalwood 46
    Thyme 48
The part of plant used 49
    Bitter orange 49
    Clove 49
    Cinnamon 49
    Lime 49
The country of origin 50
    Basil 50
    Rosemary 51
Specifying the extraction method 51
    Lavender 51
    Ylang-ylang 52
Testing the purity of the essential oil . . . 52
    Odour evaluation 53

Physical measures	53
Chemical analysis	54
Adulteration of essential oils	**55**
Other oils or their constituents	55
Its own main constituent	55
A reconstituted oil	55
A pure aroma chemical	55
Conclusion - adulteration	56
Natural versus synthetic	**57**

UNIT II ESSENTIAL ISSUES 59

6. Research 61

Introduction	**62**
For the public good	**62**
Towards an aromatherapy research policy	**63**
Defining the stages of a clinical trial	63
Aims of a clinical trial	63
Asking the right questions	63
Types of clinical trials	63
Background to the clinical trial	64
Patient selection	64
Randomised trial groups	64
Problems in pursuing good clinical research	65
Single case study research	65
Evaluation of patient response	65
Pharmacological and pharmacokinetic research	66
Experimental research	67
Ethical considerations	67
Conclusion	**68**

7. Essential Oil Chemistry 69

Introduction to organic chemistry	**70**
Sources of organic compounds	**70**
Structure of organic compounds	**70**
Isomers	71
Nomenclature	**73**
The chemistry of common essential oil constituents	**73**
Monoterpene hydrocarbons	74
Sesquiterpenes	76
Functional groups	77
Phenols	78

Alcohols	79
Aldehydes	81
Ketones	82
Esters	83
Lactones and coumarins	84
Ethers and oxides	84

8. Pharmacology of Essential Oils 87

Introduction	**88**
Defining pharmacology	**88**
How aromatherapy works	**89**
Properties of essential oils	**90**
Alterative effect	90
Anti-inflammatory effect	91
Antibacterial and antifungal effect	91
Astringent effect	93
Carminative effect	94
Diaphoretic effect	94
Diuretic effect	94
Emmenagogue effect	95
Expectorant effect	95
Granulation stimulating effect	96
Nervine effect	97
Rubefacient effect	97
Sedative effect	97
Spasmolytic effect	97
Tonic and stimulant effect	98

9. The Biology and Psychology of Essential Oils 99

Introduction	**100**
The physiology of smell	**100**
Olfaction	100
The physiology of olfaction	100
Olfaction and the brain	102
The psychology of smell	**102**
Introduction	102
Historical background	103
Psycho-aromatherapy	103
Emotion and olfaction	104
Psychophysiological effects of odour	105

10. Pharmacokinetics 109

Introduction 110
Absorption 110
    Dermal 110
    Inhalation 116
    Oral 116
    Rectal 116
Distribution 117
Metabolism 118
    Liver metabolism 118
Excretion 119
Conclusion 119

11. Essential Oil Safety 121

Introduction 122
Quality 122
    Contamination and adulteration 122
    Degradation 122
Packaging and labelling 123
Chemical composition 123
    Essential oils with ketone constituents 124
    Essential oils with phenol constituents 124
Essential oil hazards 125
    Toxicity 125
    Skin reactions 127
    Carcinogenesis 129
    Neurotoxicity 130
    Hepatotoxicity 132
    Hazards during pregnancy 132
General rules 134
Dosage and dilutions 134
Summary of contraindications 136

UNIT III THE REMEDIES 137

12. The Essential Oils 139

Introduction 140
Angelica Root 140
Aniseed 141
Basil 142
Bay 144

Bergamot 145
Black Pepper 146
Cajeput 147
Cardamom 148
Carrot Seed 148
Cedarwood, Atlas 149
Cedarwood, Virginian 150
Chamomile, German 151
Chamomile, Roman 152
Cinnamon 154
Citronella 155
Clary Sage 155
Clove 157
Cypress 158
Eucalyptus Leaf Oils 159
Everlasting 162
Fennel 163
Fir Needle 164
Frankincense 165
Geranium 166
Ginger 167
Grapefruit 167
Hyssop 168
Jasmine 169
Juniper 170
Lavender 171
Lavender, Spike 173
Lemon 174
Lemongrass 175
Lime 176
Mandarin 177
Marjoram, Sweet 178
Marjoram, Spanish 179
May Chang 180
Melissa 180
Myrrh 182
Myrtle 183
Neroli 184
Niaouli 185
Nutmeg 185

Orange, sweet 187
Palmarosa 187
Patchouli 188
Peppermint 189
Petitgrain 190
Pine 191
Rock rose 192
Rose 193
Rosemary 195
Rosewood 197
Sage 197
Sage, Spanish 198
Sandalwood 199
Spearmint 200
Tangerine 201
Tea Tree 202
Thyme 203
Vetiver 205
Yarrow 206
Ylang-ylang 207

13. Carrier Oils **209**

Introduction 210
Fatty acids 210
  Function of fatty acids 211
  Saturated fatty acids 211
  Unsaturated fatty acids 211
  Essential fatty acids 212
  Cholesterol 215
  Modified oils 216
How are vegetable oils extracted? 217
  Unrefined oil production stage 217
  Commercial refining process stage . . . 219
  What are cold pressed oils? 219
Commonly used vegetable oils 220
  Sweet almond oil 220
  Apricot kernel oil 220
  Avocado oil 221
  Canola oil 221
  Evening primrose oil 221
  Joboba oil 224
  Linseed oil 224
  Macadamia oil 225

Olive oil 225
Pumpkin seed oil 226
Rosehip oil 226
Safflower oil 226
Sesame seed oil 226
Soyabean oil 227
Sunflower oil 227
Wheatgerm oil 227
Macerated oils 228
  Arnica 228
  Calendula 228
  Carrot 229
  Hypericum 229

14. Hazardous Essential Oils **231**

Introduction 232
Ajowan 232
Almond, bitter 232
Boldo 233
Buchu 233
Calamus 233
Camphor 234
Cassia 235
Cinnamon Bark 235
Clove 235
Costus 236
Elecampane 236
Horseradish 236
Mugwort 237
Mustard 237
Oregano 238
Parsleyseed 238
Pennyroyal 238
Rue 239
Sassafras 240
Savin 240
Savory (winter & summer) 240
Tansy 241
Thuja 241
Wintergreen 242
Wormseed 242
Wormwood 242

UNIT IV PRACTICAL MATTERS 245

15. Requirements for Professional Practice 247

Introduction 248
Professionalism 248
The role of the aromatherapist 248
Professional ethics 249
Counselling skills 249
Personal hygiene and health 250
Setting up a clinic 250
Equipment and products 251
Sanitary and safety practices 252

16. The Consultation 253

Introduction 254
Introduction to the client 254
Explaining procedures and policies . . . 254
Assessment 254
    Inquiring 256
    Physical examination 257
Developing a treatment plan 257
Client files 258
Case history 258
Education of the client 258
    Understanding 259
    Motivation 259
    Discipline 259

17. Guidelines to Prescribing . . . 261

Introduction 262
Essential oil selection 262
    The physiological condition 262
    The psychological condition 263
    The practical availability of the essential oil . . . 266
Duration and frequency 266
Dosage 266
How the essential oils are used 267
Blending 268
    Enhancing 268

    Classical blending techniques 268
    Balancing 269

18. Methods of Administration . . . 271

Introduction 272
Massage 272
Inhalation 272
Bath 273
    Foot and hand baths 273
    Full bath 273
    Sitz bath 274
Compresses 274
    Hot compress 274
    Cold compress 274
    Warm and cold compresses 274
Douches 275
Ointments 275
Creams and lotions 275
Internal use of essential oils 276

19. The Aromatherapy Massage . . 277

Introduction 278
    Swedish massage 278
    Neuromuscular massage 278
    Lymphatic massage 279
    Acupressure massage and shiatsu 279
    Reflexology 279
    Polarity therapy 279
The autonomic nervous system 280
Aromatherapy massage guidelines 280
Aromatherapy massage contraindications . 280
Aromatherapy massage 282

UNIT V CLINICAL INDEX 289

20. Circulatory System 291

Introduction 292
General considerations 292
    Exercise 292
    Diet 292
    Tobacco and alcohol 293
    Stress 293

Aromatherapy considerations 293
Associated conditions 294
    Chilblains 294
    Hypertension 294
    Oedema 296
    Palpitations 297
    Varicose veins 297

21. Respiratory System 301

Introduction 302
General considerations 303
Aromatherapy considerations 303
Associated conditions 304
    Asthma 304
    Bronchitis 307
    Catarrh 308
    Coughs 309
    Hayfever 309
    Sinusitis 310
    Sore throat 311
    Tonsillitis 312

22. Musculoskeletal System 313

Introduction 314
Aromatherapy considerations 314
Associated conditions 315
    Arthritis 315
    Backaches 319
    Bruises 320
    Bunions 321
    Bursitis 321
    Cramps 322
    Gout 322
    Sciatica 323
    Sports injuries 324

23. Reproductive System 327

Introduction 328
Aromatherapy considerations 328
Associated conditions 329
    Pregnancy 329
    Menstrual problems 334
    Menopause 338
    Endometriosis 339

    Thrush 341
    Cystitis 342

24. Integumentary System 345

Introduction 346
General considerations 346
Aromatherapy considerations 346
Associated conditions 347
    Boils and carbuncles 347
    Acne 348
    Dermatitis 349
    Herpes simplex 350
    Psoriasis 351
    Sunburn 353

25. Nervous System 355

Introduction 356
General considerations 357
Aromatherapy considerations 358
Associated conditions 359
Psychological disorders 359
    Stress 359
    Anxiety 362
    Depression 363
    Insomnia 365
    Mental fatigue 366
Neurological disorders 368
    Headaches 368
    Migraines 369
    Epilepsy 370
    Shingles 372

26. Lymphatic System 373

Introduction 374
Structure of the lymphatic system 374
The functions of the lymphatic system . . 375
The effects of poor lymphatic performance 376
How aromatherapy can assist lymphatic
problems 376
Other considerations 377
Cellulite 378
Lymphoedema 381

27. Immune System **383**

Introduction 384
    Viruses 384
    Bacteria 386
    Fungi 387
    Parasites 388
The organisation of defence 388
    Non-specific resistance 389
    Specific resistance: immunity 389
Immunity and the mind 392
When immunity fails 393
    Infection 393
    Tissue inflammation 395
    Fever 396
    Allergies 398
    Candida 400
    Chronic fatigue syndrome (CFS) 401

28. Digestive System **403**

Introduction 404
General considerations 405
Aromatherapy considerations 405
Associated conditions 406
    Irritable bowel syndrome 406
    Constipation 407
    Diarrhoea 409
    Dyspepsia 410
    Flatulence 412
    Nausea and vomiting 413

29. Aromatherapy Skin Care . . . **415**

Introduction 416
Skin structure 416
    Epidermis 416
    Dermis 416
    Hypodermis 418
The skin's functions 418

Skin types 418
    Dry skin 419
    Oily skin 419
    Normal skin 420
    Combination skin 420
    Sensitive skin 420
    Mature skin 421
The effect of essential oils 421
Aromatherapy skin care 424
    Cleansing 424
    Toning 425
    Moisturising 425

APPENDICES AND OTHER INFORMATION

1. Glossary **427**

2. List of Properties **429**

3. Therapeutic Cross Reference . . **431**

4. List of Essential Oils **433**

5. Acupressure **437**

6. Useful Addresses **438**

References **440**

Bibliography **466**

Botanical Index **468**

General Index **470**

Acknowledgements

This book was born of a need to provide a complete aromatherapy training manual for people wishing to have a thorough understanding of aromatherapy. Without these people including all my past students this book would not have been possible.

It has taken me 5 years part-time to complete this book and I have drawn on many sources of information in writing it. I am grateful for all the sources of information referenced throughout the book. The sources of information for this book include:

- text books which have outlined the principles of anatomy and physiology, aromatherapy, perfumery, physiology, nutrition as well as medicine
- technical books and journals on aromatherapy, essential oils, holistic health and medicine
- personal accounts of others, and,
- my own experiences.

I gratefully acknowledge the efforts and contribution that many researchers, therapists and clinicians have made to aromatherapy. This includes people such as Robert Tisserand who has done so much to promote the professionalism of aromatherapy and who organises the International Aroma Conferences in the UK which have for me been sources of immense inspiration.

I am also indebted to the following people:

All my teachers and people who have inspired me to pursue my career in natural healing and aromatherapy. In particular Jan Jedryka who introduced me to natural therapies, and made me realise that this was exactly what I had been looking for. I am also grateful to have had the opportunity to train with Madame Micheline Arcier, a person whose dedication and commitment to aromatherapy has taught me humility and respect. She has always been a major source of my inspiration.

Simon Sparkes at Soyatech for all his expertise in the field of vegetable oils and for providing typical fatty acid profiles of each cold pressed vegetable oil.

In terms of the presentation of this book, Kevin Long, of Page People Pty Ltd, has done an outstanding job with the typesetting, design and layout of this book. Vic McKay has done a magnificent job of proof-reading in preparation for the second printing.

The staff at The Perfect Potion, for their support and dedication in ensuring the business ran smoothly while I have buried my head in the computer while writing this book.

I would like to thank Ruth Zorde, Melinda Smith and Shantal Walker for many of the illustrations.

The photograph on page 25 has been reproduced, with the kind permission of the publisher, from the book *Eucalyptus leaf oils: use, chemistry, distillation and marketing,* 1991, edited by D.J. Boland, J.J. Brophy and A.P.N. House, ACIAR/CSIRO Canberra, published by Inkata Press.

I would also like to thank all my friends and family who have also been encouraging, and last but not least my wife Carolyn, for her constant support and encouragement.

Foreword

The booksellers' shelves are crammed with aromatherapy books. Much of the information is usually recycled from earlier English or French texts. While books such as *The Art of Aromatherapy* by Robert Tisserand and Tricia Davis's book, *Aromatherapy an A-Z* have become classics and are useful reference books, the majority of books on aromatherapy are not as useful as one would wish. They provide an entertaining series of recipes and often misguided information, sometimes making unsubstantiated claims.

This makes it difficult for the modern holistic aromatherapist who needs to be a multi-disciplined practitioner with training in remedial therapies, counselling, chemistry, botany, pharmacology, anatomy, physiology and pathophysiology.

The Complete Guide to Aromatherapy addresses all the topics listed above. This is the first time a book on aromatherapy has been aimed specifically at people with a serious interest in aromatherapy and the health professional working in the field of aromatherapy. While this book covers in detail both theoretical and practical aspects of aromatherapy, I have ensured that it remains true to the main principles of holistic healing which embraces three basic concepts:

- a holistic approach to health which treats the patient as an individual;
- the wisdom of the past and the validity of traditional empirical knowledge; and
- the analytical back-up provided by modern pharmacology and biochemistry.

I believe that the future of aromatherapy as a powerful, safe and effective form of natural healing is embodied in terms of the issues that I have raised in this book and I therefore hope that this book can contribute to the achievement of that future.

Salvatore Battaglia
1995

How to Use this Book

This book is a comprehensive and practical guide to aromatherapy. It will provide all the information needed to enhance your skills and knowledge of aromatherapy. However, the book is not intended to replace formal aromatherapy training for those interested in pursuing a career in aromatherapy. For information regarding aromatherapy training please refer to Appendix 6, which lists the organisations which will advise you of the recommended teaching institutions.

The book is divided into five units:

Unit I: Background

*   A general introduction to the principles of wellbeing and wholistic health which are fundamental to the successful practice of aromatherapy.
*   The changing role of essential oils throughout history, from the ritual uses in ancient civilisations, through medieval alchemy, to modern day applications in aromatherapy.
*   The nature and characteristics of the essential oils, how they are extracted and quality control and assurance guidelines.

Unit II: Essential issues

*   Latest research and clinical trials in aromatherapy.
*   Chemical composition of the essential oils.
*   Pharmacological activity of the essential oils.
*   Psychological influence of essential oils.
*   How the essential oils are absorbed into the body.

Unit III: The remedies

*   Monographs of all the commonly available essential oils and carrier oils used in aromatherapy; including definition of botanical name, country of origin, traditional uses, essential oil constituents, properties, blending, indications, practical uses and safety.

Unit IV: Practical matters

*   The knowledge and skills required for the practice of aromatherapy:
    -   The requirements for setting up professional practice
    -   The aromatherapy consultation which allows us to assess the client's medical and social background, and helps us determine what kind of treatment should be given and which oils should be used.
    -   The aromatherapy massage.
    -   The necessary knowledge to select the appropriate essential oils.

Unit V: Clinical index

*   A clear and detailed guide to the treatment of a wide range of conditions. Each condition is listed with a description of cause and symptoms and followed by the recommended treatment - the essential oils used, their application, as well as suggestions with regards to diet, herbs, acupressure and additional therapies.

UNIT I

BACKGROUND

This unit is designed to provide the therapist with the basic knowledge of aromatherapy. We outline the history of aromatherapy, we discuss factors relating to health and well-being and identify the role of aromatherapy in healing. The methods by which essential oils are extracted are outlined and the factors that determine the quality of essential oils are identified.

Unit I includes the following chapters:

Chapter 1. Introduction to Aromatherapy

Chapter 2. History of Aromatherapy

Chapter 3. What Are Essential Oils?

Chapter 4. Methods of Essential Oil Extraction

Chapter 5. Quality Control and Quality Assurance

Chapter 1

Introduction to Aromatherapy

Natural therapies have become popular with a large segment
of the community.
Aromatherapy has emerged as one of the most popular
natural therapy modalities.
This chapter discusses what aromatherapy is, how it can be
used and investigates many of the factors that have
contributed to aromatherapy's popularity.

Defining aromatherapy

In order to begin any discussion on aromatherapy, the term 'aromatherapy' needs to be defined. It has definitely become a very popular word, however what do people mean when they use the term? It has been the failure to clearly define the term that has led to a misunderstanding and abuse of the term 'aromatherapy'. There is no doubt that the use of the term has given commercial advantage as the therapeutic implication of aromatherapy has been used to provide credibility for frivolous products. The English word 'aromatherapy' is derived from the French word 'aromatherapie' which was first coined by French chemist Gattefosse.

Whilst I do not agree with Professor Gerard Buchbauer's semantic objection to the term aromatherapy (1), I do agree that the term often implies the therapeutic use of fragrances by inhalation only. Buchbauer suggests that since aromatherapists predominantly use essential oils by other means, that more suitable names could be 'essence therapy' or 'essential oil therapy'.

However Jan Kusmirek (2) suggests:

'The word aromatherapy has a nice sound, it flows and fits the essence of the ideas it is representing'.

I believe that the blatant misrepresentation of the term has been detrimental to aromatherapy as a true form of healing as it has made licensing of genuine essential oils for use in aromatherapy more difficult. It has also led to a state of confusion for the public and for government legislators. The public may often assume that the use of the term aromatherapy has therapeutic implications and government legislators are trying to protect the public from danger that may be associated with the use of essential oils.

This is evident in Australia, where the current belief among government legislators is that all essential oils, regardless of purpose should be scheduled as poisons. This action I feel is totally unwarranted simply because the majority of the essential oils are not poisons but are very safe to use. (Please refer to Chapter 11 for a detailed discussion on essential oil safety).

While I do not wish to see the practice of aromatherapy or use of essential oils regulated by government bureaucrats, I feel that it is important that the aromatherapy industry (essential oil manufacturers, distributors, educators and practitioners) set standards which clearly prevent any misrepresentation of the word.

The broad definition of aromatherapy as defined by Jan Kusmirek (2) is:

'The use of pure essential oils to seek to influence, to change or modify, mind, body or spirit; physiology or mood.'

This statement may encompass the use of essential oils in perfumery, cosmetics, medicine both orthodox and alternative, psychotherapy, aromacology or science. Whilst it is clear that aromatherapy exists in these many forms, the focus of this book will be on what I will now define as holistic aromatherapy.

Holistic aromatherapy

We talk about aromatherapy as if we know exactly what we are referring to - but do we?

We find medical doctors in France treating chronic infections using aromatherapy and at the same time we find 'aromatherapy' being offered in beauty salons. Are the beauty salons offering the same treatment as the doctors in France?

It is about time we realised the complexity of aromatherapy. While we can remain true to our own concept of aromatherapy, we should also be exploring other aspects of aromatherapy and respect our colleagues who have different approaches.

Essential oils are often used by:

- aromatherapists
- medical practitioners
- nurses
- counsellors and psychologists
- massage therapists
- medical herbalists
- natural therapists
- beauty therapists
- perfumers.

In each of the above occupations, essential oils are used in quite different ways and for different purposes. Is there one 'aromatherapy' which incorporates all of the above? If there were, it would be the real holistic aromatherapy.

Ideally, holistic aromatherapy should incorporate:

- the pharmacological
- the psychotherapeutic
- the metaphysical

activities of the essential oils.

As more research is conducted in many of the aspects of aromatherapy, an integration of the varied aspects of aromatherapy will occur.

The popularity of aromatherapy

Fewer than 20 years ago most people outside of France had not heard of aromatherapy, even though the use of essential oils for healing had existed for some 5000 years. We often talk about how old aromatherapy is, and of course it does have very ancient origins. However it is perhaps surprising to find that one of the first books written on aromatherapy, *Aromatherapie*, was written in 1937 by Gattefosse. This book was translated into English only in 1993.

There was no book of aromatherapy published in the English language until *The Art of Aromatherapy*, written by Robert Tisserand, was released in 1977. In the 40 years that followed Gattefosse's publication only four books on the subject were published. However, in England over 40 books about aromatherapy have been published since 1988. (3)

The interest in aromatherapy has perhaps surprised even aromatherapists. The reasons for the resurgence in traditional therapies such as aromatherapy are many. I believe that this is because aromatherapy works on a holistic level, addressing the:

- body
- mind
- soul.

Often the main benefits of an aromatherapy treatment come from the pleasant smells of the essential oils, which have a predominantly psychological effect. The essential oils are usually administered by massage, in an oil vaporiser or added to baths. Used in these ways, essential oils add a sense of luxury to the treatment and have a relaxing effect.

Many people view natural therapies such as aromatherapy as 'magic potions'. You cannot just 'zap' people with the essential oils and expect them to get better overnight. It's to do with having somebody to talk to, somebody who can listen and respond to you, it's about having a hands-on treatment. There is more to holistic aromatherapy than essential oils and massage - it is a healing process.

Aromatherapy is popular because it makes use of two close range senses; those of touch and smell. It is a very pleasant therapy, with powerful medicinal applications. Some essential oils have powerful anti-bacterial properties, rivalling antibiotic drugs in their effectiveness. Other essential oils have psychotherapeutic

Aromatherapie	R.M. Gattefosse	1937
Les Produits Aromatiques Utilises en Pharmacie	A. Couveur	1939
Le Capital Jeunesse	M.Maury	1961
Die Physiologischen and Pharmakologischen Wirkungen der Atherischen Ole, Reichstoffe und Verwandten Produkte	A. Muller	1964
The Art of Aromatherapy	R. Tisserand	1977

The first aromatherapy books published (3)

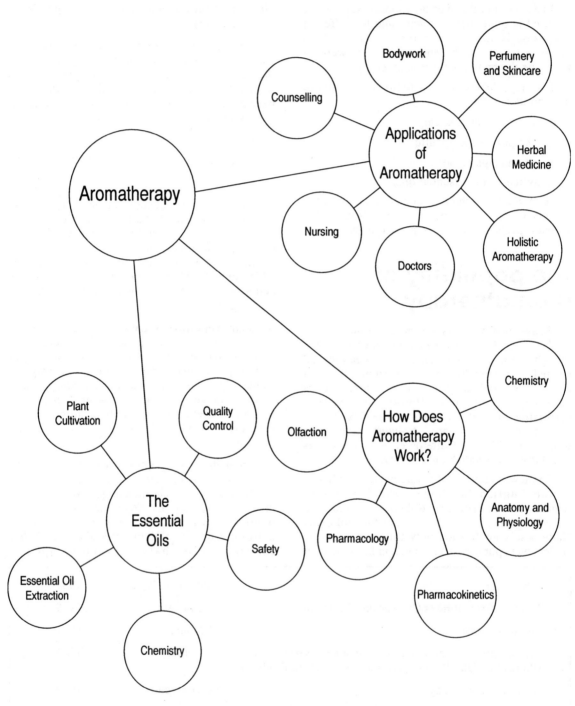

This diagram illustrates the different aspects of aromatherapy

applications, relieving stress, depression, insomnia and pre-menstrual syndrome.

The popularity of aromatherapy will continue to increase as more and more proof emerges of its real clinical value. Many people express nothing less than sheer delight at the way in which their treatment has cured problems not previously improved by conventional medical treatments.

Aromatherapy as a healing art

The scientific revolution and the subsequent professionalisation of medicine has been responsible for splitting up the components of healing. Modern medicine has been relegated to the role of being just another tool or technique for the physician to offer as part of the general service of limited treatment for specific, isolated ailments. The formalisation of scientific experimentation took medicine out of the hands of ordinary people.

When I speak to clients who come in for an aromatherapy treatment, I always ask them why they have been drawn to aromatherapy. This usually turns out to be a difficult question to answer, but all are drawn to its multifaceted nature, its combination of natural, fragrant essential oils, practical hands-on skills, and its humanistic, caring approach.

The real significance of aromatherapy is in using these elements in a holistic manner. A large number of 'natural therapies' claim to be holistic in that they aim to treat the whole person, but the process of the treatment remains prescriptive.

The distinctive strength of holistic aromatherapy as a healing art is dependent upon:

*   the pharmacology of the essential oils

*   the massage

*   the therapist/client relationship

*   realisation of the complexity of the problem of illness and ill health

*   olfaction.

The pharmacology of the essential oils

The natural chemical complexity of essential oils derived from plants makes them an ideal form of pharmacological therapy. The synergies of essential oil constituents in their natural state are easily adapted to human physiology and, when safely and well-prescribed, are free from undesirable side effects. While the essential oils carry a vital life force which assists their activity, the use of essential oils in aromatherapy must also be pharmacologically sound. Pharmacology describes the essential oils in objective, measurable and quantitative terms only.

Many pharmacological studies dealing with essential oils have been conducted using individual essential oil constituents rather than the complete essential oil. In this process there is an inherent mistake in assuming if substance X is pharmacologically active on its own, that when blended with substances Y and Z, it will continue to have similar pharmacological activities. This has clearly been demonstrated not to be the case with the antibacterial properties of lemongrass which were found to be the synergystic effect of the sum of its constituents rather than the effect of a single constituent.

'While the geranial and neral components individually elicit anti-bacterial action on gram-negative and gram-positive organisms, the third component, myrcene did not show observable anti-bacterial activity on its own. However, myrcene provided enhanced activities when mixed with either of the two main components....' (4)

Therefore any attempt to study the pharmacological interaction of the essential oils needs to consider:

*   the individual chemical constituents

*   the traditional known actions of the essential oils.

While the essential oils may have drug-like effects on the mind and body, they differ greatly from drugs because of their:

*   chemical complexity

*   synergy

*   multifaceted actions

- reduced side effects
- subtle and gentle activity.

The massage

The effect of touch clearly has a profound psychological and physical impact. Massage is possibly the only situation in which we can be touched in a caring way by someone who is not close to us, and not feel uncomfortable.

'Touch is a basic behavioural need, in much the same way as breathing is a basic physical need. When the need for touch remains unsatisfied abnormal behaviour will result.' (5)

Babies will distinguish by movements and feeding behaviour between a stranger and their mother. Premature babies held in a sling between the mother's breasts have improved growth compared with incubator managed babies.

In animal experiments, deprivation of contact at this early stage is associated with failure to thrive, and slowing of development with neuro-anatomical brain changes. It should be no surprise that early deprivation in humans leads to neuropsychological disturbances.

Dr James Prescot (6), an American neuropsychologist states:

'The absence or withdrawal of physical affection in early life, and even as an adult, may be responsible for many types of disturbed behaviour such as depression, violence, aggression and hyperactivity.'

Hooper (7) states:

'In one hospital, disturbed teenagers go through an intensive course of physical treatment, learning to appreciate the significance of touching and being touched. Since this kind of therapy has been introduced, violence at the hospital has noticeably abated.'

The physical benefits of massage are also comprehensive. It stimulates the circulation of blood and lymph, reduces high blood pressure, stimulates the immune system, reduces muscular tension, and relieves pain in muscles and joints.

The healing process in massage has often been underrated. I feel that massage is one of the truly preventative holistic therapies, as it is able to effectively induce a state of relaxation by easing muscular tension. Not only is muscular tension

directly related to physical pain, but often it relates to psychological tension and repressed emotions. The act of soothing the physical tension has a reflex effect on psychological tension.

Massage can alleviate stress and by doing so can enable patients to utilise their own healing energies. Massage has already been incorporated into the standard treatment of some hospitals to relieve muscular tension, promote sleeping, relieve pain, reduce high blood pressure, and for its comforting effect.

Field (8) discussed the benefits of using massage to reduce anxiety in children and adolescent psychiatric patients:

'Fifty two children and adolescents hospitalised for depression or adjustment disorder participated in this study, receiving a thirty minute back massage daily for five days. Self and staff reports of anxiety and depression, behavioural observations, saliva and urine samples, and time-lapse video of night sleep sessions were included in the assessment protocol.

When compared to the control group who watched relaxing video tapes, the massage group were less depressed and anxious, and had lower salivary cortisol levels. Their night sleep improved and the staff reported them as being more cooperative and less anxious. Those subjects who were depressed also demonstrated a reduction in urinary cortisol and norepinephrine levels, indicating the longer term effects were more pronounced for the depressed patients than the adjustment disorder patients.'

The therapist/client relationship

People are increasingly dissatisfied with having had their responsibility and involvement in their own treatment and healing taken away. Conventional medicine is totally prescriptive and excludes patients from an understanding of their own conditions. This has led to the development of a major gap between therapist and client, and has meant that people are looking to natural therapies, which consider physical, emotional and psychological aspects of wellbeing.

Bell (9) discussed the growing number of doctors who are turning to alternative therapies because modern medicine is only concerned with getting rid of disease and does not deal with wellbeing.

The empathy of the therapist is an important ingredient in the success of a treatment. A trial with pain killers and dental pain showed that identical tablets had widely differing effects when one group was given the tablets impersonally, and the other had a smiling nurse who briefly touched each patient's shoulder and expressed care. If such brief interventions are of value, the influence of personality of the individual administering the treatment is enormous.

It is important that the therapist be balanced. In particular the therapist needs to be able to come to terms with the dangers of eroticism, and feelings of anxiety when faced with advanced disease.

Dr Sapira (10) believes that confidence in the physician is of the utmost importance both for the wellbeing of the patient and for the doctor's success. Confidence, he explains is first gained through the impression created by the physician during the interview and physical examination.

'A physician should appear to be pleased to see the patient; to think nothing but the complaint; to be sympathetic and understanding; to be confident of effecting a cure, and if not, to take a cheerful note and inspire hope; to feel privileged to treat the patient; to be courteous and considerate; and be glad to take the time to hear the patient's problems.'

Many patients of aromatherapy may have experienced both physical and verbal isolation and the contact with a caring practitioner will itself be therapeutic. A truly holistic approach acknowledges that the therapist and the client each plays an essential part in the healing process.

The complexity of illness and ill health

There has been a growing realisation of the inherent complexity of the problem of illness and ill health - moving away from the orthodox approach of separating the ailments and symptoms towards an acknowledgment that these symptoms commonly result from inherent imbalances within the person as a whole.

According to Professor Alan Husband (11) there is now considerable anecdotal evidence that immunity and resistance to disease are linked to attitude and behaviour. Dr Anslie Meares (12) had for many years suggested that positive thinking and imagery are useful in the treatment of cancer.

Dr Andrew Malleson in *'Need your Doctor be so Useless?'* says (13):

'Roughly one third of all patients with physical illness said that they felt better after being given a completely inert substance. Modern science has traditionally sought to exclude the placebo effect from its considerations and dismissed the results. The common notion was that anyone gullible enough to react to a sugar pill as if they had been given an active chemical was an unstable, weak-minded hysteric overly concerned with body health. However according to studies by Dr Gordon Claridge, author of 'Drugs and Human Behaviour' this is untrue.'

The concept of health today has come to mean a lot more than just a lack of disease or infection at a purely physical level. Rather it is based on a notion of physical, emotional and psychological wellbeing and an ability to cope positively with a variety of pressures and stresses placed on us by our modern lifestyle and expectations.

In conclusion Dr Bach (14) best summarises our discussion:

'As long as our souls and personalities are in harmony, all is joy and peace, happiness and health. It is when our personalities are led astray from the path laid down by the soul, either by our worldly desires or the persuasion of others, that conflict arises. This confict is the root cause of disease and unhappiness.'

Olfaction

'The best recipe for health is to apply sweet scents unto the brain.'

Alexis (15)

The effect of smell alone has a powerful influence on the central nervous system. Fragrance researchers are discovering that odours can and do influence mood, evoke emotions, counteract stress and reduce high blood pressure. To explain how essential oils can affect us in this way we must explore the connection between the sense of smell and the brain.

Smell is the only sense in which the receptor nerve endings are in direct contact with the outside world. It is also interesting to know that the olfactory nerve cells are the only type of nerve cell in the body which can repair themselves if damaged.

The blood-brain barrier must also be considered. The walls of the tiny capillaries that carry blood around the brain are very selective. Although tiny nutrient and oxygen molecules can pass through the capillary walls, larger molecules, including those of most drugs, cannot. Aromatherapy bypasses this barrier by going straight to the brain through the olfactory system.

When inhaled, essential oils may have the following effects:

- stimulating memory associations
- altering mood and feelings
- influencing hormonal responses
- stimulating the cortical areas of the brain associated with memory and learning.

Medical aromatherapy

While there is no definition for the term 'medical aromatherapy', for the purpose of this book I will refer to medical aromatherapy as the style of aromatherapy practiced by medically trained doctors in France.

In medical aromatherapy, the essential oils are usually taken internally having predominantly a pharmacological effect. Medical aromatherapy is used, among other things, to treat infectious diseases by using what French doctors call aromatograms. By this process, doctors can identify the essential oil or combination of essential oils which will be most effective to fight an infection.

While the treatment of bacterial infections is well established, more attention is now focussed on research of degenerative and viral diseases. Immunological tests, with blood examination before and after the treatments, confirm the ability of the essential oils to stimulate the immune system. From a pharmacological point of view,

precise relationships between the structure of the aromatic molecules and their physiological activity have been established in many areas. In this respect, medical aromatherapy is similar to orthodox medicine.

Asked to comment on the internal use of essential oils, which is a common practice in France, Dr Lapraz (16) a prominent French Doctor who uses phytotherapy extensively in the treatment of cancer says:

'Our position with regards to the internal use of aromatherapy is very clear. As essential oils are extremely active agents having some demonstrable effects on the different organs of the body, they need to be administered under medical supervision.'

He also gives an example which stresses the importance in understanding the physiology of the body. It is not sufficient to use lavender oil for respiratory problems on an asthmatic patient without knowing whether the asthma attack is due to parasympathetic or sympathetic imbalance. For the asthmatic who has a predominant function of the sympathetic nervous system, then lavender oil will have a reducing effect on the condition, but if the patient has hyperfunction of the parasympathetic system and has an asthma attack the prescription of lavender oil would make it worse.

However it is unfortunate that a French patient suffering from stress does not have access to a holistic aromatherapy practitioner who would use aromatherapy massage. The holistic approach including lifestyle changes is rarely part of a French doctor's consultation, as it would normally be in a holistic aromatherapist's consultation.

Aromatherapy and herbalism

The practice of aromatherapy can be seen as part of the larger field of herbal medicine, since the essential oil is only one of many components of the crude herb. Although most plants which yield essential oils are used in medical herbalism, it is important to distinguish the therapeutic qualities of a particular oil from those of the herb taken as a whole or prepared in another manner.

As an example, most of us are familiar with chamomile, which when used as a tea is effective for insomnia, nervousness, and digestive problems of a nervous origin. When you prepare your chamomile tea, I am sure that it does not turn blue (If it does please let me know, you have probably discovered a new method of extracting the oil!).

German chamomile oil has a rich inky blue colour due to the presence of chamazulene, which has traditionally been reported to give the oil its excellent anti-inflammatory properties. The chamazulene is not a water soluble constituent of the herb so it will not be extracted when a herbal infusion is made.

Although the aromatic component of the plant plays a central role in its overall characteristics, the herb also contains bitter components (anthemic acid), tannins (tannic acid), mucilage and a glycoside among other substances.

Therefore, essential oils usually represent the water insoluble components of the plant. While preparing herbal infusions the water soluble components of the plant are extracted and only a very small component of volatile oils is dissolved into the tea. While the properties of essential oils and teas may overlap, one would expect they would also have properties unique to the tea or the essential oil. Because the essential oil is less concentrated in the infusion, this makes the infusion more suited to internal use.

Peppermint oil is usually recommended as an inhalation for the treatment of respiratory conditions for its antispasmodic and antiseptic properties. However for digestive disorders it is better to use herbal infusions, where the action of the volatile oil is supported by the presence of bitters and tannins.

Conclusion

Aromatherapy and its spectacular growth have contributed to some potential problems. One problem is that there is currently very little useful clinical research relating to aromatherapy.

There is also a need to set standards for training and identification of aromatherapists. Well qualified aromatherapists come from many different professional backgrounds, but all need to have several qualities in common.

- They have a sound theoretical and practical knowledge of several types of body massage.

- They have a solid grounding in anatomy and physiology.

- They can maintain a sensible balance between the intellectual and intuitive approaches to their work.

- They treat their clients holistically.

- They have a sound knowledge of the virtues of the essential oils which they use.

- They are, above all else, concerned for the wellbeing of their clients.

- They should belong to a professional organization, representing aromatherapy.

There should also be strict guidelines for the use and sale of essential oils. Some essential oils are considered toxic if ingested or if they come into contact with the skin.

Robert Tisserand (17) indicates that in the 1920s and 30s there were 427 recorded deaths from wintergreen and methyl salicylate in the USA. In Australia wintergreen is scheduled as a poison, which means it may only be legally sold in an appropriate childproof container with a warning label. It is very clear that the aromatherapy industry needs to become safety conscious and needs to regulate itself before government bodies decide to regulate for us.

For the sake of aromatherapy's future, it is vital that aromatherapists, medical professionals, the fragrance industry, the rest of complementary medicine, the essential oil industry and politicians collaborate in order to reach our goal, where aromatherapy is recognised as a professional therapy playing a vital role in the healing of our planet and its inhabitants.

Chapter 2

History of Aromatherapy

The history of aromatherapy stretches back through many ages and many civilisations.
Plants have played a part in many cultures over many centuries. On a closer study of the subject it will become clear just how great the knowledge of the use of aromatic materials was in the ancient civilisations of Egypt, China, the Middle East, India and Greece.
We also trace the development of aromatherapy during the middle ages in Europe and how it flowered into one of the most sought after forms of holistic healing.

Introduction

When discussing the history of aromatherapy we need to remember that the word 'aromatherapy' was brought into use only in the 20th century. The term aromatherapy means 'a therapy using essential oils derived from plants'. Even though herbalism involves the use of the entire plant we need to begin our study into the history of aromatherapy by tracing the use of aromatic plant extracts to the origins of herbalism.

Ancient civilizations

Egypt

Egypt was the cradle of the sciences, including medicine, pharmacy, perfumery and

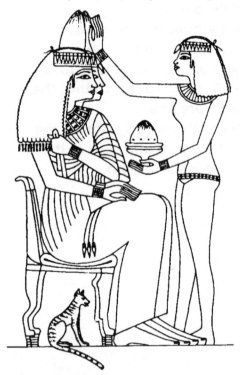

The maid-servant adds a few dabs of essential oils to the perfumed cones of aristocratic Egyptian women.
(Theban wall painting)

cosmeticology. Perfumes were used by the Egyptians as offerings to their gods. The temples all had a small room in which all the aromatic products were prepared. In the temple of Edfu, a room was discovered that contained inscriptions detailing the formulae of very expensive perfumes used by the Pharaohs and their families.

The priests, who were also the doctors, employed resins, balms and powders in many different ways for magical and religious ceremonies, for embalming the dead and in medicinal preparations. The statues of gods were covered in odoriferous oils. Different oils were dedicated to different divinities - such as styrax to Saturn, costus to Mars, myrrh to the moon, and frankincense to the sun.

One of the best known perfumes, kyphi, was used by the priests. It contained up to 16 different ingredients, including honey, myrrh, cinnamon, turpentine, juniper, cardamom and wine. The Greek philosopher Plutarch wrote about kyphi:

'Its aromatic substances lull to sleep, allay anxieties, and brighten dreams. It is made of things that delight most in the night.'

One of the ingredients of kyphi was calamus, which Tisserand (1) has described as having potent narcotic and sedative properties. Calamus contains up to 80% asorone a toxic phenol which is a precursor of TMA-2, a phenylethylamine capable of powerful narcotic effects.

The Egyptians believed in the transmigration of souls. They believed that the soul, after leaving the body, entered the body of some other animal, and, having successively passed through all the creatures of the earth, water and air, it again assumed a human shape. The journey was to be accomplished in 3000 years. This belief accounted for the great care they took in embalming the bodies of their dead, so that after the long journey, the souls might find their original body in a tolerable state of preservation.

Greece

The ancient Greeks further advanced the use of aromatic oils and ointments. The oils were used not only for their fragrance but also cosmetically and medicinally. The first treatise on scent was the study *'Concerning Odours'* by Theophrastus (2).

Not only did he take an elaborate inventory of all the Greek and imported aromatics, but he discussed ways in which they could be used. Theophrastus commented on the therapeutic nature of perfumes, saying:

'It is to be expected that perfumes should have medicinal properties in view of the virtues of their spices. The effect of plasters and of what some may call poultices prove these virtues, since they disperse tumours and abscesses and produce a distinct effect on the body and its interior parts.'

Here he has observed one of the fundamentals of holistic aromatherapy, that essential oils applied externally affect the internal organs and tissue. Pedacius Dioscorides, of Anasarca in Cicilia, wrote a magnificent treatise on herbal medicine during the first century AD. His book remained a standard medical reference work in western medicine for over a 1,000 years after his death, and much of our present knowledge of medicinal herbs originates from Dioscorides. His book contains five sections, one of which deals with aromatics. Many of the remedies he discusses are still used today in aromatherapy (3):

- **Myrrh** 'Doth strengthen the teeth and ye gummes' and is 'soporiferous'.

- **Juniper** is described as 'diureticall'.

- **Marjoram** is described as 'soporific'.

- **Cypress** 'the flux of the belly (diarrhoea). It doth also stanch the bloud.'

- **Costus** 'Provokes venerie' (aphrodisiac).

Aromatherapists are aware of the sedative properties of marjoram, that juniper is a diuretic, and that the astringent properties of cypress are useful in cases of diarrhoea. Costus, while traditionally used as an aphrodisiac, is now wisely avoided, since it can cause allergic reactions.

Hippocrates lived some 500 years before Dioscorides, about 2500 years ago. He recommended aromatic baths for the treatment of female disorders. He also promoted the benefits of massage:

'The physician must be experienced in many things, but assuredly in rubbing...For rubbing can bind a joint that is too loose, and loosen a joint that is too rigid.'

Hippocrates is referred to as the father of modern medicine, but it would be more fitting to dub him the father of holistic medicine. Some 300 years after Hippocrates, Asclepiades, a Greek physician who was perhaps closer to our concept of an aromatherapist than Hippocrates or Dioscorides, was a great believer in massage. He practised in both Greece and Rome, believed in curing his patients with as little discomfort as possible for them, and was against the excessive use of purgatives and emetics, which were then so much an integral part of medicine. Instead, he advocated the use of massage, music and perfume as soothing and healing agents.

China and India

It is known that essential oils were used in China and India at the same period as in ancient Egypt. The oldest form of Indian medicine is known as ayurvedic, meaning 'knowledge of longevity'. One of the principal aspects of ayurvedic is massage. Essential oils are often employed, especially sandalwood.

The Materia Medica of Li Shih-Chen, referred to as the *Pen Ts'ao,* described almost 2000 herbs. The essential oils of 20 of these were described, including the following:

- *Rose*: This was said to act on the liver, stomach and blood, and was employed as an anti-depressant.

- *Jasmine:* This was used as a general tonic for the whole body.

- *Chamomile:* This was given for headaches, dizziness and colds.

- *Ginger*: This was used to treat catarrhal coughs and malaria.

The Middle East

The discovery of distillation is credited to the Persians, in particular to a physician and alchemist called Ibn Sina, known in the West as Avicenna (AD 980-1037) (4). This Islamic genius, known as the 'Prince of Physicians' and as the 'Aristotle of the Arabs' was appointed physician to one of the princes of Persia at the age of 17. He wrote over 100 books and though some of them were quite short his celebrated 'Canon of Medicine'

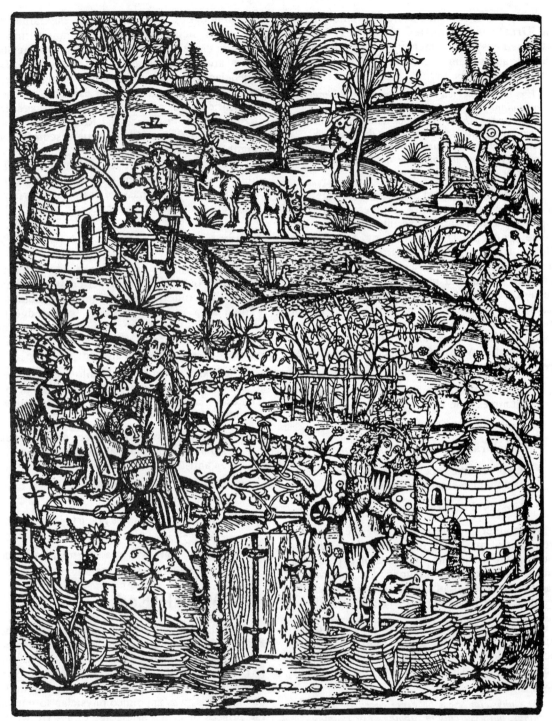

Scene of the herb garden in Hieronymus Braunschweig's *Liber de Arte Distillandi*

contained over a million words. In the pharmacological sections of the 'Canon' he lists no fewer than 760 drugs. He also expressed interest in music, physics, had considerable knowledge on mathematics and astronomy and his interest in alchemy led to the first production of distilled oils. However, distillation was not invented by this one person, but took some 100 years to develop. It was Avicenna who sophisticated and refined the process and first made it possible to extract the pure essential oil.

It is said that his first successful distillations were made from *Rosa centifolia*. In the thirteenth century Damascus became one of the major centres of rose production, giving rise to the name, Damask rose.

The Middle Ages

The rise of Christianity in the fourth century saw the use of aromatic substances denounced as decadent. This resulted in a significant reduction in the use of scents and perfumes. It would be several centuries before Christianity would gradually accept many of the traditional olfactory practices and beliefs.

Distillation was still unperfected but in the early fifteenth century the *Libellus de distillatione Philosophia* noted that tinctures of herbs in alcohol were impervious to decay, and it gave the advice that herbs should not be distilled in vessels of lead.

By the sixteenth century printed books were readily available and this gave rise to a new era of progress and the spread of knowledge. In Germany, Hieronymus Braunschweig, often referred to as Jerome of Brunswick, who was a physician, wrote several books on distillation. His last great work, the *New Vollkomen Distillierbuch* was published in 1597. It includes reference to 25 essential oils including rosemary, lavender, clove, cinnamon, myrrh and nutmeg. Braunschweig's books on distillation went through 680 editions appearing in every European language.

Other contributions to the development of aromatherapy were made by Conrad Gesner, and by Ryff, a Strasburg physician, who published his *Neu Gross Destillierbuch* in 1545.

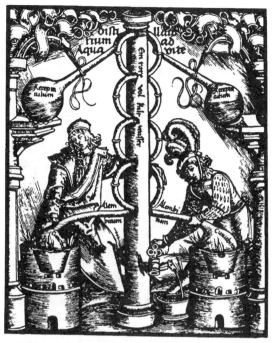

Sixteenth century distillation apparatus.

Many books on distillation were written during the sixteenth century, especially in Germany, which seems to have been the centre of this aromatherapy renaissance. The books also referred to alchemical practices. Alchemy was very popular at this time, and the distillation of all kinds of substances was one of the alchemists' favourite pastimes in their pursuit of the 'quintessence' of matter.

In *The Treasure of Euonymus* (5), published in 1559, Conrad Gesner speaks of essential oils having the power to 'conserve all strengths, and to prolong life'. His findings on the properties of rosemary oil are remarkably perceptive:

> *'It strengtheneth the harte, the braine, the sinnewes [muscles] and the hoole bodye.....members [limbs] sick of the palsy it heateth them for moste parte, and healeth them sometimes. Fistulaes and Cancars that give not place to other medicines, it healeth them throughlye.'*

Many of these comments, especially the properties ascribed to rosemary oil, would be regarded as valid by aromatherapists today.

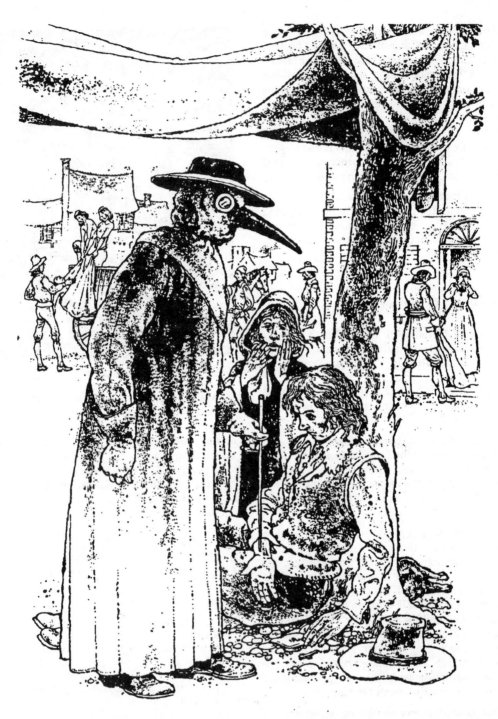

A seventeenth century doctor is wearing the protective clothing of his profession. The beak through which he breathes is filled with cinnamon, cloves and aromatic herbs.

Western medicine was next enlightened by the fiery Theophrastus Bambastus von Hehnheim, known as Paracelsus (1493-1541), who revolutionised both medicine and alchemy by diverting alchemy away from its desire to change lead into gold and opening up medicine to the materials and tools used by the alchemists.

He castigated those in the medical profession who merely followed the texts of the ancient Greek and Roman herbalists and would not test their materials and processes by experience.

It was also the time of the industrial revolution, which saw the population of many European cities increase, creating immense sanitation problems. These problems were highlighted in Suskind's novel (6):

'In the period of which we speak, there reigned in the cities a stench barely conceivable to us modern men and women. The streets stank of manure, the courtyards of urine, the stairwells stank of mouldering wood and rat droppings, the kitchens of spoiled cabbage and mutton fat ... People stank of sweat and unwashed clothes; from their mouths came the stench of rotting teeth, from their bellies that of onions, and from their bodies, if they were no longer very young, came the stench of rancid cheese and sour milk and tumorous disease ... For in the 18th century there was nothing to hinder bacteria busy at decomposition, and so there was no human activity, either constructive or destructive, no manifestation of germinating or decaying life, that was not accompanied by stench.'

It is not surprising that plagues became an unavoidable part of life in medieval Europe, occurring every few years from the fourteenth century until the end of the seventeenth century. While it is now known that these epidemics were spread primarily by rat fleas that carried the germs, many people at the time suspected that the plagues were a result of astrological influences or other more dramatic agents.

A widely accepted cause of the plague was the foul odour caused by putrefaction. This belief was reinforced by the fact that plague victims emitted a strong odour. Theories about the source of this foul odour abounded.

Some sought a theological basis, saying that evil spirits had poisoned the air, or that God had come to cleanse the unholy cities of Europe. Others held that it was the sun and the planets which fouled the air with invisible poisons. Still others argued that the corrupt air came from the earth within and was released into the atmosphere through earthquakes.

It is here that we find that measures against the plague were directed in controlling and combatting corrupt air. Municipal authorities lit bonfires of aromatic woods in the streets to purify the atmosphere. A popular device of the time was a pomander: an orange stuck full of cloves. Physicians recommended that the sickrooms have herbs at the window, an aromatic fire burning in the fireplace, and rose-water and vinegar sprinkled on the floor. Doctors often wore a nose-bag as shown in the picture opposite. The use of such smells was not without medicinal value as the essential oils used are now known to be considered powerful germicides.

By the seventeenth century essential oils had become a small but regular part of the herbalist's repertoire of remedies. For instance, Culpeper says of rosemary (7):

'The chymical drawn from the leaves and flowers is a sovereign help.... to touch the temples and nostrils with two or three drops for all diseases of the head and brain spoken of before, as also to take one drop, two or three, as the case requires, for inward diseases; yet it must be done with discretion, for it is very quick and piercing.'

Of lavender, Culpeper says (7):

'It is of especial use for pains in the head and brain, following cold, apoplexy, falling-sickness, the dropsy or sluggish malady, cramps, convulsions, palsies and faintings. It provokes women's courses, and expels the dead child and afterbirth.'

It is clear from these extracts that essential oils were successfully being used for a variety of internal and external problems. Both doctors and herbalists used them, a trend that would continue until the end of the nineteenth century. By this stage dosages had been established and the need for dilution and suitable vehicles for internal use had become clear.

The scientific revolution

By the nineteenth century the medical doctor became well established as the family physician. In spite of the regular use of essential oils by doctors, essential oils never really caught on with the medical profession, whose interests were now firmly fixed on chemical drugs and isolating the active principles.

However, the *Squire's Companion to the British Pharmacopoeia* in 1882, listed many essential oils including the following (8):

Rosemary: The oil of rosemary is a powerful stimulant. Used in hysteria and nervous headaches; externally as a rubefacient, and for its odour.

Sandalwood: The essential oil obtained from sandalwood *(Santalum album)* is described for gonorrhaea.

Lavender: An aromatic stimulant and carminative. Useful in hysteria, hypochondriasis and colic.

Somebody drew attention to the low incidence of tuberculosis in the flower-growing districts of France, especially in the south. Tuberculosis was very much a common illness in those days, however it had been noted that most of the workers who processed the flowers and herbs remained free of respiratory diseases.The most likely cause of this was believed to have been the essential oils contained in these plants. This led, in 1887, to the first recorded laboratory test on the anti-bacterial properties of essential oils.

The role of micro-organisms in disease had only been recognised in the early 1880s. Chamberland in Paris in 1887 and Cadeac and Meunier in 1888 published similar studies that showed that the micro-organisms of glandular and yellow fever were easily killed by essential oils. They noted the active properties of oregano, Chinese cinnamon, angelica and geranium. (9)

In July 1910 Rene-Maurice Gattefosse discovered the healing properties of lavender oil after severely burning his hands in a laboratory explosion. He was not the first person to use essential oils therapeutically nor the first to write about such use.

However, he was the person who coined the term *'Aromatherapy'* in 1937. Gattefosse used essential oils for treatment of soldiers in military hospitals during the First World War.

Some of his observations included (10):

'Wounds to the scalp: healed in 10 days
Firearm wound: healed in 15 days
Crushing of the thigh, open leg fracture; varices becoming ulcerated; delayed healing of an amputation stump of the thigh: healed in 21 days after failing with all other medication.'

He concluded by saying:

'It must be conceded that, while the antiseptic power of essences is of enormous interest, especially since it is not attended by any of the disadvantages found to such a large degree with all the other antiseptics used hitherto, greater attention needs to be devoted to the power they have of revitalising tissue.'

Although Gattefosse deserves full credit for his vision of aromatherapy, he was not the only person at that time to recognise the benefits of the essential oils. In 1939 another Frenchman, Albert Couvreur, published a book on the medicinal properties of the essential oils.

At about the same time Dr Penfold in Australia was discovering the benefits of tea tree oil, while in Italy Dr Giovanni Gatti and Dr Renato Cayola were researching the psychotherapeutic application of the essential oils.

Dr Jean Valnet, an army surgeon, began to use, with great success, essential oils as antiseptics in the treatment of war wounds during the Indochina war from 1948-1959. After the war he continued using essential oils in his capacity as a doctor, and in 1964 published a comprehensive text entitled *Aromatherapie* (now available in English), which has since earned him global recognition. Shortly after this he began teaching other doctors about the healing benefits of essential oils.

Doctor Valnet made the following comments in praise of essential oils:

'Essential oils are especially valuable as antiseptics because of their aggression towards microbial germs and their harmlessness to tissue - one of the chief defects of chemical antiseptics is that they are likely to be as

harmful to the cells of the organism as to the cause of the disease." (11)

It was Marguerite Maury, a French biochemist who extended the study of essential oils into the world of cosmeticology. She practised and taught aromatherapy until her death in 1964, and wrote two books on the subject. The second book was translated into English as *The Secret of Life and Youth*, a title which accurately reflects the book's preoccupation with rejuvenation. While she did not give much practical information in this book, she laid down the fundamental principles of holistic aromatherapy today. She emphasised the importance of applying the essential oils externally, diluted in vegetable oil, in combination with massage:

> *'Massage of the conjunctive, neuro-muscular or soft tissues pave the way admirably for the penetration of odoriferous substances, and the resultant rejuvenation ... It is therefore clear that preparations with a basis of essential oils with vegetable oils used as carriers, will be of great assistance.'* (12)

It is at this point that we see a clear shift in the original meaning of the French word 'aromatherapie'. Maury, who became Chairperson for CIDESCO (Pour le Comite International D'Esthetique et de Cosmetologie), forged a link between aromatherapy and the beauty industry. As a result, beauty therapists, who were already working in the context of wellbeing, were able to introduce additional benefits, such as massage and the essential oils, to their treatment. Today, some schools offering aromatherapy training in the UK are, in effect, schools for beauty therapists, although they represent themselves as aromatherapy training establishments.

At a beauty therapy conference in 1959, Micheline Arcier met Marguerite Maury. This lead to Micheline Arcier's lifelong devotion to aromatherapy. She trained with both Marguerite Maury and Dr Jean Valnet.

Micheline Arcier has developed some of the most effective aromatherapy techniques being used today. She is considered to be a leading authority in aromatherapy and has been responsible for training many aromatherapists practising today - including myself.

The work by Robert Tisserand, the author of *The Art of Aromatherapy*, has undoubtedly generated intense interest in aromatherapy. Not only has his book become a best seller in its field, but he has been involved in the establishment of two aromatherapy associations and setting training standards in the UK. He is also editor of the International Journal of Aromatherapy and the organiser of the highly successful AROMA conferences.

Chapter 3

What Are Essential Oils?

When we peel an orange, walk through a rose garden or rub a sprig of rosemary between our fingers, we inhale the scent of that plant.
What exactly is it that we can smell?
Generally speaking, it is the essential oil which gives a plant its specific scent.
This chapter explores the role of essential oils in nature, how the plant manufactures the essential oil and the factors that will determine the quality of the essential oil.

Introduction

Aromatic plants are those that contain essential oils. Essential oils are complex mixtures of individual chemical constituents, the precise nature and proportions of which determine its therapeutic and fragrant properties.

The essential oil constituents are mainly hydrocarbons and oxygenated compounds which are derived from hydrocarbons such as alcohols, aldehydes, esters, ethers, ketones, phenols and oxides. In certain plants, one main constituent may dominate the essential oil. Clove oil for example contains up to 95% eugenol, while in other oils such as rose there may be up to 300 individual constituents. The trace constituents, even those which have not yet been identified, often significantly modify the odour and the pharmacological properties of an oil.

The International Standard ISO Draft 9235.2, entitled *'Aromatic Natural Raw Materials'*, clearly defines essential oils as:

'A product obtained from natural raw material, either by distillation with water or steam, or from the epicarp of citrus fruits by mechanical processing, or by dry distillation. The essential oil is subsequently separated from the aqueous phase by physical means.'(1)

According to Drs Francomme and Penoel (2):

'Plant essences, in the physiological meaning of the term are most certainly true life essences, elaborated by the secretory cells of the plants that have tapped the photo-electro-magnetic energy of the sun and have converted it, with the intervention of enzymes, into biochemical energy under the form of highly diversified aromatic molecules.'

Essential oils are highly volatile, meaning that they readily evaporate, transforming from liquid to vapour.

Essential oils occur widely in the plant kingdom, not only in the flowers, leaves and fruit but also in the root stems and in other parts of green plants. A plant that produces an essential oil may do so in only one of its parts, such as jasmine from the flowers. However, in the case of the bitter orange tree, three different oils may be produced from the whole plant - from the leaves we obtain petitgrain essential oil, from the flowers we obtain neroli essential oil and from the fruit peel we also obtain bitter orange essential oil.

Examples of the distribution of essential oils in plants are:

Flowers:	Jasmine, neroli, rose, ylang-ylang
Leaves:	Citronella, lemongrass, petitgrain, palmarosa, patchouli
Bark:	Cinnamon
Wood:	Cedarwood, sandalwood, rosewood
Roots:	Ginger, vetiver
Entire aerial plant:	Geranium, lavender, rosemary, spike lavender
Fruit peel:	Bergamot, lemon, lime, bitter and sweet orange, tangerine, mandarin.

The more oil glands or ducts present in the plant, the higher the yield of essential oil, thus the less expensive the cost of the oil. Some examples of the yield of essential oils from plants is as follows: (3)

Essential Oil	% Yield of Essential Oil
German chamomile	0.2-0.4%
Clove leaf	2.0-3.0%
Eucalyptus	up to 10%
Everlasting	0.07-0.09%
Grapefruit	0.05-0.1%
Jasmine	rarely greater than 0.2%
Neroli	0.08-0.1%
Rose	0.02-0.05%

Each plant species has characteristic glands or cells that store the essential oil. Some examples are:

Glandular cells or glandular hairs

These are single or multi-celled protuberances on the surface of the plant epidermis. Plants from the Labiatae family such as rosemary, sage, and marjoram and the eucalyptus species store essential oils in this manner.

Oil resin canals

Inter-cellular spaces in the plant tissue store essential oils and resins. Plants from the Umbelliferae family such as aniseed, fennel and carrot seed store oils in this manner. The conifers also have resin canals. If the tree is damaged large quantities of resin often are exuded.

Oil reservoirs

Lysigenous secretory reservoirs are formed inside a plant as the walls of secretory cells gradually disintegrate. Plants from the Rutaceae family such as lemon, orange and bergamot store the essential oils in lysigenous cavities.

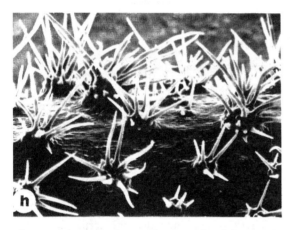

A scanning electron micrograph of the leaf surface of a eucalyptus leaf showing the stellate hairs associated with the oil glands. *(Picture courtesy of The Australian Centre for International Agricultural Research)*

Origin of essential oils

The exact origin of the essential oils is not known with any clarity. Evidence shows that the essential oil forms in the region of photosynthetic activity in the cells surrounding the oil glands. It then passes through the cell wall into the interior of the gland. (4)

The physiological rationale for the specific aspect of the relationship between photosynthesis and essential oil production is poorly known at present. Monoterpenes have been demonstrated to utilise sugars as a carbon source. (5)

Recent studies have confirmed the possible influence of photosynthesis and photorespiration on the terpene metabolism of peppermint oil (6). The results of these studies indicated that photosynthetic inhibition by the use of herbicides caused a decline in the content of monoterpene alcohols.

Photosynthesis

The chloroplasts of plants capture light energy from the sun and convert it to chemical energy stored in the bonds of sugar and other organic molecules made from water and carbon dioxide. This process is called photosynthesis.

Cells cannot create their own energy, but as open systems they are able to absorb energy from their surroundings. Photosynthetic cells aquire their energy in the form of light, which they use to make the organic compounds that provide energy to other cells. Hence photosynthesis nourishes almost all the living world directly or indirectly.

The energy-collecting cells of plants are called chloroplasts. All green parts of a plant, including green stems and unripened fruit have chloroplasts, but the leaves are the major sites of photosynthesis in most plants. The colour of the leaf is due to a green substance known as chlorophyll.

Scientists tried for centuries to piece together the process by which chloroplasts convert light energy to the chemical energy stored in organic molecules. Although some of the steps are still not understood, the overall photosynthetic equation has been known since the early 1800s. It has only been in the twentieth century that scientists have begun to understand how plants trap sunlight and convert it to chemical energy.

Photosynthesis can be summarised with this chemical equation:

$$6CO_2 + 12H_2O + \text{light energy} = C_6H_{12}O_6 + 6O_2 + 6H_2O$$

A more detailed account of photosynthesis may be found in any biology text book.

The carbohydrate $C_6H_{12}O_6$ is glucose, a major product of photosynthesis. The free energy from the sun has thus been stored in the form of a complex molecule, glucose.

Biological activity of the essential oils

Research indicates that the essential oils play an important role in mediating the interaction of plants with their environment. However, traditional theories suggested that the essential oils were regarded as toxic waste products of the plant's metabolic processes with no practical value to the plant. (7)

The lack of transport of the oils from the leaves back onto the stem immediately prior to shedding the leaves in winter, as happens with the sugars and starches, and the storage of essential oils in highly specialised secretory structures has been used as evidence to support these traditional theories.

I find it hard to believe that essential oils, which are such highly complex substances, are merely waste products. Dietrich Gumbel (8) suggests that the essential oils have multiple biological-ecological functions:

* to excrete toxic substances in the course of catabolism

* to protect against pest infestation

* as 'ectohormones' for social behaviour in plants, or as stimulation for the ripening of fruit

* to activate their own metabolism

* to use as a sexual attractant in animals or as an attraction, inducing insects such as bees and moths to pollinate plants.

Essential oils play important roles in the continuous molecular activity necessary to plant life. They have different functions, some acting as chemical messengers from cell to cell, others going to make up the structure of the plant in the formation of new cells and others are used in the defence of the plant against predators, or to attract insects for pollination purposes.

In various plants, plant feeding studies with radio-labelled carbon dioxide and terpenes have shown that essential oils provide a 'metabolic'

pool for the synthesis of indispensable plant components such as pigments, sugars, amino acids and other respiratory coenzymes (9).

The essential oils must also be segregated from other plant tissues because they can be extremely toxic. Pine oil, for example, can damage plant tissue in as small a ratio as 1:50 000. This toxicity will keep away predators, but it must not harm the plant that compounds it.

If the metabolic requirements of a plant have been met, essential oil production can be considerable. The gas plant, *Dictamnus alba* secretes so much volatile oil on hot days that it can actually self ignite. The peel of an orange, when pressed near a flame, will release oils which will similarly combust. This shield of oils emitted into the air often serves to ward off grazing animals as the oil irritates the mouth and thus protects the plant. (10)

The goats that scourge the forests around the Mediterranean normally spare many of the pungent herbs such as wild thyme and wild marjoram. Citronella and camphor oil repel certain insects, and sandalwood is impervious to termites. Sage, wormwood, tansy and thuja all contain thujone, which is so powerful against parasites that it has been used as vermifuges in traditional medicine. The essential oils manufactured by the plant to ward off pests are also powerful antimicrobial and antifungal agents.

There is evidence that the terpenes in the leaves of eucalyptus and pine contributes to allelopathic effects on the forest floors inhibiting the germination and growth of competitors (11).

Factors affecting the essential oils

There are many factors that can affect the quality of the essential oil, including:

* ecological variables eg soil type, climate and use of chemicals

* harvesting time

* genetics

* chemotype

* type and age of leaf.

These factors must be considered when comparing the essential oil status (yield and composition).

Ecological variables

Among the Labiatae (Lamiaceae) family there are a number of botanical species which produce essential oils of distinct difference. Most of these plants have developed in the temperate regions of the Mediterranean, or in similar climates around the world. Apart from this preference, each genus has its own preferred variables, which are specific.

For example, mild and moderate water stress increases *Ocimum basilicum* essential oil content and alters the oil composition. Linalool and methyl chavicol increase as water stress increases, while the relative proportion of sesquiterpenes decreases. (12)

Experiments were also conducted to study the response pattern of *Pelargonium graveolens* to fertilizers and the variation of essential oil constituents under varied agroclimatic regions. The essential oil yields were greater at lower altitudes than at higher altitudes. The oil produced from plants grown in the temperate climate of high altitude locations was richer in menthone, citronellol, nerol and geraniol, while the oil produced from the plants grown at lower altitude locations was richer in isomenthone, linalool and citronellyl formate. The variations in these growing conditions brings about a change in the quantity and quality of the essential oils produced. (13)

The effect of mineral fertilisers was evaluated on the basis of the fresh plant and essential oil yields. A study involving *Salvia officinalis* found that the concentrations of various chemical constituents were significantly affected by the various concentrations of fertilisers. An increase in fertilisers caused a reduction in the ratio of oxygenated components to hydrocarbons. (14)

Harvesting time

Many studies have been conducted to determine the optimum time for harvesting. The conclusions were as follows:

- The volatile oil content of the leaf increases with time, and also with leaf size.

- The maximum leaf yield was measured at the same time for most species: late summer, but the maximum oil yield varied from species to species. Thus it is important to know at what time in the plant's cycle the plant matter has been harvested.

Chamomile recutita is one of the medicinal plants whose use is increasing from year to year. Because some of its constituents have high therapeutic value, much attention has recently been given to its cultivation. Investigations of the influence of several extrinsic factors (daylight length, temperature, air and soil humidity, etc.) and sowing and harvesting times were conducted to determine the changes in the quantity and quality of the essential oil produced. It was found that the essential oil content was significantly higher if it were sown in spring rather than autumn. (15)

Another example is *Salvia officinalis*, which contains varying amounts of α-thujone depending on when it is harvested. It contains more after it has flowered, so it is better harvested before it flowers as α-thujone is one of the more harmful constituents in essential oils.

It was also found that *Ocimum basilicum* essential oil distilled from the whole plant gave an oil with a higher percentage of methyl chavicol whereas the flower spikes produced an oil richer in linalool (16). For aromatherapy purposes it is better to use basil with the least amount of methyl chavicol as this constituent is considered a skin irritant and has possible carcinogenic effects.

It was found that the essential oil of peppermint accumulates in the aerial parts of the plant and attains a maximum level in the growing period and then diminishes rapidly. The best harvesting time for maximum yield was found to be when the flowers were only barely visible at the stem extremity. (17)

Genetics

Plants belonging to the Labiatae family are prone to hybridisation, which makes defining species and subspecies a difficult task. Hybridisation is when two different species cross-pollinate, and the offspring is usually sterile.

There are over 150 subspecies of the genus thymus (18). A subspecies occurs when a particular plant produces others like itself, usually with some marked difference between it and the parent species.

Some of the different thymus species investigated include the following.

Thymus Species	Main Constituents
Thymus vulgaris	thymol, carvacrol, p-cymene, linalool
Thymus zygis	thymol, carvacrol
Thymus capitatus	carvacrol, thymol
Thymus satureoides	borneol, camphene, γ-terpineol
Thymus mastichina	linalool, 1,8-cineole

Chemotype

Another type of classification which is used nowadays is chemotype, which refers to subspecies which have the same morphological characteristics, but which produce different quantities of chemical constituents in their essential oils.

This phenomenon that chemical differences exist in morphologically identical species is widespread among the Lamiaceae family. Two examples in which chemotypes exist are thyme and rosemary. There are six chemotypes of *Thymus vulgaris*: (19)

- thymol
- carvacrol
- linalool
- geraniol
- α-terpinyl acetate
- thuyanol-4.

It was found that there is a correlation between chemotype, sexual polymorphism and the environment. It is noticed that the phenol containing species of thyme often show two chemotypes, a thymol type, as well as a carvacrol-type. Their common precursor p-cymene leads to either thymol or carvacrol, even though both substances can be found in many phenol-containing species, usually with one dominating.

Rosemary essential oil from *Rosmarinus officinalis*, has three main chemotypes (20):

- camphor-borneol type
- 1,8-cineole type
- verbenone type.

More information on the difference between the various chemotypes of rosemary oil can be found in Chapter 5.

When purchasing certain essential oils it is therefore important to know which chemotype you are buying, as the differences in the composition of the oil will affect the therapeutic properties of the oil. It is useful to know the geographic and ecological origin of the essential oil, as this will give you information about its chemotype.

It has been suggested that for those cases where there is actually more than one oil from a plant, the terminology used be the Latin name of the plant followed by the name of the predominant chemical component.

Overview

The factors affecting the quality of essential oils highlight some of the qualitative and quantitative variations found in essential oils and draw attention to some of the principal sources of this variation. The essential oil industry and aromatherapists would benefit from more carefully controlled experiments aimed at pinpointing these key factors.

Chapter 4

Methods of Essential Oil Extraction

Essential oils are complex plant extracts.
In order to understand the nature and characteristics of the
essential oils it is important that the aromatherapist
understands how the essential oils are produced.
This chapter defines some of the extraction procedures which
require highly specialised skills and equipment.
An understanding of these procedures gives the
aromatherapist an appreciation of the final cost of some of
the essential oils.

Introduction

We must be grateful to the practitioners of alchemy for what we know about essential oil extraction today. While the art of extracting essential oils has its roots in the ancient cultures of China, India and Egypt, it is the famous Arab alchemist and physician Ibn Sina, commonly known as Avicenna (AD 980-1037), who perfected the process of steam distillation to produce pure essential oils.

In order to understand the extraction of pure essential oils from plants I refer to E.J. Holmyard who discusses the ancient 'spagyric' preparation (from the Greek word spagyria - to gather, bind or join) of plant remedies in his book *Alchemy* (1). He discusses the works of Paracelsus (AD 1493-1541) who said that the creation of a spagyric plant remedy was based on the liberation and joining of the three philosophical principles of the plant. The three principles that he mentions are sulphur, mercury, and salt which are referred to as soul, spirit, and body.

The first substance is 'sulphur' (the essential oil component of the plant), which was represented as the very 'soul' or consciousness. 'Sulphur' is fiery, radiant and a masculine active principle which would be liberated via steam distillation.

The plant residues would be fermented with yeast to produce ethanol or grain alcohol. This was distilled to create the pure 'mercury' which represents the principal 'lifeforce' known as Qi. It represents the feminine or passive principle. Lastly, the remaining plant residue would be completely burnt, the ash washed with water and water evaporated to liberate the water soluble minerals or 'salt', which represents the 'body' or vehicle of the first two principles.

The three 'principles' were then combined to give a finished preparation. These spagyric preparations, according to alchemists, 'open' the plant, and liberate stronger curative powers. As in homeopathy and other forms of vibrational medicine, spagyric preparations are based on their synergistic effects rather than simply the pharmacologically active components.

In aromatherapy therefore we have an entire therapeutic approach based on the 'sulphur' of the alchemists. We can understand why the term 'essential oil' was derived from 'essence' meaning the 'soul' of the plant.

Aromatherapy employs essential oils created through a variety of extraction processes which are discussed below.

Why are many extraction processes needed to obtain essential oils?

The choice of extraction depends on the nature of the raw plant material. The basic methods of extraction are:

- expression processes
  - sponge
  - écuelle à piquer
  - machine abrasion
- distillation processes
  - water
  - steam
  - water and steam
  - hydro-diffusion
- solvent extraction processes
  - enfleurage
  - solvent
  - hypercritical CO_2.

Expression processes

With most citrus fruits the essential oil of interest to aromatherapists is contained in the large cells of the flavedo. These, being close to the surface, are readily ruptured by lateral compression of the peel or puncturing by scarification or grating. Only essential oils from citrus fruits are extracted by expression processes.

The sponge process

This is one of the two, original manual processes by which citrus oils were obtained before the development of mechanical methods for their mass production. Small amounts of lemon and orange oils are still produced by this method.

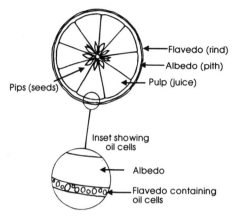

Transverse section of a typical fruit peel

sponge against its surface, causes rupture of many of the oil cells and consequent release of the oil, which is absorbed by the sponge. The sponge is periodically squeezed into a collecting vessel, from which the essential oil is decanted.

The écuelle à piquer process

The whole fruit is rotated against the spikes around the rim in order to puncture the oil cells. These cells contain not only essential oil, but also cell sap and protoplasm, so the essential oil released is mixed with cell contents from these and surrounding cells which were punctured in the process. The mixture of essential oil, other cell contents, including pigment is then emptied into a collecting vessel, from which the oil is decanted after separation from the aqueous layer.

The fruit is cut transversely into two halves, from which the pulp is then removed. The hemispheres are soaked in warm water for a short time in order to allow the pith to absorb a proportion of water, which softens it and renders it more elastic. The softening process is completed by exposing the peel to the air for several hours, after which it is ready for the removal of essential oil.

The diagram below shows how the peel is everted by the sponge, so that the flavedo is now on the inside of the hemisphere and is laterally compressed. This process, coupled with that of the

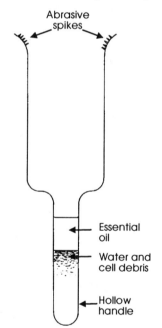

The écuelle à piquer process

Machine abrasion

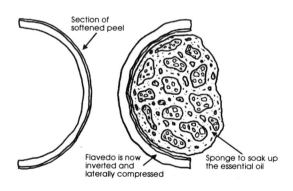

Eversion of fruit in sponge method

The machine abrasion method is no different in principle from the ecuelle process. The whole fruit are fed from a hopper into a rotating drum within which are rows of spikes. As the fruit tumble over the spikes, they are stripped of their outer peel, which, in the form of a finely divided mixture of cell debris, essential oil and other cell contents, is washed away by running water into a centrifugal separator. This machine performs a very rapid separation of the essential oil from the aqueous matter. It should be noted, however, that in this process the essential oil is mixed with other cell contents, so that the chance of alteration of the quality of the oil by enzyme action is higher.

Distillation processes

Distillation is the process of converting a volatile liquid into a vapour, condensing the vapour by cooling and collecting the condensed liquid in the same vessel or in a different one. Most essential oils are extracted by the distillation processes.

Principles of distillation

Steam distillation for the extraction of essential oils from plant matter is a very simple process. The process is so simple that until recently no one has investigated how steam liberates the essential oil.

Because saturated equilibrium between a liquid surface and the overlying vapour space occurs almost instantly, it has been assumed since the early 1900s that oil bearing plants had to merely be enveloped in an atmosphere of steam for any exposed oil to vaporise instantaneously into the steam in the vapour space.

For distillation, the oil bearing plant matter is placed into a still. Steam is then passed through the still, and this causes the oil to vaporise. The mixture of steam and oil vapour then passes through a condenser, where it returns to a liquid phase in which the oil separates spontaneously from the water.

To understand how this is done we need to review simple thermodynamic principles. Firstly, to convert any liquid into a vapour, energy in the form of heat is required. This is called the latent heat of vaporisation. Conversely, if any vapour is converted back into liquid, its energy is reduced and the latent heat is surrendered and released.

Secondly, all compounds with determinable boiling points will emit fast moving vapour molecules from their surfaces. These vapours exert a pressure on their surroundings which increases with rising temperature. If heat is applied to a liquid until its temperature attains the point where its vapour pressure becomes equal to the surrounding atmospheric pressure, the temperature will rise no further. If heat continues to be applied, the liquid will merely take up this energy as latent heat and vaporise at the appropriate rate. The liquid is then said to boil and the temperature at which this occurs is the boiling point under the prevailing pressure.

If two mutually insoluble compounds such as oil and water are present in the same vapour space, each will exert the pressure appropriate to the concentration of its own molecules, as though the other were not there. The total pressure exerted by the mixed vapour then becomes the sum of the partial pressures exerted by each constituent present. It follows that a liquid mixture will boil when its temperature is raised to the point where the combined vapour pressure of its components becomes equal to the surrounding pressure.

The basic principle of distillation, therefore, consists of bringing two mutually insoluble liquids (in this case, one of these liquids is water) into contact at a temperature very close to the boiling point of the more volatile of the two, the water. Then the addition of a small amount of vapour pressure from the oil will make the combined pressure equal to the surrounding pressure. The mixture will then boil and the oil will vaporise into the passing steam as fast as its requirement of latent heat can be applied.

Water distillation

In this process the plant material is completely covered with water. The still is brought to boil. This method of distillation can be carried out at reduced pressure and lower temperature as the oil should not under correct distillation conditions be subjected to a temperature much above 100°C.

Thus the presence of water safeguards the quality of the essential oil by preventing it from being overheated. This method is particularly useful for oils that are heat sensitive such as neroli and rose.

Because water distillation is a slow process, it can only be applied to those oils that are not damaged by long contact with hot water, which is particularly aggressive towards essential oils containing a high percentage of esters, breaking them down to the corresponding alcohols and carboxylic acids. Because of this, lavender requires the much faster process of steam distillation.

Steam distillation

As described, the equipment for water distillation consists of a distillation vessel, a vapour pipe leading to a downward sloping water-cooled condenser and a receiver for the collection of the distilled oil. Distillation of essential oil will proceed, but at a much faster rate.

The steam is under pressure greater than that of the atmosphere, thus the water from which it is produced is boiling at a temperature above 100°C. The object of steam distillation is to complete the process as quickly as possible, as certain essential oil compounds are thermolabile or heat sensitive.

Therefore damage to the essential oil through the effect of the hot steam is minimised.

Constituents such as linalyl acetate found in lavender will decompose back to linalool and acetic acid and the matricin found in German chamomile will decompose into the intensely blue chamazulene.

Steam distillation usually favours only the most volatile compounds from monoterpenes through to diterpenes. This is of importance to us as it has been found that clary sage normally contains only a small percentage of the diterpene alcohol, sclareol. This can be anywhere from trace to 2% of the total. (2)

Holmes (3) mentions that the sclareol is known to contribute to clary sage's oestrogenic like effects. The solvent-extracted clary sage was found to contain 70% sclareol (4).

Cohobation

Rose oil is one of the most expensive oils produced. One of the major constituents of rose oil is phenyl ethyl alcohol, a colourless, rose-smelling substance which is water soluble.

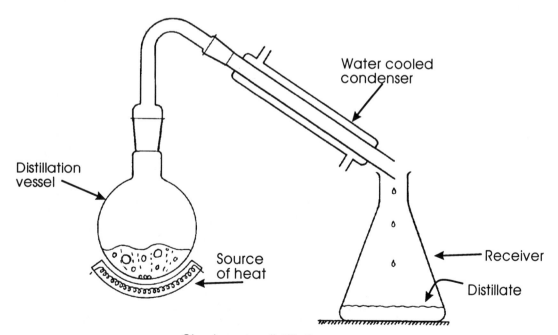

Simple water distillation process

When rose is distilled much of the phenyl ethyl alcohol is dissolved in the distilled water.

This means that rose oil produced by this method is deficient in this important constituent. It is therefore necessary, in order for the producer to be able to offer a complete and pure essential oil of rose, for the phenyl ethyl alcohol component to be recovered. This is done by returning the distilled water to the distilling vessel, where, on further distillation, the phenyl ethyl alcohol separates from the distilled water.

This separated phenyl ethyl alcohol is then mixed with the original distillate in the correct proportion to form the rose oil known as Otto of Rose. This process is known as cohobation and it is used only for the production of Rose Otto.

Rectification

Any essential oil containing 'impurities' may be purified by redistillation, either in a vacuum or in steam. Redistillation is known as rectification and the products are known as rectified oils. Eucalyptus oil often sold as 'double-distilled' is the result of rectification.

Water and steam distillation

In the water and steam distillation process, live steam is generated in a separate apparatus and then led through the still, which is filled with plant material and water. This method is a compromise between water distillation and pure steam distillation.

Fractional distillation

The process is conducted as per normal distillation, however the essential oil is collected in batches as distillation proceeds, instead of being continuously collected. These batches of the essential oil are called fractions.

Ylang-ylang is subjected to fractional distillation, yielding in succession ylang-ylang oils extra, No. 1, No. 2, and No. 3.

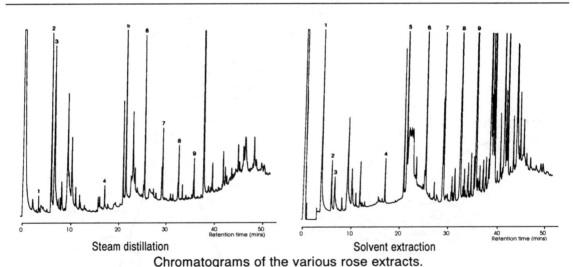

Steam distillation   Solvent extraction

Chromatograms of the various rose extracts.
1. Phenyl ethyl alcohol, 2. Citronellol, 3. Geraniol, C17-C27 Hydrocarbons. Notice that the main body of the rose extract 'Phenyl ethyl alcohol' is lost in the steam distillation process.
(Courtesy of Allured Publishing)

Hydro-Diffusion

Hydro-diffusion is a variation on direct steam distillation. The main difference is that the steam is introduced at the top of the still and not at the base. Condensation of the oil/steam mixture occurs inside the still directly below the grill or perforated tray supporting the material being processed. The advantages over direct steam distillation are lower steam consumption and shorter processing time which increases the essential oil yield.

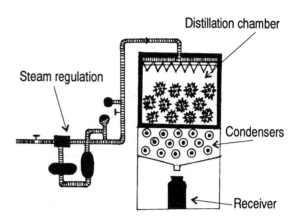

Hydro-Diffusion process

Solvent extraction processes

For raw materials with a very low concentration of essential oil (eg jasmine) or others with mostly resinous constituents (eg oakmoss), extraction with volatile solvents is the best way of isolating the essential oil.

Compared with steam distilled essential oils, extracted products have a finer fragrance. The disadvantage with this process is that not only the essential oil components of the plant but also the non-volatile constituents such as waxes and plant dyes are extracted.

There are many liquid solvents used by industry, especially petroleum ether, hexane, toluene, methanol and ethanol. There are also gases such as butane and carbon dioxide which become liquid under pressure.

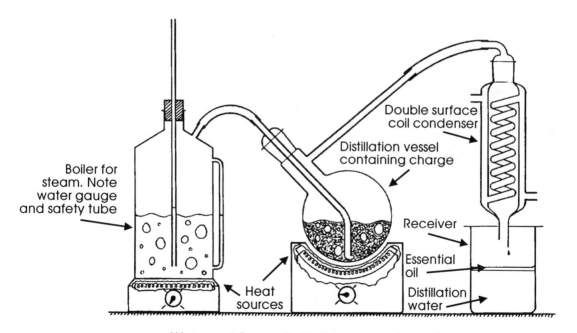

Water and Steam distillation processes

Animal and vegetable oil fats are also used as 'solvents' in the traditional enfleurage process which is rarely used today.

Solvent extraction

Solvent extraction is a very gentle production method. This process tends to create less 'rearrangement' of the essential oil compounds compared to distillation methods and will also extract the heavier constituents.

This complex mixture of volatile and non-volatile substances dissolved out by the solvent, usually an ether or hydrocarbon, comprise the 'extract'. The extract solution is then placed into a distillation vessel, to which very

gentle heat is applied, just enough to boil off the solvent, but insufficient to drive off the more volatile constituents from the essential oil contained in the extract. It is important to remember that although the process is distillation, its purpose is to recover the solvent, not to distill the essential oil.

The concentrated extract solution removed from the distillation vessel is known as a 'concrete' if it is not resinous and a 'resinoid' if it is resinous. The preparation of absolutes from concretes follows the principles of the Distribution Law. The essential oil present in the concrete is soluble in both the non-volatile material of the concrete and in alcohol.

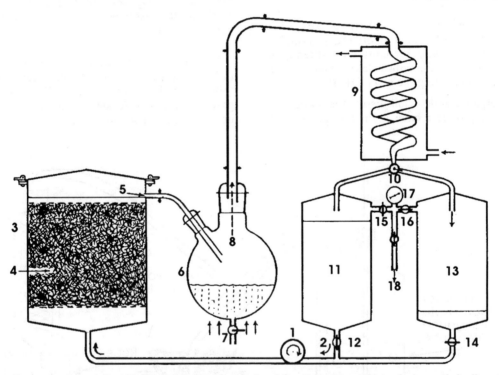

This diagram shows the basic equipment required for the extraction of essential oils with a volatile solvent, coupled with a vacuum still for recovery of the solvent after extraction.

1: Solvent pump; 2: Solvent to extraction vessel; 3: Extraction vessel; 4: Material for extraction; 5: Extract solution to distillation vessel; 6: Distillation vessel; 7: Drainage tap for recovery of concrete after extraction; 8: Solvent vapour to condenser; 9: Water-cooled condenser; 10: Two-way tap; 11: Receiver containing recovered solvent being recirculated to extraction vessel; 12: Solvent outlet tap; 13: Receiver being filled with recovered solvent; 14: Solvent outlet tap; 15 & 16: Vacuum taps; 17: Vacuum gauge; 18: To vacuum pump.

The concrete is warmed with some alcohol to a temperature just sufficient to melt it, and the mixture is then stirred. Essential oil from the molten concrete will dissolve into the alcohol as will a small amount of the waxes, fats and fixed oils found in the concrete.

The alcoholic solution is chilled and this precipitates much of the poorly soluble, non-volatile matter. The alcoholic solution is then filtered and the alcohol removed by distillation in a vacuum still at the lowest possible temperature.

The final result is the 'absolute', which is frequently described as the highest concentration of natural fragrance that can possibly be obtained.

There is a certain amount of 'hype' on absolutes regarding the use of solvents. Some of the solvents that are used are:

Alcohol (ethanol)

The problem with alcohol is that being a polar solvent, it will not only dissolve the essential oils, but also mix with the water naturally present in the plant matter, thus dissolving many vegetable pigments. For this reason alcohol is not regularly used for the extraction of aromatic materials, and is only used for certain resinous materials.

Ether (diethyl ether)

While ether is immiscible, it does have the problem of being extremely flammable and the toxicity of the vapour requires most careful handling.

Volatile hydrocarbons

The hydrocarbons that are used or have been used include liquefied butane gas, benzene and hexane. Benzene is no longer recommended as it is carcinogenic. The hydrocarbons are extremely useful solvents for the extraction of aromatic substances from their natural sources. They have a very low viscosity, and readily penetrate vegetable matter provided it is not too compact, because of their high volatility and are readily distilled off from the extract solutions, especially under reduced pressure.

Recent studies have been conducted proving that the composition of solvent-extracted jasmine and enfleurage-extracted jasmine is relatively the same (5).

Some of the problems have resulted from the use of benzene as a standard solvent in the past.

Pressure from governments and safety organizations led to the alternative use of hexane.

Nowadays, it is industry policy to limit the solvent residue to less than 10ppm (parts per million) - such a low concentration that even the safety organisations admit that a person would have to consume thousands of kilograms of an absolute before the solvent could do any harm. It has also been confirmed that solvent-extracted oils are relatively similar in chemical composition to enfleurage-extracted oils.

Enfleurage

'Jasmine season began at the end of July, August was for tuberoses. The perfume of these two flowers was both so exquisite and so fragile that not only did the blossoms have to be picked before sunrise, but they also demanded the most gentle and special handling. Warmth diminished their scent; suddenly to plunge them into hot macerating oil would have completely destroyed it. The souls of these noblest of blossoms could not be simply ripped from them, they had to be methodically coaxed away.

In a special impregnated room, the flowers were strewn on glass plates smeared with cool oil or wrapped in oil soaked clothes, there they would die slowly in their sleep. It took three or four days for them to wither and exhale their scent into the adhering oil. Then they were carefully plucked off and new blossoms spread out.

This procedure was repeated a good, ten, twenty times, and it was September before the pomade had drunk its fill and the fragrant oil could be pressed from the clothes. The yield was considerably less than with maceration. But in purity, it was unequalled, the jasmine oil radiated the sticky sweet, erotic scent of the blossoms with lifelike fidelity.'
From *Perfume: The Story of a Murderer* by Patrick Suskind (6)

Suskind has eloquently described the enfleurage extraction process in which the essential oil naturally released by fragrant flowers is absorbed by highly purified and odourless, solid fat or oil.

Fresh blossoms, gathered in the early morning, are placed by hand upon a thin layer of fat spread on a sheet of glass surrounded by a wooden frame

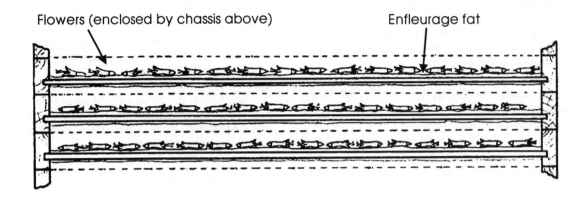

Flowers (enclosed by chassis above)   Enfleurage fat

Enfleurage

known as a chassis. During the course of the following 24 to 48 hours, depending on the nature of the flowers being processed, essential oil is transferred from the flowers to the fat, which absorbs it.

After the correct period of time the flowers are removed from the chassis and are replaced by fresh, recently-picked blossoms. This process is repeated every morning or every second morning, until the enflueurage fat is saturated with the dissolved fragrance. The product is called an enfleurage pomade, and consists of the original fat, plus the absorbed essential oil.

An enfleurage absolute is now produced from the pomade by a process of washing with alcohol similar to that used for the production of ordinary absolutes. Being a manual process, enfleurage demands the employment of large numbers of skilled work people. It is rarely used today, but continues sometimes for the extraction of tuberose and jasmine.

Hypercritical carbon dioxide extraction

Extraction with carbon dioxide is a relatively new process that has been hailed as a major breakthrough for the essential oil industry. Any substance can exist in three different states: gas, liquid and solid, depending on its temperature and pressure. In addition, certain substances can be found in the hypercritical state. They are neither liquid nor gas, but rather they are both. The hypercritical fluids disperse as readily as gases and also have solvent properties.

Carbon dioxide is one gas that becomes hypercritical. Its hypercritical temperature is 33°C. Hypercritical carbon dioxide then becomes an excellent solvent of essential oils. The advantage is that the whole operation takes place at a low temperature, and therefore the essential

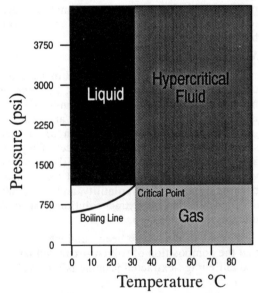

Physical states of carbon dioxide

oil is not affected by heat, as may occur in the distillation process.

The extraction process is almost instantaneous and because the solvent (carbon dioxide) is virtually inert, there are no chemical reactions between the solvent and the aromatic substances. The solvent can be removed simply by releasing the pressure. The whole process takes place in a closed chamber.

Unfortunately there is one catch: the hypercritical pressure for carbon dioxide is over 200 atmospheres (that's right, 200 times that of regular atmospheric pressure!). This requires very heavy and expensive stainless steel equipment. Only small amounts of hypercritical essential oils have been produced so far, but commercial production may not be too far down the line.

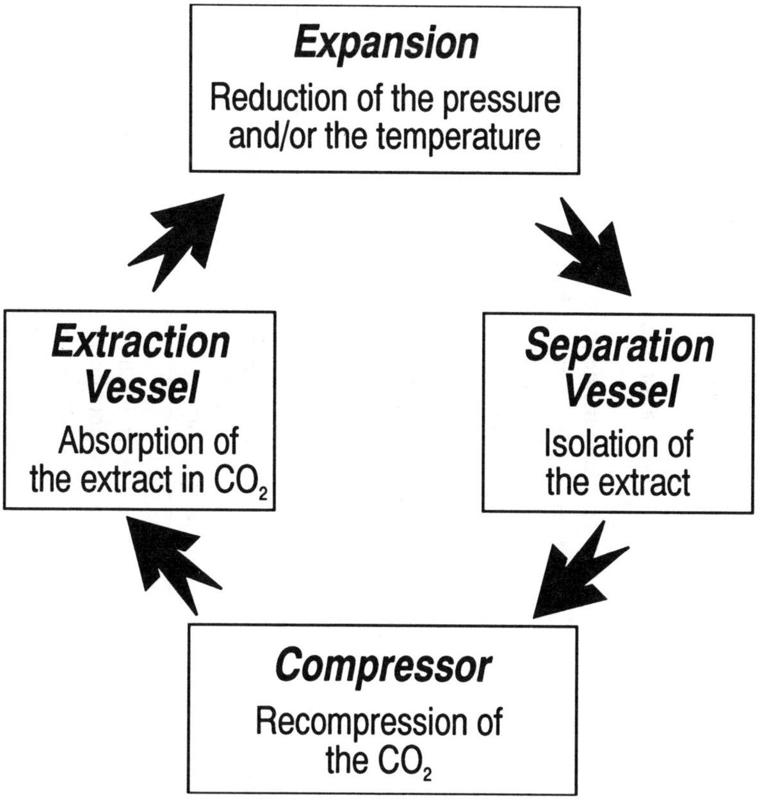

Expansion
Reduction of the pressure
and/or the temperature

Extraction Vessel
Absorption of
the extract in CO_2

Separation Vessel
Isolation of
the extract

Compressor
Recompression of
the CO_2

Hypercritical CO_2 extraction process

Extraction process	Advantages	Disadvantages
Cold pressed	• essential oil is not subjected to heat	• only possible for citrus oils
Distillation	• economical process for extracting oils • less labour intensive • large quantities can be processed in relatively short periods • very simple apparatus required	• essential oils liable to modification by the effect of heat and water
Enfleurage	• less rearrangement of essential oil constituents because low temperature is used • no concern regarding solvent residues	• labour intensive, time consuming
Solvent extraction	• less rearrangement of essential oil constituents because of low temperature	• possibility of solvent residues
CO_2 extraction	• less rearrangement of essential oil constituents because low temperature is used • no concern regarding solvent residues	• expensive equipment required due to high pressure needs

Summary of essential oil extraction processes

Chapter 5

Quality Control and Assurance

The essential oil industry is very large, catering to the needs of the food flavouring, perfumery, pharmaceutical and aromatherapy industries.
The standard of essential oils produced for food flavouring or other industrial applications, however, is not suitable for aromatherapy.
This chapter details the requirements and standards necessary to ensure that the aromatherapist is using the highest quality essential oils suitable for aromatherapy.

Introduction

Whether for professional or home aromatherapy use, essential oils which are of the highest quality should be used. With approximately five percent of the essential oils produced in the world being used for aromatherapy, the majority of essential oils are used in the food flavouring, perfume, and pharmaceutical industries.

While essential oils produced for the food flavouring and perfume industry are pure and natural, they have in most cases been purified by subsequent distillation processes such as rectification. In this process only the essential oil is distilled with the purpose of regaining more volatile constituents and discarding the minor constituents. This refining usually yields a colourless, clear oil which is perceived by some as having an improved lighter fragrance.

To standardise the quality of essential oils, it is a common practice to comply with the British Pharmacopoeia (BP) standards. This is the case with eucalyptus oil. The BP standards for this oil require it to have a 1,8-cineole content of 70%. As most eucalyptus oils have a cineole content less than this, the oil must be rectified or redistilled to achieve this standard. From a holistic aromatherapy viewpoint it is recognised that the synergistic action of all components of an essential oil is far superior to that of the redistilled oil.

The term 'Pure and Natural' used by many suppliers of essential oils indicates that there are no synthetic materials added. However it is important that essential oils used in aromatherapy be 'Genuine and Authentic'. In order for an essential oil to be definable as genuine and authentic the following information should be readily available for the oil in question:

- the botanical name
- the part of plant used
- the country of origin
- the extraction method
- quality specification.

The botanical name

If the essential oil is being used for therapeutic purposes it makes sense that it has been sourced from the proper botanical origins. Often suppliers refer to the essential oils by their common names only. The following examples show that this can often be very misleading and it is of utmost importance to specify the true botanical source of the essential oil.

First of all we must know the exact botanical species of the plant used for the production of the essential oil. The term 'lavender oil' for instance, is inadequate, because there are many species of lavender. The correctly defined name of lavender gives the genus 'lavendula' in Latin, followed by an adjective which defines the species. (eg angustifolia, spica, stoechas, hybrida). It is sometimes necessary to define the variety, if such exists. In the case of *Lavendula vera* for example, we need to mention the variety, because there are so many varieties eg *Lavendula vera* var. *fragrans* or *Lavendula vera* var. *maillette*, the former being of wild origin and the latter a cultivated clone.

The name of the variety narrows the description of the botanical species and its origin. The knowledge whether it is 'wild' or 'cultivated' is also important as far as the quality of the essential oil is concerned.

Some examples of the importance of identifying the essential oil by its correct botanical name follow.

Chamomile

- *Anthemis nobilis* or *Chamaemelum nobile* (Roman chamomile)

- *Matricaria chamomilla* or *M. recutita* (German or Blue chamomile)

- *Ormensis mixta* or *Anthemis mixta* (Moroccan chamomile).

There are three main chamomile essential oils, each of which corresponds to a plant with its own chemical profile and hence different action. All three species belong to the Compositae (Asteraceae) family and are similar in appearance.

Roman Chamomile
(Anthemis nobilis or chamaemelum nobile)

Roman chamomile is also known as English chamomile. It differs greatly from German chamomile oil - composed predominantly of aliphatic esters such as iso-butyl-angelate and iso-amyl-angelate. This oil is largely influenced by its high ester content. The essential oil has been used topically to reduce inflammation and to accelerate healing (1).

It has anti-inflammatory and antispasmodic properties, though to a lesser degree than that of German chamomile. However, due to the more pleasing aroma, Roman chamomile may be more suitable for its effects upon inhalation, for its sedative, and calming properties.

German Chamomile *(Matricaria chamomilla or M. recutita)*

Also known as blue chamomile, the major constituents are (-)-α-bisabolol (up to 50%), a sesquiterpene alcohol, bisabolol oxides and a sesquiterpene lactone chamazulene (formed during distillation from its precursor matricine). The oil has a deep blue colour and a strong, herby medicinal smell. German chamomile is well known for its anti-inflammatory properties which have been extensively documented. The (-)-α-bisabolol found in German chamomile also promotes granulation and tissue regeneration (2). Roman chamomile does not contain any (-)-α-bisabolol. German chamomile also exhibits antispasmodic, cholagogue and choleretic activity. The essential oil has demonstrated liver regenerating properties (3). Recent studies have also found German chamomile to demonstrate antibacterial activity against candida (4).

Moroccan Chamomile
(Ormensis mixta or Anthemis mixta)

While this chamomile belongs to the same family as the German and Roman chamomiles, it has very little in common with either of the true chamomiles. A typical chemical composition of Moroccan chamomile is (5):

α-pinene (15.0%), camphene (0.4%), sabinene (0.2%), yomogi alcohol (2.4%), 1,8-cineole (0.5%), limonene (0.8%), santolina alcohol (3.2%), artimesia alcohol (2.3%), trans-pinocarveol (3.0%), borneol (1.0%), bornyl acetate (2.2%), bisabolene (2.5%), germacrene (5.0%), δ-cadinene (0.8%), caryophyllene oxide (0.8%), caryophylladienol (0.7%).

According to Lavabre (6) it has antispasmodic, sedative, cholagogue, emmenagogue and soothing properties which can be used for treating depression, irritability, colitis, amenorrhoea, dysmenorrhoea and liver and spleen congestion.

In aromatherapy, *Ormensis mixta* may be used as an economical substitute for the more expensive Roman chamomile.

Juniper and cedarwood

* *Cedrus atlantica* (Atlas cedarwood)
* *Cedrus deodorata* (Himalayan cedarwood)
* *Juniperus virginiana* (Virginian cedarwood)
* *Juniperus oxycedrus* (Cade)
* *Juniperus communis* (Juniper)
* *Juniperus sabina* (Savin)
* *Thuja occidentalis* (Thuja).

There are many more varieties of cedars and juniper trees than are listed above. Some belong to the Pinaceae family and others to the Cupressaceae family. Both these families belong to the conifer class.

Atlas Cedarwood
(Cedrus atlantica)

Believed to have originated from the famous Lebanon cedars (*C. libani*), which grow wild in Lebanon and on the island of Cyprus. It is a close botanical relative of the Himalayan cedarwood (*C. deodorata*), which produces a very similar essential oil.

Himalayan Cedarwood
(Cedrus deodorata)

Produces an oil which is very similar to Atlas cedarwood. The oil has a rich, herbaceous, camphoraceous, pleasant woody-balsamic undertone and is used in aromatherapy for the treatment of acne, dandruff, dermatitis, eczema, bronchitis, catarrh, for urinary tract infections and for nervous tension and stress related conditions.

Virginian Cedarwood
(Juniperus virginiana)

The wood from this tree has been used for making pencils. The tree is botanically related to the Texas cedarwood. and the East African cedarwood *(J. procera)*. It is commonly used in aromatherapy for the treatment of respiratory infections, for genito-urinary tract infections and for nervous tension and stress related disorders.

Cade
(Juniperus oxycedrus)

The oil of cade is obtained by destructive distillation from the branches and wood. A rectified oil is then produced from the crude by steam or vacuum distillation. The oil has traditionally been used for the treatment of cutaneous diseases such as chronic eczema, parasites, scalp problems and allergic skin conditions.

Juniper
(Juniperus communis)

The oil from this tree is extracted from the berries, twigs and leaves. The essential oil is commonly used in aromatherapy for its detoxifying and diuretic properties. It is often classified as a kidney irritant, however recent studies have shown that the essential oil extracted from the ripe juniper berries may be considered safe.

Savin
(Juniperus sabina)

Native to North America, and parts of Europe, it is closely related to the common juniper *(J. communis)*. The essential oil has a high percentage of sabinyl acetate which contributes to savin's toxic properties. It is considered a powerful emmenagogue and rubefacient but is an oral and dermal toxin and should not be used in aromatherapy either externally or internally.

Thuja
(Thuja occidentalis)

Native to north eastern America, it is cultivated in France. While the twigs are currently listed in the British Herbal Pharmacopoeia, used specifically for bronchitis with cardiac weakness and for warts, the essential oil of thuja contains over 60% thujone and is considered an oral toxin, not to be used in aromatherapy.

Lavender

- *Lavendula officinalis* or *L. vera* or *Lavendula angustifolia* (French Lavender)

- *Lavendula burnatti* or *L. hybrida* (Lavandin)

- *Lavendula latifolia* or *L. spica* (Spike lavender).

Whereas true lavender ideally grows at high altitudes (above 600 metres) lavandin and spike lavender grow abundantly on much lower coastal grounds making them easier to cultivate.

True Lavender
(Lavendula officinalis, or L. angustifolia)

Although lavender has been classified as lavender vera de Cadolle; *L. officinalis* Chaix or *L. angustifolia* Miller, it is the latter name which is the correct derivation for the most common commercially grown aromatic member of the labiatae family.

The true lavender plant is easily distinguished by its small delicate flowerheads and there are no side shoots from the main stem. This has the most pleasant and subtle of fragrances. There are about 15 sub-species grown in France and Tasmania. It is the lavender most commonly referred to in aromatherapy texts.

Spike Lavender
(Lavendula spica, L.latifolia)

This is a large plant that has close-knit flowerheads with two small side stems. It yields an oil with a camphoraceous scent. The essential oil yield is very high, making it an inexpensive oil, and the fact that it grows at much lower altitudes, makes farming easier.

Spike lavender has a natural camphor and 1,8-cineole content which makes it useful as an inhalant for respiratory infections, for muscular aches and pain and it is also useful as an insecticide.

Lavandin
(Lavendula fragrans, L. burnatii)

The lavandin plants yield almost twice as much oil as true lavender and are easier to grow.

Lavandin is a hybrid of true lavender and spike lavender. Lavandin essential oil has a lower ester content and contains some camphor.

The fragrance is not as refined as that of lavender, and has often been referred to by most aromatherapy authors as being an oil of inferior quality and only suitable for soap making.

According to a recent randomised double-blind trial on post-cardiotomy patients using *Lavendula angustifolia* and *L. burnatii* topically, both oils aided respiration and their effects on mood and coping ability were similar. However, lavandin was nearly twice as effective as *L. angustifolia* in alleviating anxiety. It was also noted that lavandin was rarely used therapeutically and was not supplied to hospital pharmacies. (7)

My concern is that lavandin, being an oil produced specifically for the fragrance industry, may be prone to adulteration. This would make it totally unacceptable for aromatherapy purposes.

Marjoram

- *Marjorana hortensis* or *Origanum marjorana* (Sweet marjoram)
- *Thymus mastichina* (Spanish marjoram)
- *Thymus capitus* (Spanish oregano).

The most common types are French marjoram (*Origanum onites*) which is a hardier plant than sweet marjoram (*Marjorana hortensis*), Spanish marjoram (*Thymus mastichina*), and wild or common marjoram or oregano (*Origanum vulgare*) which is used to produce oregano oil.

Sweet Marjoram
(Origanum marjorana, Marjorana hortensis)

This is the marjoram oil most aromatherapy books write about. This oil is useful for respiratory tract infections, muscular aches, anxiety, depression and insomnia. It can also be used as an emmenagogue for the treatment of amenorrhea and dysmenorrhea. It is a hypotensive and is used for digestive spasms.

Chemical constituent	*Origanum marjorana*	*Thymus masticina*	*Thymus capitus*
methyl chavicol	trace	-	-
terpinen-4-ol	10.7 - 28.5%	0.7%	0.66%
1,8-cineole	3.7 - 6.4%	55%	-
linalool	1.0 - 2.6%	11.1%	2.0%
sabinene	2.4 - 4.5%	1.1%	-
terpinolene	1.9% - 3.3%	trace	0.07%
α-terpinene	8.4 - 10.1%	trace	1.2%
caryophyllene	2.1 - 4.0%	-	trace
α–terpineol	trace	8%	trace
α–pinene	trace	2.6%	0.84%
cymene	trace	1.3%	15%
myrcene	-	-	2.0%
thymol	-	-	0.12%
carvacrol	-	-	62%

A typical chemical composition for *Origanum marjorana* (9), *Thymus masticina* (11) and *Thymus capitus* (8)

Spanish Marjoram
(Thymus mastichina)

This is not a true marjoram and in fact is a species of thyme and as can be seen below the oil is chemically quite different to sweet marjoram oil. It has a high 1,8-cineole content, which gives the oil an aroma reminiscent of eucalyptus.

Lavabre (10) recommends *Thymus mastichina* be used for its antispasmodic properties for digestive and respiratory spasms, as an analgesic for migraines, arthritis and rheumatism and as a sedative for nervous tension and insomnia.

Due to the higher cymene component, Spanish marjoram is preferable for muscular aches and pain and because of its higher 1,8-cineole content it is preferable as an inhalation for respiratory problems. (Refer also to Thyme on page 48.)

Spanish Oregano
(Thymus capitus)

Thymus capitus is found mainly in Spain, Greece, Portugal, Turkey, Italy and Morocco. Its principal constituent is carvacrol (70-85%) and its composition is similar to that of oregano *(Origanum vulgare)*.

Pine

- *Pinus mugo var. pumilio* (Dwarf pine)
- *Pinus palustris* (Longleaf pine)
- *Pinus sylvestris* (Scotch Pine).

There are numerous species of pine which yield an essential oil from their heartwood as well as the twigs and needles.

Scotch Pine
(Pinus sylvestris)

The oil from the needles of the scotch pine is one of the most useful and safest therapeutically.

Longleaf Pine
(Pinus palustris)

It is this species of pine that provides the largest source of turpentine essential oil. Turpentine refers to both the crude oleoresin formed as a physiological exudate from the trunk of *Pinus palustris* or the distilled and rectified essential oil of other *Pinus* species. Turpentine is not commonly used in aromatherapy.

Dwarf Pine
(Pinus mugo var. pumilio)

Also known as Swiss mountain pine. This is the favoured pine fragrance for perfumery use due to its very pleasant, balsamic unique scent. The unusual scent is due to its aldehyde content. Dwarf pine is often the cause of contact dermatitis, although it is very likely that all pine oils are potent irritants when oxidised, but not when fresh.

Sage

- *Salvia officinalis* (Dalmatian sage)
- *Salvia lavendulaefolia* (Spanish sage).

Julia Lawless (12) indicates that there are several species and cultivars of sage such as Mexican sage *(S. azurea grandiflora)* and red sage *(S. colorata)* both of which are used medicinally. Essential oils are also extracted from Spanish sage *(S. lavendulaefolia)* and clary sage *(S. sclarea)*.

Dalmatian Sage
(Salvia officinalis)

The principal source of *Salvia officinalis* is the Balkans. Sage contains thujone, a substance which is considered toxic in high doses. Traditionally sage has been used for a variety of disorders such as respiratory infections, menstrual difficulties and digestive complaints.

Spanish Sage
(Salvia lavendulaefolia)

Spanish sage is often mistaken for eucalyptus because of its high 1,8-cineole content. It does have very little thujone making it less toxic than the true sage, but it should not be used in place of the true sage oil. The oil is chemically quite different from true sage oil.

Sandalwood

- *Santalum album* (Sandalwood)
- *Santalum spicatum* (Australian sandalwood)
- *Amyris balsamifera* (Amyris or West Indian sandalwood).

Chemical constituent	*Salvia officinalis*	*Salvia lavendulaefolia*
α–thujone	28.0%	-
β–thujone	8.52%	-
1,8-cineole	11.16%	54%
borneol	13.18%	4.3%
camphene	3.53%	4.0%
caryophyllene	7.15%	-
α–pinene	3.98%	6.0%
β–pinene	trace	7.0%
camphor	0.90%	1.0%
limonene	1.42%	1.5%
terpinen-4-ol	5.09%	-
linalool	-	1.0%

A typical chemical composition for *Salvia officinalis* (13) and *Salvia lavendulaefolia* (14)

Sandalwood is produced from various species of santalum genus but the oil from *Santalum album* is the most sought after of the sandalwood oils.

Indian Sandalwood *(Santalum album)*

Belonging to the Santalaceae family, this is the true sandalwood, native to Maharastra, Kerala, Andra Pradesh, Karnataka, and Tamil Nadu (India). Of these Indian states, the last two produce most Indian sandalwood.

The sandalwood from India is the most prominent and sought after of the wood oils. The sandalwood industry has been under the threat of shortages due to lack of availability, lack of replanting and illegal logging of young trees. For the manufacture of quality sandalwood oil the heartwood of mature trees (aged 30 years or more) is preferred.

The Indian government has introduced tougher legislation to control the production of sandalwood and reduce the illegal felling of young trees so that it can sustain its sandalwood production in the long term.

Santalum album contains 10% santalene (α and β) and 90% santalol (α and β).

Australian Sandalwood
(Santalum spicatum)

The Australian sandalwood *(S. spicatum)* produces an oil very similar to the oil of *Santalum album*, but with a dry bitter top note.

According to Lassak (15), *S. spicatum*'s slow regrowth has resulted in a cessation of oil production and it is quite unlikely that it will ever restart on any commercial scale. This is a pity, as essential oil suppliers will find it more and more difficult to obtain quality sandalwood oil as the preferred Indian oil becomes less available.

Australian sandalwood oil was found to be effective against the 'golden staph' whereas Indian sandalwood oil was reported to have negligible activity. (16)

Santalum spicatum contains α and β santalol.

West Indian Sandalwood
(Amyris balsamifera)

The West Indian sandalwood is a poor substitute for the oil of *Santalum album* and bears no botanical relationship to the East Indian sandalwood. Preferably called amyris oil, it belongs to the Rutaceae family. The oil, which is commonly obtained from Haiti, possesses a weak woody sandalwood-like odour which is used as a fixative in soap fragrances.

Amyris contains methyl alcohol, diacetyl, furfural, β-caryophyllene, α-candinene and α-cadinol.

Thyme

- *Thymus vulgaris* (Red thyme)
- *Thymus zygis* (Spanish thyme)
- *Thymus serpyllum* (Wild thyme)
- *Thymus capitatus* (Conehead thyme or Spanish oregano)
- *Thymus mastichina* (Spanish marjoram).

There are more than 80 Thymus subspecies from 27 different countries all over the world (17). The common thyme is believed to be derived from the wild thyme *(Thymus serpyllum)*.

Researchers have found it difficult to categorise the oil botanically. The analyses done on many species were quite varied and difficult to evaluate accurately. Depending on which book you read, you will get conflicting reports on which constituents could and should be found in the different species.

The predominant species is *Thymus vulgaris*, of which there are six different chemotypes. The two most common, thymol and carvacrol (phenols), are located close to the Mediterranean Sea, at a low altitude. (18)

Elisabeth Stahl-Biskup (19) found, that for phenol-containing thyme oils, the phenol content peaks at the onset of flowering or when the plant is in full bloom.

At higher altitudes between 1000 and 1200m, the linalool chemotype is found. Of all the species of thyme, only five have been found with concentrations of linalool greater than 50%. These oils smell quite different from the phenol-containing oils. The linalool-rich thyme oils have antibacterial properties, are immunostimulants, tonics to the nervous system

Constituent	*Thymus vulgaris*			*Thymus serpyllum*
	thymol chemotype	carvacrol chemotype	linalool chemotype	
α-thujene	4.6%	4.9%	0.26%	1.53%
α-pinene	0.75%	4.3%	0.3%	0.7%
camphene	0.3%	0.8%	0.27%	0.2%
β-pinene	0.34%	0.35%	-	0.17%
p-cymene	26%	33.9%	2.0%	25.0%
α-terpinene	24%	44.85%	0.28%	4.85%
linalool	4.2%	4.2%	77.5%	3.4%
borneol	0.65%	0.8%	0.2%	-
β-caryophyllene	3.55%	2.5%	2.8%	2.5%
thymol	34%	5.5%	2.2%	8.3%
carvacrol	4.7%	24.5%	trace	14.2%
geraniol	-	-	-	9.0%

The chemical constituents of several varieties of thyme (20)

and are not considered dermal irritants or sensitisers.

These three chemotypes, thymol, carvacrol and linalool, are the most commonly used in aromatherapy.

Red thyme
(Thymus vulgaris)

The most commonly available oil originates from either *T. vulgaris* or *T. zygis*. Even though the phenol content of Red thyme is much lower than wild thyme it still must be used with care as it may irritate the skin.

Wild thyme
(Thymus serpyllum)

Wild thyme has a higher percentage of phenols than Red thyme so should be used with extreme care as it will irritate the skin.

Spanish thyme
(Thymus zygis)

Spain produces great quantities of *Thymus zygis*, which has a high thymol content (50-75%).

Spanish oregano
(Thymus capitus)

Spanish oregano is found mainly in Spain and Greece, but also in Portugal, Turkey, Israel, Italy and Morocco. It has a high carvacrol content (70-85%) and its composition is similar to that of *Oregano vulgare*.

Spanish marjoram
(Thymus mastichina)

Spanish marjoram is cultivated mainly in Spain, Portugal and Morocco. It contains mostly 1,8-cineole (60-75%) and linalool (5-20%). Its odour is similar to that of 1,8-cineole eucalyptus, making it very different from other thyme species.

The part of plant used

There is little concern when the entire plant is distilled as is the case with peppermint, marjoram or rosemary. However, for some oils the part of the plant used must be specified as the essential oil produced varies qualitatively according to the part of the plant used.

Bitter orange

The bitter orange tree is a classic example of a tree from which four different essential oils are produced:

- neroli, from the flowers
- petitgrain, from the leaves
- bitter orange, from the rind
- an oil from the juice of the fruit (used in food flavouring only).

Clove

- clove bud
- clove leaf
- clove stem.

Clove oil can be extracted from both the leaf and the bud. Both the clove bud and clove leaf oils have similar chemical constituents. However the clove bud oil is of superior quality as it has a sweet, rich, warm, spicy, fruity top note and a woody base note, compared with the crude somewhat harsh phenolic odour of the leaf oil.

Cinnamon

- cinnamon bark
- cinnamon leaf.

Cinnamon oil is available from both the bark and the leaf. Cinnamon bark oil has a sweet, warm and spicy aroma with approximately 70% cinnamic aldehyde content.

Cinnamon leaf oil is warm and spicy, but lacks the depth and body of cinnamon bark oil. It has a eugenol content of about 75% (eugenol is also found in clove oil).

Unfortunately cinnamic aldehyde is a skin irritant so while the bark oil has a superior fragrance it is not recommended for topical use in aromatherapy.

Lime

- distilled lime oil from the whole fruit
- cold pressed lime oil from the rind.

Lime essential oil is extracted by two methods:

- cold expression of the peel of the unripe fruit which results in an oil with a fresh citrus peel odour

- steam distillation of the whole ripe crushed fruit which produces an oil with a sweet, fruity odour (a product used by the juice industry).

The country of origin

It may be surprising but plants from a single botanical species can produce essential oils of distinctly different compositions. The reasons for this are not fully understood. Obvious factors of influence are the geographic location and the prevailing climate, but genetic factors may also contribute.

Basil

There are four principal types of basil essential oils, two of which are extracted from *Ocimum basilicum*:

- Exotic or Reunion basil, which is distilled in the Comoro Islands, Malagasy Republic, Thailand and occasionally in the Seychelles contains a high percentage of methyl chavicol.

- The French basil oil, also known as European or sweet basil, has a higher percentage of linalool and is safe to use in aromatherapy.

- Methyl cinnamate basil is distilled in various countries of the world including India, Haiti and Guatemala.

- Eugenol basil is distilled in Russia, Egypt and Morocco. True basil and exotic basil

Constituent	Origin		
	Comoro Is.	France	Egypt
α–pinene	0.18%	0.11%	0.25%
camphene	0.06%	0.02%	0.07%
β–pinene	0.25%	0.07%	0.43%
myrcene	0.12%	0.13%	0.35%
limonene	2.64%	2.04%	4.73%
cis-ocimene	2.52%	0.03%	0.63%
camphor	0.37%	1.43%	0.57%
linalool	1.16%	40.72%	45.55%
methyl chavicol	85.76%	23.79%	26.56%
α–terpineol	0.84%	1.90%	1.09%
citronellol	0.65%	3.57%	1.76%
geraniol	0.03%	0.38%	0.2%
methyl cinnamate	0.05%	0.34%	0.25%
eugenol	0.74%	5.90%	5.90%

A comparative chemical composition of *Ocimum basilicum* oil (21)

are obtained from *Ocimum basilicum.* Methyl cinnamate and eugenol basil are thought to be derived from *Ocimum gratissimum.*

Methyl chavicol is considered a skin irritant and a possible carcinogen. For this reason it would be safer not to use basil from the Comoro Islands in aromatherapy.

Rosemary

Rosemary is another plant which has several chemotypes. Three principal chemotypes of *R. officinalis* can be found growing in Europe:

- camphor-borneol
- 1,8-cineole
- verbenone.

Due to their different compositions, these oils can be applied for different purposes to achieve maximum efficiency. Chemotypes with a high camphor content are more effective in cases of muscular aches and pain. The 1,8-cineole chemotype is best used for respiratory congestion, while the verbenone chemotype has excellent regenerative properties and is used in skincare preparations.

Specifying the extraction method

Genuine and authentic oils should be extracted correctly. With distillation, this usually means lower distillation temperatures to protect the essential oils from being oxidised and the molecules from being destroyed by too much heat.

Lavender

Distillation at lower temperature takes longer. Lavender, for example, is distilled rapidly in the first 25 minutes of the process and this usually accounts for 75% of the total yield. However the bulk of the natural coumarin content takes another 50 to 80 minutes to be distilled.

This final fraction does not add considerably to the fragrance of the essential oil, but it does make a difference to the therapeutic properties of the essential oil. Distillers are paid by the kilogram. As a result, commercial grade lavender oil usually contains the first half hour of distillate only.

Compound	Origin		
	Tunis	**Spain**	**France**
α-pinene	17.1%	18.1%	14.7%
borneol	3.0%	3.1%	6.3%
β-pinene	5.5%	4.8%	5.7%
camphor	14.8%	23.2%	13.1%
bornyl acetate	1.3%	3.4%	1.5%
camphene	6.63%	9.4%	3.6%
1,8-cineole	32.5%	19.2%	25.0%
verbenone	0.4%	0.5%	1.5%
limonene	3.7%	4.0%	7.8%

A typical chemical composition of the major rosemary oils available (22)

Ylang-ylang Constituents	Extra	1st grade	2nd grade	3rd grade
linalool	13.6%	18.6%	2.8%	1.0%
geranyl acetate	5.3%	5.9%	4.1%	3.5%
caryophyllene	1.7%	6.0%	7.5%	9.0%
p-cresyl methyl ether	16.5%	7.6%	1.8%	0.5%
methyl benzoate	8.7%	6.4%	2.3%	1.0%
benzyl acetate	25.1%	17.4%	7.0%	3.7%
benzyl benzoate	2.2%	5.3%	4.7%	4.3%
other sesquiterpenes	7.4%	28.8%	54.5%	97.0%

A typical chemical composition of the various grades of ylang-ylang (23)

This commercial grade lavender is commonly referred to as:

Lavender 40/48.

The 40/48 refers to the percentage of linalool and linalyl acetate present in the essential oil.

Ylang-ylang

The large flowers of ylang-ylang are subjected to fractional steam distillation or fractional steam and water distillation, thus yielding, in succession, ylang-ylang extra; No. 1; No. 2; and No. 3. A complete essential oil is also available by non fractional steam distillation of the flowers or by combining the first three fractions.

In the production of ylang-ylang the first proportion of the distillate is collected over several hours and becomes the 'extra' quality oil which is rich in oxygenated constituents but poor in the high boiling point terpenes known as sesquiterpenes.

The operators of the stills producing ylang-ylang oils grade the different qualities by specific gravity and by odour. Since there is no agreed standard, the quality of a given grade varies from one producer to another, a fact that has to be borne in mind when ylang-ylang is purchased.

Passing from ylang-ylang extra oil through No. 1 and 2 to No. 3 the following observations may be made:

- There are decreases in specific gravity, volatility, floral odour character, proportion of oxygenated constituents and price;

- There are increases in sesquiterpene content and oiliness of odour character.

From a perfumer's aspect, ylang-ylang extra is the best grade and the most highly valued of the four grades. The traditional use of ylang-ylang in aromatherapy as a relaxant and anti-depressant indicates that the extra or 1st grade would be more suitable than 3rd grade, as esters are chemical constituents which traditionally have such qualities. Ylang-ylang complete is the ideal oil for use in aromatherapy as it is non-fractionated.

Testing the purity of the essential oil

To certify the authenticity of an essential oil, it must undergo a series of tests such as:

- odour evaluation

- physical measures

- chemical analysis.

While odour evaluation is purely subjective, it is nevertheless essential. With an experienced nose, one is able to appreciate the intrinsic qualities, the balance of composition and the specific nature of an essential oil.

Various physical measures carried out on essential oils allow them to be compared with official standards. The density and the refractive index are two constant specific values of a pure essential oil which can be measured to establish its consistency with a corresponding standard. Optical rotation specifies whether the sample is dextrorotatory or laevorotatory. However, frauds cannot be absolutely detected with these physical characteristics because of the essential oils' complex chemical compounds.

We must therefore turn to chemical analysis. That is why gas chromatography linked to mass spectrometry (GC/MS) remains the most thorough analysis technique available, as it is able to separate, measure and identify chemical constituents found in essential oils.

Odour evaluation

The most economical method of testing the oils is organoleptic analysis. This means using your nose. Smelling oils is both an art and a science, and it can take some time to develop your sense to be able to evaluate the aromatic compound. However it is important to remember that some of the constituents found in the oil may not have an odour, and that smell alone will not define purity or quality. The composition of an essential oil can be quite complex.

Most essential oils have 20 to 50 readily-accessible chemical components; some up to 200. So organoleptic testing tends to be subjective and cannot be regarded as a test to determine purity. At best it is merely a useful guide.

Some points to consider when smelling the oils:

- Choose an area free from odours, foods or household smells.

- The room should be moderately warm and free from draughts.

- Prepare to smell the oil by using a paper blotter.

- Clear the nose before you start, by breathing rapidly in and out through the nose several times.

- Don't attempt to evaluate more than six oils per session and clear the nose between sessions.

Write down your impressions using descriptive words. Include the name of the oil, its botanical name, its origin, supplier and any other notes. This will allow you to compare the quality of oils from other sources or those you obtain at a later date.

Physical measures

Specific gravity

The specific gravity of a substance is defined as the ratio of the mass of a given volume of the substance to the mass of an equal volume of water at a stated temperature.

$$\text{S.G. (at stated temp.)} = \frac{\text{Mass of a given volume of substance}}{\text{Mass of an equal volume of water}}$$

To measure specific gravity a clean, dry specific gravity bottle of a nominal capacity is accurately weighed. Let us assume that the mass of the bottle and stopper is m_1 g.

The bottle is then filled with freshly boiled and cooled distilled water (usually at 20°C). The bottle and contents are then accurately weighed (mass = m_2 g).

The bottle is then emptied and thoroughly cleaned before it is filled with the test sample material at the same temperature and weighed with its contents (mass = m_3 g.).

$$\text{Then S.G.} = \frac{m_3 - m_1}{m_2 - m_1}$$

This can be a time-consuming and demanding technique for obtaining reproducible results, but can sometimes detect adulteration that would normally go undetected by the nose. For example genuine rosewood oil has a specific gravity of 0.872-0.887, while pure linalool has a specific gravity of 0.87. Approximately 84-93% of rosewood essential oil is linalool. If the specific gravity of rosewood is much less than 0.872 it would be suspected of having been diluted with the much cheaper synthetic linalool.

Refractive index

When a ray of light passes from one medium to a denser medium, the ray is partially reflected, but most of it takes a different path by changing direction at the interface and entering the denser medium at a smaller angle to the normal at the point of incidence than the angle of incidence.

This simply means that angle p is always smaller than angle q, whatever the value of the angle q, and that angles p and q are measured perpendicularly to the interface at the point of entry of the ray of light into the denser medium, in this case the essential oil.

Each essential oil has a specific refractive index and while the testing procedure is quite simple, the test must be done at the same temperature as the standard which is used as a reference.

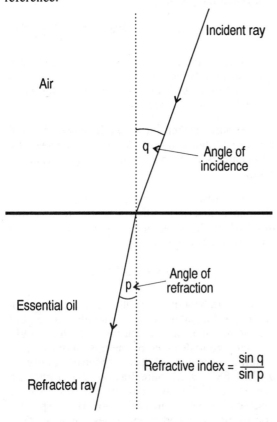

Measurement of Refractive Index

Optical rotation

Certain substances have the ability to rotate a plane of polarised light. Those substances which cause anti-clockwise rotation of the polarised light are said to be laevo-rotatory, symbolised 'l-', and those which cause clockwise rotation are said to be dextro-rotatory, symbolised 'd-'. Thus we have, for example:

- l-citronellol, which has a fine rose odour

- d-citronellol, which has a rose odour less fine than the l-type.

Optical activity is conferred upon a substance by the presence in its molecule of a carbon atom which is bonded to four different atoms or chemical groups. Such a carbon atom is said to be asymmetric.

As many essential oils contain optically active components, the measurement of optical rotation using a polarimeter can provide some information on the concentration of those components in the oil and hence can indicate the quality of the oil. It can also be used to help differentiate between natural and synthetic oils.

Chemical analysis

Gas chromatography linked to mass spectrometry (GC/MS)

The more expensive, but qualitative and quantitive method of determining the composition of an essential oil is gas chromatography. This is the most important method used to analyse essential oils.

Gas chromatography (GC) is used to separate an essential oil into its individual constituents. While the GC analysis shows the relative concentrations of the chemical components, their identification remains impossible until mass spectrometry (MS) is used to identify each peak of the gas chromatograph.

While GC/MS equipment is able to identify and quantify the chemical compounds of an essential oil, it cannot detect fraudulently-added synthetic compounds. These can be detected only with marginal and very costly techniques using liquid scintillators or isotopic NMR.

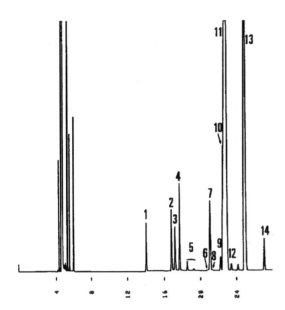

Gas chromatogram of a genuine
cold-pressed mandarin essential oil
(Courtesy of Allured Publishing)

1 = α–thujene
2 = α– pinene
4 = myrcene
5 = sabinene
6 = α–phellandrene
7 = β–pinene

9 = p-cymene
10 = (-)-limonene
11 = (+)-limonene
12 = octanol
13 = γ-terpinene
14 = terpinolene

Adulteration of essential oils

According to Dr Brian Lawrence (24) there are four ways of adulterating an essential oil. These methods involve the blending of an essential oil with:

- other oils or their constituents

- its own main constituent

- a reconstituted oil

- a pure aroma chemical.

Other oils or their constituents

A publication recently addressed the adulteration of spike lavender. It was found that when Spanish sage oil was blended with spike lavender oil, the blend appeared to have an acceptable odour quality. Nevertheless, the presence of Spanish sage oil (greater than 5%) could be detected by the marked increase in ratio of:

camphor:1,8-cineole:linalool,
and the decrease in the ratio of:

1,8-cineole: α–pinene: β–pinene.
Other oils such as lavandin oil could have been used to blend with spike lavender. This would have been detected by a marked increase in linalyl acetate, whereas the use of rosemary or eucalyptus as 'blender oils' was considered to be easily detected even by odour quality.

Its own main constituent

This procedure was considered to be a 'sound method which may be difficult to detect'. An optimum blend for spike lavender was reported as being a mixture of camphor:1,8-cineole:linalool in a 1:2.5:3 ratio. The only way to successfully detect this type of blending was to examine the physical and chemical constituents, such as solubility and optical rotation.

For example, the addition of camphor to spike lavender oil can be detected by the reduction in solubility (in 70% aqueous ethanol) of the oil plus the increase in optical rotation.

A reconstituted oil

It was noted that the blending of an essential oil with a reconstituted or modified essential oil was the most effective and proper solution from technological and olfactory points of view. Unfortunately no comment was made on the detection of this type of blending.

A pure aroma chemical

This refers to a pure aroma chemical which is either present in the original oil in a small quantity or absent from the original oil. The authors felt that this method of blending was easy to detect by the smell, and by gas chromatography. This type of blending has little to do with the aesthetic side and can never be recommended because it inevitably impairs the characteristic note of the pure oil.

Conclusion - adulteration

In conclusion, it was noted that the major constituents of an oil cannot be used to grade an essential oil for its quality. Furthermore the determination of the combined qualities of trace substances is not very useful.

Dr Wladyslaw Brud (25) states that the availability of true, natural steam distilled oils that are not blended or treated is very scarce. Due to the high level of blending, mixing and adulteration

it is difficult to examine and differentiate a true product from a treated product. He cites several examples where essential oils have been blended with inferior oils.

The first example is geranium oil *Pelargonium graveolens*. The most sought after geranium oil is from Bourbon, however this oil is often blended with other, less expensive geranium oils from other countries. Some people refer to the Bourbon geranium as rose geranium, because of its 'rosy' aroma. Most essential oils sold as rose geranium however are inexpensive geranium oils distilled over roses, or a blend of geranium and rose odorants.

Often patchouli oil is blended with other oils such as gurjun balsam oil, copaiba balsam oil, cedarwood oil, castor oil and aroma chemicals such as 8-camphene, menthanol or isobornyl

Compound	Algeria	Egypt	Morocco	Bourbon	China
α-pinene	0.56%	0.45%	0.57%	0.76%	0.35%
cis-rose oxide	0.69%	1.04%	1.31%	0.52%	2.25%
trans-rose oxide	0.31%	0.4%	0.56%	0.28%	1.04%
menthone	1.28%	0.78%	0.95%	1.09%	1.94%
isomenthone	5.33%	6.05%	5.63%	8.12%	4.51%
linalool	6.25%	9.9%	5.63%	8.12%	4.51%
citronellyl formate	9.4%	7.43%	7.64%	12.39%	17.45%
geranyl formate	6.49%	3.89%	4.33%	5.92%	2.2%
citronellol	27.87%	32.1%	18.59%	23.24%	44.39%
geranyl propionate	0.98%	1.69%	1.61%	1.7%	0.6%
citronellyl propionate	2.62%	2.1%	2.49%	1.74%	2.2%
geraniol	24.97%	19.7%	18.59%	20.67%	6.4%
geranyl butyrate	2.4%	1.72%	1.64%	1.68%	0.73%
10-epi-gamma-eudesmol	5.41%	4.62%	5.2%	1.04%	2.03%
geranyl tiglate	1.56%	1.44%	1.54%	0.45%	1.64%

A quantitative comparison between Bourbon (Reunion), Chinese, Algerian, Egyptian and Moroccan geranium oils (26)

acetate. These adulterants, however are easily detectable by gas chromatography.

It is my belief that the practice of extension or adulteration of the essential oils may present no great problem when the oils are being used merely for the purpose of fragrances. However this practice should be condemned when the essential oils are being used for aromatherapy.

> **Only 100% pure, natural and authentic essential oils should be employed for use in aromatherapy.**

The only way to obtain true oils for aromatherapy purposes is to have reliable suppliers, either by having direct contact with the manufacturer of the oils or by keeping in contact with a dealer who has enough contacts with producers to offer a full range of the best quality oils available.

Natural versus synthetic

Essential oils such as eucalyptus and lavender are readily available in sufficient quantities at rather reasonable prices. These oils are usually not duplicated in the chemical laboratory. The synthetic substitute would be more expensive than the natural distillate! The common problem with these oils is adulteration (with even less expensive similar essences). However this situation is reversed in the case of jasmine or rose. It may take one tonne of rose petals to produce 500 grammes of rose oil. Most of the essences of rose and jasmine found on store shelves almost invariably are synthetic.

Given this situation and the high demand for these essences in perfumery it is not surprising that chemical research has succeeded in producing rather good imitations of these oils. Usually these products smell very nice, and may sometimes be even closer to the fragrance of the actual flower than the true essence. The objective of the artificial fragrance is to duplicate the scent of the flower and not that of the essential oil. It has to be emphasised that the synthetic fragrance does not

have any of the therapeutic qualities of the essential oil.

The following comment by Tisserand (27) summarises the way most aromatherapists feel about using essential oils.

> *'Why natural oils? Why not anything that smells nice whether it is natural or synthetic? The answer is simply that synthetic or inorganic substances do not contain any 'life force'; they are not dynamic. Everything is made of chemicals, but organic substances like essential oils have a structure which only mother nature can put together. They have a life force, an additional impulse which can only be found in living things.'*

On the other side of the coin the following comment summarises the perfume industry's attitude to the use of essential oils. (28)

> *'The nose of the civilised human being has become more fastidious and demanding. All the rose, mint and lavender fields in the world would not be able to fulfil the needs of the hygiene and body care industries alone. The extraction of natural fragrances is difficult and expensive....The nature identical products which are synthetic substances duplicate their natural counterparts completely in terms of chemical structure as well as fragrance.'*

According to Professor George H. Dodd (29), perfumer and lecturer in chemistry at the University of Warwick the aromatherapeutic argument is completely faulty. He states that:

> *'The chief defect is that aromatherapists are not willing to consider the chemical evidence and so remain in ignorance about current concepts of molecular structure and their relationships to cellular dynamics.'*

He claims that this belief impeded the development of biological chemistry until Wohler synthesised urea in 1828, at which stage it became evident that the chemical substances of living tissues were in all physiological respects identical to the same molecules synthesised in the laboratory.

This argument is valid for the purpose of either perfumery or olfactory experiments. It does not matter whether we use linalool from a laboratory synthesis or a sample which has been isolated from lavender oil, provided that sufficient attention has been given to impurities. Dodd (30) also comments on aromatherapists' vitalistic approach to essential oils:

'These impurities may affect the odour of the oil, but we cannot expect them to contribute the "vibrations" cited by Tisserand.'

The vibrations of which Robert Tisserand speaks are well documented. The life force is a very old concept. The Chinese call it *Qi*, the Japanese *Ki* and the Indians *Prana*. Some years ago a Russian scientist, Semyon Kirlian, developed a method of photographing this energy field. Anything which is alive, whether plant or animal, shows an energy field around it when photographed in this way. What the photographs show is the electrical field of the living organism.

A form of diagnosis has recently been evolved based on Kirlian photographs of patients' hands.

Recent research has now proven that individual components of a plant do not always behave in the way we expect when they are isolated and they only display their therapeutic properties in synergy with all the other components of the oil. While there is now extensive evidence to compare the medicinal properties of the essential oils with the properties of synthetic drugs, I feel that we are about to enter a new phase in healing which will involve energy. It is here that we find the greater healing value of essential oils and aromatherapy becoming apparent.

UNIT II

ESSENTIAL ISSUES

"Quintessence they name to be, the chief and the heavenliest power or vertue in any plant.... which by ye force and puritie of the hoale substance....conserveth the good health of mans body, prolongeth a mans youthe, differeth age, and putteth way all manner of diseases."
Conrad Gesner, 1559

What is it about the essential oils that gives them so many virtues? The major theme of this unit is:
'How do essential oils work?'
It is now possible to piece together from a diversity of sources an account of the pharmacological activity of the essential oil constituents. This will provide strong circumstantial evidence for the clinical effectiveness of the essential oils. There is no doubt that the subject of essential oil pharmacology will develop rapidly in the coming years.

Unit II includes the following chapters:

Chapter 6. Research
Chapter 7. Essential Oil Chemistry
Chapter 8. Pharmacology of Essential Oils
Chapter 9. Biology and Psychology of Essential Oils
Chapter 10. Pharmacokinetics
Chapter 11. Essential Oil Safety

Chapter 6

Research

References are cited for a considerable amount of research work into the pharmacology of medicinal plants. This highly academic research does much to reassure aromatherapists that essential oils contain many constituents with real effects on the body. However it is clear that what is lacking is any substantial scientific research into the effect of the whole essential oil on the human being.

If it is accepted that the plant is a vast complex of pharmacologically active chemicals, then it is obvious that the whole essential oil will have different properties from that of any single constituent acting alone.

However, if aromatherapists make certain claims, it is fair to ask why they have provided so little evidence of genuine clinical effects.

The obvious point to make is that many people have found aromatherapy effective, and most users of essential oils have strong anecdotal evidence of their apparent benefits.

Therefore the challenge has been put forward:

If what we say about aromatherapy is true then it should be able to stand up for itself in any forum.

It is in this spirit that the following discussion of the prospects for research into aromatherapy is offered.

Introduction

Through experience, many people take for granted that aromatherapy works based on the observed actions of the essential oil. I have been to many conferences presented by researchers and scientists who discredit the claims made by aromatherapists because of the lack of scientific evidence. The simplest point to make in introducing a review of the scientific validation of aromatherapy is that some of those practising aromatherapy have not understood the requirement for research.

It may also be maintained that investigating the mechanisms behind proven oils only serves to distract those who could be searching for new ones. However, without proving the properties of essential oils by clinical experiments we will never increase our knowledge of how aromatherapy works. We need an experimental framework to back our empirical knowledge.

There are many problems in pursuing good clinical research. One is that to produce results carrying sufficient statistical weight is expensive and laborious. Another is that there is considerable doubt about the applicability of conventional, technological, scientific pursuit and analysis to the healing event in general and to aromatherapy in particular.

Healing involves an element of purely human contact - the therapist stepping outside his or her own position and into the life of the patient - and is not an event which can be subjected to analysis by independent observers. Nor can predictions or general conclusions be made from such an exercise. Current medical research generally concerns itself only with measuring events and data divorced from the human being, ignoring the practitioner's immensely powerful influence in the treatment of the patient.

According to Benor (1) psychological and psychosomatic contributions to health and disease can explain aspects of many illnesses, but these concepts have not been fully integrated into Western medicine.

Excellent research has been conducted, for example, demonstrating that aromatherapy massage can reduce heart and breathing rates in patients in intensive care and coronary care units.

According to a senior nurse involved in the clinical trial (2):

> *`This study demonstrates what we all intuitively know: that patients benefit from a caring touch. This is particularly appropriate in the high-tech environment of intensive care. As the research shows, benefits of aromatherapy are ultimately longer lasting than massage without essential oils.'*

Yet most surgeons are either unaware of these methods or find these subjects are so alien to their belief systems that they are usually unwilling to consider them.

For the public good

Although real insights into the characteristics of remedies come from practical clinical experience, there is a need to reassure the public and legislature that aromatherapy is at least safe, and preferably effective. In Australia this has been a concern pursued by the natural therapies industry in discussion with the government under the terms of the Therapeutic Goods Act 1989.

It happens that for the treatment of minor self-limiting disorders remedies have been allowed to be sold to the public on the basis of bibliographic evidence of traditional usage alone, and the authorities have not significantly encroached upon the right of the therapist to use whatever remedies he or she considers appropriate. Nevertheless, the licence to market essential oils or herbs as registered therapeutic goods for what are considered moderate to severe ailments is dependent on providing conventional clinical evidence for such a claim. The double-blind clinical trials and experiments on animals, to name two areas of contention in research, will therefore remain essential as evidence as long as legislative and medical authorities consider them so.

This causes aromatherapists real concern. Apart from the cost of undertaking effective clinical trials, it is disturbing to know that the legal future of a remedy is more likely to rest on the results of animal testing than on the testimony of patients and practitioners.

At the Aroma '93 conference held at the University of Sussex, England it was revealed that there are now signs that patient assessment may be increasingly used in calculating efficacy in clinical research. However it is most likely that the great weight of scientific and medical opinion will insist on playing the same rules as before.

Towards an aromatherapy research policy

The following guidelines will be useful in developing research methods that can be applied for investigating the efficacy of aromatherapy.

Defining the stages of a clinical trial

In order to conduct valid clinical trials, there are several stages which are necessary:

- *Planning* (defining the precise purpose of the clinical trial)
- *Design* (how to conduct the clinical trial)
- *Conduct* (doing the experiment or clinical trial)
- *Analysis* (making sense of the data)
- *Interpretation* (drawing conclusions).

Aims of a clinical trial

Despite the fact that most aromatherapists and others believe that aromatherapy works, there is little objective evidence that it actually does work. If aromatherapy does work, a better way of convincing others would be to show them objective evidence, allowing them to see for themselves that it works, rather than having them accept your word for it.

Careful and clearly defined procedures must be carried out to collect and present the objective evidence to people. Of course, the clearly-defined procedures of which we speak are known as the 'scientific method'.

It is essential that the aims of a clinical trial or study be clearly determined before starting. Unless the aims of the clinical trial are clearly and precisely stated, it will be difficult to identify suitable patients for the clinical trial, devise appropriate evaluation parameters and calculate the necessary sample size for a clinical trial.

Asking the right questions

Most research is designed and carried out to answer questions that are comparative in nature. This means instead of saying 'Is lavender a good oil for people with high blood pressure?', which is an unclear question and open to idiosyncratic interpretation of the word 'good', we should be asking 'Is lavender oil better than nothing at all, or is it better than, say, hypotensive tablets, or better than sweet marjoram in helping people with high blood pressure?'.

The word 'better' here can be defined in terms of observed differences in objective measures of the actual blood pressure in clients under two or more different situations. In every case, the question needs to be answered by comparing the objective measures with the variables or aspects of the problem identified as being relevant to the clinical trial.

Types of clinical trials

Most clinical trials can be classified as either observational studies or experimental studies. In observational studies the researcher simply observes what is happening to a population and has no control over the conditions. In general, observational studies take the form of either surveys or case-control studies. Experimental studies are generally clinical trials in which the researcher needs to specify the conditions under which the clinical trial is conducted. They are designed to evaluate the effects of various treatments, or preventative measures.

Both types of clinical trial use results from a limited population sample on which decisions are made or inferences drawn about the general population. For example decisions about how to treat the general population of patients who have the same ailment are made using data derived from a clinical trial involving a small number of patients. Since future patients are unlikely to be identical in all respects to the patients in the clinical trial, there will be some uncertainty associated with claims that are made regarding the treatment. The credibility of claims that are made on the basis of a clinical trial depends critically on the various features of that trial.

Background to the clinical trial

The initial intention for conducting a clinical trial may be to fill the gaps in present knowledge. The trial will therefore need to specify how it will begin to fill these gaps and contribute to that knowledge. This is not only based on the researcher's clinical knowledge and that of other practitioners, but also on existing literature.

Reviewing existing literature can be a research study in itself. It demands a great deal of application to search, collect and read the relevant material. Reading about other researchers, who too have been excited by ideas and have attempted to demonstrate those ideas in practice, will bring much satisfaction and encouragement.

There are numerous databases available for searching the literature. These searches are made easier if the categories to be searched, the range of publications, the language and duration of publication are identified.

Once literature research is complete, then papers must be critically reviewed, notes made and conclusions written. This will act as a pilot study of ideas where new research builds on previous clinical trials. It may be advantageous to contact the authors of the clinical trials to ask how they would further investigate their fields.

By reviewing the literature it is possible to see exactly what is required as a next step in terms of preparing clinical trials, avoid the mistakes of others and construct a trial which builds upon what has been done before.

Patient selection

Who is eligible for inclusion in the clinical trial? It is important that the patients included in a trial are representative of the population to whom the trial's findings will be applied. Whether the clinical trial recruits its patients from hospitals or from volunteers, careful consideration needs to be given to the final conclusions which may not be of great significance to the wider population.

For example, a clinical trial of depressive illness which studies hospital inpatients sees a special group of patients tending to be the more severe cases. Consider a clinical trial of an essential oil for premenstrual syndrome. If an advertisement is placed in a health magazine it is very likely to produce a biased subset of the population of women who suffer from PMS. However an advertisement in a women's magazine with a broader range of readership might be more reasonable. Volunteers from self-help groups, such as those who read health magazines, are likely to be very compliant and the drop-out rate low.

In determining the selection criteria it is important to clearly define the condition to be studied. This would be a problem for a trial involving PMS, as there is still no precise definition hence there would be great difficulty in determining which patients are eligible.

Randomised trial groups

The purpose of randomised trials is to safeguard against selection bias. For the result of any clinical trial to be considered statistically valid, it is important that each patient could have received, during the trial, any one of the treatments being compared. Selection bias refers to the process in which the therapist consciously or subconsciously encourages or discourages a patient to take part in a trial because the therapist is aware of the treatment the patient will receive.

Therefore the simplest and most commonly used clinical trial design is a two-group comparison in which patients are randomly allocated, perhaps using random number tables, to one of the treatment groups. One treatment group receives 'treatment A' and the other 'treatment B.'

It is also important for the clinical trial to be double blind; that is, both the patient and the therapist are unaware of which treatment the patient is receiving. This is desirable as it allows assessment of response and side effects to be unbiased. When it is not possible for a therapist to be 'blind', it is desirable for the person assessing the patient's response to be different from the person who is administering the treatment; the assessor can then be kept 'blind' to the treatment the patient received.

Problems in pursuing good clinical research

To produce results that carry sufficient statistical weight is expensive and laborious. Some of the problems associated with pursuing good clinical research in natural therapies and aromatherapy are:

- There is a lack of the necessary infrastructure of teaching institutions, funding from a wealthy industrial sector and hospitals all of which are a part of conventional medicine.

- Because the essential oils are complex pharmacologically active chemicals, the whole essential oil will have different properties from that of any single constituent acting alone. Most pharmacological studies involve the use of individual chemical constituents. (3)(4)

- The application of essential oils and their effect on the body are not always the same as is usual for conventional medicines. Clinically, essential oils are often used to evoke healing responses in the body rather than attack symptoms. This is not a simple concept to put on a product label.

Single case study research

According to David Aldridge (5) single case study research is becoming a part of a spectrum of research methods. This usually relies on the monitoring of individual case histories rather than on comparing treatment and control groups. When clinicians of whatever therapeutic persuasion gather for their clinical discussions, they usually focus on individual case studies. Even research scientists at conferences adopt a style, usually when away from the podium, which reflects the human story as epitomised by the single case study. Single case studies bring an important facet to clinical research - that of personal application.

Single case studies have always been used as guides to the study of rare clinical situations, for the reporting of new information about side effects of treatment or for introducing views which challenge the existing theories of disease. While the clinical account of single case studies was once the primary form of medicine, it is now often unfairly dismissed as 'unscientific'.

The use of single case studies is an attempt to formalise clinical stories. The case study uses as its basis the clinical process where the illness is assessed and diagnosed, a treatment is prescribed, the patient is monitored during the application of the treatment, and the success of the treatment is then evaluated. The main concern about a single case study is that it cannot credibly select real effects from confusing variables, treatment effects from placebo effects and so on. In some cases, the disease may have run its course and improvement would have occurred without therapeutic intervention.

The account of each participant is assembled individually, and then it should be brought back for a case study conference discussion at a later date to cross check and combine so as to produce a final report of the treatment. Each report can be examined by a coordinating researcher or assistant. As each case is thus graphically characterised, it can be used for comparative purposes with other cases to see whether a pattern occurs and can be sustained.

Evaluation of patient response

Essential oils are usually applied in a qualitatively different way from conventional drugs. Whereas drugs are primarily designed to directly affect a specific disability without the context in which the disability occurs, essential oils are usually used to support the individual's recuperative capacities, where the main complaint is seen as only one feature in a wider and unique pattern of disturbance. The character of the essential oil therefore reflects this broader, interactive and often supportive action. It is apparent clinical effect is not entirely measured by purely analytical investigative methods.

To give an example let us use a clinical trial conducted in the intensive care unit of Middlesex Hospital (6) using foot massage with neroli oil on heart surgery patients. This research took the form of a randomised control trial group involving 100 post-cardiac surgery patients divided into four groups. The groups were as follows:

- Nothing Group: control group with no intervention
- Chat Group: control group receiving a general chat, not designed to be counselling
- Plain Group: group receiving a foot massage with plain apricot kernel oil
- Aromatherapy Group: group receiving a foot massage with neroli essential oil.

Throughout the clinical trial an independent recorder assessed the physiological and psychological changes of each trial group. The physiological measurements taken were heart rate, blood pressure and respiratory rate. A questionnaire was used to measure the patient's state psychologically, looking at pain, anxiety, tension, calm, rest and relaxation. The questionnaire gave the subjects four options with regard to how they felt in each category:

- not at all
- slightly
- moderately
- very.

While the clinical trial was not perfect in its design, it was interesting to examine the differences, if any, to be found in the short term benefits between aromatherapy massage and plain massage. In general the patients perceived themselves as having benefited more from the neroli foot massage than from the plain massage in a variety of ways, including reduction of anxiety and from the oil's calming, relaxing and restful effects.

It is hoped that clinical trials such as this will encourage aromatherapy practitioners to use their skills in this field alongside the orthodox medical treatments, such as cardiac surgery, where the patient can benefit from the best of both worlds, and thus slowly close the gap between the two.

Pharmacological and pharmacokinetic research

The aromatherapist insists on the uniqueness of the individual patient, and on the right to provide a unique combination of essential oils in each case. Apart from the objection to participation in randomised blind trials, there is the impression that essential oils are interactive with the patient ie their actual effect varies with the nature of the condition being treated.

Traditional views of the essential oils emphasise their primary influence on transient body functions eg, expectorants, circulatory stimulants, diuretics, diaphoretics and so on. Many essential oils also encourage self-correcting processes. The requirement is to devise a process in which such properties can be verified.

Emphasis needs to shift from isolated observation to simultaneous recording of several parameters of change. All events that occur influence each other and are equally related to each other and to the effect that is observed. These events are usually excluded in conventional trials as distracting variables. Acceptance of these variables as important data is a key feature of such work and would profoundly change the nature of the information gathered.

Instead of trying to eliminate all the variables that might cloud the specific issue in question, the aim, according to Simon Mills, should be to define all the factors which determine the substance's influence on the course of disease.

'The task would in some ways resemble the homoeopathic 'proving'. This information would be better suited to systems, rather than casual analysis, and any conclusions drawn from it will be qualitative rather than quantitative.' (7)

Rather than stating that it is statistically likely that an essential oil is effective against bronchitis, asthma or other disease state, it would be more useful to state that an essential oil, in certain individuals at least, changes the constitution of phlegm, of urine, or alters circulatory activity to one or other tissues or over the body as a whole.

There can also be no long term future for aromatherapy unless it examines the processes by which the body interacts with, metabolises and eliminates essential oils. The factors that influence the movement of an essential oil through the body and its availability to the body tissues allow the aromatherapist better insight into the ideal conditions in which to apply any prescription.

It must be emphasised, however, that most factors are highly variable so that total bioavailability is very much an individual matter, to be assessed, if at all, only as a result of years of practical diagnostic experience.

Experimental research

Apart from clinical trials already discussed, the question of research models for studying the action of essential oils is the most difficult. As part of the modern move away from animal experimentation, increasing attention is being paid to techniques for assessing the effects of drugs on cultures of cells, tissues and organs in vitro. Conventional drug research is switching to this direction for preliminary screening in drug discovery programs.

The problems are the limited application of such observations to the in vivo situation and the need to confirm any in vitro findings anyway. It is also impossible to actually know which plant constituents have actually reached internal tissue after absorption. Nevertheless, in vitro techniques could provide valuable supplementary information to other research, as in the following suggested projects:

- the absorption of essential oils on epithelial tissue cultures (to reduce the possibility of skin irritation)

- the influence of essential oils on microbiological cultures (Much work has already been done in this area, but there are still many questions that remained unanswered.)

- alteration in the migratory behaviour and internal metabolism of macrophages as a result of exposure to essential oils (There are many claims that the essential oils improve resistance to infection by general enhancement of defensive mechanisms; looking directly at macrophage response is an established screening technique.)

- using psychophysiological changes such as sweat, saliva, blood and urine, to measure emotional responses to the odour of essential oils (This might also include the measurement of electrical potentials generated within the brain which are recorded using an electroencephalograph [EEG]).

There can be no doubt about the problems of using animals to support research into essential oils. Apart from the difficulty of applying such findings to the human situation, there are extremely strong ethical objections from almost all of those that support the use of aromatherapy. Perhaps we need to develop research along the lines of a therapy system that aims to support the vital functions. If the intention of any trial was to assess the effects of essential oils applied in the approximately therapeutic doses adjusted for body weight and metabolism, there could be little complaint that the animals would be harmed, and that they would in fact be likely to actually benefit. This type of experimentation has already proved to be successful in finding evidence of the sedative properties of neroli when mice were exposed to the neroli vapours (8).

Feasible studies might include observing behavioural and social changes after administering the essential oils, and the effects of antimicrobial remedies on normal resistance of diseases among large populations. These studies would be valuable in veterinary practice.

Ethical considerations

It is often necessary for a researcher to obtain approval for a clinical trial. If the researcher's professional group has a code of ethics then it will be necessary to consider these ethics. Mention of such a code of ethics should be made in the research paper. If the researcher is working for an institution then there will be an ethics committee which will need to see the research submission.

The consent of the patients and cooperating practitioners must also be obtained. The researcher must be clear how this consent is to be obtained, and what information will be given to patients in the trial. The rights of the patient to refuse to participate in, or withdraw from, the trial must be observed. It is also essential that any risks to the patient be made clear.

Conclusion

Modern medicine chooses to make an in-depth physiological analysis of the human body in order to find a cause for the illness. Side by side with this very symptom-orientated and analytical approach the pharmaceutical industry makes particular drugs which are known, subject to precise analysis, reproducible and always conform to norms in context of experimentation. So conventional medicine can now correlate, with utmost precision, the medication to the symptom. We are however becoming aware of the vast limitations of such a purely analytical approach as we know that disease is multifactorial, with many different aspects that come into play.

Clinical pharmacologists have discovered that as far as the patient is concerned predictability is an illusion. The aromatherapist should view the essential oils as stimulating vital responses, without producing extraneous toxic side effects. Although there is variability, it is within workable limits, and quality control can reduce it even further. In recording the action of the essential oils, the aromatherapist can constantly renew the impression that the complete oil is much more than the sum of its constituents.

The issues discussed in this chapter provide guidelines for possible further work that might appropriately test many of the claims made by those using essential oils. At this stage only a few claims have been validated. However as the momentum for the use of essential oils grows, it is inevitable that the scientific spotlight will focus more on this subject.

Most of the scrutiny will be by those whose role it is to act as medical advisers to the Government. Politicians, like most of the public, have a generally detached view about scientific arguments in general, and the demands for research proof in particular. Their concern is public safety. The drive for evidence comes primarily from those who see themselves as the medical guardians of the public good, the large lobby of advisers who help the politicians declaim in this area.

These so-called medical guardians sometimes see natural therapies as fiendish, complex, dubious and antiquated forms of medicine full of hidden perils for the unsuspecting public. In many cases they are simply protecting an established, wealthy and powerful medical interest. If such scrutiny which can be harsh in its requirements for evidence, continues to grow, then as aromatherapists we will need to develop research principles similar to the ones outlined above, or else face the possibility of being denied our rights to treat people holistically using essential oils.

Chapter 7

Essential Oil Chemistry

The purpose of this chapter is to establish basic scientific criteria in which the action of the essential oil can be identified.

However, any assumption that the action of the essential oil relies solely on a single constituent should be resisted. The action of the complete essential oil is more than the action of its parts, therefore the study of essential oil chemistry should aim at:

• Providing possible explanations for the already perceived action of the essential oil.

• Highlighting the possible actions, beneficial or harmful, that might have been missed out because of the context of traditional use.

• Finding evidence for the particular therapeutic approach traditionally applied to the use of essential oils.

• Illustrating the full diversity of essential oil pharmacology.

Introduction to organic chemistry

In the early days of chemistry, scientists said that there were two classes of compounds. One class was produced by living organisms - these substances were called 'organic'. The other class, found in minerals and rocks was called 'inorganic'.

It was also a belief of the time that organic compounds could not be synthesised from inorganic compounds. It was believed that the 'vital force' possessed only by living organisms was necessary to produce organic compounds.

Unfortunately this theory was disproved in 1828 by Friedrich Wohler. He heated an aqueous solution of two inorganic compounds, ammonium chloride and silver cyanate, and to his surprise obtained urea.

$$NH_4Cl + AgNCO \rightarrow NH_2CONH_2 + AgCl$$
$$\text{heat} \qquad \text{urea}$$

This fits the old definition of 'organic', because the urea has been isolated from human urine. This single experiment of Wohler's was enough to disprove the 'doctrine of vital force'. This meant that the words organic and inorganic no longer had real definitions, since, for example, urea could be obtained from both sources. A few years later Friedrick Kekule assigned the modern definition - organic compounds are those containing carbon.

The chemistry of living organisms is no longer called organic chemistry; today that branch of science is called biochemistry.

Sources of organic compounds

The key to the chemical characteristics of an atom is in its configuration of electrons, which determines the kinds and number of bonds it will form with other atoms. Carbon has a total of six electrons, with two in the first electron shell and four in the second shell. Having four valence electrons in a shell that holds eight, carbon has little tendency to gain or lose electrons to form ionic bonds. It completes its valence shell by sharing electrons with other atoms thus acting as an intersection point from which a molecule branches off in up to four directions.

This electron configuration makes carbon, of all the 108 known chemical elements, unique in the ability of its atoms to catenate; that is, to bond or link up with one another in seemingly endless arrangements of chains, branched chains, rings, multiple rings, combinations of chains and rings and so on.

The possible number of these arrangements that exist in the essential oils is staggering and carbon's ability to form so many compounds is due to:

- Carbon atoms form stable bonds with other carbon atoms, so that both long and short chains of carbon atoms, and even whole networks, are possible.

- Carbon atoms also form stable bonds with certain other atoms, including hydrogen, oxygen, nitrogen, the halogens, and sulphur.

- The valence of carbon is four, which can be made up in many different ways so that many combinations and arrangements of atoms are possible.

Besides carbon atoms, a carbon-based molecule contains hydrogen atoms, and may contain atoms of other elements, such as oxygen, nitrogen and sulphur. The branch of this chemistry that is concerned with the study of carbon-based chemicals is known as organic chemistry, from its original association with substances from living things. Despite this, innumerable carbon compounds that are known today do not occur in plants and animals.

Structure of organic compounds

Organic chemistry molecules are made up of hydrocarbon structures. These hydrocarbon structures are called the backbone of the molecules. The carbon and hydrogen atoms in a hydrocarbon structure are very strongly bonded and do not have a pronounced polarity. They are chemically inert or stable. Even with only two elements, there are many thousands of known hydrocarbons. Hydrocarbons are also the major components of the fossil fuel petroleum. Our interest in hydrocarbons is in the diversity of their carbon skeletons, which is the basis of most essential compounds.

Isomers

Variations in the architecture of organic molecules can be seen in the form of isomers. These are compounds that have the same molecular formula but different structures and hence different properties. According to Shirley Price (1), at the EOTA conference (June 1990) held at Brunel University:

> 'Dr K. Tyman said that there are 4 different thujones and a change in molecular shape means a change in effect. This is an interesting comment, which possibly explains why sage, supposedly very hazardous because of its high thujone content, does not in practice appear to be so.'

Dr Tyman explained that because the thujone molecule can arrange itself in different ways (eg α–thujone, β–thujone, etc.) it is possible that the different isomers of thujone have different pharmacological effects, therefore it may be that not all thujone molecules will necessarily be a hazard.

However, until further evidence is at hand, caution should be maintained using sage or any essential oil containing thujone. Let us examine the principal types of isomerism that occur in essential oil constituents.

Structural isomerism

Structural isomers differ in the covalent arrangements of their atoms. The number of possible isomers increases tremendously as carbon skeletons increase in size. There are only two butanes, but there are 18 variations of C_8H_{18} and 366,319 possible structural isomers of $C_{20}H_{42}$. Structural isomers may also differ in the location of double bonds.

$$CH_3-CH_2-CH_2-CH_3$$

Butane

iso-Butane

Example of structural isomers

Positional isomerism

Positional isomers differ in the position of the same functional group in their molecules. For example:

Thymol (eg thyme, ajowan)   Carvacrol (eg oregano, thyme)

Example of positional isomers

Functional group isomerism

Functional group isomer molecules contain the same numbers of the same atoms (as they must to be isomers), but the functional groups are different. For example, the molecular formula for ethyl alcohol is C_2H_6O.

- A molecular formula shows which atoms, and how many of each are present in a molecule.

- A structural formula shows not only all the atoms present in the molecule, but also all the bonds that connect the atoms to each other.

The structural formula for ethyl alcohol is:

$$H - \overset{\overset{\displaystyle H}{|}}{\underset{\underset{\displaystyle H}{|}}{C}} - \overset{\overset{\displaystyle H}{|}}{\underset{\underset{\displaystyle H}{|}}{C}} - O - H$$

However, ethyl alcohol is not the only compound whose molecular formula is C_2H_6O. An entirely different compound, dimethyl ether, is also C_2H_6O. The ether functional group is simply an oxygen atom bonded to two hydrocarbons. The structural formula for dimethyl ether is:

$$H - \overset{\overset{\displaystyle H}{|}}{\underset{\underset{\displaystyle H}{|}}{C}} - O - \overset{\overset{\displaystyle H}{|}}{\underset{\underset{\displaystyle H}{|}}{C}} - H$$

Comparison of the properties of ethyl alcohol and dimethyl ether		
Property	**Ethyl Alcohol**	**Dimethyl Ether**
Physical state at room temperature	Liquid	Gas
Boiling point (°C)	78	-23
Melting point (°C)	-117	-138
Reaction with sodium	Yes	No
Poisonous (in moderate amounts)	No	Yes
Anaesthetic (in small amounts)	No	Yes

Cis-trans isomerism

One of the properties of molecules is that different parts of a molecule which are joined by a single bond are free to rotate with respect to one another. An example is geraniol and nerol, two essential oil constituents.

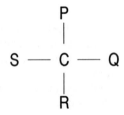

Nerol   **Geraniol**

Optical isomerism

Some organic compounds have the power of rotating the plane of polarised light. The carbon molecules which are optically active are those that contain one or more asymmetric carbon atoms, that is, carbon atoms which are bonded to four different atoms or groups of atoms.

For simplicity, let us consider P, Q, R and S to be four different functional groups. C represents a carbon atom to which these groups are bonded. The compound is represented by the following formula:

$$S - \overset{\overset{\displaystyle P}{|}}{\underset{\underset{\displaystyle R}{|}}{C}} - Q$$

This molecule will be optically active, and can exist in two forms, the molecules of which are mirror images of each other, and cannot be superimposed. The central carbon atom, being bonded to four different atoms or groups, is the assymetric carbon atom in this molecule.

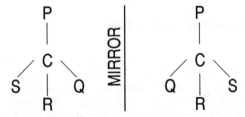

The concept of optical isomers is important in the chemistry of essential oils. Cells can tell the difference between two forms of optical isomers and usually one form is biologically active and its mirror image is not. Worse, the inactive isomer may produce harmful side effects. This may have been the case with thalidomide, the sedative that caused many birth defects in the early 1960s. The drug was a mixture of two optical isomers, only one of which has since been demonstrated to cause birth defects in rats.

Nomenclature

In aromatherapy, the older names for essential oil constituents are used. It would be almost incomprehensible to say, for example, '1-iso-Propyl-4-methylcylclohexan-2-ol' when 'menthol' is all that is required. There is no need to utter what most people would consider scientific gibberish when the simple terms are available. The complexity of the essential oils needs not be further complicated by adding the unnecesary use of long chemical names where short ones will do, provided that the latter are known to, and understood by, all concerned.

The advantage of the I.U.P.A.C (International Union of Pure and Applied Chemistry) nomenclature is, of course, that it is systemic, and can be used to name any molecule, whether or not the substance has a short name. It is not in the scope of this book to discuss the procedure of naming aroma chemicals according to the I.U.P.A.C.

The chemistry of common essential oil constituents

Almost all of the molecules found in essential oils are composed of carbon, hydrogen and oxygen. The chemistry of the essential oils is usually determined by two factors:

- the extraction process
- the biosynthesis of the constituent molecules by the plant.

Steam distillation is a process that extracts only volatile and water insoluble constituents of the plant such as the terpenes and terpenoid compounds and phenylpropane derived compounds. Many other constituents in the plant do not find their way into the essential oil. Among them are all the molecules that are soluble in water, like acids, sugars and molecules that are too large or too high in polarity to evaporate with steam, such as tannins, flavenoids, carotenoids, and polysaccharides.

Most of the constituents found in essential oils are terpenoid molecules. This name comes from turpentine, which in turn comes from the French word 'terebinth', which means 'resin'. From a chemical perspective, terpenoid compounds are chemical compounds whose carbon backbone consists of either 10,15, 20 or 30 carbon atoms (multiples of the 5-carbon isoprene unit). Isoprene is the common name for 2-methyl-1,3-butadiene:

$$CH_2 = \overset{\overset{\displaystyle CH_3}{|}}{C} - CH = CH_2$$

The Isoprene Unit

Isoprene itself is not a terpene, however all terpenes are made up of isoprene units - that is the carbon atoms of any terpene molecule can be divided into pieces, each having the following skeleton:

$$C - \overset{\overset{\displaystyle C}{|}}{C} - C - C$$

Because of this, the number of carbon atoms a terpene will have is always a multiple of five. Terpenes can have 10 carbon atoms, or 15 (sesquiterpenes), or 20 or 30 or 40. They are found in nature in a bewildering array of structures. The following diagram, by using dashed lines to divide the isoprene molecules, illustrates how the isoprene rule works.

Two examples of isoprene units joined to form monoterpene compounds. Geranial is a major constituent of geranium and menthol is found in peppermint

The complete list of terpenoid compounds is as follows:

Type	Number of isoprene units	Occurrence/Example
Hemiterpenes	1	Combined with other compounds
Monoterpenes	2	Essential oils, Iridoids
Sesquiterpenes	3	Essential oils, bitter principles
Diterpenes	4	Essential oils(esp. from resins), Vitamin A
Triterpenes	6	Sterols, Steroids, Saponins
Tetraterpenes	8	Carotenoids
Polyterpenes	n	rubber

In some essential oils, terpenes are original constituents which are synthesised by the living tissues of the plant and survive the processing of the essential oils; an example is the expressed citrus oils, all of which contain high proportions of natural terpenes.

In other essential oils, such as rose and lavender, the bulk, or the whole, of the terpene content is formed during processing by the action of hot water and steam upon the thermolabile constituents of the essential oil as it exists in its natural state. It has been found that when the essential oils are extracted with solvents instead of being distilled, the absolutes so obtained are either very low in terpenes or do not contain them at all.

There are two principal kinds of chemical constituents present in essential oils:

- Unsaturated hydrocarbons having a molecular structure based on the isoprene unit known as terpene hydrocarbon compounds.

- Compounds having oxygen atoms, which are refered to as 'oxygenated' compounds. Oxygenated constituents of essential oils include alcohols, esters, aldehydes, ketones, lactones and ethers.

As the methods and instrumentation of chemical analysis become more sophisticated, trace chemical constituents that are not classified into any of the above categories may be found. Trace constituents with an unusual chemical structure often have a strong effect on the overall olfactory impression of a particular oil. Trace constituents may have a pronounced pharmacological effect, however these will not be discussed.

Monoterpene hydrocarbons

Terpenes are known as hydrocarbons. Monoterpenes have 10 carbon atoms, (two isoprene units), with at least one double bond.

Monoterpene hydrocarbons are present in almost every essential oil. Their presence is dependent on the parameters of distillation. Studies have shown that the pH at which the distillation is carried out influences the quantity of monoterpene hydrocarbons present.

Monoterpenes will react with oxygen from the air, so it is important to keep them tightly sealed, and away from sources of free energy, such as heat and light, which speed up the decomposition time. This is typical of many citrus oils which form the

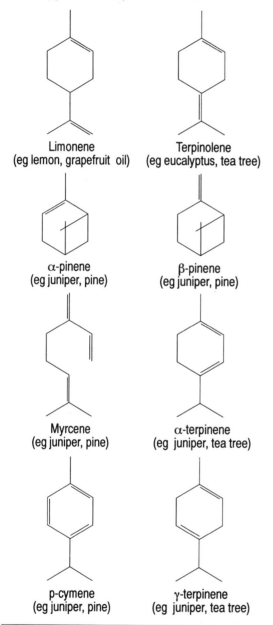

Limonene
(eg lemon, grapefruit oil)

Terpinolene
(eg eucalyptus, tea tree)

α-pinene
(eg juniper, pine)

β-pinene
(eg juniper, pine)

Myrcene
(eg juniper, pine)

α-terpinene
(eg juniper, tea tree)

p-cymene
(eg juniper, pine)

γ-terpinene
(eg juniper, tea tree)

Some monoterpene hydrocarbon structures found in essential oils

most important group of essential oils in this category.

While most citrus oils such as lemon, orange, grapefruit and mandarin consist of over 90% of the monoterpene hydrocarbon limonene, it is the traces of other highly aromatic compounds that gives each citrus oil its unique odour.

The oxidation is often so considerable that ozone forms. The antiseptic power of terpenes vapourised in the air is often attributed to this property. This spontaneous reaction with oxygen present in air is accelerated by sunlight, hence, essential oils kept for prolonged periods of time in only partly filled bottles of clear glass tend to darken in colour and thicken at the same time. Lassak (2) compares the effects of oxidised, melaleuca oil having cleared up tinea, whereas the fresh unoxidised tea tree acted slowly.

It is the oxidation of monoterpene hydrocarbons which could also account for the occasional reports of monoterpenes being irritants. However limonene, when it is present at 20% in a blend with 80% citral, has been shown to quench the ability of citral (an aldehyde) to cause sensitisation (3).

Juniper oil contains up to 80% monoterpenes, and is thought to be nephrotoxic due to its high monoterpene content. However a paper presented at the 24th International Symposium on Essential Oils by B.M. Heil and H. Schilcher challenged this assumption. It is known that high dosages of juniper oil cause clouding of urine which might be a sign of renal irritation. But this clouding disappears on dilution with ethanol, indicating that it is not due to irritation, that it may in fact be caused by the excretion of juniper oil metabolites.

A recent toxicological study found that juniper oil with low levels of α and β-pinenes did not irritate the kidneys. The authors hypothesised that the reputation for juniper oil as a renal irritant may have come from using juniper oils with high levels of α and β-pinenes which are known irritants to the urinary tract. High levels of pinenes result from the distillation of needles, branches and unripe berries. It was concluded that ripe juniper berries should be used for the distillation of juniper oils. (4)

Monoterpenes are general tonics and stimulants, particularly of the mucous membranes, and are thus considered beneficial as decongestants. Monoterpenes such as limonene, α-sabinene and γ-terpinene have all been found to possess antiviral properties in concentrations low enough not to be toxic to the host cell (5).

All monoterpenes have names ending in "ene".

Sesquiterpenes

The second most important molecular size in essential oils is that of the sesquiterpenes. These are hydrocarbon molecules which have 15 carbon atoms (three isoprene units), and a varying number of hydrogen atoms. Sesqui- means one and a half. There has been recent interest in the large number of derivatives of sesquiterpenes because of their complex pharmacological activity.

To assess the sesquiterpene hydrocarbons and their derivatives, they need to be discussed separately. This means that when we discuss the functional groups, there will be a separate discussion of mono and sesquiterpenoid compounds. Monoterpene alcohols and sesquiterpene alcohols will be discussed within their own subgroups because of their different properties.

The functional group of monoterpenoid compounds is employed as a principal method of classifying the essential oils and their effects. With sesquiterpenoids the individuality of the whole molecule rather than the influence of the functional group is the determining factor of the oil's pharmacological effects. Many biological properties such as anti-inflammatory, antiphlogistic, antitumour, choleretic, cholagogue, hypotensive, sedative and spasmolytic have been observed in sesquiterpenoid compounds.

From this array of properties and the high degree of activity that many of these compounds have, it becomes clear that even low concentrations of sesquiterpenoids found in essential oils contribute profoundly to the overall properties. Being terpenes, their names also end in "ene", and like the monoterpenes the rest of the name is derived either from its source plant or country.

Sesquiterpene hydrocarbons

Sesquiterpene hydrocarbons are a group of compounds that do not enjoy much recognition outside aromatherapy. Anecdotal evidence suggests that the anti-inflammatory or antiphlogistic effect is a feature common to most sesquiterpene hydrocarbons. The one compound for which there is much information is chamazulene found in German chamomile. It has

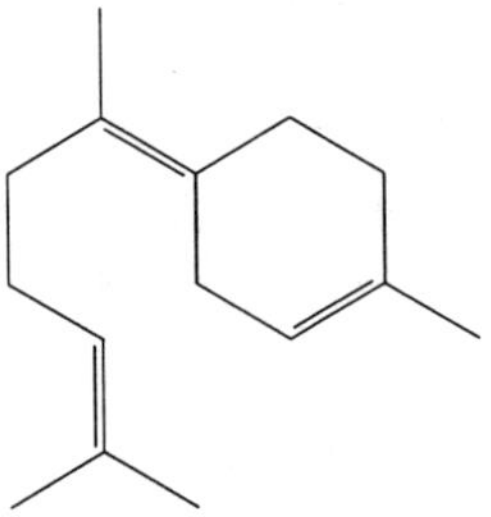

Bisabolene
(eg German chamomile)

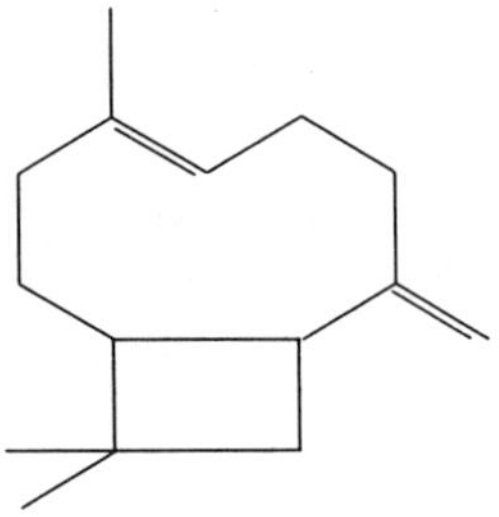

Caryophyllene
(eg Clove)

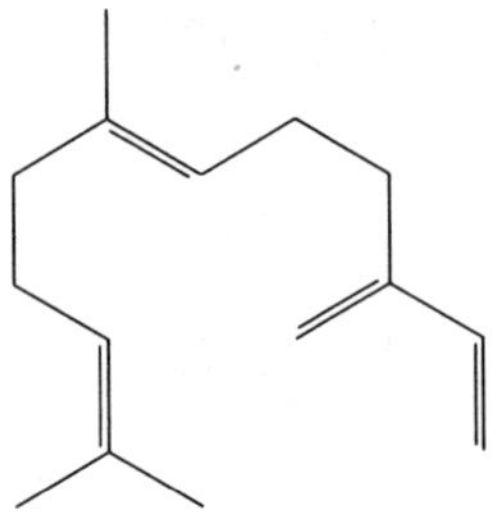

Farnesene
(eg Rose)

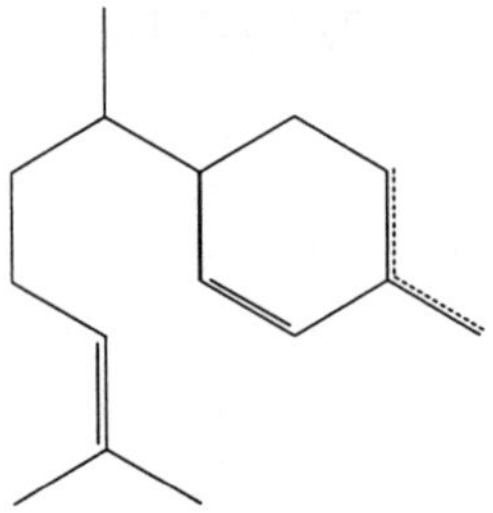

Zingiberene
(eg Ginger)

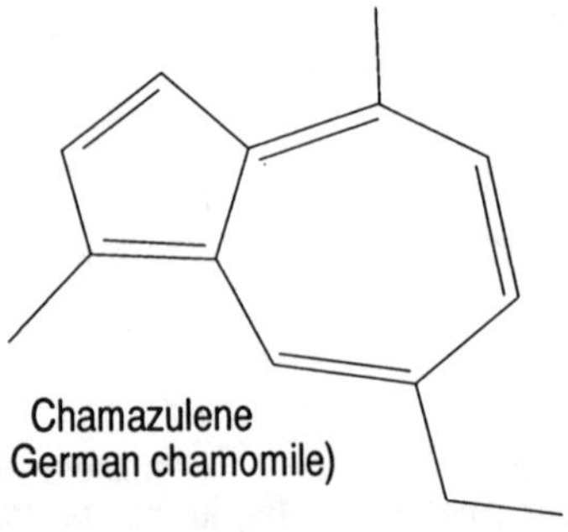

Chamazulene
(eg German chamomile)

Some sesquiterpene hydrocarbon constituents found in essential oils

soothing anti-inflammatory, antiphlogistic and possibly anti-allergenic qualities. Everlasting is an essential oil with up to 50% sesquiterpene hydrocarbons. It has been used extensively in regenerative skincare in France.

Caryophyllene exhibits a strong sedative effect. Recent research has shown it to be effective against viruses at low concentration ranges that were non-toxic to the host cells of the viruses. Caryophyllene is found in clove oil and in many other oils in low concentrations.

Other sesquiterpene hydrocarbons commonly encountered in essential oils include farnesene (found in chamomile, rose and many flower oils) and β–caryophyllene which is found, among others, in clove oil at a concentration of about 10%.

Functional groups

A functional group is a small part of an organic molecule consisting of a single atom or group of atoms that substitutes for a hydrogen atom and has a profound influence upon the properties of the molecule as a whole. It is the chemically active centre of the molecule.

Many properties of essential oils can be accounted for by the functional groups made up of different combinations of oxygen-containing molecules such as alcohols, aldehydes or ketones. Generalisations can be made, but specific actions of the constituents will be as varied as their structure.

As the physiological properties of molecules are strongly dependent on their functional groups, the different constituents of essential oils will be discussed in these terms.

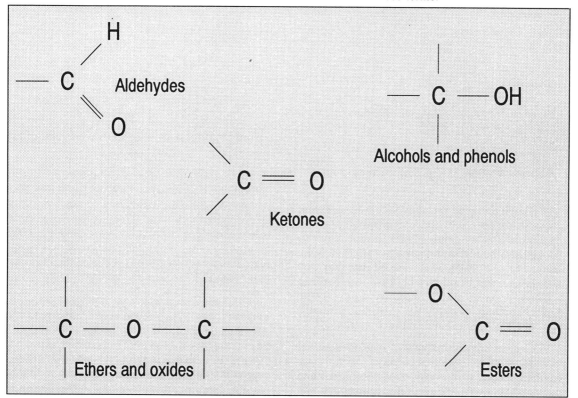

Functional groups found in essential oil constituents

Phenols

Phenols are compounds where an alcoholic hydroxyl group (-OH) is attached to the aromatic benzene ring system. The term aromatic refers to the structure of the ring system with a special configuration of six electrons. The aromatic quality is represented in a ring formula through a circle symbol.

The aromatic ring has the effect of amplifying the electronegativity of the oxygen atom, so the hydrogen atom of the hydroxyl group is strongly electro-positive.

Benzene

Phenol

Representation of the structure of phenol

Pure phenol as in the above formula does not occur in nature. The simplest phenol is phenol itself which is a solid that is fairly soluble in water. An aqueous solution of phenol is called carbolic acid. This solution was one of the earliest antiseptics used in surgery because it is toxic to bacteria. Today it is no longer used directly on patients because it burns the skin, but it is still used to clean surgical and medical instruments.

The most common phenols found in essential oils are phenols which also have carbon side chains attached to the ring such as thymol and carvacrol. Phenols are powerful antiseptics and bactericides and are considered to be the most stimulating of all the constituents. Phenols will prevent most micro-organisms from growing, and in most cases will kill them.

According to experiments by Karl Knobloch (6) the phenolic alcohols, such as thymol, carvacrol and eugenol and the aromatic aldehydes such as cinnamic aldehyde were the most powerful antiseptics.

Phenols should be used in low concentration and for short periods of time as long term use of all phenolic compounds may lead to toxicity. In order for the body to excrete them, the liver has to convert them into sulfonates, and massive doses would cause damage to the liver cells by overworking them (7). Phenols are classified as the most irritant of the constituents to the skin and mucous membranes.

Thymol
(eg thyme, ajowan)

Carvacrol
(eg oregano, thyme)

Some monoterpenoid phenol constituents

In essential oils, some phenols have a three carbon chain attached to them which makes them phenyl propane derivatives. They can occur as esters or ethers or with a free hydroxylic group as in eugenol. The antiseptic power of those esters bonded with a free hydroxylic group is stronger than in those where the oxygen is bonded between two carbons.

Cinnamon and clove are highly antiseptic essential oils. They cause severe skin reactions and must be used with caution. Eugenol, the main constituent of clove oil, is antiseptic and fungicidal and also has local anaesthetic properties. It has also been reported to inhibit certain carcinogenic processes. Other essential oils containing phenyl propane derivatives are aniseed oil, basil and tarragon. While they are not

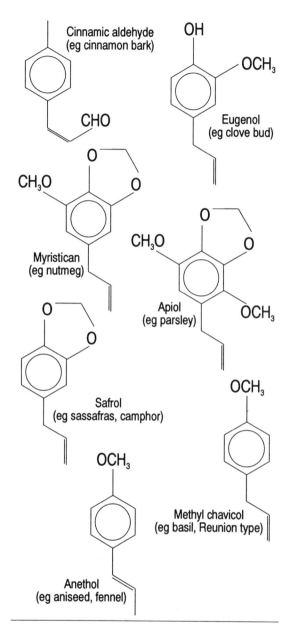

Some phenyl propane derivatives found in essential oils

as aggressive as cinnamon or clove they all share that certain sweet character in their fragrance.

The main constituents of basil and aniseed (methyl chavicol and anethol respectively) also warrant some caution as they are considered to be

skin irritants. While most of these essential oils can be beneficially used in aromatherapy, it is important to keep in mind their potential hazards.

Alcohols

A molecule which is an alcohol will have an hydroxyl group attached to one of its carbon atoms. An hydroxyl group is also known as an -OH group, because it is exactly that: an oxygen atom, bonded on the one hand to a carbon atom in a chain and on the other hand, to a hydrogen atom. Phenols are also a type of alcohol, but due to their aromatic ring, are classed differently from other types of alcohols.

Alcohol constituents are considered to be the most beneficial molecules found in essential oils. Linalool and terpineol are examples of terpene-alcohols. Some alcohols are remarkably germicidal, yet exhibit zero toxicity. Thus essential oils rich in terpene-alcohols are used frequently in everyday skincare preparations. Alcohols often provide very agreeable fragrances and energising antiseptic properties. Blends containing lavender, geranium or bergamot have a natural deodorant effect since they inhibit the proliferation of odour causing bacteria.

Monoterpene alcohols

Monoterpene alcohols all have the monoterpenoid carbon chain of ten atoms, and may contain an hydroxyl group anywhere along the chain. The terpene alcohols found in essential oils are mildly electropositive molecules giving them antiseptic, antifungal and antiviral properties with very little toxicity and irritating effects on the skin. Some alcohols such as terpineol-4-ol found in tea tree and juniper, because of the strained configuration of the terpenoid ring system, exhibit a markedly stronger electropositive character which explains their superior bactericidal properties.

According to tests done by Knobloch (8), citronellol was shown to possess antibacterial properties. Citronellol is a major constituent in rose and geranium oils.

Essential oils containing a high proportion of terpene alcohols often contain the respective esters of these alcohols. In lavender most of the linalool is present in an esterfied form, linalyl acetate. In its pharmacological testing linalool has exhibited a distinct sedative effect which is not generally found with other terpene alcohols. (9)

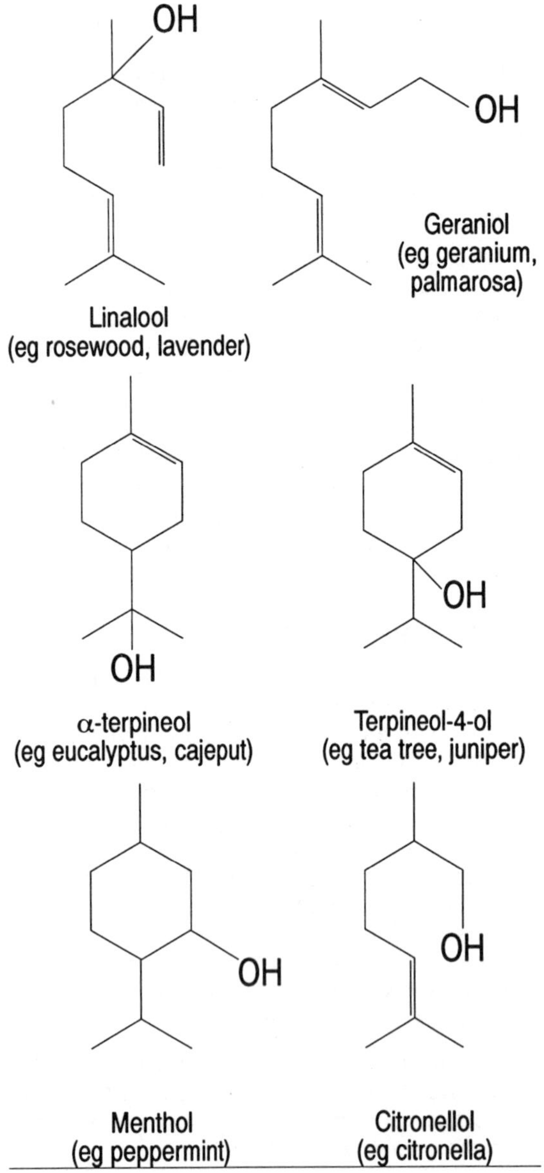

Sesquiterpene alcohols

The pharmacological properties of sesquiterpene alcohols are varied. Properties include anti-allergenic, liver stimulant, glandular stimulant, antiphlogistic and anti-inflammatory. Some of the sesquiterpenes demonstrate more interesting features such as anti-tumour or immune stimulant properties. These sesquiterpenes are not found in the most common essential oils.

Farnesol, a sesquiterpene alcohol, has been found to be effective as a bacteriostatic agent and is ideally suited as an active ingredient in deodorants. Being bacteriostatic, it does not eliminate healthy flora on the skin yet it inhibits the proliferation of odour-causing bacteria. At the same time it is considered non-irritant.

Bisabolol, a natural sesquiterpene alcohol, is known as the most effective antiphlogistic and anti-inflammatory principal in the oil of German chamomile. Extensive pharmacological tests (10)

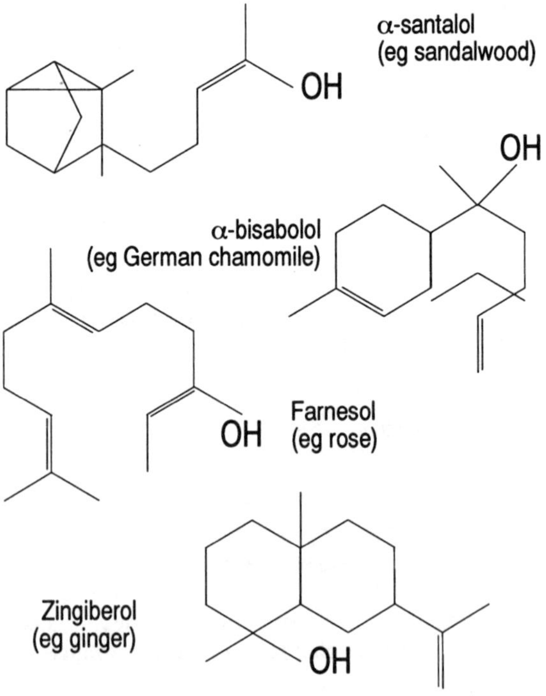

Linalool
(eg rosewood, lavender)

Geraniol
(eg geranium, palmarosa)

α-terpineol
(eg eucalyptus, cajeput)

Terpineol-4-ol
(eg tea tree, juniper)

Menthol
(eg peppermint)

Citronellol
(eg citronella)

Some monoterpene alcohol constituents found in essential oils

α-santalol
(eg sandalwood)

α-bisabolol
(eg German chamomile)

Farnesol
(eg rose)

Zingiberol
(eg ginger)

Some sesquiterpene alcohol constituents found in essential oils

have shown that its action is even stronger than the effect of the hydrocarbon chamazulene, which gives chamomile oil its characteristic blue colour. The main constituents of blue chamomile are the hydrocarbons farnesene, chamazulene and, about 50%, (-)-α-bisabolol. In order to use the most effective chamomile oil it is desirable to use an oil with as high a content of (-)-α-bisabolol as possible.

Sandalwood oil consists almost exclusively of the sesquiterpene alcohol α-santalol. It is traditionally used as a urine antiseptic and to alleviate heartburn. Its antiseptic properties have been controversial as on one hand there is ample anecdotal evidence for its usefulness in urinary tract infections (11). On the other hand it has not been possible to scientifically confirm its antiseptic properties. It may be tempting to speculate that searching for an outright bactericidal effect of α-santalol may be incorrect in light of the fact that sesquiterpenes can be effective immune stimulants. The effect of the oil may result not through direct bactericidal action but rather through stimulation of the body's immune system.

Other oils with high proportions of sesquiterpene alcohols are ginger, patchouli, vetiver, carrot seed, everlasting and valerian. Not much is known in terms of modern pharmacological research on the constituents of such oils.

Aldehydes

Aldehydes consist of an oxygen atom double bonded to a carbon atom, at the end of a carbon chain. The fourth bond is always a hydrogen atom.

$$—C=O$$
$$|$$
$$H$$

The -CHO chemical grouping which is common to all aldehydes is readily oxidised to the -COOH (carboxylic acid) group and when this happens heat is given out during the reaction. This is consistent with observations that essential oils

such as lemongrass can be skin irritants if used undiluted.

The aldehydes are responsible for the citrus-like fragrance in melissa, lemongrass and citronella. Essential oils with a high aldehyde content are calming and anti-inflammatory. These effects are best when the oils are used in low concentrations (1% or less).

The sedative effects of citronellal have been confirmed by Buchbauer (12) in a series of experimental procedures. Under standardised experimental conditions the motility of female mice was reduced from an arbitrarily graded 100% for untreated animals to 50.18% by citronellal. In the serum of the animals exposed for one hour, the concentration of citronellal was analysed and found to be 2.53 ng/mL (ng=nanogram). The citronellal was evaporated in the cage of the animals.

Lemongrass, an aldehyde-rich essential oil, was found to be particularly effective in inhibiting *Candida albicans* organism (13). Repeating the tests with individual constituents of lemongrass showed that citral and citronellal were active

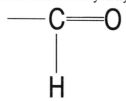

Citronellal
(eg *Eucalyptus citriodora*, citronella)

α-citral (geranial) β-citral (neral)

Citrals (eg lemongrass, lemon)

Some monoterpene aldehyde constituents found in essential oils

against the fungi whilst dipentene and myrcene had no activity.

Aldehydes are not as effective as phenols for their anti-bactericidal properties. The major exception is cinnamon aldehyde, from cinnamon. Aldehydes are very unstable and will readily oxidise to acid form in the presence of oxygen and a little heat. Aldehydes will be either called by their common name, followed by "aldehyde", for example cinnamic aldehyde; or the name will end in "al".

Ketones

The word 'ketone' is derived from the name 'Aceton'. Ketones have an oxygen atom double bonded to a carbon atom, but always on a carbon atom which is bonded to two other carbon atoms.

The most prominent property of ketones is their mucolytic effect, or their ability to ease the secretion of mucus. Some neurotoxicity is associated with certain ketones, so essential oils containing ketones should be used in their proper dosages. It is important to remember that not all ketones are necessarily toxic. The most toxic ketones are thujone and pinocamphene. Essential oils with high ketone content that should be avoided include wormwood and thuja.

On the other hand oils such as hyssop, eucalyptus and rosemary, in which their ketone content is only moderate, can be used advantageously for their mucolytic properties. Essential oils containing ketones are also known for their ability to stimulate the formation of new cells and tissues (14).

Helichrysum italicum, commonly known as everlasting, is one such oil which is valuable in regenerative skin care. A number of unusual compounds have been found in everlasting. These compounds have anti-inflammatory and anti-allergenic properties. One, Italidone (a di-ketone having 20 carbon atoms) has been found

Some monoterpene ketone constituents found in essential oils

to have strong mucolytic (mucous thinning), expectorant and cicatrisant properties. It may also be used to treat prostatitis in men.

Everlasting has excellent cicatrisant properties, speeding cellular growth and assisting in wound healing of all types. It reduces old scar tissue, stretch marks and loosens adhesions after injuries. It has both anti-inflammatory and anti-allergenic properties, being useful for treating eczema and dermatitis. Its mucolytic and expectorant properties coupled with its antispasmodic effects make it useful for treating asthma, bronchitis and catarrhal conditions. Ketones will either be known by their common name, such as camphor, or will have names ending in "one".

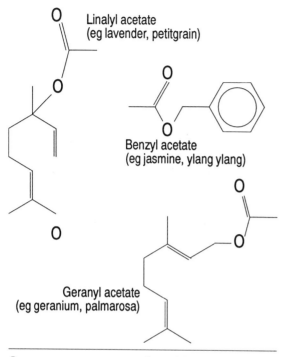

Some common esters found in essential oils

Esters

Esters are formed through the reaction of alcohols with acids. Most acids from plants are so soluble in water that they do not occur in essential oils, but are found in the waters of distillation. However, they are easily combined with alcohols to make esters. Esters are made from alcohols and acids, and are named after both parent molecules thus: the alcohol drops the 'ol', and gains a 'yl', and the acid drops the 'ic', and gains an 'ate' (see diagram below).

They are usually very fruity and fragrant. A characteristic quality of esters found in essential oils is that they are sedative. They exhibit a direct calming effect on the central nervous system and some of them can be powerful spasmolytics. Roman chamomile contains a number of esters such as iso-butyl-angelate and iso-amyl-angelate. It is highly likely that the antispasmodic property of this oil is largely influenced by its ester content. The intensity of the spasmolytic effect of the ester depends on the structure and number of carbons in the parent acid.

The number of different esters found in essential oils is larger than that of the representatives of any of the other functional groups. There are not many essential oils with esters as a main component, but even small amounts of esters are crucial to the finer notes in the fragrance of the essential oil.

Essential oils with a large percentage of the ester linalyl acetate include lavender, clary sage and petitgrain. Some esters have been found to be active against candida. Geranium oil contains esters which gives it considerable antifungal properties.

linalool + acetic acid ⇌ linalyl acetate + water

The formation of esters from an alcohol

Lactones and coumarins

A chemical compound is called a lactone if it contains an ester group integrated into a carbon ring-system.

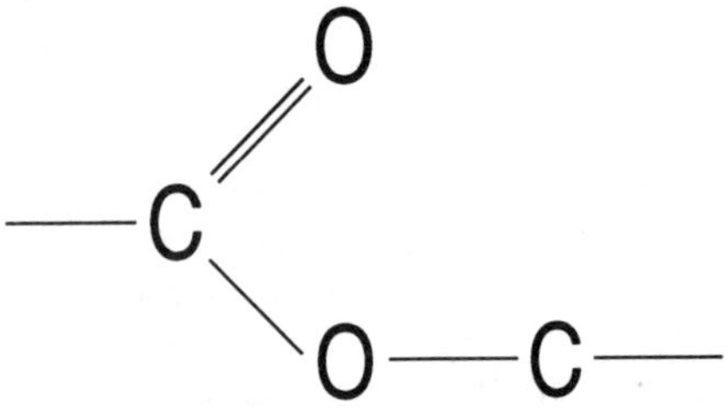

Coumarins are types of lactones, and both are known by their common names, as the chemical name is too lengthy. They tend to end in '-in', but can also end in '-one', eg umbelliferone which is also known as 7-hydroxy-coumarin. Lactones and coumarins tend to have the same neuro-toxic effects as ketones, and are also known to cause skin allergies. Fortunately they exist in small amounts in essential oils.

The well known UV sensitising effect of bergamot oil on the skin is due to the presence of a furocoumarin, bergaptene, which is thought to interfere with the DNA of the cells responsible for the production of melanin. This means that the skin is not protected from damage by UV rays via the production of melanin, and skin cancers can be started. (15)

The sesquiterpene lactone helenalin has been found to be one of the principal constituents responsible for the anti-inflammatory properties of arnica. Lactones are very effective mucolytic agents due to the heightening of the ketone function by the oxide group. Lactones are even stronger mucolytic constituents than ketones. Elecampane *(Inula helenium)* which contains lactones, is traditionally used for chronic bronchitis and coughs.

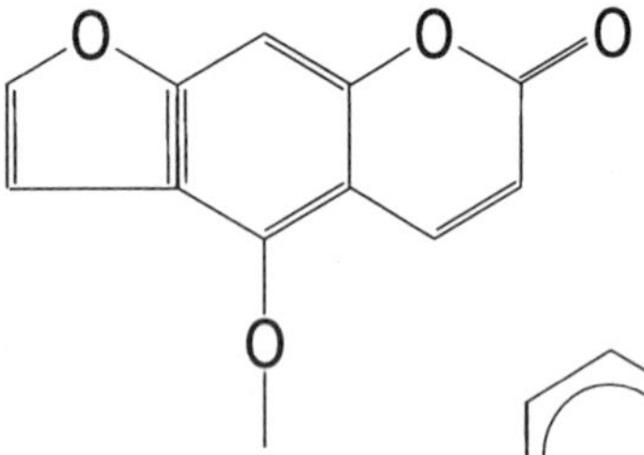

Ethers and oxides

Ethers

Most ethers occurring in essential oils are phenolic ethers. They are derived from the hydroxyl group of the phenol (or alcohol), the hydrogen of which is replaced with a short carbon chain, either a methyl group ($-CH_3$), or a two carbon ethyl group ($-CH_2-CH_2$).

If oxygen is not integrated in a ring system but linked between two unconnected carbon chains then the resulting molecule is called an ether. In aromatherapy the only ethers of importance are anethol found in aniseed oil and methyl chavicol found in basil and tarragon. These oils have been discussed in the phenylpropane derivative group. Ethers are predominantly spasmolytic and carminative and affect the body organs below the diaphragm.

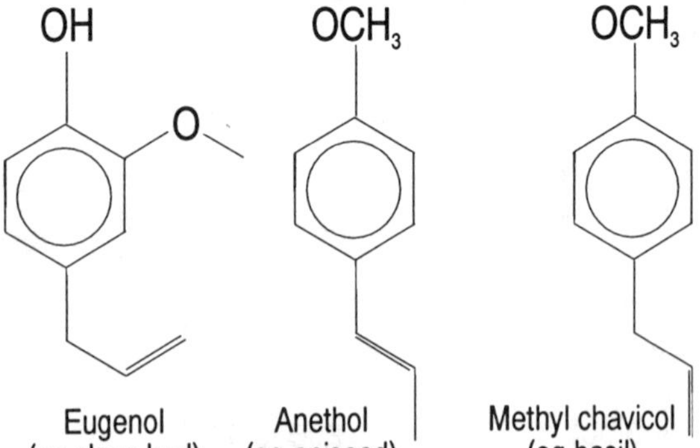

Bergaptene

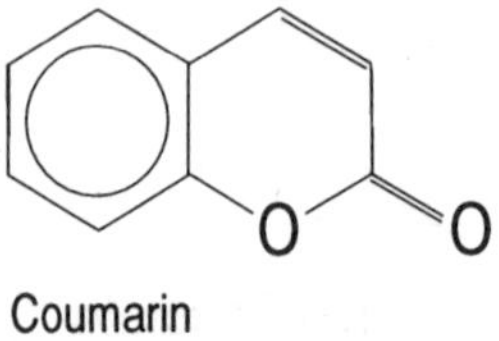

Coumarin

Typical lactone constituents found in essential oils

Eugenol (eg clove bud)

Anethol (eg aniseed)

Methyl chavicol (eg basil)

Example of ether essential oil constituents

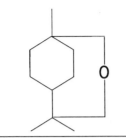

Structural diagram of the most common
oxide; 1,8-cineole

Oxides

These molecules occur where an oxygen atom
is included in the structure to make a ring. As they
are usually derived from alcohols, they keep their
alcohol name, and just add 'oxide', eg linalool
oxide.

However, there are a few which go by their
own special names, the most common being

1,8-cineole, commonly known as 'eucalyptol'.
The 'ole' ending is indicative in this case of the
oxygen atom in the structure. This compound is in
a group of its own.

As a chemical compound it is an oxide. It
stimulates the mucous glands of the respiratory
tract, which results in its strong expectorant effect.
It is particularly prolific in many oils from plants
belonging to the myrtaceae family.

According to Dr Penoel (16) 1,8-cineole has
two main pharmacological properties:

- It is an exocrinostimulant for the glands of
  the respiratory system and digestive
  organs.

- It is an expectorant because it stimulates
  mucin-secreting cells and activates the
  cilia of the respiratory mucous membrane.

Essential oil constituent classification	Example of essential oil constituent	Example of essential oils containing the constituents	Property	Naming
Monoterpene alcohols	linalool, geraniol, terpineol-4-ol, menthol	lavender, peppermint, petitgrain, rosewood, tea tree, sweet marjoram	antiseptic, bactericidal, antiviral, diuretic, immunostimulant	-ol
Aldehydes	citronellal, geranial, neral	lemongrass, citronella, melissa, eucalyptus citriodora	anti-inflammatory, sedative, antifungal	-al
Esters	linalyl acetate, geranyl acetate, methyl salicylate	Roman chamomile, clary sage, lavender	spasmolytic, sedative, antifungal, mildly anti-inflammatory	-yl -ate
Ethers	eugenol, anethol, methyl chavicol	tarragon, aniseed, basil	balancing, spasmolytic and carminative	-ol
Ketones	pinocamphone, thujone, pulegone, camphor, verbenone	everlasting, sage, hyssop, pennyroyal, thuja, wormwood	promote tissue formation, mucolytic, potentially neurotoxic	-one
Lactones	bergaptene, coumarin	bergamot	phototoxic, mucolytic	-
Oxides	1,8-cineole, 1,4-cineole	Eucalyptus oil and most oils belonging to the myrtaceae family.	expectorants, immuno-stimulants	-ole
Monoterpene hydrocarbons	limonene, pinene, myrcene, terpinene, p-cymene	most citrus oils eg lemon, grapefruit, orange and juniper, pine	antiseptic, possible skin irritants	-ene
Phenols	thymol, carvacrol	thyme, oregano, savory	bactericidal, immunostimulants, skin irritants, potentially toxic, tonifying, warming	-ol
Sesquiterpene hydrocarbons	chamazulene, caryophyllene, bisabolene, farnesene	German chamomile, yarrow, everlasting	anti-inflammatory, antiviral, anti-allergenic, cooling	-ene
Sesquiterpene alcohols	bisabolol, santalol, farnesol	German chamomile, sandalwood, rose	bactericidal, anti-inflammatory, anti-allergenic, possibly immunostimulant	-ol

Summary of essential oil constituents

Chapter 8

Pharmacology of Essential Oils

In pharmacology, nature is effectively disintegrated so that the actions of isolated chemicals on isolated pieces or functions of the body can be observed as precisely as is possible in a variable world. These observations are then stuck together to make a jigsaw picture of the effect of that substance on the body. On this basis drugs are given to real people.

Any pharmacology suited to the application of aromatherapy must be different. At no time must the view of the whole be lost. Traditional pharmacology's role is therefore to draw from human experience and the effects on the mind and the body to enable the aromatherapist to better predict the action of each essential oil in the infinitely variable circumstances that will be encountered in practice.

Introduction

Aromatherapists cannot afford to ignore the growing interest in aromatherapy from within the medical sector which insists on asking many questions such as:

- Is there any evidence of the therapeutic benefits claimed by aromatherapists?

- Have clinical trials been done to prove the properties of essential oils?

- Do essential oils pass through the skin?

- Are the effects of essential oils anything more than a placebo effect?

- Does the body metabolise the essential oils?

- Why do the effects of aromatherapy vary from person to person?

As mentioned in Chapter 6, if we are unable to provide suitable answers to such questions, we may eventually be denied the right to treat people holistically because the so-called medical guardians will see aromatherapy as a fiendish and dubious form of medicine full of hidden perils for the unsuspecting public. Perhaps I should bring to your attention an article recently published in the Nursing Standard Journal, called *Alternative roads to hell?*. The author ridicules a statement commonly made by aromatherapists about essential oils: *'... elixirs from aromatic oils represent the soul of the plant.'* (1). She states that it is un-Christian and contravenes the UKCC Code of Professional Conduct.

In an interview (2) a spokesperson for the Australian Medical Association said:

'General AMA policy is that if something is scientifically valid, then we will support it'

He continued by saying:

'If it hasn't undergone some degree of validation, then we're basically against it, in the patient's interest.'

It is with this in mind that this chapter addresses research that has already been conducted which confirms traditionally-held beliefs of aromatherapy, and also highlights the urgency for further clinical trials.

Defining pharmacology

Pharmacology is defined as the study of the manner in which the function of living organisms can be modified by drugs. This fascinating exploration has been dominated by modern medical science, so that pharmacology often represents a narrow, fragmented investigation.

Pharmacognosy is a branch of pharmacology concerned with the study of crude drugs of plants. Modern pharmacognosy is concerned with analysing natural medicinal substances and defining their therapeutic activity according to the chemical constituents.

Drugs are standardised and have a predictable action so that the manipulative and invasive action of the remedy on the body can be controlled as tightly as possible. However, essential oils extracted from plants consist of an immense array of chemical constituents, each liable to be interacting with others, most with little known pharmacological action.

Faced with this fiendish complexity and infinite variability found in the essential oil, the pharmacologist hungers for the identifiable 'active constituent', which, whilst reflecting the useful action of the plant, can be isolated and ultimately synthetically derived, and of course one can patent synthesised medicines but not plants.

These scientific analytical studies provided by the modern pharmacognosist will define the properties of the natural remedy according to its 'action'. This approach which defines the remedy in accordance with physically quantifiable properties is mechanistic, reductionist, and analytical.

As a result each essential oil is individually labelled with a string of qualifiers such as sudorific. hepatic, etc., - which according to Holmes (3) are worn out labels which are meaningless to the practitioner who is unaware of the meaning of its treatment strategies.

Today most texts use these terms to describe remedies. Unfortunately the original action of the remedy has been abandoned. This has been due partly to the rise of anatomical-clinical medicine and partly due to the impact of experimental pathology and pharmacology.

However with the introduction of traditional Eastern medicine in the West, the appreciation of using remedies according to their vitalistic and energetic principles has once again grown.

With this in mind it has been suggested by Simon Mills that the pharmacology of natural remedies should be defined as follows:

'The interpretation of the observed action of the remedy in practice;
The process of developing the character of each remedy so that it can be used more creatively and informatively in support of the healing processes, rather than searching for the actions of constituents per se.' (4)

If we are therefore to maintain a holistic system of aromatherapy which is not only based on analytic pharmacological studies, it is necessary to integrate three basic elements:

- the holistic context in which the remedy shall by used

- the empirical context which draws on centuries of traditional use

- the analytical back-up provided by chemistry of the essential oil.

How aromatherapy works

In some respects the word 'aromatherapy' can be misleading because it suggests that it is a form of healing which works exclusively through the sense of smell, and on the emotions. This is not the case, for apart from the fragrance of the essential oil, each essential oil has a unique combination of constituents which interacts with the body's chemistry in a direct manner, which then, in turn, affects certain organs or systems as a whole.

There are two principal approaches to the practice of aromatherapy:

- the medical, and

- the holistic.

Medical aromatherapy usually recommends *oral* dosages of essential oils, for example for the treatment of infections. The essential oils selected depend on the micro-organism present and the dosage used will be determined by the amount of oil necessary to obtain sufficient antimicrobial action to treat the patient. Thus the essential oil clearly has a pharmacological effect.

Holistic aromatherapy usually involves *massage* and *inhalations* and the following questions need to be asked about its benefits:

- Are externally applied or inhaled oils absorbed into the bloodstream?

- If they are, do they have a pharmacological effect?

Recent clinical trials have confirmed that small concentrations of essential oil constituents have been detected in the blood within minutes, following either massage or inhalation (5) (6). The amount of essential oil absorbed into the bloodstream from dermal or inhalation application was significantly less than from oral administration, and these same clinical studies confirmed that linalool, the main chemical constituent found in lavender, had a pharmacological sedative affect.

Therefore, if lavender oil is known to be a sedative pharmacologically then it should always reliably have a sedative effect no matter how it is applied and to whom it is applied.

However, at the second Psychology of Perfumery Conference held at Warwick University, England (7) a number of interesting conclusions were reached. There was a general agreement that it is impossible to predict the effect of an odour on humans because its effects when inhaled may be subject to the many factors as described:

A. How the odour or essential oil is applied

B. Quantity applied

C. The circumstances in which it is applied

D. The person to whom it was applied (age, sex, personality type)

E. The person's mood

F. Previous memory associations the person may have with the odour

G. Anosmia

If factors A,B and C are controlled, the control of factors D, E and F is difficult. Therefore the extent to which a psychological effect can override one that is pharmacological, or a pharmacological effect can override its psychological counterpart, has yet to be researched. Some would say that there are no predictable psychological or pharmacological effects at all.

Properties of essential oils

Essential oils have many properties such as:
- alterative effect
- anti-inflammatory effect
- antibacterial and antifungal effect
- astringent effect
- carminative effect
- diaphoretic effect
- diuretic effect
- emmenagogue effect
- expectorant effect
- granulation stimulating effect
- nervine effect
- rubefacient effect
- sedative effect
- spasmolytic effect
- stimulant effect
- tonic effect.

These properties will be discussed in terms of traditional use and current pharmacological studies.

Alterative effect

Alteratives are remedies that cleanse and purify the blood. The terms now commonly used are 'detoxifiers' or 'blood-purifiers'. The concept of blood cleansing is difficult for a person with a medical or pharmacological background to understand or agree with.

Alteratives assist the body's natural eliminatory response by stimulating the liver, lungs, lymphatic system, kidneys, bowels and sweat glands therefore excreting injurious or toxic matter that may cause irritation such as:

- mucous
- faeces
- urine
- menstrual blood
- other toxins.

Any essential oil which has one or more of the following properties is classified as an alterative.

- lymphatic (assists the tissue-cleansing action of the lymphatic system)
- diaphoretic (promoting sweating, thus assisting the excretory functions of the skin)
- expectorant (promoting expulsion of mucus, thus assisting the respiratory system)
- diuretic (promoting urination, thus assisting the excretory functions of the kidneys)
- hepatic (enhancing liver function, thus assisting the liver's detoxifying function)
- laxative (promoting bowel movement, thus assisting the excretory functions of the large intestine)
- emmenagogue (promoting menstruation, thus assisting in the elimination of menstrual blood)

All of the above properties will help promote detoxification for the treatment of general toxaemia. Please refer to the appropriate sub-headings in this chapter for more information on the individual properties.

Remedies which promote one or more of the body's eliminatory functions have always been an important treatment strategy in holistic therapies. Essential oils most commonly used as alteratives include: angelica root, aniseed, black pepper, carrot seed, cypress, everlasting, fennel, grapefruit, geranium, juniper, lemon, orange, peppermint, rosemary.

Anti-inflammatory effect

There are many reasons for the anti-inflammatory effect of essential oils, and it varies for different oils. Essential oils with scientifically documented anti-inflammatory properties include German chamomile and oils with thymol as a constituent. German chamomile is considered anti-inflammatory due to its chamazulene and the α−bisabolol content.

In recent studies, Professor Della Loggia (8) from Trieste, Italy evaluated the anti-inflammatory activity of essential oils. He states that anti-inflammatory activities have been falsely attributed to many essential oils and their components. Of the 31 essential oils investigated which have traditionally claimed to be anti-inflammatory only three can be said to have such properties. The most acknowledged anti-inflammatory oil is German chamomile, however here we find some surprises.

The accepted wisdom is that the anti-inflammatory activity of chamomile is mainly due to chamazulene. This blue compound is formed from matricine by steam distillation. In other words the compound found naturally in chamomile is matricine, and this is converted into chamazulene by the action of the steam. When chamazulene was tested for topical anti-inflammatory activity, eg skin and digestive tract, it was found to be inactive. In contrast, matricine found in the herb was found active topically. However it must be noted that bisabolol, found only in the essential oil, is active topically.

The antiphlogistic effects of (-)-α-bisabolol found in German chamomile have been proven in experiments on adjuvant arthritis in rats (9). Experiments showed that (-)-α-bisabolol had a greater effect than bisabolol oxides A and B. It was suggested that in standardising chamomile preparations for antiphlogistic effectiveness the content of (-)-α-bisabolol was important, but that standardising the amount of oxides present was not necessary.

Thyme oil is a skin irritant, however it also has an anti-inflammatory effect using mechanisms different from chamomile's. While the mechanisms have not been fully explained, it seems that through skin irritation the skin reflexes release binding endogenous substances, whereby the local inflammation process is influenced.

Some antirheumatic compounds are known to inhibit the synthesis of prostaglandins, important factors in the occurrence of inflammation. The inhibitory effectiveness of plant extracts in prostaglandin synthesis was investigated using the cyclo-oxygenase system in sheep cells. (10)

Clove oil and cinnamon oils displayed strong inhibitory effects. Dwarf pine, eucalyptus and chamomile oils produced a weak inhibitory effect, whilst juniper berry had no effect. The weak inhibitory effect of German chamomile showed that its known antiphlogistic properties were due to a different process.

The anti-inflammatory properties of clove oil were examined in the case of a wasp venom sensitisation. A significant reduction of the inflammatory response was observed. Further studies confirmed that the main component of clove oil, eugenol, showed a dose dependent induction of NADP(H) quinone reductase. This indicates that the inflammatory activity may, in part, be caused by action upon oxygen metabolism. [11]

Antibacterial and antifungal effect

The role of infection by micro-organisms such as bacteria is often overemphasised. The terrain on which the micro-organism falls is equally important. To understand the principles of phytomedical infection treatment it is important to look at the cause and progression of infection according to current understanding of the mechanisms of the immune system.

The onset of an infection is often seen in metabolic imbalances in the intestinal tract. The intestinal tract is a complex ecological site with several hundred species of bacteria. Of these, more than 80% are anaerobic. These anaerobic bacteria play an important part in the sugar, fat, protein and vitamin metabolism. Some of them also destroy foreign bacteria. The cells of the intestines as well as a healthy intestinal flora form an excellent first line defence against invading foreign bacteria.

Any disturbances in a healthy anaerobic intestinal flora caused by stress, diet, antibiotics, drugs and many other factors can allow the pathogenic bacteria to increase. As a consequence, necessary detoxification and elimination processes are reduced and toxins reach the liver. Usually this goes unnoticed, as cells in the liver neutralise and eliminate such toxins. When these detoxification functions are unable to cope with the toxins, they are diverted towards the mucous membranes and other emergency elimination sites. This discharge through the mucous membranes provides the breeding ground for the proliferation of bacteria and consequent inflammation of the mucous membranes such as the sinuses and bronchi. This simplified scenario

Essential oil	R-W Coefficient
Melaleuca alternifolia	11
Eucalyptus dives	8
Eucalyptus citriodora	8
Eucalyptus polybractea	5

Essential Oil Constituent	R-W Coefficient	Functional Group
1,8-Cineole	3.5	ether
Geraniol	21	alcohol
Citronellol	14	alcohol
Linalool	13	alcohol
Terpinen-4-ol	13	alcohol
α-terpineol	16	alcohol
Menthol	19	alcohol
Citral	19.5	aldehyde
Citronellal	13.5	aldehyde
Anethole	11	phenolic ether
Thymol	25	phenol
Eugenol	15	phenol

R-W Coefficient of some essential oils and some constituents according to Penfold and Grant (13)

assists us to understand the application of essential oils in the treatment of an infection.

Valnet has verified the antibacterial properties of many essential oils. According to his studies the bactericidal action in their vaporised state appears in the following decreasing order:

lemon, thyme, orange, bergamot, juniper, clove, citronella, lavender, niaouli, peppermint, rosemary, sandalwood, eucalyptus and *Chinese anise.* (12)

His observation was that this order almost exactly corresponds with the strength of essences studied in respect of their terpene content. According to Valnet's studies the bactericidal potency of these vapours was experienced in relation to meningococcus, staphylococcus and the typhus bacillus. He found the diphtheric bacillus more strongly resistant, and the spores of anthrax bacillus not affected at all.

Australian researchers Penfold and Grant determined the phenol coefficients of a number of essential oils and their components by the Rideal-Walker method using *Salmonella thypi* as the test micro-organism (13). The Rideal-Walker test (R-W) compares the germicidal power of a substance with a well-known germicide, phenol (carbolic acid=1).

They were surprised to find many essential oils were indeed powerful disinfectants. The R-W test is now superseded by the Sykes-Kelsey test, due to the introduction of new germicidal compounds such as quaternary ammonium salts, however it still remains a valid test. Some of Penfold and Grant's results are shown in the tables on this page.

Knobloch et al. (14) investigated the antibacterial and antifungal properties of essential oil components. According to the authors the antimicrobial activity of essential oils is due to their solubility in the phospholipid bilayer of cell membranes. The terpenoid constituents have been found to interfere with enzymatic reactions of energy metabolism. In general, essential oils cause damage to a biological membrane due to their lipophilic properties; however specific functional groups such as the phenols and alcohols revealed the strongest inhibitory effects, followed by aldehydes and ketones.

The antifungal effects of essential oils seem to be of increasing interest, as infections such as *Candida albicans* and other fungal or yeast organisms become a widespread problem. There is much research showing beneficial effects of fennel, clove, cinnamon, thyme and tea tree on fungi.

Another study found that quite a large number of aromatic constituents found in essential oils such as aldehydes and esters had a strong effect against *Candida albicans* and other fungi or yeasts.

Larrondo (15) found melissa oil had 100% inhibition on *Candida albicans*, while rosemary oil had no effect and lavender had little effect. An article in the Lancet (16) reports a case of a woman suffering from anaerobic vaginosis who refused to take antibiotics and treated herself with tea tree pessaries. Re-examination by her doctor a month later showed normal vaginal secretions and bacterial flora. It was indicated that tea tree may be a preferable treatment for the condition rather than nitroimidazoles.

Pena (17) investigated the effect of tea tree oil in the treatment of vaginal infections in a total of 130 cases. Results were compared with a control group of 50 cases treated by 'standard' methods. A combination of essential oil impregnated tampons and daily douches of the diluted oil proved to be highly effective in the treatment of trichomonal vaginitis, moniliasis, cervicitis and chronic endocervicitis. The clinical evidence supported laboratory tests which showed that *M. alternifolia* oil has penetrating antibacterial and antifungal actions, and had dissolved pus and debris.

While on the topic of tea tree, Basset et al. (18) reported, in the Medical Journal of Australia, that a single blind randomised trial was conducted on 124 patients with mild to moderate acne to evaluate and compare the efficacy and skin tolerance between 5% tea tree oil gel and 5% benzoyl peroxide lotion. It was concluded that both had a significant effect by reducing the number of inflamed and non-inflamed lesions. Tea tree acted more slowly, but fewer side effects were experienced by those treated with the oil.

Hmamouch et al. (19) investigated the antibacterial and antifungal properties of 12 different eucalyptus oils. To their surprise *E. citriodora* was found to be the most active, affecting all organisms. From the experiments, the most active components were citronellal and its derivatives, but when the components were tested separately they showed little activity. They therefore assumed that the antibacterial and antifungal activity is related to the synergy of all the constituents and is not necessarily due to the amount of 1,8-cineole as previously thought.

Astringent effect

Astringents are remedies that have a firming and healing action on the mucous membranes or exposed tissues. They bring about contraction, they firm and dry up secretions and generally make tissues more dense. Although primarily drying, astringents also prevent moisture loss. In traditional Chinese medicine astringents are remedies which would be used to treat 'damp' conditions.

Astringents may be used symptomatically to stop bleeding or to treat diarrhoea, however it must be remembered that they often do not correct the cause of the problem.

Astringents are often classified as:

- those which arrest bleeding (haemostatics)

- those which tonify and restore venous circulation (eg; for the treatment of varicose veins and hemorrhoids)

- those which stop excessive discharge of waste materials (eg; for the treatment of menorrhagia, diarrhoea, excessive perspiration)

- those which restrain infection and promote the healing of tissues (vulnerary).

Essential oils which arrest bleeding and restore venous circulation include cypress, geranium, lemon and yarrow.

Essential oils which stop excessive discharge of waste materials include cypress, frankincense, myrrh, rock rose, sage and sandalwood.

Essential oils which promote the healing of wounds and prevent infection and swelling are everlasting, frankincense, myrrh and rock rose.

Carminative effect

Carminatives are essential oils that relieve intestinal gas, pain and distension. They will settle digestion, increase absorption and promote normal peristalsis, thus promoting digestion and assisting in dispelling accumulation of undigested food materials.

Many carminatives tend to have warm and dry qualities and are also known as digestive stimulants. Carminatives consist mostly of the essential oils extracted from the umbelliferae plant family such as angelica, aniseed, coriander, caraway, fennel and dill.

Other carminative essential oils include basil, bay, cardamom, cinnamon, chamomile, clove, ginger, neroli, nutmeg, peppermint, spearmint and thyme.

Carminatives' mechanism of action occurs via:

- a reflex that causes a toning of the intestinal walls with increased resorption and passing through of gases
- a local irritating effect on the lining of the stomach or the gastric mucosae
- a spasmolytic effect and relief of flatulence
- a cholagogic effect.

Rangelov et al (20) studied the choleretic action of essential oil constituents such as menthol, camphene, anethol, borneol and fenchone. In guinea pigs, only menthol caused an increase in bile production, while cholesterol excretion was increased by menthol and camphene. Nerol and anethol increased the production of bile acids. Nerol had a choleretic effect on both rats and guinea pigs. The authors' interpretation of the results was that firm conclusions were difficult to form, because some of the chologogic and choleretic actions appeared to be species specific. Rangelov (21) also found peppermint, fennel and lavender to have pronounced choleretic properties.

Diaphoretic effect

Diaphoretics induce perspiration and by this action restore circulation, dispel fever and chills, while eliminating toxins from the body via the skin. Strong diaphoretics are referred to as sudorifics.

Diaphoretics will assist the body in the following ways:

- assist the excretory function of the skin
- resolve the development of local congestion or inflammation resulting from cold
- relieve muscular tension and aching joints
- relieve headaches due to cold and congestion.

The initial or acute stages of colds and febrile diseases inhibit the circulation of 'defensive energy' which in turn inhibits sweating. Therefore diaphoretic essential oils will stimulate and restore the defensive energy of the body.

In traditional medicine there are two kinds of diaphoretics:

- warming diaphoretics
- cooling diaphoretics.

Warming diaphoretics are used to treat the common cold by dispersing wind, cold and dampness. Some are also stimulants and expectorants. Essential oils which are warming diaphoretics include angelica, basil, cardamom, cinnamon, clove, eucalyptus, ginger, rosemary, thyme.

Cooling diaphoretics are more effective for treating high fever, sore throats and other inflammatory conditions involving toxins. They are generally also alteratives and may possess diuretic properties. Essential oils which are cooling diaphoretics include: German chamomile, everlasting, peppermint, spearmint and yarrow.

Treatment involving diaphoretic remedies should include hot baths, sleeping under a warm blanket and fasting.

Diuretic effect

A diuretic is an agent which causes increased production of urine. Diuretics either: (22)

- stimulate the blood flow to the kidneys, or
- reduce the resorption of water from the filtrate in the kidneys' nephrons.

Those which stimulate the blood flow to the kidneys are referred to as circulatory stimulants and cardioactive remedies and include substances such as coffee and tea.

Diuretics have the following therapeutic properties:

- They assist in the removal of waste products and toxic materials.
- They promote the excretion of waste fluids from the tissues and cavities of the body.
- They maintain kidney action by stimulating the normal excretory function.
- They help eliminate urine solids, and lessen irritation of the genito-urinary tract when the urine contains an excessively high concentration of irritant substances.
- They have an antiseptic effect, reducing urinary infections.

It should be noted that diuretics should not be used when the kidneys are deficient in functioning power. Essential oils with diuretic properties include black pepper, fennel, carrot seed, geranium, juniper berry, parsley seed.

Emmenagogue effect

Emmenagogues are essential oils which help promote and regulate menstruation and therefore are used to treat many special disorders of the female reproductive system such as:

- painful menstruation (dysmenorrhoea)
- mucous discharge (leucorrhoea)
- absence of menstruation (amenorrhoea)

Emmenagogues may also be antispasmodics, thus relieving uterine cramps and pain.

More specific triggers of amenorrhoea should be examined. These include emotional shock, ceasing use of the contraceptive pill, ovarian tumours and cysts, early menopause, hormone imbalances, poor nutrition, adrenal disease, thyroid insufficiency, or structural impairment of the reproductive organs.

Typical emmenagogues include angelica, basil, chamomile (German and Roman), cinnamon, ginger, jasmine, juniper, lavender, myrrh, peppermint, rose, rosemary.

It needs to be mentioned that emmenagogues are not necessarily abortifacients. Only some are contraindicated during pregnancy.

Expectorant effect

Expectorants promote the discharge of phlegm and mucus from the bronchopulmonary mucous membrane.

The stimulating action on the bronchi makes coughing easier, thus encouraging the natural eliminatory response that brings bronchial secretions and other airborne matter up to the throat. In this cleansing process there are two main problems:

- excessive mucous secretion which causes an overload of the mucociliary escalator and results in congestion in the lungs
- an inflammatory response or hypersensitivity which results in a tight, dry, unstable condition as seen in dry coughs and asthma.

Essential oils with expectorant properties work in two different ways:

- Some generate warmth, thus removing mucus by their drying action. These are often referred to as 'stimulating expectorants', because they stimulate activity of the 'mucociliary escalator' leading to a more productive cough.

    Typical expectorants that will generate warmth and expel phlegm include aniseed, angelica, basil, cardamon, cinnamon, ginger, hyssop, pine, eucalyptus, fennel, marjoram, rosemary, thyme, myrrh, frankincense.

- Some have a soothing and demulcent effect, ideal for dry and irritable conditions, and are known as relaxing expectorants. They appear to act by reflex to soothe bronchial spasm and loosen mucous secretions.

    Essential oils for treating dry and irritable conditions include chamomile (German and Roman), cypress, cedarwood and sandalwood.

It is very important that the cough be identified as either productive or unproductive and that the client be treated with the appropriate essential oils. It is inappropriate to use relaxing expectorants for a congested bronchial condition and conversely may be contraindicated to use stimulating expectorants for asthmatics.

Many expectorants possess cough-relieving actions. These are known as antitussives and may possess more specific nervine or antispasmodic properties. Antitussive essential oils include angelica, eucalyptus, clary sage, cypress, hyssop, myrtle and pine.

When mucus blocks the nasal passage making breathing difficult, essential oils such as chamomile (German and Roman), eucalyptus, lavender, marjoram, peppermint, rosemary and thyme may be used in inhalations.

Clinical trials have confirmed the expectorant effect, after inhalation, of some essential oils (23). As a measure for expectoration the amount and the consistency of bronchial liquid was determined. According to clinical trials performed by Boyd the following essential oils and essential oil constituents have been found to be effective expectorants when inhaled: lemon, citral, citronellal, geraniol, limonene and α-pinene.

It is important to note that high concentrations of essential oils dried up respiratory fluids, whereas low concentrations increased fluid, creating an expectorant effect. Boyd's conclusion was that only low concentrations of oils should be used in vaporisers for treating lung conditions. Assuming that the results obtained by Boyd from animal experiments can be applied to humans, essential oils can be used for stimulating the secretion of condensed thick mucus in the respiratory tract.

It was also observed that oral application often did not have a pronounced effect whereas inhalation showed good results in very low dosages. A further observation was that the desired effect of the inhaled essential oils was greatly reduced or even absent when dosages were applied which gave a pronounced aroma to the inhaled air. According to Reichelmann (24), it is therefore advantageous to use concentrations which make the inhaled air only faintly aromatic

as the secretion stimulating effect seems to change to a suppressant effect with higher doses.

Application of essential oils to the skin has also been found to be effective for the treatment of chronic obstructive bronchitis. The expectorant effect of certain essential oils and their constituents has been traditionally utilized in chest rubs and inhalations to improve bronchial secretion and reduce bronchial spasms. (25)

Granulation stimulating effect

Traditionally some essential oils have been used to promote the healing of wounds. These essential oils have been used successfully and extensively to keep wounds antiseptic and to promote healing and are defined as cicatrisant, promoting granulation and preventing formation of scar tissue.

Such essential oils include bergamot, chamomile (German and Roman), frankincense, geranium, lavender, myrrh, neroli, palmarosa, rose and sandalwood.

The effects of chamomile on wound healing was tested on 14 patients after dermabrasion of tattoos. The period of the healing and drying process was noted. The decrease of the weeping wound area as well as the drying tendency was statistically significant. (26)

Calendula, the flower of the marigold, is traditionally known as an agent which promotes healing and skin repair. The effects of calendula extracts on wound healing was investigated in a Romanian study in 1982. Two fractions of calendula were combined in a study; an aqueous extract and one made from 70% ethanol. This combination accelerated healing, but when it was further combined with allantoin a dramatic increase in repair occurred. (27)

Gattefosse (28) claims that the cytophylactic properties of essential oils are not only due to the antiseptic power of the essences. He reports of cases:

'of the healing by the application of essential oils of wounds which were not bacterial and in which suppuration was insignificant, which had not responded to any of the usual medication and had hitherto remained atonic.'

Nervine effect

Nervines are substances which strengthen and tone the activity of the nervous system. They can actually be stimulants or sedatives. Many nervines are also antispasmodics or relaxants. These essential oils relax the whole body, not only mentally, but also in terms of visceral neuromuscular function.

Relaxants are indicated whenever it is desired to reduce the effects of tension or overactivity of a body system. Therefore in cases of nervous indigestion, bowel problems, bronchial spasms, menstrual spasms and any other physiological disorders where tissue tension is elicited, relaxant essential oils will be useful.

Essential oils with relaxant nervine properties include: bergamot, chamomile (German and Roman), clary sage, geranium, jasmine, lavender, neroli, sweet marjoram and ylang-ylang.

Essential oils with stimulant nervine properties include: basil, black pepper, cardamom, cinnamon, clove, fennel, ginger, lemon, nutmeg, peppermint, pine, rosemary, thyme.

Rubefacient effect

Essential oils with rubefacient properties usually increase local blood circulation, which can be observed by a redness of the skin, but they also influence the inner organs. The local skin irritation, the 'primary irritation', sets free mediators in the body which in turn cause vasodilation. The local skin irritation can also have an analgesic influence on the inner organs. The primary irritation also causes humeral reactions, the results of which can be observed as anti-inflammatory effects. Thus, besides an agreeable feeling of warmth and relief of pain, anti-inflammatory effects can be observed.

Essential oils with rubefacient properties include: black pepper, cinnamon, clove, ginger, lemon, nutmeg, peppermint, pine, rosemary, thyme.

Sedative effect

According to Guillemain (29), lavender essential oil diluted 1:60 with olive oil was given orally to mice, and the sedative effects observed by performing a number of tests. It was found that a significant interaction existed with pentabarbital; the sleeping time was increased and the asleeping time was shortened.

Buchbauer (30) found that under standardised experimental conditions lavender significantly decreased motility, and hyperactivity which had been induced by caffeine injection was reduced almost to normal. It was concluded that the effectiveness of the traditional aromatherapy use of lavender as a sedative was proven and that the use of lavender could facilitate and minimise stressful situations.

Jager (31), investigated the sedative effects of neroli, citronellal and phenyl ethyl acetate in a series of experimental procedures involving mice. Under standardised experimental conditions the motility of mice was reduced from an arbitrarily graded 100% for untreated animals to 34.73% by neroli, to 50.18% by citronellal and 54.94% by phenyl ethyl acetate. The method of application was inhalation.

At Newholme Hospital, Balewell, England the effects of lavender oil being diffused at night time in a ward of dementia sufferers was investigated. The results concluded that lavender oil was found to be beneficial in improving the time spent sleeping. One resident involved in the trial who regularly had disturbed nights, was observed to be more relaxed and sleeping undisturbed throughout the night. As a result he was brighter in the morning without the obvious 'hangover' symptoms, usually apparent following the use of night sedation. (32)

There is much evidence that essential oils, being aromatic, lipid soluble and electrically active compounds, have a profound psycho-physiological effect when inhaled. This will be discussed in Chapter 9.

Spasmolytic effect

Spasmolytics, also known as antispasmodics, reduce spasm or tension, especially in the visceral smooth muscle, the muscle of the gut wall, bronchial tubes and blood vessels. Essential oils with this property are used to control functional tensions in these areas.

Antispasmodics may also serve as broncho-dilators, preventing spasms of the bronchial tubes, thus being beneficial for asthma and other respiratory problems.

The spasmolytic activity has been found and pharmacologically proven for a number of essential oils, such as chamomile, caraway seed, fennel, orange and peppermint. According to McKenzie (33), peppermint oil was used to relax the smooth muscle of the bowel for patients with colostomies. This was found to reduce colonic pressure and reduce the frequency of bag changes and postoperative colic.

Leicester (34) found that peppermint oil reduced colonic spasms during endoscopy. Colonic spasms had been shown to cause discomfort and physical hindrance during flexible sigmoidoscopy and intravenous antispasmodic drugs had been used to counter this. In 20 patients, peppermint oil was injected along the biopsy channel of the colonscope and in every case colonic spasm was relieved within 30 seconds.

Tonic and stimulant effect

Tonics increase body tone. They primarily act on the digestive system and therefore benefit the entire physiology. Organs acting in conjunction with the stomach can be directly influenced by the use of tonics. Tonics have nourishing, supportive and restorative properties. Essential oils that are digestives, hepatics, circulatory stimulants and rubifacients have nourishing and supportive actions on specific organs and body systems and are known as tonics.

Stimulants temporarily increase the functional activity of the human body or any one of its organs. Many stimulants will help to improve circulation. Stimulants are mainly 'warming' by nature and include most spice oils such as cinnamon, clove, black pepper and ginger. Their action usually increases the body's warmth, strengthens metabolism and circulation, warms the stomach and increases the appetite. They often have antibacterial properties and stimulate the immune system.

Many of the digestive stimulant essential oils are carminatives and stomachics. Others have diaphoretic properties.

In promoting circulation, many stimulants may also possess some blood-purifying properties and may help dispel mucus from the stomach, lungs and nasal passages.

Simon Mills warns that stimulants may increase the activity in body function without regard for the inherent capacity of the system to support that activity. In other words they may be intrinsically exhausting (35). This is particularly true of substances such as nicotine, caffeine and alcohol.

Many of the 'stimulants' used in aromatherapy are actually 'restorative' remedies and will assist the body's physiological functioning.

Typical stimulant essential oils are basil, black pepper, cardamom, cinnamon, clove, fennel, ginger, lemon, marjoram, nutmeg, peppermint, rosemary, thyme.

Chapter 9

The Biology and Psychology of Essential Oils

The late Marguerite Maury, a well-known aromatherapist who wrote one of the first books on aromatherapy, describes the effects of essential oils on the psyche:

'The greatest interest is the effect of fragrance on the psychic and mental state of the individual. Powers of perception become clearer and more acute and there is a feeling of having, to a certain extent, outstripped events. They are seen more objectively, and therefore in truer perspective.'

This chapter will investigate the effect of fragrance on the psyche and mental state of the individual.

Introduction

The sense of smell (olfaction) was one of the earliest senses to arise in evolution. It is well developed in lower animals and nocturnal animals. Olfaction for example, is used to detect odours of foods, enemies, territory and the opposite sex. In humans and animals alike, olfaction evokes, perhaps more than any other sense, emotional reactions resulting in strong behavioural changes. The scent of a rose can bring pure pleasure; the smell of rotten eggs can cause nausea and vomiting. Although humans are not known for their olfactory keenness, memories of odours carry deep and emotionally rich associations. The sense of smell is also very important for regulating appetite and food intake. As a result congested sinuses usually cause a loss of appetite.

The following examples highlight the effects that olfaction has on human behaviour and performance. Investigations at universities in Washington and Cincinnati were performed whereby subjects took a 40 minute vigilance computer test whilst breathing through oxygen masks. The persons given intermittent doses of peppermint performed 25% better than those given pure air only. (1)

A study in Japan monitored 13 keypunch operators eight hours a day for a month. When the air was scented with lavender, errors per hour dropped by 21%, with jasmine by 33% and with lemon by 54%. The Japanese have now developed an environmental fragrancing system that delivers scents through air conditioning ducts under computer control. (2)

According to John Steele (3) fragrances can be used to create 'an environmentally induced positive effect'. The benefits of this effect are:

- better memory, organisation and cooperation

- higher self-set goals

- greater job satisfaction

- anticipation of higher outcomes in negotiation, but also a willingness to be flexible.

When fragrance was coupled with pleasant lighting and music the 'positive effect' was amplified.

Dr Alan Hirsch, a neurological director at the Smell and Taste Treatment and Research Foundation in Chicago, noted that customers not only bought more, but paid for the higher priced athletic shoes in a floral scented sales room, even when the scent in the room was so low it was not consciously detected. He predicts that scent will become the marketing tool of the future. (4)

The physiology of smell

Olfaction

Interest in the effect of odours has arisen only recently and it seems such a shame that society has generally neglected scent and its effects on people, both psychological and physiological. Most text books on anatomy and physiology contain no more than one page on the mechanisms of smell. It is obvious that this poor understanding of smell and its effects is based on the fact that so little information is available on its mechanisms. In this chapter I discuss the latest research on olfaction, emotion and aromatherapy.

The physiology of olfaction

In order for a substance to be smelled it must be volatile, that is, capable of entering a gaseous state so that the molecules can enter the nostrils. The substance must be water soluble, so that it can dissolve in the mucus to make contact with the olfactory cells, and it must be lipid-soluble, since the plasma membranes of the olfactory fibres are largely lipid, and the substance to be smelled must dissolve in the lipid covering to make contact with olfactory cilia in order to initiate a response.

The sense of smell is located in two regions of the nasal mucous membranes, each about 3-4 cm^2 in area, on the roof and the upper part of both walls of the nasal cavity. This region consists not only of cells that secrete mucus like the rest of the nasal mucous membrane, but also of slender nerve cells called olfactory cillia, covered with a thin film of mucus. In the 8 cm^2 area of the olfactory mucous membrane regions, humans carry some 10 million olfactory nerve cells.

It is here that the complex mechanism of smell begins. Two principal theories have been formulated to explain how olfaction works: (5)

- The chemical theory assumes that there are different receptor chemicals in the membranes of the olfactory hairs, which are capable of reacting with a particular olfactory substance. The interaction between chemical receptor and substance alters the permeability of the plasma membrane so that a generator potential is developed, followed by initiation of a nerve impulse.

- The physical theory holds that there are physical receptor sites on the plasma membranes of olfactory hairs that react with olfactory substances. This interaction then causes a change in membrane permeability, development of a generator potential, and initiation of a nerve impulse.

As soon as an odour molecule that has penetrated into the mucous layer is caught in a matching depression (receptor), a signal is sent to the brain. The individual fine processes of the nerve cells are bundled in the nasal area and extend through the cribriform plate of the ethmoid bone behind the septum and into the interior of the skull. Here they enter part of the brain known as the olfactory bulb. It is in the olfactory bulb that the olfactory impressions are initially processed. There is evidence for some mapping of odours in the olfactory bulb: eg stimulation with a single odour (eg peppermint) enhances metabolic activity in a circumscribed region of the bulb. The olfactory messages are then sent, via the olfactory tract, to the higher olfactory areas of the brain.

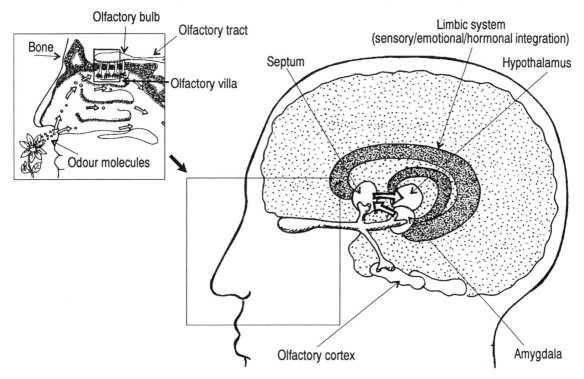

A schematic of the olfactory system with its primary and secondary paths to other regions in the brain

Olfaction and the brain

The olfactory output from the bulb to the brain has two targets. One is the thalamus which then transmits to the neocortex and the other is the hypothalamic region. The neocortex is the cognitive part of the brain where sensory processing occurs. The neocortex area is the site of olfactory discrimination, perception and memories which, for example allows us to perceive the scent of a rose and correctly identify its specific variety.

The second target, the hypothalamic region, forms part of the limbic system. This is a series of central and basal structures, which was given its name over a century ago because it forms a threshold or limbus, around which the higher centres of the brain are built. In evolutionary terms it is the oldest part of the brain, referred to in the past as the 'rhinencephalon' or the 'smell brain'. In recent years it has become clear that a complex set of structures and their pathways in the brain, referred to as the 'limbic structures', is where olfactory signals activate smell-related emotions and behaviours.

The areas of the brain associated with emotional responsiveness are also concerned with visceral function: regulation of heart rate, blood pressure, respiration, digestive activity and levels of various hormones. Regulation of visceral functions depends on two systems. One is called the sympathetic nervous system. It prepares the body for fight or flight, raising heart rate and the blood pressure and decreasing digestive activity, since the blood is needed elsewhere. The parasympathetic nervous system does the reverse, preparing the body for more vegetative activities. The 'head office' for these two systems is located in the hypothalamus. The hypothalamus is also responsible for the regulation of hormones through its control of the pituitary gland activity.

This direct effect that smell can have on the hypothalamus perhaps suggests why aromatherapy is considered one of the most valuable tools in the treatment of stress and anxiety related problems which can be seen as an overload of the sympathetic nervous system.

Damage to the hypothalamus in experimental animals not only disturbed the regulation of their visceral functions, but also altered their emotional responsiveness. When a small area of the outer part of the hypothalamus is destroyed, cats change from being easily handled to responding with blind rage to all contact. (6)

The psychology of smell

Introduction

In the novel, *Perfume: The Story of a Murder*, by Patrick Suskind (1986) the central character is obsessed by the fact that he has no body odour of his own. This obsession forces him to become a mass murderer and he extracts the body odours of people he has killed in order to concoct for himself the perfect odour, the very essence of beauty, the source of all excitement and total contentment. The chilling feeling that emanates from this novel is not from the cold blooded murders, as they are not described in any detail - but from the unconscious awareness of the evil act of psychological vandalism which is inflicted on the victims as they are drained of their scent. Suskind writes about the significance of scent:

> '...people could close their eyes to greatness, to horrors, to beauty, and their ears to melodies or deceiving words. But they could not escape scent. For scent was a brother to breath. Together with breath it entered human beings, who could not defend themselves against it, not if they wanted to live. And scent enters into their very core, went directly to their hearts, and decided for good and all between affection and contempt, disgust and lust, love and hate. He who ruled scent ruled the hearts of men.'

Thoughts such as these have been in the minds of philosophers throughout the ages. Odours seem to penetrate to the deepest levels of the unconscious mind, to where only the greatest philosophers are able to explore and from where most of humanity is barred. There is much to learn from the writings of philosophers and other people who probe the unconscious about odour symbolism, and about the special relationship which exists between the nose and the psyche. Research into the psychology of olfaction is still in its infancy because of the difficulties associated with scientific analysis of that most temperamental of human attributes - emotions.

Fragrances are often applied to the body in controlled emotional settings. A person who applies a perfume or cologne, may be doing so for a number of reasons. When people are asked why they apply perfume or fragrances, they will often say that it makes them feel good and promotes a sense of wellbeing. Essential oils may be used for their sensory role; the initial intake of the fragrance evokes positive feelings and pleasant emotions.

Knasko (7) reported that 90 subjects were divided into three groups (of equal distribution of sexes) and each group placed for one hour in a room which contained a hidden source of lavender, lemon or dimethyl sulphide. Questionnaires on mood, health and the environment were then completed by the individuals of the groups, and personality and creativity tests performed. The experiment was repeated a week later with no odour present in the room. It was found that exposure to malodour tended to lower mood ratings but that the pleasant odours had no effect on the mood.

However lemon was found to decrease health symptoms reported, possibly due to the association with cleanliness and freshness. There was a relationship between personality traits and the effect of odour on mood and performance. It was suggested that associations and expectations regarding odours may be important in the effect of ambient odour on health and mood.

Historical background

The therapeutic use of aromatic plants and oils dates back to earliest times. In Egypt, infused oils and unguents were employed over 5000 years ago for both spiritual and medicinal uses. Early civilisations burnt aromatic herbs and woods to drive out 'evil spirits', which we now might interpret as mental sickness. In many parts of the world fragrant plants have been and still are, an integral part of the ritual in sorcery, healing and religious practices.

In the old testament, God instructs Moses in the creation of a 'holy perfume', based on frankincense, myrrh and other exotic gums.

'Take sweet spices: storax, onycha, galbanum, sweet spices and pure frankincense in equal parts and compound an incense such a blend as the perfumer might make, salted, pure and holy. Crush a part of it into a fine powder, and put some of this in front of the testimony in the tent of meeting, the place appointed for my meetings with you. You must regard it as most holy..'

Such holy perfumes were probably used to evoke a spiritual atmosphere, or to heighten spiritual awareness. The Greek philosopher Plutarch wrote about an ancient Egyptian perfume known as 'kyphi':

'Its aromatic substances lull to sleep, allay anxieties and brighten dreams.'

One of the 16 ingredients of kyphi was calamus, a potent narcotic and sedative. Hines (8) comments that:

'odours are capable of creating an emotional and ecstatic state of consciousness that renders individuals more susceptible to religious experience.'

Incense and other aromatic substances were employed in ritual practices for the following reasons: (9)

- as a way of uplifting and altering one's state of mind - to create the correct mood

- as a means of 'communion' between the earthly and divine realm

- as a protection against evil and to ensure favour

- as a purifying agent for the psyche or soul of an individual

- as a cleansing agent for physical body and the environment .

The basis of using aromatic substances may be described in terms of its physiological and psychological effect on the human psyche.

Psycho-aromatherapy

In Italy, in the early 1920s, there appeared the first review of psycho-aromatherapy, written by two medical doctors, Giovanni Gatti and Renato Cayola (10). In 1923 they published *'The action of essences on the nervous system'*, explaining clearly how odours influence mood and emotion, and defining the two opposing states of anxiety and depression.

Two methods of application for the essential oil were suggested - inhalation or ingestion. In digestive absorption the essential oil is introduced like other medicines, and arrives at the nerve cells by the slow transmission of the blood stream. In respiratory absorption the essences exert an influence on the brain via the nerve endings of the olfactory mucosa. The authors noted, immediately following inhalation, changes in pulse rate, blood circulation and depth of respiration. They concluded by saying:

'The sense of smell has, by reflex action, an enormous influence on the function of the central nervous system.'

Essential oils such as chamomile, melissa, neroli and petitgrain were identified as sedatives and therefore of use in treating anxiety. Stimulating essential oils included angelica, lemon, fennel, cinnamon and clove. In recent years Gatti and Cayola's early research has been taken one step further by Professor Paolo Rovesti of Milan University (11). According to Rovesti, 'green notes' such as bergamot, lime, neroli, petitgrain, lavender, marjoram, violet leaf, rose and cypress are usually anxiety-relieving and sedative.

He suggests that blends of essential oils are more pleasant than single oils. To treat depression he suggests the use of lemon, orange, verbena, jasmine, ylang-ylang and sandalwood. Rovesti does not give any details of controlled experimentation, but he does state that

'very conclusive experiments have been carried out in various clinics for nervous diseases, on patients affected by hysteria or psychic depression.'

Rovesti also describes the response of psychiatric patients to aromatherapy:

'It may be said that the patients felt as if transported by the perfume or by the essential oil into a different, more agreeable and acceptable world, so that many of their reactive instincts are curbed and they gradually return towards normality.'

Very often a patient's response to the first treatment is simply 'I feel better' or 'I feel brighter' or 'I am much more relaxed'. We should not underestimate the importance of this effect, whatever the complaint may be, physical or psychological. A positive mental attitude is important for the patient's full recovery.

Many researchers have detected physiological changes in response to odour stimulation in areas such as blood pressure, muscle tension, skin temperature, skin conductance and brain wave patterns. (12) (13) None of these responses are under conscious control, and the subjects are often unaware of their response to an odour.

Emotion and olfaction

How does fragrance influence our emotional state? In recent years it has become clear that the limbic system (an important and complex set of structures and their pathways) relates to emotion. The major function of the limbic system is to combine the many parts of the brain as shown schematically in the diagram on page 101. It should also be remembered that the limbic system has an influence on the hormones and autonomic nervous system which influences behaviour and emotions.

According to Watts (14) the limbic system also determines the total sensory input into the brain as either 'pleasant' or 'unpleasant'.

While literature surveys in perfumery suggest that there is a special relationship between emotion and odour, there has been very little evidence to verify this. After many years of research, International Flavors and Fragrances have made the following observations (15):

- Fragrance-evoked mood changes are small, but beneficial to our wellbeing.

- Fragrance can be used to reduce the stress response in humans, but its physiological effects on a non-stressed subject are minimal and difficult to measure.

- Measurement of fragrance-evoked mood change by psychological methods is feasible and yields intriguing results.

It seems that fragrance-evoked emotional changes do not have any significant influence on human behaviour. Humans are the only mammals to exhibit sexual and social behaviour that is not under olfactory control. Dr Michael Stoddart suggests that the loss of olfactory controlled sexual and social behaviour was necessary for the development of the human race. Stoddart explains:

> *'During the Miocene epoch, man's prehominid ancestors started to band together in order to hunt the large ungulates, which evolved in association with the grassy plains. This gregarious habit posed a threat to the integrity of the pair-bonds which existed between males and females ... To retain the sociobioligical advantages which the pair-bonds afford the young, it was necessary for the information present in the signal to be scrambled by the brain until it was meaningless.'* (16)

It is not known how the ability to perceive oestrus odours (odours associated with ovulation) was lost, but Stoddart assumes that it occurred when the cerebral cortex was gaining ascendancy over the smell brain (rhinencephalon).

Humans do not depend upon odours as a primary source of information about their environment as do other animals. In many animals, sexual and emotional behaviours are governed largely by the limbic system. In contrast, in humans odours no longer control sexual and social behaviour, rather, they create small changes in feeling states.

If odours do not cause overt changes in our sexual and emotional behaviours, what do they do? Ehrlichman and Bastone (17) suggest that odours can influence cognitive and behavioural patterns in similar ways to mood states.

> *'in contrast to strong emotions, these feeling states do not interrupt our thoughts, but subtly colour and redirect them often without our notice'.*

The authors' research suggests that odours are likely to influence particular types of cognitive processes such as creative performance, evaluation and personal memories. Compared with unpleasant odours, pleasant odours tend to:

- enhance creative performance
- generate more positive evaluation of words and pictures of people
- elicit more happy memories.

Baron found that subjects working in the presence of pleasant ambient odour set higher goals, and were more likely to employ an efficient strategy, than subjects working in an unscented room. (18)

The results of Baron, Ehrlichman and Bastone suggest that pleasant odours stimulate pleasant thoughts and positive mood states and odours are less dependent on high cognitive pressures to produce these effects than are auditory or visual stimuli.

It has also been shown that the social setting was an important determinant of emotion. In terms of olfaction a beautiful perfume will elicit the learned response of turning round to look for a beautiful woman. In this response the perfume has a set of attributes, some of which are emotional. However, a sufferer of allergies would be wary as the smell of the perfume is likely to trigger an allergic response.

Children may also dislike the smell; it seems that perfumes are too sophisticated for the young, who lack aesthetic dimension. If children do like perfumes, those they prefer tend to be single notes or simple floral perfumes. There is of course the added complication that children respond through learned behaviour. In the home the smell of perfume can mean that their parents are going out for the evening, thus there is some resentment.

Psychophysiological effects of odour

In recent years there has been much attention paid to how aromatic substances, including essential oils, exert their action upon the mind and body through inhalation. Is it how the brain processes the information about odours that leads to an alteration in awareness, mood or physiological response? Or is it in fact a result of a cascade of reactions created by aromatic compounds exerting a more pharmacological mode of action by working on a molecular level?

Attempts have been made over the years to measure the psychophysiological effects of odour using a variety of means. How can we measure emotional response to an odour?

Psychophysiology is the study of covert physiological responses that accompany behavioural changes. Psychophysiological changes which are long term can be measured using bodily fluids such as sweat, saliva, blood

An electroencephalogram (EEG) records the continuous neural activity of the neurons. An EEG can be made by placing electrodes at various locations on the scalp and then connecting the electrodes to an apparatus that measures electrical potential differences between the various cortical areas. The resulting patterns of neural activity are called brain waves.

Because of the differences in individuals, everyone has a brain wave pattern that is as unique as fingerprints. However, a pattern of four frequency classes has been identified.

- **Alpha waves** are low-amplitude, slow, rhythmic and synchronous waves with an average frequency of 8-13 Hz (hertz or cycles per second). In most cases alpha brain wave activity indicates a calm relaxed state of wakefulness.

- **Beta waves** are also rhythmic, but they are more regular than alpha waves and have a higher frequency of 14-25 Hz. Beta waves occur when we are awake and mentally alert, or when we concentrate on a problem or visual stimulus.

- **Theta waves** are irregular, and they have a frequency of 4-7 Hz. Theta waves are common in children and in adults in the early stages of sleep. They are considered abnormal in adults when awake.

- **Delta waves** are high amplitude waves with a frequency of 4 Hz or less. They occur during deep sleep and when the reticular activating system is sedated, such as when under anaesthesia.

Brain waves have a normal frequency range of 1-30 Hz, a dominant rhythm of 10 Hz, and an average amplitude of 20-100 microvolts. The amplitude reflects the number of neurons firing simultaneously, not the degree of electrical activity of individual neurons. When the brain is active and neurons are involved in different activities, complex low-amplitude brain waves are seen. When the brain is inactive, during sleep, meditation or deep state of relaxation, large numbers of neurons fire simultaneously, producing similar, high-amplitude brain waves.

Brain wave patterns and the EEG

and urine. Short term changes often involve the amplification and recording of the minute bioelectrical potentials that are found in the body. These may include muscle potentials and heart rate as well the electrical potentials generated within the brain. The latter are recorded by the electroencephalograph (EEG) which measures brain wave activity.

Thus the subject's reaction to an odour may be measured by using psychophysiological techniques. The advantage of using these techniques is that they overcome problems associated with subjective responses.

John Steele carried out experiments using an EEG to evaluate the effects of various oils on the brain's rhythm patterns. His results were as follows (19):

'As predicted, the cephalic oils such as basil, rosemary, black pepper and cardamom, induced beta predominant patterns. Beta brain rhythms (38-13 hertz) are correlated with aroused attention and alertness. At the other end of the spectrum, orange blossom, jasmine and rose induced an unusual amount of delta rhythms (4-0.75 hertz) with some alpha(12-8 hertz) and theta (7-5 hertz). These lower frequencies indicate a quietening of mental chatter (alpha), with the mind going into reverie and intuitive flashes (theta and delta).

Professor Torii (20) of Toho University, Japan studied changes in the contingent negative variation (CNV) to ascertain whether odours were stimulant, sedative or neutral. CNV is an average of many EEG readings and is a very sensitive measure for determining the effects of odours on brain electrical activity. Torii was able to confirm many of the traditional properties of the essential oils, eg lavender was sedative and jasmine was a stimulant. Of interest were geranium and rosewood which were shown to be either stimulating or sedative.

This confirms the traditional role of these two oils as 'adaptogens'. That is, they are said to have a balancing effect, whether the individual is prone to hyperactivity or listlessness.

Torii's study, suggested that the measurement of CNV was an accurate method for assessing the response of the brain to odours as it was 'almost independent' of the subject's mood, expectations or level of arousal.

Other studies using CNV measurements and essential oils as odorants disagree, concluding that CNV changes are very much subject to cognitive mediation - dependent on the person's expectations and experiences of the odours presented. Odours presented during sleep and at subliminal levels are unlikely to be subject to cognitive mediation and have been shown to cause alterations in the central nervous system, including EEG changes.

In another study using essential oils (including lavender, lemon and jasmine) little correlation was found between the different odours and the EEG changes that they produced. What is more, many subjects found lavender was one of the most arousing and least pleasant of the test odours. This demonstrates that subjectivity exists with the sense of smell. (21)

Van Toller (22) also studied the effect of fragrance on the two hemispheres of the brain. The right hemisphere deals with imagination, emotion and aesthetic awareness, and the left hemisphere is more concerned with reasoning, words and logic. Normally, both hemispheres of the brain work harmoniously to integrate all incoming data, yet the researchers found that when a fragrance which was considered pleasant was inhaled, a wave of electrical activity was noticed in the right hemisphere which then spread to areas of the left hemisphere, as if the brain confirmed that the smell had been pleasant.

However in the same test, another subject who was presented with a pleasant smell did not show any right hemispheric burst of electrical activity, but showed continuous left hemispheric activity throughout the odour presentation. The electrical

activity appeared to be around the speech area of the cortex. It was later confirmed that the subject, whose native language was not English, knew the name of the oil being used, but was not able to think of the English name. It seems that the cognitive part of the brain was able to override the emotional response.

In an experiment conducted by Buchbauer (23) the effect of the inhalation of lavender essential oil, linalool and linalyl acetate on the activity of mice was observed. All three substances caused a significant reduction in motility, and hyperactivity induced by caffeine injection was reduced almost to normal. It confirmed the traditional use of lavender as a sedative.

With regard to using aromatic substances in the field of stress management, fragrances have a proven role to play in those individuals who are stressed, but the effects upon non-stressed subjects are more difficult to measure.

Research into this field has been conducted over several years by International Flavours and Fragrances in conjunction with stress researchers at Yale University. Fragrance-enhanced relaxation as advocated by King (24) appears to be more effective than using the fragrance alone, and utilising the concept of pairing an emotional state with an odour is an important contribution to the field of stress management. Aromatherapy massage could be regarded as a form of fragrance-enhanced relaxation.

The results obtained in the studies mentioned above have a direct relevance in the field of aromatherapy. It is possible to conclude that:

- The fragrance does not have to be intense in order to be effective. Changes are measurable even at subliminal levels. The more intense the odour, the less pleasant it becomes.

- Odour perception and its subsequent psychophysiological effects are extremely subjective and will vary from person to person according to the following factors:

  - how much odour is applied

  - how the odour is applied

  - the circumstances in which it is applied

- the person to whom it is applied (age, sex, personality type)

- the mood the person was in to start with

- what previous association the person may have with the odour

- anosmia or inability to smell

- expectations or cognitive thought about the odour.

• As a person's expectations of an odour affects the physiological response, the way in which the odour is presented to them by the therapist is an important consideration.

• If a paired emotional response with an odour is desired, the same fragrance should be used until odour conditioning occurs.

Chapter 10

Pharmacokinetics

This chapter investigates the processes by which the body interacts with, metabolises and excretes essential oils. The name for the study of this is pharmacokinetics, the science of the movement of drugs. The factors that influence the movement of an essential oil or its constituents through the body allow the aromatherapist to have a better insight into the ideal conditions in which to apply essential oils.

Introduction

Pharmacokinetics is generally considered under the following headings:

- absorption
- distribution
- metabolism
- excretion.

Absorption

There are several ways in which essential oils are administered for use in aromatherapy:

- dermally
- by inhalation
- orally
- rectally.

Dermal

Aromatherapists often take for granted that essential oils are absorbed into the skin. It is surprising that very little research has been conducted to address the absorption of essential oils and vegetable oils into the body via the skin. However, the absorption of drugs and cosmetic substances through the skin has been studied in great detail (1).

Recent studies involving lavender essential oil diluted in peanut oil massaged over the stomach area for 10 minutes indicated that traces of linalool and linalyl acetate were detected in the blood after 20 minutes. After ninety minutes most of the lavender oil had been eliminated from the blood. (2)

Surprisingly Buchbauer (3) suggests that it is nonsense to apply essential oils by massage!

'Massage application is wrong because of the high concentration in which the fragrant molecules evoke unspecified effects, in particular irritation by destruction of cell membranes. On the other hand, essential oils reaching cells in very low concentrations as in inhalation where the resultant plasma concentrations of the essential oil compounds are 100- to 10,000 fold smaller, are integrated in special areas of cell membranes and evoke specific effects by influencing the enzymes, carriers, ion channels and receptor proteins which are in these localised areas.'

Whether you agree with Buchbauer's comments on massage application or not, he has been one of the few researchers to determine the amount of essential oil in the blood plasma as a result of inhalation and massage.

Essential oils and vegetable based carrier oils, being composed of fat soluble molecules, tend to be absorbed easily into the skin. There are many aspects that need to be addressed in order to study the factors that will affect absorption of the essential oils into the skin and how they find their way into the circulatory system.

Skin's functions

Although the skin excretes wastes, receives sensory stimuli and helps regulate body temperature, its principal function is to protect the sensitive protoplasmic jelly of the body's interior from an environment that can be very harsh. The skin prevents various microbes, chemicals and some forms of radiation from penetrating the body, and prevents body fluids and tissues from spilling out.

Until the late 1800s, the skin was considered by many to be totally impermeable. By the beginning of this century enough work had been done for scientists to realise that the skin was relatively permeable to fat-soluble substances and relatively impermeable to water soluble substances such as salts and, indeed, water itself. The impermeability to water and salts lies in the paper-thin outer layer of the skin called the stratum corneum or horny layer.

Skin's structure

The stratum corneum is a layer of dried, dead, elongated cells (corneocytes) at the surface of the skin. Keratin, deposited within the corneocytes, provides strength and chemical resistance. Resistance to transport through the stratum corneum depends on the properties and arrangement of its alternating hydrophilic and hydrophobic layers, as well as their thickness, which varies from individual to individual. Additional variables are the local concentration of

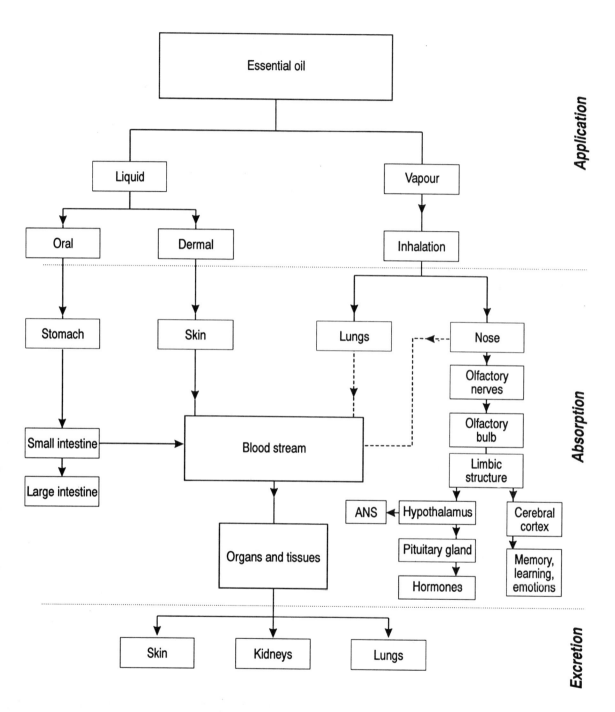

Pathway to illustrate how essential oils are absorbed into the body. The dotted lines indicate only trace amounts of essential oils being absorbed.

hair follicles and sweat glands; these provide possible alternative pathways for absorption.

Experimentally, different rates of absorption have been demonstrated depending on the skin location (4). The permeability of skin at various body sites has been rated as follows:

Relatively permeable: genitals, head areas such as forehead and scalp, soles and palms, armpits, mucous membranes

Relatively impermeable: trunk, abdomen, limbs, buttocks

The stratum corneum is manufactured by the next skin layer down, the epidermis. The epidermis has many cells in various stages of biochemical alteration. There is a constant movement of newly generated cells upward, from the basal layer towards the skin surface.

Hair follicles and associated sebaceous glands are structurally part of the epidermis. The follicles are lined with epidermal tissue. The sebaceous glands are holocrine glands which produce a lipid mixture (sebum) that is deposited onto the skin surface. The glands and the upper sections of the follicles are potential locations for the absorption of essential oils.

The epidermis has no blood vessels. Nutrients must diffuse into this tissue from the dermis, a much thicker layer that contains many fibres and is responsible for the skin's mechanical strength and feel. Blood vessels and nerve endings are also found here.

The dermis is supported by a layer of fatty tissue, called the hypodermis or subcutis, which provides insulation and mechanical cushioning. The thickness of this layer varies greatly from one body site to another.

Principal absorption pathways

When essential oils are applied to the skin surface, two major thoroughfares exist:

- through the stratum corneum

- via 'shunts' - the hair follicles and sweat gland ducts.

Absorption through the latter is faster than the route across the stratum corneum. However, the stratum corneum is considered to be the major pathway for most substances. (5)

Within the stratum corneum itself, two penetration pathways exist: one crosses the cells and intercellular spaces (polar pathway) while the second involves passage only through the intercellular lipid domain (lipid pathway). This explains the ability of molecules with a wide disparity in physiochemical properties to permeate the skin. The polar pathway accommodates primarily water and ions and has a smaller capacity and so contributes less to the total penetration while the lipid pathway handles everything else.

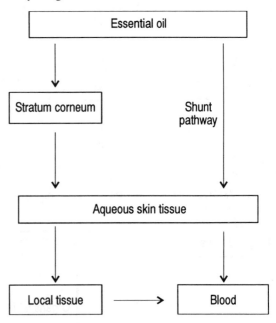

Schematic diagram showing principal absorption pathways (5)

Factors affecting absorption into the skin

The following factors have been demonstrated to influence the rate of essential oil absorption:

- integrity of the stratum corneum

- skin hydration

- occlusion

- viscosity of base oils
- temperature
- the use of surfactants.

Integrity of the stratum corneum

Conditions such as eczema, which results in thickened skin with maintenance of an intact structure, may retard absorption because of the increase in absorptive path length (6). On the other hand, absorption through psoriatic skin is enhanced (7). This may be secondary to altered epidermal structure as well as to changes in vascular perfusion.

Systemic disease states could also potentially alter the rate of topical absorption. For example, diabetes is known to alter the structure of epidermal basement membranes and capillary functions such that compound diffusion out of cutaneous capillaries is enhanced in chronic diabetes. (8)

Skin hydration

Skin hydration occurs through bathing, sweating, being in an area of high humidity, occlusion or application of a film-forming product such as a moisturiser.

Water influences the barrier performance of the stratum corneum more than any other non-irritating substance and it has been found that skin hydration which may result from a bath or shower could enhance essential oil absorption. (9)

Taking a hot bath or shower could also stimulate the blood flow to the dermis, which can increase the absorption of essential oils. Using a massage oil after bathing is also a way of increasing essential oil absorption.

Hydration is known to accelerate the passage of drugs through the skin and is the basis of cosmetic skin claims made about moisturisers.

Topically-applied drugs such as nicotenic acid (10), salicylic acid (11) and aspirin (12) have all been shown to be enhanced in terms of absorption on hydrated skin versus normal skin. The mechanism through which absorbed water affects skin penetration has not been investigated in any detail.

Occlusions

A common method of increasing skin hydration is by the use of occlusive dressings.

Occlusion prevents surface evaporation resulting in stratum corneum hydration.

Occlusion of the skin can result from wearing clothes, bandages, plasters, masks and materials such as petroleum jelly. Not only will the occlusion increase the temperature of the skin but it will also increase the hydration of the skin, and these factors will increase absorption.

Cosmetic facial masks are a form of occlusion in which the skin's percutaneous hydration is increased. Fragrances under occlusion have also been found to double the percutaneous absorption rate of unoccluded fragrance materials (13).

Viscosity of base oils

Viscosity refers to the thickness of the carrier oil being used. For instance olive oil which is viscous is slowly absorbed through the skin whereas apricot kernel oil which is much less viscous, is rapidly absorbed. Because essential oils are highly soluble in vegetable oils it is very likely that the viscosity of the vegetable oil will determine the rate of absorption of the essential oil.

The degree of unsaturation of an oil also affects the rate of cutaneous penetration: linseed oil which is rich in polyunsaturates traverses the skin much better than its low viscosity would lead one to expect; on the other hand, olive oil which is rich in monounsaturated fatty acids is not easily absorbed by the skin.

According to studies conducted by Loth (14), fatty acids such as caprylic, capric, stearic acid, oleic acid and α-linoleic acid were found to be penetration enhancers. All these fatty acids are abundantly found in cold pressed vegetable oils.

Temperature

Either a rise in ambient room temperature or the use of warm oil will lead to an enhanced absorption. Such conditions would also increase vaporisation, thus increasing the amount of essential oil inhaled. No doubt the increased rate of absorption is due to enhanced capillary circulation.

Biological factors	thickness of stratum corneum
	age
	blood flow
	metabolism
	hydration
Environmental factors	temperature
	climate
	time
Trauma factors	mechanical disease
	chemical disease
Vehicle factors	penetrating properties
	occlusivity
	surfactant
Permeant factors	molecular weight
	solubility
	binding
	molecular size

Factors affecting absorption (5)

The use of surfactants

Surfactants (surface active agents) are widely used in skin products to serve a variety of functions. It has been found that many surface active agents such as soaps and detergents can increase the permeability of the skin (15).

The mechanisms of action appear to be protein denaturation (permanent), membrane expansion, hole formation and loss of water binding capacity. It has been demonstrated that the use of surfactants with certain antimicrobial agents has increased the absorption of the antimicrobial agent into the skin. (16)

The physiology of the skin

Apart from its structural role, the skin is a dynamic organ with a myriad of biological functions such as neurosensory reception, endocrinology, immunological affector and effector axes, glandular secretions, and keratin, collagen, melanin, lipid and carbohydrate metabolism. The skin's complex biological functions may alter the absorption of topically-applied substances such as essential oils.

A large percentage of topically-applied substances may never penetrate the rate-limiting stratum corneum barrier. If the compound is volatile as are essential oils, part of it will be lost through evaporation. Topically-applied substances may chemically bind to the stratum corneum and thus may be lost due to desquamation.

However, if the substance has entered the stratum corneum, there are three possible fates:

- complete absorption into the cutaneous microcirculation

- formation of a reservoir by binding to the stratum corneum or subcutaneous fat where it subsequently may be slowly released into the capillaries

- metabolism by cutaneous enzymes.

In some cases, the route of entry into the skin may be via appendages such as hair follicles or sweat ducts. The ability of the stratum corneum and the lower dermal strata to act as a reservoir for topically-applied agents such as essential oils is well known (17).

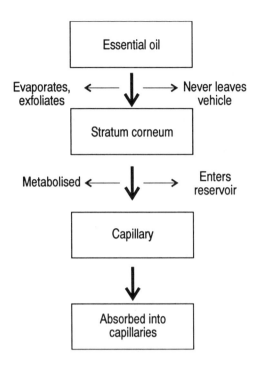

Possible fate of a topically applied essential oil

Other physiological activities of the skin are the metabolism of an essential oil and the removal of the essential oil from the skin via the vascular and lymphatic pathways or the circulatory system.

The skin is a site of extrahepatic metabolism for certain types of chemicals such as drugs and carcinogens, not to mention carbohydrates, lipids and proteins (18). Recent studies have indicated that cutaneous metabolism may be an important component for permeation of some chemicals. It has become clear that various factors will influence the amount of essential oil which, after penetrating the stratum corneum, is absorbed intact or as a metabolite due to epidermal metabolism.

Some essential oil constituents are believed to be converted into potentially carcinogenic compounds. This seems to be the case with cytochrome P450 enzymes which convert essential oil constituents such as safrole and methyl carvracrol into potentially carcinogenic compounds. (19)

Often if the essential oil is not metabolised, the vascular and lymphatic systems are still involved in actively clearing it from the surface of the skin.

Metabolism is not the only physiological function of the skin which has a major impact on the absorption of a substance into the skin. Binding of a substance to protein in the skin is critical for the occurence of certain responses, such as allergic contact dermatitis. Here binding of the penetrant to a cutaneous or serum protein is crucial to the formation of an allergen before induction can begin and cutaneous sensitisation can result. (20)

The question:

'Is an essential oil more readily available for systemic absorption via cutaneous or gastrointestinal routes?'

surprisingly is now reversed! Unfortunately, the answer to this question is simply not known at this time.

Entry into the blood

Molecules which have passed through the epidermis are carried away by the capillary blood circulating in the dermis below. The dermis of the skin has a large network of capillaries which modulates cutaneous blood flow in response to thermoregulatory needs. When the environmental temperature exceeds body temperature, cutaneous blood flow increases so that heat is lost through the skin. In contrast, blood flow is reduced or totally shunted in cold temperatures to prevent surface heat loss.

In vivo topical absorption of methyl salicylate was increased threefold in humans when they were exposed to high ambient temperatures or underwent strenuous exercise. Increased blood flow was presumed to be a major factor, although increased skin hydration or sweating also contributed. (21)

Because the blood flow in the skin is low compared to that in the muscle, it could well be that for easily absorbed substances, cutaneous blood flow will limit the rate of absorption into the blood stream. In such cases massage can be expected to increase the rate of systemic absorption because massage greatly enhances blood flow.

Inhalation

Whether essential oils are inhaled directly from a bottle, a vaporiser, a bowl of steaming water or from an aromatherapy massage, a significant concentration of odoriferous molecules will pass down the trachea into the bronchi, and then into the bronchioles and finally the alveoli, where essential oil molecules pass into the blood stream. It is also assumed that substances absorbed via the nasal mucosa have very easy access to the central nervous system.

The essential oils' lipophilic nature means that they easily pass the blood-brain barrier. Their affinity for lipid-rich tissues like those of the central nervous system facilitates an exchange of essential oil constituents from the blood into the lipid rich nervous system.

According to Buchbauer (22) *Lavendula angustifolia*'s sedative action is due to a direct pharmacological action on the brain, rather than its pleasing aroma and consequent subjective response through the sense of smell. It is now known that essential oils are readily absorbed into the bloodstream through inhalation. They have a high solubility in blood and excellent absorption takes place through the nasal mucosa and pulmonary system.

Falk-Filipsson (23) demonstrated a high uptake of d-limonene (a major constituent of lemon and other citrus oils). 70% of the supplied amount was absorbed after two hours, and traces of d-limonene were found in the blood only minutes after inhalation.

A correlation was made between peak blood levels of an inhaled substance and locomotor activity (stimulation or sedation). Inhaled *Rosmarinus officinalis* (24) increased locomotor activity of the brain. The particular component of rosemary oil causing the stimulating effect was not investigated.

Buchbauer (25) compares inhalation to someone eating a cube of sugar. Not only will one sense a sweet pleasant feeling as they taste the sugar, but the ingested sugar molecules will induce the whole cascade of insulin reactions. Why should the fragrance molecules not act similarly via a molecular interaction as well as producing feelings of wellbeing?

Oral

As already mentioned, the oral ingestion of essential oils is unnecessary and carries risks which are absent when they are applied to the skin or inhaled. Oral administration is most popular for drugs which are formulated so that they have little or no taste and gastro-intestinal irritation is minimal or non-existent.

Tony Balacs (26) suggests that extra care would be required when administering the essential oils orally because a significantly higher percentage of oil would reach the circulation, and the liver would receive a relatively large dose via the portal circulation, which takes blood from the gastrointestinal tract to the liver.

It also needs to be noted that almost all recorded cases of serious poisoning by essential oils has occurred by oral self-dosing of small quantities of undiluted essential oil. Other disadvantages of oral administration include:

- possibility of nausea and vomiting
- irritation of the gastrointestinal tract
- much of the essential oil will be metabolised by the liver
- destruction of essential oil constituents by stomach acidity or enzymes in the intestines.

Rectal

Suppositories are often used by doctors in France in aromatherapy treatments because:

- The essential oils can be administered in higher doses than in oral administration for the treatment of acute infectious conditions.

- There is the absence of the interaction between the essential oil and the gastrointestinal tract or the liver which possibly breaks down the essential oil.

- There is a more rapid absorption of the essential oil into the body.

- They reduce the possibly hazardous effects on the liver of essential oils containing phenol constituents (which are very commonly used in France orally). In order to excrete phenols the liver has to convert them into sulphonates which may cause damage to the liver by overworking it.

• They are an easier method of administering essential oils than oral administration.

Suppositories are a common method of essential oil application by French medical doctors. However, it needs to be stressed that similar safety issues to those of oral administration need to be considered. Being lined with mucous membrane, the rectum is highly sensitive to irritation and there may be the risk of occasional irritations.

Distribution

The distribution of a substance once it has entered the body depends on the affinity it has for the various components of the tissues. Many essential oil constituents, being fat soluble, can enter the CNS through the blood-brain barrier. The blood-brain barrier is not a physical structure as such, but represents the lack of permeability in cerebral blood capillaries when compared to peripheral capillaries and the presence of cells through which these constituents must pass if they are to reach the brain's nerve tissue. This is to protect the brain from many potentially toxic chemicals.

The brain is very rich in lipids, and so fat soluble molecules will have a natural affinity for it. Conversely, highly water soluble molecules will tend to linger in the watery environment of the blood. The essential oils are distributed to the tissues in accordance with the extent of blood flow, the ease of passage across cell membranes, and the extent of binding to plasma and tissue proteins.

The body tissue most perfused by blood will also be the tissue most exposed to the action of the essential oil, whilst the tissue with little active circulation will have less chance to respond to treatment. The following list details the different body tissues in decreasing order of blood perfusion (27):

• endocrine glands, heart, lungs, brain, liver and kidneys

• lean tissue as skin and muscle

• fat tissues

• bone, teeth, ligaments and tendons.

The presence of disease also plays a considerable role, such as inflammation in which the blood flow to the area is increased considerably, improving access of the essential oil to that affected tissue.

Another appreciable factor inhibiting access to tissues is obesity. The presence of large fat stores creates a sink wherein much remedial benefit is likely to disappear.

Substances bound to plasma proteins and those with a very low fat-solubility do not readily pass through the barrier into the brain. Molecules such as phenyl acetic acid (found in rose oil), ketones, esters and aldehydes, all of which are extremely common in all essential oils, tend to hydrogen bond with plasma albumin. Essential oils often have electrically charged functional groups. This means that essential oil molecules will easily attract other molecules which are electrically charged, such as proteins and that they will also bind to plasma albumin.

It may be advisable therefore to reduce the dosage of essential oil given to patients with kidney diseases or cirrhosis of the liver whose plasma albumin levels are low. These people have less protein available to bind the oil and so the concentration of oil in the bloodstream may be higher than expected.

A protein-bound constituent will have a much longer effective life in the tissues, but its free levels will never get very high.

Unfortunately, there is little information on the fate of essential oil constituents, however overall changes in the amount of plasma protein can affect the dosages required.

When treating pregnant and nursing mothers it should be assumed that the placental membrane is no different from any other tissue, and therefore that essential oils will reach the foetus unhindered. Also, during breast feeding, the very high perfusion of the lactating mammary glands means that the infant receives a proportionately high dose of any remedy that the mother is taking so care is necessary.

Metabolism

The skin is very effective at transporting small, relatively fat-soluble molecules like oils into the body's interior, especially when aided by a massage. Once in the body, all sorts of transformations occur in the essential oil. What happens to an essential oil once it has been absorbed into the bloodstream?

Because essential oils are small organic molecules, like drugs in this respect, it seems likely that the changes which drugs undergo happen to essential oils as well. As many essential oil constituents are fat soluble, they will behave more like fat soluble drugs in terms of their distribution, metabolism and elimination, rather than behaving like highly water-soluble drugs.

I am also concerned with the possible effects of the essential oil on drug metabolism. A study by Jori (28) investigated components of essential oils such as 1,8-cineole, menthol, α-pinene and β-pinene to determine their effect on drug metabolism. Inhalation of aerosols and subcutaneous injections of the components were evaluated against the pentabarbitol effect (sleeping time) in rats.

The enzymatic activity of three reactions was measured in vitro on liver homogenate of treated and control rats. It was found that 1,8-cineole produced a significant decrease in pentabarbitol effect both by injection and inhalation, and that this effect was dosage related. The liver enzyme activity of the treated rats was significantly increased. It was concluded that 1,8-cineole increases the activity of microsomal enzyme systems.

Other studies have also confirmed that essential oils and essential oil constituents have been shown to influence the absorption of drugs.

Several cases have demonstrated the potentiating effect of topically-applied salicylates on the action of warfarin and the symptoms this can cause (29). Therefore any essential oil with salicylates such as wintergreen or sweet birch oil should not be used at all for patients using warfarin as it may increase the risk of haemorrhage.

Myristicin, which is found in nutmeg, parsley leaf and parsley seed oil, has been found to inhibit monoamine oxidase (MAO) in rodents (30). According to the Martindale Pharmacopoeia, MAO inhibitors should not be given in conjunction with pethidine: (31)

> '*Very severe reactions, including coma, severe respiratory depression, cynanosis and hypotension have occurred in patients receiving monoamine oxidase inhibitors and given pethidine*'.

Tisserand therefore suggests that oral dosages of the myristicin rich oils must be avoided by persons given pethidine. (32)

Liver metabolism

Many substances which are introduced into the body undergo biotransformation in the liver. If they are pharmacologically active, this process usually results in loss or reduction of their activity. However some substances are actually activated by biotransformation, often into toxic metabolites.

The liver contains glutathione which is responsible for detoxifying reactive chemicals that can damage DNA or protein. If the glutathione is completely depleted, the reactive chemicals are able to attack and destroy liver cells. It is very unlikely that any essential oils would be absorbed dermally in sufficient amounts to cause glutathione depletion.

However pennyroyal, which contains pulegone, is metabolised in the liver into menthofuran, a highly reactive metabolite which irreversibly binds to the cells of the liver in which the metabolism takes place, destroying the liver. (33)

A similar process of biotransformation is responsible for the hepatotoxicity of methyl chavicol, eugenol and cinnamaldehyde which may also reduce the level of glutathoine in the liver. (34)

The liver is the most important organ for metabolising chemicals which have found their way into the body. In general, the aim of such 'detoxification' reactions is to make the chemical less lipid and more water soluble, allowing its excretion into the watery environment of the urine much easier.

The types of chemical reactions involving the metabolism of drugs and other compounds are classified as:

- oxidations
- reductions
- hydrolyses
- conjugations.

Most of these reactions are carried out by microsomal enzymes in the liver.

Often a lipid soluble substance is changed into one that is water soluble so that it is more easily excreted. This reaction is known as a 'Phase I' reaction and usually involves oxidation. Compounds such as aldehydes and alcohols are oxidised by nonmicrosomal enzymes. Esters are typically metabolised by hydrolysis.

If the products of biotransformation are still pharmacologically active, they often undergo a second reaction which will render them inactive. Essential oil constituents containing a hydroxyl group (-OH) may undergo this second reaction and end up being eliminated from the body as glucuronides. This process is known as a conjugated reaction or a 'Phase II' reaction . The conjugates that are formed are excreted in the urine if the molecular weight of the essential oil constituent is 300 or less. (The maximum molecular weight of essential oil constituents is about 225).

Excretion

As soon as an essential oil enters the body, it begins to be excreted. Excretion occurs at the kidneys, via the bile and bowel and to a variable extent through the sweat glands and other body secretions.

The kidney is usually the most important organ of excretion for many substances. However the essential oils, being extremely volatile, are also excreted by being exhaled through the respiratory system.

The kidneys are the main organ of excretion and any essential oil in the blood stream will have

to be filtered by them. On this basis one would expect the smaller molecules such as aldehydes and alcohols to be filtered out more rapidly than the larger terpene molecules.

Many of the lipid-soluble molecules are known to diffuse passively back through the tubule walls of the kidneys into the bloodstream. Therefore the liver would usually attempt to render fat-soluble substances such as terpenes, terpenoid ketones and ethers into more water-soluble components in readiness for excretion.

Conclusion

It is perhaps understandable that very little work has been done on the essential oils as they are made up of so many individual constituents that would make a detailed pharmacokinetic study impossible. However, we need to be able to relate the current knowledge to our practice as aromatherapists, so that we can accurately determine the length of time that oils remain active after application, in what dosage and how often the oils should be applied.

Chapter 11

Essential Oil Safety

It is important to point out that because the essential oils are natural substances it does not automatically guarantee that they are safe. A number of hazards do exist, but users of essential oils are most likely to do harm through ignorance of these hazards.

The purpose of this chapter is to ensure that the user of essential oils is aware of these hazards so that aromatherapy is practised with the absolute minimum of risk to the client.

Introduction

The recent interest towards natural health therapies including aromatherapy and the realisation that one's wellbeing is a personal responsibility, has led to a growth in over-the-counter sales of natural remedies such as essential oils.

This growing interest in aromatherapy has raised a number of important issues regarding the efficacy and safety of the essential oils. The safety of essential oils is a concern to all aromatherapists and other individuals who use them and raises several issues of fundamental importance to the practice of aromatherapy such as:

- quality
- packaging and labelling
- chemical composition
- essential oil hazards.

Quality

The use of the highest quality essential oils is of the utmost importance in ensuring that aromatherapy is practised safely.

Most of the essential oils produced are used by the fragrance or flavouring industries. The aromatherapy sector accounts for only 5% of the world's total consumption of essential oils. It is therefore important that essential oils that are used in aromatherapy meet standards set by the aromatherapy industry and not other industries using the essential oils.

The following issues need to be considered when determining the quality of an essential oil:

- contamination and adulteration
- degradation.

Contamination and adulteration

Contaminants may include pesticides; adulterants may include synthetic constituents similar to those normally found in essential oils. Contamination and adulteration may potentiate toxicity of an otherwise safe essential oil. It is believed that some of the reported allergic reactions to essential oils have been due to the pesticide or herbicide residue and not the essential oil (1). However, it is interesting that the permissible levels of biocides in foods are much higher than for essential oils (2). Biocides, which by definition are toxic, are not welcome in either food or essential oils, even in trace amounts.

Adulteration is usually easily detected by performing a series of tests. The best advice in purchasing essential oils is to buy from reputable suppliers who carry out their own quality control testing.

Degradation

Chemical degradation is the process by which the quality of the essential oil is reduced over time. This usually occurs with essential oil because of prolonged storage, or poor storage conditions. The main factors responsible for essential oil degradation are:

- oxygen
- heat
- light.

The effect of oxygen on essential oils is called oxidation and tends to occur in essential oils rich in monoterpenes such as citrus and pine oils. Limonene and pinene, two relatively major constituents of citrus and pine oils are both reactive terpenes. Oxidation is accelerated by both heat and light.

Not only do many essential oils lose their therapeutic properties (3) but also the chemical changes that occur may make the essential oil more hazardous. An example is oxidised pine oil which is more likely than fresh pine oil to cause dermal sensitisation (4).

To avoid degradation of essential oils:

- Ensure that oils are not stored in clear glass bottles.

- Small amounts of essential oils remaining in large bottles should be transferred to smaller bottles to reduce the risk of oxidation.

Packaging and labelling

As most essential oils are sold undiluted, it is important that they carry the appropriate warnings and instructions for use. These instruction should include:

- Keep out of reach of children.
- Skin irritation may arise from contact with undiluted essential oils.
- For external purposes only.

An essential oil scheduled as a poison is required by Australian law to carry a label giving appropriate first aid advice if poisoning occurs. This advice is as follows:

If poisoning occurs get to a doctor or hospital quickly. If swallowed do not induce vomiting. Give a glass of water.

At the time of writing the following essential oils or constituents are scheduled as poisons (5):

- camphor oil, except:
  (a) in preparations containing 10% or less of camphor
  (b) when enclosed in an inhaler device which prevents ingestion of its contents
- cineole, except in preparations or oils containing 25% or less of cineole
- eucalyptus oil, except in preparations containing 25% or less of eucalyptus oil
- melaleuca oil (tea tree oil) except in preparations containing 25% or less of melaleuca oil
- methyl salicylate in liquid preparations containing 25% or more of methyl salicylate
- sassafras oil or safrole, except:
  (a) for internal use (sic); or
  (b) in preparations containing 1% or less of safrole.

This means that these essential oils may be sold only in a ribbed-poison bottle with a child proof lid.

While there may be specific risks associated with the above essential oils, any move to schedule all essential oils as poisons is not necessary considering that the majority of essential oils are extremely safe to use.

However I believe that the use of integral dropper-dispensers is very important in limiting the quantity of essential oil that a child could ingest accidentally. Essential oils in open neck bottles probably represent the greatest risk of accidental ingestion in aromatherapy today.

The following information on a label would also be very useful from a safety point of view:

- the botanical name of the originating plant
- the concentration of the essential oil, eg 'undiluted' or the percentage the product is diluted
- a use-by date, or other indication of useful lifespan
- the part of the plant the oil came from, if relevant, eg cinnamon bark or leaf.

Chemical composition

A typical essential oil may have 100 or more different essential oil constituents, which in combination give the essential oil its unique odour, therapeutic properties and in some cases, its toxicity.

The chemical composition varies not only from one oil to another obtained from different plants, but also between oils obtained from the same botanical species. These variations may be due to factors such as geographical location, elevation, part of the plant used, time of harvesting, weather conditions and soil types and when they occur are referred to as chemotypes.

For example thyme oil is often classified as a dermal irritant because of the high percentage of thymol and carvacrol constituents found in the oil. However another thyme oil chemotype exists which is rich in the constituent linalool and does not carry the same dermal irritant risks associated with the thymol/carvacrol chemotype.

Basil oil is another example in which more than one chemotype exists. The basil chemotype methyl chavicol is considered not only a dermal irritant but also a potential carcinogen. Basil chemotype linalool is safer to use in aromatherapy.

One cannot assume that if a particular constituent is found to be hazardous that it means that the essential oil is hazardous. It has been observed that many pure constituents particularly aldehydes isolated from a natural source, proved to be strong sensitisers. The essential oils from which they were isolated did not induce sensitisation even when the specific aldehydes were present in concentrations as high as 85%.

For example lemongrass contains around 85% citral, the irritant effect of which can be quenched by making a 50% blend with an essential oil containing dextro-limonene. Two citrus oils containing around 90% d-limonene are sweet orange and grapefruit. (6)

This phenomenon is recognised as the quenching effect. Quenching seems to be a consistent behaviour of natural essential oils.

Essential oils with ketone constituents

As previously discussed ketones are among the most common toxic constituents. However to assume that all essential oils containing ketones are toxic is simply not correct. Essential oils with non toxic ketone constituents are jasmine (jasmone) and fennel (fenchone).

The most common toxic ketone is thujone. This ketone is found in high concentrations in oils such as mugwort, sage, thuja, wormwood and tansy. The essential oil of sage varies distinctly in its chemical composition depending on its geographic origin.

Most sage oil comes from the Balkans and is commonly known as Dalmatian sage. The thujone content of this oil can vary from 35-60%. This alone would certainly render sage toxic. This contradicts most of the research on and experience with this oil which clearly does not indicate the toxicity one would expect from such a thujone content.

Independent studies have shown that the LD_{50} of sage is much lower than the toxicity of an equivalent amount of thujone by itself (7). The reason for this behaviour is thought to be the different isomers of thujone that exist, not all of which are known to be hazardous. As a result it can be concluded that the traditional use of sage should not be considered hazardous. However, it would be wise to exercise extra care when using sage. It should be avoided during pregnancy.

Another toxic ketone is pulegone. It is found (up to 85%) in pennyroyal oil. Essential oil of pennyroyal is considered toxic and should not be used.

Pinocamphone is the primary constituent found in hyssop. Hyssop, according to LD_{50} values, is distinctly more toxic than sage. Hyssop should always be used carefully in low doses and should not be used continuously for more than four weeks.

Essential oil	Toxic ketone	Oral LD_{50} (g/kg)
Pennyroyal	pulegone	0.4
Mugwort	thujone	0.37
Sage	thujone	2.6
Tansy	thujone	1.15
Thuja	thujone	0.83
Wormwood	thujone	0.96
Hyssop	pinocamphone	1.4

Toxicity of essential oils with ketone constituents (8)

Essential oils with phenol constituents

Phenols are considered valuable essential oils in aromatherapy. However, 50% of essential oils containing phenols are classified as irritants, 30% are classified toxic and approximately 18% are considered carcinogenic (9).

Thyme, oregano and savory are very useful essential oils in aromatherapy because of their antimicrobial activity. However they are dermal and mucous membrane irritants.

There are a number of essential oils, such as calamus, camphor and sassafras, known to be carcinogenic, and which contain phenolic compounds such as safrole and asarone.

Essential oil	Phenol	Comment	LD$_{50}$ (g/kg)
Savory (summer)	carvacrol/ thymol	caution	1.37
Savory (winter)	carvacrol/ thymol	caution	1.37
Oregano	carvacrol	caution	1.85
Thyme	carvacrol/ thymol	skin hazard	4.70
Clove Bud	eugenol	skin hazard	1.37
Basil (Comoros Is.)	methyl chavicol	skin hazard	1.40
Calamus	asarone	carcinogenic	0.84
Sassafras	safrole	carcinogenic	1.90
Camphor (brown)	safrole	carcinogenic	-
Camphor (yellow)	safrole	carcinogenic	-
Parsley Seed	apiol	abortifacient	-
Cassia	cinnamic aldehyde	skin irritant	2.80
Cinnamon	cinnamic aldehyde	skin irritant	3.40

Toxicity of essential oils with phenol constituents (10)

Essential oil hazards

The undesirable side effects of essential oils are organised into the following categories:

• toxicity

• skin reactions

• carcinogenesis

• neurotoxicity

• hepatotoxicity

• hazards during pregnancy.

Toxicity

Toxicity is what we commonly call poisoning, and at a certain level may become fatal. In aromatherapy, the degree of toxicity depends to a certain extent on the method of application. Therefore toxicity is often classified as either:

• oral toxicity, or

• dermal toxicity.

Oral toxicity is the degree of toxicity of a substance when it is ingested by swallowing.

Dermal toxicity is the degree of toxicity of a substance when it is absorbed through the skin. Both types of toxicity are determined by the lethal dose, which is the amount necessary to kill the organism.

The greatest hazard is associated with oral administration. The majority of incidents involving toxicity result from oral dosing. Toxicity is dose-dependent. The risk of injury increases when larger doses of essential oils are used.

There are two categories of toxicity:

• acute toxicity, and

• chronic toxicity.

Acute toxicity occurs with short-term use of a toxic essential oil, usually involving a single dose and may result in death. When the amount administered is less than a lethal dose, damage may occur to the liver and/or the kidneys.

Chronic toxicity describes the result of the long-term use of a toxic essential oil. For an example of chronic toxicity see Chapter 12, Eucalyptus leaf oils, Precautions.

The result of chronic toxicity is usually organ tissue damage, most commonly degenerative changes in the liver and kidneys. Death may eventually result, but the problem here is one of slow tissue damage, rather than fatality. Chronic toxicity usually involves oral administration and it would be reasonable to assume the same applies to dermal administration.

A common method of establishing a measure of toxicity is the LD$_{50}$ experiment. LD$_{50}$ is the dose of a specific substance that has been lethal for 50% in a group of test animals. This is usually not given as an absolute value but in grams of toxin per kilogram body weight. For example:

$$LD_{50} = 1 \ [g/kg]$$

means that 1 gram of essential oil per kilogram of body weight induces death in 50% of the test animals. Using this value as a guide to toxicity in humans, it would mean, assuming the body weight to be 70 kg, that

$$1[g/kg] \times 70 \ [kg] = 70 \ [g]$$

70 grams of essential oil would be a lethal dose in humans. LD$_{50}$ values generally refer to oral toxicity. LD$_{50}$ values are commonly accepted in establishing toxicity of a given substance in humans.

Essential oil	LD$_{50}$ g/kg	Actual lethal dose for 70kg person	Comment
Boldo	0.13	9.1g	toxic
Hyssop	1.40	98.0g	caution
Sage	2.52	176.0g	safe
Chamomile	8.56	600.0g	safe

LD$_{50}$ values and corresponding lethal doses (11)

Apart from the ethical issues involving animal testing to determine the LD$_{50}$ value, I am concerned about the assumption that human toxicity levels are similar to rodent toxicity levels for essential oils.

Clearly the toxicity of the same substance in animals and humans can be quite different. The following table indicates the gross errors that are often assumed in using animal toxicity data to determine lethal doses for humans (12).

Essential oil	Type of toxicity	Animal toxicity (g/kg)	Human toxicity (g/kg)
Eucalyptus	acute oral	2.5	0.4-0.8
Wintergreen	acute oral	1.2	0.23-0.37
Camphor	acute oral	0.5-15	0.005-0.5
Pennyroyal	acute oral	0.4	0.4

The RIFM (The Research Institute of Fragrance Materials) often conducts acute dermal toxicity studies on rabbits. It has been shown that human skin and rabbit skin do not absorb the same essential oils at the same rate. According to Sharon Hotchkiss, lecturer in biochemical toxicology at St Mary's Hospital Medical School, London, absorption is usually higher through rat or rabbit skin (13). Therefore existing information regarding dermal toxicity probably gives no useful indication of the toxicity of dermally applied essential oils for human skin.

Cases of poisoning

There are many recorded cases of poisoning from essential oils and all arose from oral ingestion. In every case the amount taken was much higher than normal therapeutic amounts. The following oils have frequently appeared in cases of poisoning (14):

camphor
cinnamon
citronella
clove
eucalyptus
hyssop
nutmeg
parsley
pennyroyal
sage
thuja
sassafras
wintergreen

wormwood
wormseed.

This does not mean that oils not appearing here are necessarily safe. It is very likely that any essential oil, ingested in sufficient quantities, may cause serious problems.

Skin reactions

The most common method of applying the essential oils in aromatherapy is massage. It is therefore not surprising that the most common hazard in aromatherapy is skin reactions. Skin reactions that often occur are classified as:

- irritation
- sensitisation
- phototoxicity
- idiosyncratic.

Compared with toxicity, skin reactions may vary considerably from one individual to another, and are therefore very difficult to predict.

Irritation

Irritation is a reaction to a substance by an organism resulting in local inflammation, affecting the skin or mucous membranes. Of all the hazards, acute irritation is the least harmful. Like toxicity, irritation is dose-dependent. Skin irritation is one of the most difficult hazards to effectively analyse and classify. Many animal tests, which are of little relevance, are performed. This is due to the fact that the results of the tests show discrepancies between human and animal testing.

The tests are conducted by the IFRA (International Fragrance Research Association), which also makes recommendations for the safe use of essential oils. The tests are normally conducted on 25 volunteers. Even though this gives us reliable projections for only 89% of the population it is considered to be an adequate representation of the population. Preparations of fragrant materials are diluted in a petroleum jelly at percentages calculated at ten times greater than the maximum concentration used in perfumes.

Testing for primary irritation is conducted by applying the diluted fragrance material on a patch of skin (usually the forearm or back) under occlusion with cotton gauze for 24-48 hours, after which the patch is removed and the skin examined for indications of a reaction.

Even though IFRA's standards have become international, variations among population groups do occur and recent research by Japanese universities has shown that Asian skins tend to be more sensitive to irritant substances than the skins of caucasians (15).

A Japanese study by the Department of Dermatology of Toho University Medical School in 1979 involving approximately 200 human volunteers over an eight year period using 270,000 close patch tests has shown that the following factors affect the skin's sensitivity to irritation (16):

Change in season
Most sensitivities occurred among the test volunteers in October when the season was changing from summer to autumn and in March when the season was changing from winter to spring.

Sex
Men are 2.5 times more sensitive than women.

Illness and stress-related situations
Individuals experiencing stress related problems or illness experienced an increase in the skin's sensitivity; the same individuals were less sensitive when not ill or less stressed.

Many aromatherapists associated the irritation of an essential oil to the skin or the mucous membrane with the terpenes, thus suggesting that deterpenated oils were considered safe. Marguerite Maury wrote (17):

'When we tried to administer by the digestive tract we found we had to employ essences which had been deterpenated owing to the sensitivity of the mucous membranes to pure essences and essential oil.'

Robert Tisserand concluded that essential oils with the highest terpene content such as lemon, grapefruit and orange are in fact amongst the least irritating oils (18).

It has become clear from many studies that the most irritating essential oils are those with a percentage of phenols as can be seen from the table following:

Essential oil	Irritant constituent
Clove	Eugenol
Oregano	Carvacrol/thymol
Thyme	Carvacrol/thymol
Savoury	Carvacrol/thymol
Cinnamon bark	Cinnamic aldehyde
Cassia	Cinnamic aldehyde

Dermal sensitisation

Dermal sensitisation reactions are induced when applying an essential oil to the skin. Even diluted essential oils can cause sensitisation reactions, and repeated applications increase the chances of such a reaction from a sensitising oil. The skin normally reacts in the form of a rash, blotchy redness, often accompanied by irritation or slight blistering. Chronic contact with a sensitising substance can lead to a form of dermatitis, known as contact dermatitis.

There are five oils likely to cause sensitisation reactions in normal individuals which should not be used in aromatherapy (19):

Essential Oil	Number of people who reacted out of 25 tested	Dilution of oil used
Costus	25/25	4%
Elecampane	23/25	4%
Cinnamon bark	18/25	8%
Fennel (Bitter)	3/25	4%
Cassia	2/25	4%

Sensitisation is an allergic reaction to a substance by an organism that involves the interaction of its immune system with a substance. Substances that are capable of inducing an immune response from an organism are called antigens. The antigens interact with the lymphocytes causing the formation of antibodies that will in turn react with the antigen rendering it harmless. When an antigen induces an immune response at first exposure, the organism will experience altered body reactivity to subsequent exposure to the same or similar antigens. This may cause exaggerated reactions like sneezing and itching. This is defined as the allergic reaction. (20)

Recent research on sensitisation has found that sensitisation is the response of the immune system and not an antigen antibody reaction. Skin sensitisation is a delayed type humoral immune response mediated by the T-cells. The incomplete allergen bonds with a protein in the skin. Cells in the stratum germinativum of the skin interact with this allergen, migrate to the thymus gland and prime the other initiated thymus T-cells. When the sensitised T-cells leaving the thymus gland come into contact with the allergen, they liberate lymphokines, attracting other leucocytes to the area and this process raises the temperature in an attempt to be rid of the material, thus producing the inflammation (21).

The allergen that causes allergic reactions in some essential oils is usually not known, with the exception of some substances such as cinnamic aldehyde found in cinnamon oil and cassia oil. If an essential oil causes an allergic reaction, its use should be discontinued immediately. Generally no further consequences may be expected. The Research Institute of Fragrance Materials has halted all animal testing for skin sensitising as the results were unsatisfactory for predicting human susceptibility.

Photosensitisation

Photosensitisation is a skin reaction that occurs in the presence of ultra violet light. Certain constituents of essential oils are capable of absorbing energy from ultraviolet light much more effectively than the skin. Essential oils listed as photosensitisers are hazardous only in this context. To simply apply these oils to the skin diluted or undiluted will not in itself produce a photosensitisation, which can only be achieved if the skin is covered in a photosensitising oil, and then exposed to the sun or any other source of ultraviolet light.

Citrus oils extracted by direct expression without distillation are the major group of essential oils to be phototoxic. Bergamot and other expressed citrus oils contain small quantities of bergaptene or 5 methoxypsoralen also known as 5-MOP. This furocoumarin has been identified as the phototoxic constituent. The table below indicates the phototoxic potential of citrus oils.

As can be seen from the table, the phototoxic potential of citrus oils is neutralised when the furocoumarin content is reduced to 0.0075% and below. According to these results we can make the following conclusions:

Phototoxic oils include: Bergamot, cold pressed lime, cold pressed bitter orange, angelica.

The following oils may be mildly phototoxic: Cold pressed grapefruit, cold pressed or distilled lemon, distilled lime, cold pressed sweet orange, cold pressed tangerine.

It is suggested that skin which has had any phototoxic essential oil applied to it should not be exposed to sunlight or UV lamps for at least 12 hours (22).

Idiosyncratic sensitisation

Idiosyncratic sensitisation is an allergic reaction to a substance that is generally not known to be an allergen. Like a food allergy it is a phenomenon which can appear and disappear again with no apparent logic. The allergic reaction may be induced by dermal application, inhalation, or any other means. As with other types of sensitisation the substances responsible can produce a severe reaction even in quite low dilutions, especially if the subject is already sensitised.

Carcinogenesis

This is defined as the stimulation of the formation and growth of cancerous cells in the body by a particular substance. It is well known that certain chemicals, and even physical or emotional irritation can lead to the onset of cancer.

Tests have shown that carcinogens require repeated application, usually for several weeks or months, before any cancerous growth can be detected. Studies on the carcinogenesis of essential oils include calamus oil and all oils containing significant amounts of safrole, which is found in sassafras and the yellow and brown fractions of camphor.

Expressed citrus oil	Furocoumarin average content	Phototoxicity at 100%	Level when not phototoxic
bergamot	0.44%	severe	1-2%
lime	0.25%	strong	2-3.5%
bitter orange	0.072%	moderate	3.5-7%
lemon	0.0032%	weak	5-10%
grapefruit	0.0012%	weak	10-20%
sweet orange	0.00005%	mild	no limit
tangerine	0.00005%	mild	no limit
mandarin	trace	mild	no limit

Phototoxic potential of citrus oils (23)

Essential oil	Constituent	Concentration
Cade	benzo (a) pyrene	8 p.p.m
Sassafras	safrole	90%
Basil (methyl chavicol)	methyl chavicol	87%
Tarragon (French)	methyl chavicol	87%
Tarragon (Russian)	methyl chavicol and methyleugenol	46%
Camphor (yellow)	safrole	20%
Camphor (brown)	safrole	80%
Calamus (Indian)	beta-asorone	80%

Essential oils to be avoided in aromatherapy, due to their carcinogenic properties (25)

Miller reported on the possible carcinogenic compounds found in essential oils (24). It was found that the alkenylbenzene compounds found in some essential oils are responsible for the carcinogenic effect. The constituents concerned were methyl chavicol, found in basil; safrole, found in sassafras and brown and yellow camphor; and asorone, found in calamus. Two points need to be emphasised:

- Most of the studies required daily application of high concentrations over many months to induce tumour growth.
- Camphor and sassafras have already been banned from human consumption.

In light of this I do not believe basil should be considered an essential oil 'not to use'. I do think it is imperative that the therapist select the basil with the lowest methyl chavicol content and the highest linalool content.

It is also worth noting that some essential oils such as garlic, Virginian cedarwood and thyme have been shown to have anti-carcinogenic actions in low dilutions (26).

Massage and cancer

There is a common belief that massage will spread cancer cells from one part of the body to another, by stimulating lymph flow. However, there is no clinical evidence that massage can spread cancer or that it can't.

It would be reasonable to assume that gentle massage would stimulate the lymph flow no more than gentle exercise or normal body movement. However the following precautions should be observed before massaging a client with cancer:

- Avoid deep massage of any kind, over or near the lymph glands
- Avoid areas of the body which have been treated with radiation therapy, as the skin is usually very fragile.
- Massage should also be avoided over areas of skin cancer.

Any health professional who decides to use massage should have a very good understanding of both massage and cancer.

Neurotoxicity

A neurotoxic substance is one which has a toxic or destructive effect on nervous tissue. It is highly unlikely that essential oils may cause physical damage to nerve tissue, except in cases of acute oral toxicity. Because many essential oil constituents are lipid-soluble, they may be readily absorbed into the CNS through the blood-brain barrier.

The known neurotoxic effects of essential oils on the central nervous system are:

- convulsant effects
- psychotropic effects.

Convulsant effects

A convulsant is an agent which produces a convulsion. The following essential oils and their constituents have potential convulsant effects (27):

Constituent	Essential oils
fenchone	fennel
pinocamphone	hyssop
camphor	camphor, spike lavender, rosemary, common sage
thujone	common sage, tansy, thuja, wormwood

This means that those suspected of being vulnerable to seizures, such as people who suffer from epilepsy, anyone with strong family history of epilepsy, and anyone with a fever should not use the above oils. It needs to be noted that many of the above essential oils are not used in aromatherapy because of their toxicity.

The essential oil constituents believed to be responsible for the convulsant effects are ketones. Some consider that all ketones are highly stimulating to the CNS, and therefore are a risk to those prone to epilepsy. I believe that there is no reason to assume that all other ketones found in essential oils present any danger to people prone to epilepsy.

Psychotropic effects

A psychotropic substance is one which affects the brain in such a way that it alters mood or behaviour. The following have been reported as having psychotropic effects:

- nutmeg
- thujone.

Some of the psychotropic effects reported after having used the above include hallucinogenic effects. These substances may also be classified as hallucinogens which are described as (28):

'Chemicals which, in non-toxic doses, produce changes in perception, in thought, and in mood, but which seldom produce mental confusion, memory loss, or disorientation for person, place and time.'

'Absinthe' which contained wormwood, whose neuroactive constituent is thujone, was a popular drink of the nineteenth century. Oscar Wilde explicitly describes the effects of absinthe (29):

'After the first glass you see things as you wish they were. After the second, you see things as they are not. Finally you see things as they really are, and that is the most horrible thing in the world.'

Many artists, writers, actors and sculptors, including Maupassant, Toulouse-Lautrec, Degas, Gauguin, Van Gogh, Manet, Baudelaire and Verlaine, drank it.

Some paintings of the period show absinthe drinkers, mostly depicted with the glazed expression that absinthe elicited. In small amounts it was said to stimulate the mind and the sexual appetite, however in excessive amounts it produced terrifying hallucinations and a condition referred to as 'absinthism'. Many addicts showed signs of mental derangement, and most died young, or like Van Gogh, committed suicide.

The hazards of absinthe did not go unnoticed, and in 1915 France finally banned absinthe. The mode of action of thujone has not been confirmed. It has been suggested that thujone and delta-9-tetrahydrocannabinol, the most active constituent found in cannabis, interact with the same receptor in the CNS, and so have similar psychotropic effects. (30)

The psychotropic effects often associated with nutmeg are believed to be due to the myristicin and elemicin found in the nutmeg (31). It is possible that myristicin and elemicin are metabolised to TMA (3,4,5-trimethoxyamphetamine) or MMDA (3-methoxy-4,5-methylenedioxyamphetamine), both of which are hallucinogenic substances. (32) However, closer investigation has revealed the following (33):

Component	Psychotropic effect
whole nutmeg	highly active
whole nutmeg less the essential oil	no activity
nutmeg oil	weakly active
myristicin on its own	no activity

It appears that the psychotropic properties are due not only to the myristicin and elemicin but to other constituents found in the nutmeg.

While ground nutmeg is moderately to strongly psychotropic when taken in high doses, the effect of the essential oil is very weak, and it appears that non-oral doses will not have any effect at all.

Hepatotoxicity

The liver has a wider variety of functions than any other organ in the body. Apart from its major roles of carbohydrate and lipid metabolism, protein synthesis and secretion of bile, it is responsible for the detoxification of the blood.

Some essential oil constituents have been shown to cause liver damage. While it is unlikely that any of the essential oils could be absorbed in sufficient quantities through dermal application to damage the liver, oral administration may be considered hazardous. The following table lists the essential oils and their corresponding constituents which are potentially hepatotoxic.

Constituent	Essential oil
trans-anethole	aniseed, fennel
cinnamaldehyde	cassia, cinnamon bark
methyl chavicol	basil (methyl chavicol), tarragon
eugenol	West Indian bay, cinnamon leaf, clove
pulegone	buchu, pennyroyal
safrole	camphor (brown and yellow), sassafras

Hazards during pregnancy

There is often a concern that some essential oils may not be safe to use during pregnancy and some aromatherapists even suggest that no essential oil should be used during pregnancy (34). In my opinion this is being over cautious, as aromatherapy can be immensely beneficial in maintaining the general health of the expectant mother and in minimising the various discomforts of pregnancy.

The main concerns during pregnancy in using some essential oils are that they:

- may have a hormone like activity, disturbing the normal, finely tuned balance of hormones
- may cause injury to, or malformation of, the foetus
- may cause abortion.

Hormone properties

The two most important female hormones are oestradiol, which is an oestrogen, and progesterone, which is a progestogen. Oestradiol controls the development and maintenance of the female sexual organs and gives a woman her essentially feminine shape and physiology. Progesterone prepares the uterine lining for pregnancy each month.

Some essential oil constituents have hormone-like behaviour because their structure is similar to the hormones, so they interact with the same receptors that identify hormones.

Oestrogenic activity has been found in essential oils of aniseed and sweet fennel. Anethole which is a methyl ether of oestradiol is responsible for the oestrogenic activity of these oils. There are no essential oils which have progesterone-like activity, nor are there any oils used in aromatherapy which have androgen-like activity.

The essential oils with oestrogenic activities influence the menstrual cycle, lactation and secondary sexual characteristics.

Since there is no conclusive data available on the effects of oestrogenic oils on the pregnancy it would be advisable to be cautious and not use anethole-rich essential oils such as fennel and aniseed during pregnancy.

Injury to the foetus

There are many problems in studying the effect of essential oils during pregnancy. Results of animal studies often do not correlate well with the results of human studies unlike in other fields of research. Associating to humans the results of animal toxicity studies is very difficult. For example, the effects of the sedative thalidomide on human foetuses is still not understood.

There are very few studies on the distribution and fate of drugs within the human embryo, because it is almost impossible to design safe clinical experiments. It is often assumed that drug or essential oil concentrations in the embryo would reach similar levels to that in the mother's serum. This may be inaccurate and the truth is that it is not known whether essential oils circulating in the mother's blood stream reach the developing child.

However it can be assumed that if essential oil molecules can cross the blood-brain barrier into the central nervous system they are likely to reach the foetus.

Teratogenesis is the effect a substance or an agent has which causes developmental malformation in a foetus. There is no evidence that essential oils possess any potential hazards of teratogenesis.

It would however be strongly recommended during pregnancy, to avoid the use of any essential oil which is scheduled as: 'not to be used at all' or 'not to be used on the skin at all' on page 136 of this chapter.

Abortifacient oils

There is no clear evidence that essential oils are abortifacients. Most of the essential oils that have traditionally been labelled as abortifacients are potentially toxic and therefore are not used in aromatherapy.

All the so-called 'abortifacient' oils are known to have a strong emmenagogue action. However, not all emmenagogues will induce abortion, and not all emmenagogue oils are toxic.

Many essential oils such as clary sage, cedarwood, cypress, sweet marjoram, peppermint and rose are classified as contraindicated during pregnancy, however they are not abortifacients. It has been suggested that these essential oils present no danger in pregnancy as long as they are not used orally (35). However it would be prudent to avoid using these essential oils as there is anecdotal evidence which indicates that they may be unsafe to use during pregnancy.

The following is a summary of essential oils known as abortifacients:

Mugwort Because of its specific action on the uterus, it has the reputation of being abortive, at least for high doses over a period of time. Should not be used in aromatherapy.

Parsley seed Preparations made from parsley seed oil have been used to induce abortion for many years (36). It appears that the constituent apiol is responsible and that any other apiol-rich essential oil should also be avoided during pregnancy.

Pennyroyal Pennyroyal, which has been marketed as an insect repellent, has been known to induce abortions for at least 2,000 years. There have been many documented cases where pennyroyal has been intentionally ingested or applied to the skin to induce abortion. In all cases, toxicity and poisoning occurred. In some of the reported cases death occurred due to the high dosages of essential oil taken. Should not be used in aromatherapy.

Rue Rue oil is reported to cause abortion in pregnant guinea pigs and pregnant women. Should not be used in aromatherapy.

Sage An essential oil which should not be used because of its high thujone content is sage *(Salvia officinalis)*.

Sassafras It has the property of stimulating the uterus, and this stimulation could be strong enough to provoke abortion.

Savin It should never be used in pregnancy as it produces abortion. Should not be used in aromatherapy.

Thuja The twigs may produce abortion, like those of savin, by reflex action on the uterus from severe gastro-intestinal irritation. Should not be used in aromatherapy.

Tansy Tansy *(Tanacetum vulgare)* contains 66-80% thujone. In large doses, tansy is extremely irritant to mucous membranes and also causes seizures. Other toxic effects include cramps, irregular heart beat, hepatitis and uterine bleeding. Tansy's thujone content has given it a use as a vermifuge, emmenagogue and abortifacient. Should not be used in aromatherapy.

Wormwood Wormwood *(Artemisia absinthium)*, often referred to as 'absinthe', contains up to 70% thujone. Its toxic effects are similar to tansy's. Should not be used in aromatherapy.

The following table summarises which essential oils to avoid during pregnancy, either because they are toxic and will possibly harm the mother and foetus, or because they may involve some risk of miscarriage.

Due to abortifacient and toxic effects:	pennyroyal, rue, savin, mugwort, sage, tansy, thuja, wormwood.
Due to toxicity:	boldo, mustard, horseradish, wormseed.
Due to oestrogen stimulant activity:	aniseed, fennel, basil.
Moderately toxic oils:	clove, hyssop, savory, thyme, wintergreen.
Due to emmenagogue properties:	cedarwood, clary sage, jasmine, juniper, marjoram, myrrh, peppermint, rose, rosemary.

General rules

1. Do not take essential oils internally.

2. Essential oils should not be used undiluted on the skin. The only exception to this rule is an emergency measure when a tiny amount of lavender or tea tree essential oil could be used on a sting, small burn or tiny wound.

3. Essential oils should not be used directly on the eyes to treat eye conditions. If someone accidently gets any essential oil or massage oil in the eye or eye area, wash thoroughly with cold clean water for 5 minutes. If the stinging has not subsided after 15 minutes seek medical attention.

4. Essential oils should always be used in the correct dosages. If used in excess, they can often lead to skin irritations, headaches, nausea, and a feeling of unease.

5. Asthma often responds well to aromatherapy. However, inhaling the steam from a basin of hot water with essential oils, is contraindicated as it could have the reverse effect and make breathing more difficult.

6. The following safety precautions must be observed when treating children:

a) Rules 1 through to 3 apply, and observe all toxic and possibly hazardous oils mentioned in the previous section.

b) When blending an oil for massage or for a bath, use less oil. Instead of the standard 3% dilution use between 1% and 2% dilution.

c) If using a steam inhalation with a bowl of hot water, never leave the child unsupervised.

d) Give inhalation for only a few seconds to 1 minute at the most. If the child tolerates this, inhalations may be increased to 2 minutes.

Dosage and dilutions

Most essential oils destined for therapeutic use are sold in bottles which dispense the oils by the drop. The size of the drop dispensed by these bottles hardly varies at all. For the purpose of this manual we will assume that the standard drop is equal to one twentieth of a millilitre.

1ml = 20 drops

For aromatherapy massage treatments essential oils are generally diluted in a base of vegetable oil. The recommended dilutions are always between 1% and 5%. I usually recommend a dilution of 3% for most essential oils.

A simple way to calculate how much essential oil to add to a base oil is to measure the amount of base oil in millilitres and then add half that number of drops of essential oils.

For example: to a 50 ml bottle of base oil, add 25 drops of essential oil - this gives a 2.5% dilution.

- For babies (0 to 12 months) use 1 drop of lavender, Roman/German chamomile, neroli, dill or mandarin to 10 ml of carrier oil. This is equivalent to 0.5% dilution.

- For infants (1-5 years) use 2-3 drops of the safe essential oils, ie. those that are non-toxic and non-irritant to 10 ml of carrier oil.

- For children (6 to 12 years) use half the recommended dosage for adults.

The frequency of the treatment is perhaps of more concern than the dosage. Much depends on the extent of the skin area covered, and how efficiently the essential oils are absorbed, since this does vary from one individual to another. For a whole body massage, twice a week is sufficient for a regular treatment. For facial treatments, or anything involving only a small part of the skin tissue, daily application is regarded as quite safe.

It is important to remember that the reaction of different individuals to essential oils when applied to the body varies enormously, and some hypersensitive individuals will often be allergic to even the smallest amounts. This does not make the essential oil hazardous. If there is a possible sensitivity, start with a very low concentration and gradually increase to the recommended 2-3%.

Summary of contraindications

Toxic essential oils which should not be used at all

The following list is of essential oils considered the most hazardous of all essential oils, having very high oral and dermal toxicity.

> Almond (bitter), boldo leaf, buchu, camphor, sassafras, calamus, horseradish, mugwort, mustard, European and North American pennyroyal, rue, savin, savory, southernwood, tansy, thuja, wintergreen, wormseed, wormwood.

Essential oils which should not be used on the skin at all

The following list is of essential oils which are the most hazardous when applied to the skin. The list takes into account dermal toxicity, skin sensitisation and skin irritation.

> Ajowan, cinnamon bark, cassia, clove leaf, clove stem, clove bud, costus, elecampane, fennel (bitter), oregano, pine (dwarf).

Note that the *toxic* oils listed above should also be avoided dermally.

Essential oils which should be used on the skin with caution

These oils may irritate the skin when used in baths or massage. Do not use at all on anyone who is known to have sensitive skin, or who is susceptible to reactions.

> Basil (all varieties), cinnamon leaf, fennel (sweet), fir needle (Siberian), lemongrass, lemon, lemon verbena, melissa, orange, peppermint, red and wild thyme.

Essential oils which should not be used during pregnancy

The following oils should not be used during pregnancy, nor should any of the toxic oils listed above.

> Aniseed, basil, birch, cedarwood, clary sage, cypress, fennel, jasmine, juniper, sweet marjoram, myrrh, peppermint, rosemary, sage, thyme.

Essential oils which should not be used by people prone to epilepsy

The following oils should not be used by any one suffering from epilepsy.

> Fennel (sweet), hyssop, sage.

Wormwood of course should not be used in therapy at all. These essential oils are thought to stimulate an epileptic fit in people who have epilepsy and should be avoided.

Essential oils which should not be used by people with high blood pressure

The following oils should not be used by anyone suffering from high blood pressure.

> Hyssop, rosemary, sage, thyme.

For people with high blood pressure, gentle massage using relaxing essential oils is beneficial.

UNIT III

THE REMEDIES

This unit provides you with an extensive and systematic survey of commonly available essential oils and carrier oils. Unit III contains monographs of over 60 essential oils including botanical names; country of origin; traditional uses; chemical constituents; properties; blending; indications for use and safety.

Unit III includes the following chapters:

Chapter 12 The essential oils

Chapter 13 The carrier oils

Chapter 14 Hazardous essential oils

Chapter 12

The Essential Oils

This chapter is an extensive survey of the most commonly available essential oils. Each essential oil is defined by:
Exact botanical origin
Synonyms
Other species
Description
Characteristics
Part of plant used
Country of origin
The traditional uses for each essential oil
The methods of extraction
Essential oil constituents
Properties
Blends well with
Indications
Safety.

Introduction

This chapter can be used as a reference guide to the essential oils according to the common name of the plant from which the oil is derived. It includes detailed information on each essential oil including its botanical origins, history of use, principal constituents and therapeutic uses.

Angelica Root

Botanical name   *Angelica archangelica.*

Family   Apiaceae (Umbelliferae).

Place of origin   Native to Europe, cultivated mostly in Eastern Europe.

Other species   There are two subspecies of angelica, *Angelica archangelica* subsp. *litoralis Thell* and *Angelica archangelica L.* The former of these subspecies has a harsher, pungent odour whereas the latter is the one that has been used for flavouring and medicinal purposes for centuries.

Description   Grows up to two metres with fern like leaves and umbels of flowers. It has a strongly aromatic and large root.

Characteristics   An earthy, rich herbaceous, pepper-like, spicy and strong fragrance.

Part of plant used   Roots.

Method of extraction   Steam distillation.

History   Angelica has been praised since the middle ages as a plant of many virtues. It was used to strengthen the heart, stimulate circulation and Paracelsus used it during the bubonic plague to strengthen the immune system. The liqueur Benedictine derives its distinctive flavour from angelica. The candied stalks and roots were traditionally taken as a tonic to combat infection and improve energy levels. *Angelica sinensis* is one of the most important Chinese tonic herbs.

Chemical constituents   A typical chemical composition of angelica root is reported as follows (1):

α-pinene (21.12-25.24%), camphene (1.42-1.43%), β-pinene (1.28-1.48%), sabinene, d-3-carene (7.94-10.38%), α-phellandrene (2.38-9.58%), myrcene (4.00-4.62), limonene (8.54-11.53%), β-phellandrene (14.04-16.03%), cis-ocimene (0.24-0.28%), trans-ocimene (0.9-2.12%), p-cymene (6.25-11.3%), terpinolene (0.28-0.38%), copaene (0.93-1.29%), bornyl acetate (1.5-1.55%), terpinen-4-ol (0.12-0.15%), cryptone (0.44-0.99%), β-bisabolene (0.09-0.19%), rho-cymen-8-ol (0.14-0.35%), humulene monoxide (0.18-0.21%), tridecanolide (0.58-0.81%), pentadecanolide (0.87%)

Blends well with   aniseed, bergamot, clary sage, cardamom, eucalyptus, lemongrass, lemon, lavender, juniper, pine, rosemary, sandalwood, vetiver.

Properties   antispasmodic, carminative, depurative, diaphoretic, digestive, diuretic, emmenagogue, expectorant, febrifuge, nervine, stimulant, stomachic and tonic.

Indications

Mind and spirit   The plant is often referred to in medieval and renaissance herbals as Angel's herb or the *'Root of the Holy Spirit'*. These names were given to the plant because of its almost miraculous healing properties at a physical level, for purifying the blood and curing almost every conceivable malady; it was held to be a sovereign remedy for poisons, and all infectious diseases.(2)

According to Susanne Fischer-Rizzi (3), angelica oil is ideal for fatigue and stress-related disorders;

'Angelica aids people with an upset nervous system who urgently need to rebuild body and soul. The oil helps soothe all kinds of weakness. It's like super-growth fertiliser you might feed a sickly plant. The essential oil of the angelica root will help you rediscover your own inner strength and stamina',

and suggests using angelica for people who need grounding or who search for reality.

Body   The oil is well known as a carminative, stomachic and tonic and is recommended for treating a weak stomach or digestive system, lack of appetite, anorexia, flatulence, chronic gastritis and chronic enteritis.

It is also valuable as an expectorant and is used for chronic bronchial asthma, sinus infections, chronic respiratory problems and coughs.

According to traditional Chinese medicine, angelica can be used to 'scatter wind cold'. Thus it would be valuable for the treatment of the onset of a cold and for swollen glands in the neck. (4)

The oil is also used to reduce accumulation of toxins, arthritis, gout, rheumatism and water retention.

Precautions The oil is non-toxic and non-irritant, however the root oil is phototoxic. If applied to the skin, the skin must not be exposed to sunlight or sunbed rays for at least 12 hours. Angelica has not been shown to stimulate uterine contractions, but, given its traditional uses to induce menstruation, it would be prudent for pregnant women not to use the oil.

Aniseed

Botanical name *Pimpinella anisum.*

Family Apiaceae (Umbelliferae).

Synonyms *Anisum officinalis, A. vulgare.*

Place of origin Native to Greece and Egypt, now widely cultivated in Spain.

Other species There are several different chemotypes of aniseed according to the country of origin. *Pimpinella anisum* is not to be confused with star anise *(Illicium verum)*, which belongs to the Illiciaceae family.

Description An annual herb, less than a metre high, with delicate leaves and white flowers.

Characteristics Spicy-sweet scent similar to fennel.

Part of plant used Seeds.

Method of extraction Steam distillation.

History Anise seeds were a highly prized commodity in ancient Egypt, Greece, and Rome. The Greeks used the seeds for the treatment of coughs, colds and even bad dreams. Commonly used as a domestic spice. The essential oil has long been used for the treatment of dry irritable coughs, bronchitis and whooping cough.

Pliny recommended taking aniseed with honey and myrrh in the morning as a 'pick-me-up'.

Aniseed tea was used for infant catarrh, flatulence, colic and griping pain. In Turkey a popular alcoholic drink, *raki*, is made from the seed.

In Tibetan medicine a blend of aniseed and nutmeg oil is used in a lotion for anxiety, depression and other neurotic symptoms.

Chemical constituents A typical chemical composition of *Pimpinella anisum* oil is reported as follows (5): α–pinene (0.17%), camphene (0.07%), β–pinene (0.01%), linalool (0.18%), cis-anethole (2.29%), trans-anethole (85.00%), safrole (0.58%), anisaldehyde (0.91%), acetoanisole (0.94%).

A typical chemical composition of *Illicium verum* oil is reported as follows (6): trans-anethole (71.19%), feniculin (14.56%), estragole (5.04%), limonene (1.68%), linalool (0.69%), β–caryophyllene (0.63%), trans-α–farnese (0.68%), anisaldehyde (0.41%), nerolidol (0.3%), cinnamyl acetate (0.25%), cis-ocimene (0.32%).

The two plants have the common name aniseed, but belong to totally different families. Both aniseed plants yield chemically similar essential oils and have similar properties.

Blends well with Bay, cedarwood, eucalyptus, dill, fennel, ginger, mandarin, petitgrain, peppermint, rosemary, spearmint.

Properties Antiseptic, antispasmodic, carminative, diuretic, expectorant, galactagogue, stimulant, stomachic.

Indications

Mind and spirit The warm spicy scent has a comforting effect to the mind. Julia Lawless (7) suggests that it is good for introverted, melancholic or fearful people who tend to be withdrawn or frigid.

To clear the head and strengthen the nerves a few drops may be used in a vaporizer. Use up to 5 drops in a bath for nervous headaches, anxiety, stress, insomnia and general exhaustion.

Body Well known for its effect on the digestive system. Aniseed oil may be used to relieve dyspepsia, colic and flatulence. For a soothing massage to relieve digestive problems blend with the antispasmodic properties of peppermint and nutmeg.

Aniseed oil is also recommended for nauseous migraines, palpitations of the heart and any breathing difficulty which is due to bronchial spasms.

Peter Holmes (8) describes aniseed as increasing Qi, restoring cardiac and respiratory functions and stimulating the lungs and expelling phlegm. For coughs where expectoration is difficult, such as bronchitis and spasmodic asthma, aniseed is valuable. For the full therapeutic range he suggests using the essential oil.

According to the well known German herbalist Weiss (9) the expectorant action of *Pimpinella anisum* is better than that of caraway or fennel, on the other hand the carminative effect is much less than that of fennel or caraway.

It can be used to increase the milk flow of nursing mothers. For this purpose it is preferable that the mother use a herbal infusion of the crushed anise seeds.

Precautions   Its major constituent, trans-anethole, is known to cause dermatitis in some individuals, so it is advised to avoid in allergic and inflammatory skin conditions.

Due to trans-anethole's oestrogen-like action, it is advisable to avoid the use of aniseed oil during breast feeding and pregnancy and anyone with endometriosis or oestrogen-dependent cancers until conclusive safety data is available (10).

Basil

Botanical name   *Ocimum basilicum.*

Family   Lamiaceae (Labiatae).

Synonyms   Sweet Basil.

Place of origin   Native to tropical Asia and Africa, it is now widely cultivated in France, Italy, Bulgaria, Egypt, Hungary, Australia and South Africa.

Other species   There are four principal types of basil essential oils, two of which are extracted from *Ocimum basilicum*:

- Exotic or Reunion basil, which is distilled in the Comoro Islands, Malagasy Republic, Thailand and occasionally in the

Seychelles contains a high percentage of methyl chavicol.

- The French basil oil, also known as European or sweet basil, has a higher percentage of linalool and is safe to use in aromatherapy.

- Methyl cinnamate basil is distilled in various countries of the world including India, Haiti and Guatemala.

- Eugenol basil is distilled in Russia, Egypt and Morocco. True basil and exotic basil are obtained from *Ocimum basilicum*. Methyl cinnamate and eugenol basil are thought to be derived from *Ocimum gratissimum*.

Description   A tender annual herb, with a powerful aromatic scent.

Characteristics   A very pleasant, sweet, herbaceous, light refreshing odour.

Part of plant used   Flowering tops and leaves.

Method of extraction   Steam distillation.

History   Basil takes its name from Latin for a royal 'Basileum', possibly because the plant was so highly prized that it was considered a king amongst plants.

Basil is also considered one of the sacred herbs of India, where it is dedicated to Krishna and Vishnu. According to Ayurvedic medicine, basil opens the heart and mind, bestowing the energy of love and devotion. It is said to strengthen faith, compassion and clarity. (11)

Basil was recommended by Pliny against jaundice and epilepsy, and as a diuretic. It was also known as an aphrodisiac. In the middle ages it was prescribed for melancholy and depression.

The 16th century herbalist John Gerard wrote;

'The smell of basil...taketh away sorrowfulness and maketh a man merry and glad.'

Chemical constituents   A comparative chemical composition of basil oil was reported (12) as:

Compound	Origin		
	Comoro Is.	France	Egypt
α-pinene	0.18%	0.11%	0.25%
camphene	0.06%	0.02%	0.07%
β-pinene	0.25%	0.07%	0.43%
myrcene	0.12%	0.13%	0.35%
limonene	2.64%	2.04%	4.73%
cis-ocimene	2.52%	0.03%	0.63%
camphor	0.37%	1.43%	0.57%
linalool	1.16%	40.72%	45.55%
methyl chavicol	85.76%	23.79%	26.56%
γ-terpineol	0.84%	1.90%	1.09%
citronellol	0.65%	3.57%	1.76%
geraniol	0.03%	0.38%	0.2%
methyl cinnamate	0.05%	0.34%	0.25%
eugenol	0.74%	5.90%	5.90%

Blends well with Bergamot, black pepper, cajeput, eucalyptus, frankincense, geranium, ginger, hyssop, lavender, lemon, sweet and Spanish marjoram, neroli, niaouli, rosemary, peppermint, pine, thyme, tea tree.

Properties Analgesic, antidepressant, antiseptic, antispasmodic, carminative, cephalic, diaphoretic, digestive, emmenagogue, expectorant, febrifuge, nervine, sudorific.

Indications

Mind and spirit Basil is one of the most useful cephalics. Used as an inhalation in a vaporizer, it is reputed to clear the head, relieve intellectual fatigue, and give the mind strength and clarity. It may be used in all types of nervous disorders, especially those associated with weakness, indecision, or hysteria.

Julia Lawless (13) suggests basil is good for those who need protection, due to a debilitating illness, low resistance levels, nervous exhaustion or a change in life resulting in feelings of vulnerability.

Body Basil's antispasmodic property has a beneficial action on the respiratory system and is used for the relief of sinus congestion, asthma, bronchitis, influenza and whooping cough. Its sudorific and febrifuge properties mean it may be used for all types of fever. In ayurvedic medicine it is combined with black pepper for malarial fever.

Peter Holmes (14) describes the properties of basil as stimulating the lungs, dries damp, expels phlegm and relieves wheezing. Basil should be used to support the body's yang energy for asthmatic and bronchial conditions when constant fatigue, cold and depression are prominent.

Basil is also useful in digestive disorders such as vomiting, gastric spasms, nausea, dyspepsia and hiccups.

The antispasmodic and emmenagogue properties make basil effective for treating menstrual problems such as scanty periods.

Skin and hair I do not recommend using basil in baths as it may cause skin irritations. However, sweet basil has traditionally been used to soothe insect bites.

Precautions Because it is an emmenagogue it is best to avoid in pregnancy. Avoid using Basil which has a high content of methyl cinnamate and methyl chavicol as it will be an irritant to people with sensitive skin.

According to research conducted by Miller (15), it may be prudent to avoid basil with a high methyl chavicol content as it may be carcinogenic.

However, research at St Mary's Hospital Medical School in London has shown that the results of animal testing of basil oil cannot be directly extrapolated to humans. Ingestion of basil in its normal dietary form would be several million times less hazardous than the doses used in animal testing. The amounts used in aromatherapy massage would be 100,000 times less. (16)

Bay

Botanical name   *Laurus nobilis.*

Family   Lauraceae.

Synonyms   Sweet Bay, laurel, Mediterranean bay.

Place of origin   Southern Europe, Morocco and Spain.

Other species   There are several related species of bay: Californian bay *(Umbellularia california)*, West Indian bay *(Pimento racemosa)* and the cherry laurel *(Prunus laurocerasus)*, which is poisonous.

Description   An evergreen tree up to 20 metres high with dark green, glossy leaves and black berries; often used as a culinary herb.

Characteristics   Sweet and spicy, somewhat resembling cloves or cinnamon.

Part of plant used   Dried leaves and the berries.

Method of extraction   Distillation.

History   Extensively used by the ancient Egyptians and popular with the Romans who saw bay as a symbol of wisdom, protection and peace. Apollo, the god of healing, was associated with the bay tree. Its Latin name is derived from 'Laudis' meaning to praise. Hence the presentation of the laurel wreaths to victors at the Olympic games.

Culpeper says of bay:

'The oil takes away the marks of the skin and flesh by bruise, falls, and dissolveth the congealed blood in them.'

It has long been used in soups and sauces since it aids digestion by increasing salivary secretion. In the middle ages bay was thought to be a protector against evil and it is still traditional to plant a bay tree by the door of the house.

Chemical constituents   A typical chemical composition of *Laurus nobilis* oil is reported as follows (17):
α-pinene (0.3%), β-pinene (0.1%), myrcene (31.6%), limonene (1.4%), linalool (3.0%), methyl chavicol (0.3%), neral (0.5%), α-terpineol (0.8%), geranyl acetate (0.8%), eugenol (38.6%), chavicol (11.0%).

A typical chemical composition of *Pimento racemosa* oil is reported as follows (18): α-pinene (1.1%), β-pinene (0.1%), myrcene (5.7%), limonene (2.2%), 1,8-cineole (26.0%), linalool (1.9%), terpinen-4-ol (0.1%), eugenol (20.0%).

Blends well with   Bergamot, atlas or Virginian cedarwood, eucalyptus, fennel, ginger, juniper, lavender, lemon, sweet or Spanish marjoram, orange, patchouli, rosemary, thyme, ylang-ylang.

Properties   Analgesic, antiseptic, antispasmodic, cholagogue, emmenagogue, febrifuge, stomachic, sudorific, tonic.

Indications

Mind and spirit   The essential oil of bay is stimulating in small doses and acts as a sedative in larger doses, having a warm yet refreshing quality. According to Julia Lawless (19) the oil is best suited to writers, poets, painters, musicians and creative artists - those with psychic tendencies who depend on intuition and inspiration for their work. It promotes confidence, insight and courage - which is required to complete any innovatory project. The oil should be used in a vaporizer.

Body   Because of the high amount of phenols, the essential oil is a good antiseptic for the respiratory system. It has a pronounced effect on the digestive system and may be useful as an appetite stimulant. It expels wind, settles the stomach pain and has a tonic effect on the liver and kidneys. The oil may be used for sprains and bruises.

Skin and hair   The major use of West Indian bay is as a tonic for the hair and scalp. A recommended formula for hair loss, greasy hair or flaky scalp is:

perfume grade alcohol	75ml
purified water	25ml
West Indian bay	2ml
rosemary	1ml

Precautions   Both *Laurus nobilis* and *Pimento racemosa* are relatively non-toxic and non-irritant. However *Pimento racemosa* should be used with caution due to its eugenol content.

Bergamot

Botanical name   *Citrus aurantium* subsp. *bergamia.*

Synonyms   *Citrus bergamia.*

Family   Rutaceae.

Place of origin   Calabria in southern Italy.

Other species   Not to be confused with the herb bergamot *(Monarda didyma).*

Description   The bergamot fruit is not edible because the pulp is far too sour. As a result, the bergamot tree is primarily cultivated for its valuable essential oil. The tree cannot be propagated by seed; it has to be grafted onto bitter orange trees.

Characteristics   Light, delicate and refreshing. Similar to lemon and orange with a slight floral overtone.

Part of plant used   A small yellowish pear shaped fruit.

Method of extraction   Expression.

History   We have the perfume industry to thank for the existence of bergamot oil. Bergamot is named after the Italian city of Bergamo in Lombardy, where the oil was first sold. The oil has been used in Italian folk medicine for many years, primarily for the treatment of fever and worms.

Bergamot imparts that unusual flavour to Earl Grey tea. Also considered one of the most popular essential oils for use in perfumery. It was and still is an important ingredient in the classic Eau de Cologne formula, being blended with neroli, rosemary and rectified spirits.

Chemical constituents   A typical chemical composition of bergamot is reported as follows (20):
α–pinene (1.0%), β–pinene (5.7%), myrcene (0.9%), limonene (33.0%), α–bergaptene (0.23%), β–bisabolene (0.57%), linalool (13.45%), linalyl acetate (31.3%), nerol (0.1%), neryl acetate (0.42%), geraniol (0.05%), geraniol acetate (0.46%), α–terpineol (0.13%)

Blends well with   Basil, German and Roman chamomile, cypress, eucalyptus, geranium, grapefruit, juniper, jasmine, lavender, lemon, lime, Spanish and sweet marjoram, neroli, orange, palmarosa, patchouli, peppermint, petitgrain, rosemary, rosewood, rose otto, rose absolute, sandalwood, ylang-ylang.

Properties   Analgesic, antidepressant, antiseptic, carminative, cicatrisant, deodorant, digestive, febrifuge, sedative, stomachic, tonic, vermifuge, vulnerary.

Indications

Mind and spirit   Almost everyone likes bergamot's fresh, and lively but gentle, flowery fragrance. Its sedative and yet uplifting characteristics make it an ideal oil to use in an oil burner, bath or in massage for anxiety, depression and nervous tension.

Its cooling and refreshing quality seems to soothe anger and frustration probably by decreasing the action on the sympathetic nervous system. Susanne Fischer-Rizzi (21) ideally describes bergamot:

'Thanks to bergamot's sunny and warming disposition, the oil helps people regain self confidence, and it uplifts and refreshes the spirit. The gentle fragrance, like a bouquet of flowers, evokes joy and warms the heart'.

Body   It is a valuable antiseptic for the urinary tract and infections and inflammation such as cystitis. It may be used as an inhalation for respiratory tract infections such as tonsillitis, bronchitis and tuberculosis. Combined with tea tree it is used as a treatment for cold sores, chicken pox and shingles.

Used in douches and hip baths bergamot oil has proved successful in gonococcal infections, leucorrhoea, vaginal pruritis and urinary infections. Add no more than 2-3 drops to some warm water.

Its action on the digestive tract is carminative and digestive, and is useful in relieving colic, flatulence and indigestion. Peter Holmes (22) suggests using bergamot:

'to restore the stomach and liver and awaken the appetite'.

He describes bergamot as having a pronounced stimulating effect on the liver, stomach and spleen. Gastric stagnation due to weakness and deficiency is mobilised. Not only is the heaviness and distension relieved, but also the despondency which is usually associated with this condition is banished, since bergamot is an effective antidepressant.

Skin and hair   Its antiseptic properties make it ideal for treating wounds, herpes, acne and oily skin conditions. It is an effective deodorising agent.

Precautions   Certain furocoumarins, notably the chemical bergaptene have been found to be phototoxic on the skin. Avoid exposure to the sun after having used bergamot in massage or bath.

According to the the International Fragrance Association (IFRA) the average furocoumarin content is quite high at 0.2 to 0.5%. Bergamot's phototoxicity is classified as severe and it should be used in dilutions of less than 1% to avoid phototoxicity (23).

Black Pepper

Botanical name   *Piper nigrum.*

Family   Piperaceae.

Place of origin   Native to south west India; cultivated in most tropical countries. Major producers are India, Indonesia, Malaysia, China and Madagascar.

Other species   Not to be confused with cayenne pepper or paprika which is from the capsicum species.

Description   A perennial woody vine up to 5 metres high with heart shaped leaves and small white flowers. The berries turn red to black as they mature. Black pepper is the dried fully-grown unripe fruit.

Characteristics   A fresh, dry-woody, warm and spicy scent.

Part of plant used   Dried and crushed black peppercorns.

Method of extraction   Steam distillation.

History   A very old and highly revered spice, used in India for over 4,000 years, mainly for urinary and liver disorders. The root word comes from the Sanskrit 'pippali', changed to the Latin 'piper'. It was so popular with the Romans that taxes were paid with it instead of coins. The Greeks used it extensively for combatting fever.

In medieval England, black pepper was used in charms and amulets for protection, probably because it was used as an antidote to poison and used to prevent the spread of infection.

Chemical constituents   A typical chemical composition of black pepper is reported as follows (24):
α–thujone (0.22-3.59%), α–pinene (1.11-16.20%), camphene (0.23-1.44%), sabinene (0.14-13.78%), β–pinene (4.92-14.33%), α–phellandrene (0.46-27.37%), myrcene (1.66-2.53%), limonene (16.41-24.36%), caryophyllene (9.39-30.94%), β–farnesene (0.03-3.26%), β–bisabolene (0.09-5.18%), linalool (0.04-0.25%), terpinen-4-ol (0.01-0.18%)

Blends well with   Basil, bergamot, cajeput, cypress, eucalyptus, frankincense, eucalyptus, geranium, ginger, grapefruit, hyssop, lavender, lemon, sweet and Spanish marjoram, nutmeg, palmarosa, pine, rosemary, sandalwood, tea tree, ylang-ylang.

Properties   Analgesic, antiseptic, antispasmodic, aphrodisiac, carminative, diaphoretic, diuretic, febrifuge, laxative, rubefacient, stomachic, tonic.

Indications

Mind and spirit   The warming and penetrating odour is very stimulating and strengthens the nervous system. Black pepper is useful for stimulating the mental faculties and energising the body.

According to Julia Lawless (25) black pepper has a warming, comforting quality which makes it useful for extreme cold, either of a physical or emotional nature. Patricia Davis (26) suggests using black pepper to help us to 'get a move on' at times when our lives feel stuck.

Body   Black pepper's rubifacient and analgesic properties make it useful for muscular aches and pain, tired and aching limbs and muscle stiffness. Also useful as a massage oil for arthritic aches and pains. It may be of value in supporting the immune system, as it is a stimulant of the spleen, which serves as a site of immune defence against antigens in the blood. Black pepper may be added to a massage oil to treat severe bruising.

Its stomachic effect increases flow of saliva and stimulates appetite, expels wind, encourages peristalsis and is useful in bowel problems and restores tone to colon muscles.

Peter Holmes (27) describes black pepper as supporting the yang, generating warmth and dispelling cold. He suggests that the essential oil be used as a treatment for the onset of infections with headache, chills and fatigue. To make full use of black pepper's properties it should be used with a carrier oil and be massaged into the skin. Its warming property is beneficial in the treatment of respiratory illnesses particularly where there is a feeling of coldness.

Skin and hair   Helpful for dispersing bruises.

Precautions   Excessive use may over-stimulate the kidneys. Use only in moderation. Non-toxic, non-sensitising, irritant in high concentrations.

Cajeput

Botanical name   *Melaleuca leucadendron.*

Family   Myrtaceae.

Synonyms   *Melaleuca cajuputi,* White tea tree, swamp tea tree.

Place of origin   Malaysia, Australia.

Other species   Several other varieties of melaleuca are used to produce cajeput oil, such as *M. quinquenervia.*

Description   A tall evergreen tree up to 30 metres high. The flexible trunk has a whitish spongy bark which flakes off easily. In Malaysia it is called 'caju-puti', meaning 'white wood', due to the colour of the timber.

Characteristics   Sweet eucalyptus like, sharp odour.

Part of plant used   Young twigs, leaves and buds.

Method of extraction   Steam distillation.

History   Cajeput has been traditionally used for its antiseptic, antihelminthic, carminative and local analgesic properties by Australian aborigines.

'Cajeput has been used by local aborigines on Groote Eylandt for the treatment of aches and pains. The leaves are crushed in the hand and rubbed on. Sometimes young leaves and twigs are crushed and steeped in hot water; the liquid is used to bathe the affected area and the rest is poured over the head. Crushed leaves are sniffed to cure headache.' (28)

The oil made its appearance in Europe in the early seventeenth century, while in Malaysia and other Indonesian islands it has long been used for its therapeutic values. It was considered particularly valuable for colds, flu and chronic rheumatism and was prescribed for cholera.

One of the first French books that mentions the essential oil was *The Natural History of Simple Drugs* by Dr G Guibourt in 1876. He described its properties as antiseptic for intestinal problems, dysentery, enteritis, urinary complaints, cystitis and infections of the urethra. It was considered useful for the respiratory system and for viral infections such as the flu.

Chemical constituents   A typical chemical composition of cajeput is reported as follows (29):
α–pinene (38.9%), β–pinene (1.5%), myrcene (0.5%), α–terpinene (0.2%), limonene (2.9%), 1,8-cineole (21.1%), γ–terpinene (1.0%), p-cymene (3.1%), terpinolene (0.8%) linalool (0.3%), terpinen-4-ol (1.9%), α–terpineol (3.3%)

Blends well with   Bergamot, black pepper, geranium, eucalyptus, ginger, spike lavender, lemon, hyssop, myrtle, niaouli, nutmeg, peppermint, pine, rosemary, tea tree, thyme.

Properties   Analgesic, antiseptic, antispasmodic, expectorant, febrifuge, stimulant, sudorific, vermifuge.

Indications

Mind and spirit   Useful as an inhalation because of its stimulating property, helps clear thoughts and dissipates sluggish feelings.

Body   Cajeput's antiseptic and expectorant properties make it excellent for respiratory tract infections such as colds, laryngitis, bronchitis and it may be helpful for asthma. It is recommended for the onset of respiratory infections with aches and pains, chills, nasal and sinus congestion.

Its pain relieving properties make it useful in massage for neuralgia, headaches, toothaches, gout, chronic rheumatism, muscle stiffness and general aches and pain. The antispasmodic properties of cajeput make it useful for treating painful periods, delayed menses and spasmodic dysmenorrhoea.

Skin and hair   Its antiseptic properties make it useful for treating acne and psoriasis. The oil is also reputed to have insect repellent properties.

Precautions   Considered non-toxic, but may irritate the skin in high concentrations; when this occurs the use of niaouli, considered a non-irritant, is recommended.

Cardamom

Botanical name   *Elettaria cardamomum.*

Family   Zingiberaceae.

Place of origin   Asia.

Other species   There are three types of cardamom which are known commercially: the Malabar, Mysore and Sri Lanka types. The Malabar and Mysore types have been classified as originating from the same variety.

Description   A leafy stemmed shrub up to four metres high with very long leaves bearing small, yellow flowers with purple tips. The oblong, grey fruit contain many seeds and are gathered just before they are ripe.

Characteristics   A sweet-spicy, warm fragrance with a woody-balsamic note.

Part of plant used   Dried ripe fruits (seeds).

Method of extraction   Steam distillation.

History   Cardamom has long been used as a condiment and medicine in India and was generally used for digestive complaints. The Romans and Arabs both used it to settle gastrointestinal problems.

Hippocrates recommended it for sciatica, coughs, abdominal pains, spasms, nervous disorders and for bites of venomous creatures.

In Chinese medicine, cardamom has long been described as a Qi tonic, not only warming and invigorating to the lungs, spleen and nerves, but also having an effect on the spirit or mind similar to that of basil, removing listlessness and depression often found in chronic Qi deficiency conditions.

Chemical constituents   A typical chemical composition of cardamom is reported as follows (30):

α-pinene (1.5%), β-pinene (0.2%), sabinene (2.8%), myrcene (1.6%), α-phellandrene (0.2%), limonene (11.6%), 1,8-cineole (36.3%), γ-terpinene (0.7%), p-cymene (0.1%), terpinolene (0.5%), linalool (3.0%), linalyl acetate (2.5%), terpinen-4-ol (0.9%), α-terpineol (2.6%), α-terpinyl acetate (31.3%), citronellol (0.3%), nerol (0.5), geraniol (0.5%), methyl eugenol (0.2%), trans-nerolidol (2.7%).

Blends well with   Bergamot, black pepper, cajeput, eucalyptus, fennel, frankincense, geranium, ginger, juniper, lemon, myrtle, peppermint, pine, rosewood, tea tree, thyme.

Properties   Antiseptic, antispasmodic, carminative, cephalic, digestive, diuretic, expectorant, stimulant, stomachic, tonic.

Indications

Mind and spirit   The uplifting, refreshing and invigorating aroma of cardamom warms the senses and is ideal when there are feelings of weakness and fatigue.

Body   Cardamom is particularly beneficial with digestive problems. It warms and invigorates the stomach, stimulates the appetite, settles the stomach and eases nausea.

Cardamom also assists in stimulating the lungs, expelling phlegm and can be used for easing coughs and bronchitis.

Precautions   Non-toxic, non-irritant and non-sensitising.

Carrot Seed

Botanical name   *Daucus carota.*

Family   Apiaceae (Umbelliferae).

Synonyms   Wild carrot.

Place of origin   Europe.

Other species   An infused oil is produced by solvent extraction from the red fleshy root of the common edible carrot (*D. carota* subsp *sativus*) mainly used as a vegetable.

Description Annual or biennial herb, with a small, inedible, tough whitish root.

Characteristics Slightly sweet and dry.

Part of plant used Seeds.

Method of extraction Steam distillation.

History The carrot was considered of great medicinal value in ancient Greece and the name stems from the Greek word 'Carotos'. In France in the sixteenth century, carrots were prescribed as a remedy because of their carminative, stomachic and hepatic properties. They were grated and used on ulcers, and have been thought of ever since as a blood purifier and for liver and skin problems.

Chemical constituents A typical chemical composition of carrot seed is reported as follows (31):

α–pinene (11.4-13.0%), camphene (0.7%), β–pinene (2.3-2.6%), sabinene (9.4-11.0%), myrcene (1.0-1.4%), γ–terpinene (0.1%), limonene (1.1-1.3%), γ–terpinene (0.1-0.2%), β–bisabolene (2.6%), geranyl acetate (3.9-4.1%) and Carotol (22.3-23.00%)

Blends well with Bergamot, cypress, fennel, geranium, grapefruit, juniper, lavender, lemon, lime, mandarin, orange, rosemary, rose otto, rose absolute, sandalwood.

Properties Carminative, cytophylactic, depurative, diuretic, emmenagogue, hepatic, stimulant.

Indications

Mind and spirit A cleansing effect on the mind may help to relieve feelings of stress and exhaustion.

Body Used in massage oils and baths, carrot seed essential oil is considered an excellent blood purifier, due to its detoxifying effect on the liver. Can be useful for treating jaundice and hepatitis. Also reputed to increase red blood corpuscles, so it has traditionally been used to boost the general action of all organs. Possibly helpful for treating anaemia and general symptoms of weakness and exhaustion.

Skin and hair In skin care it improves the complexion due to its stimulating effect on red

blood cells, adding tone and elasticity to the skin. Both the depurative and cytophylactic properties of carrot seed oil make it useful for problems such as weeping sores and ulcers, vitiligo, pruritis, boils, carbuncles, eczema and psoriasis.

Precautions Non-toxic, non-irritant and non-sensitising. Best to avoid during pregnancy.

Cedarwood, Atlas

Botanical name *Cedrus atlantica.*

Family Pinaceae.

Synonyms Atlantic cedar, Moroccan cedarwood.

Place of origin Native of Atlas mountains of Algeria mainly produced in Morocco.

Other species Believed to have originated from the famous Lebanon cedars (*C. libani*), which grow wild in Lebanon and on the island of Cyprus. It is a close botanical relative to the Himalayan cedarwood (*C. deodorata*), which produces a very similar essential oil. (NB the oil is quite different from the Texas or Virginian cedarwood).

Description A pyramid shaped evergreen tree, up to 40 metres tall.

Characteristics *Cedrus atlantica* produces a deep amber viscous oil with a warm, camphoraceous top note and sweet tenacious, woody-balsamic base note.

Part of plant used Wood.

Method of extraction Steam distillation.

History It was used by the ancient Egyptians for embalming purposes, cosmetics and perfumery. The Lebanon cedar was prized as a building wood. The cedar trees were mentioned in the Bible, symbolising everything that was fertile and abundant. Later, Dioscorides and Galen referred to cedar's resin being used to preserve the body from putrefaction.

In 1698, Nicholas Lemery mentioned the therapeutic nature of the oil as a urinary and pulmonary antiseptic. In 1925 Doctors Michel and Gilbert in France recorded the good results obtained in cases of chronic bronchitis.

Chemical constituents   Known to contain atlantone, caryophyllene, cedrol, cadinene.(32)

Blends well with   Bergamot, cinnamon, cypress, frankincense, jasmine, juniper, lavender, lemon, neroli, patchouli, rose, orange, sandalwood, rosemary, ylang-ylang and vetiver.

Properties   Antiseptic, astringent, diuretic, expectorant, insecticide, sedative.

Indications

Mind and spirit   The essential oil of Atlas cedarwood is warming, harmonising and its calming and soothing actions benefit nervous tension and anxiety.

Susanne Fischer-Rizzi (33) suggests that the oil may provide comfort and warmth, and help stabilize energies thrown out of balance. For exhaustion, nervous tension, anger and other stress-related conditions, add to a bath or blend with other wood oils such as sandalwood to make a massage oil blend.

Its sedative effects are similar to sandalwood, and it is suggested for conditions associated with anxiety and nervous tension.

Atlas cedarwood and Virginian cedarwood share similar properties and can be used with equal effectiveness for reducing stress, tension and anxiety. The scent of both cedarwoods promotes spirituality.

Body   Its main benefits are on the respiratory system due to its expectorant properties, easing conditions such as bronchitis, coughs and catarrh.

Cedarwood oil may be beneficial in the treatment of kidney and bladder disorders. Its antiseptic properties make it an ideal remedy for bladder and kidney infections and for cystitis. The oil may be added to a sitz bath and to compresses.

Skin and hair   Its astringent and antiseptic properties on the skin are of greatest benefit to oily skin conditions. Helps to clear chronic conditions such as dermatitis and psoriasis. A good hair tonic and effective for treating seborrhoea of the scalp, dandruff and alopecia.

Precautions   Non-toxic, non-irritant and non-sensitising.

Cedarwood, Virginian

Botanical name   *Juniperus virginiana.*

Family   Cupressaceae.

Synonyms   Red Cedar.

Place of origin   Native to North America.

Other species   There is a shrubby red cedar (*J. sabina*) also known as savin. Texas Cedarwood (*J. mexicana*) is a small alpine evergreen tree up to 7 metres tall. It has little use as timber as it has an irregular shaped trunk and branches and the wood tends to crack easily. It is botanically related to the Virginian cedarwood.

Description   A coniferous, slow growing, evergreen tree up to 35 metres high with a narrow, dense pyramidal crown, a reddish heartwood and brown cones.

Characteristics   A mild, sweet balsamic pencil-like scent.

Part of plant used   Wood.

Method of extraction   Steam distillation.

History   The North American Indians used it for respiratory infections, especially those involving an excess of catarrh. Decoctions of leaves, barks, twigs and fruit were used to treat a variety of ailments such as menstrual delay, rheumatism, arthritis, skin rashes, venereal warts, gonorrhoea, pyelitis and kidney infections. It is an excellent insect repellent and can be used with citronella for this purpose.

Chemical constituents   A comparative chemical composition of cedarwood oil is reported as follows (34):

Constituent	Virginiana	Texas
α–cedrene	20.0	21.2
β-cedrene	6.6	4.9
thujopsene	18.9	29.0
other sesquiterpene	13.3	15.5
cedrol	31.60	25
widdrol	4.8	4.2

Blends well with   Bergamot, cypress, frankincense, juniper, lavender, lemon, lime, neroli, rose, rosewood, sandalwood,vetiver.

Properties   Antiseborrhoeic, antiseptic, antispasmodic, astringent, diuretic, emmenagogue, expectorant, insecticide, sedative (nervous system).

Indications   Refer to Atlas Cedarwood for details of indications as the properties of *Juniperus virginiania* oil are similar to *Cedrus atlantica*.

Precautions   Non-toxic, non-irritant and non-sensitising. Best avoided during pregnancy.

Chamomile, German

Botanical name   *Matricaria recutita.*

Family   Asteraceae (Compositae).

Synonyms   Although it has been commonly thought that the botanical origin of blue or German chamomile was *M. chamomilla,* the true botanical origin of this oil is *M. recutita.*

Place of origin   Native to Europe, it is cultivated extensively in Hungary, Egypt, Eastern Europe and France.

Other species   There are many varieties of chamomile, such as the pineapple weed *(Chamaemelum suaveolens),* Roman chamomile *(C. nobile)* and Maroc chamomile *(Ormensis multicaulis* or *O. mixta).*

Description   An annual, strongly aromatic herb, up to 60 cm tall with a hairless, erect, branching stem. It has delicate feathery leaves and simple daisy-like white flowers on single stems.

Characteristics   An inky blue viscous liquid with a strong, sweet warm herbaceous odour.

Part of plant used   Flower heads.

Method of extraction   Steam distillation.

History   This herb has a long standing medical tradition, especially in Europe. The fragrance of chamomile flowers has often been likened to that of apples, and it was called kamai melon (ground apple) by the Greeks, which gave rise to the English name. Chamomile used to be regarded as the 'plant's physician', and was thought to keep other plants in good health.

Chemical constituents   A typical chemical composition of German chamomile is reported as follows (35):
Chamazulene (2.16-35.59%), α–bisabolol (1.72-67.25%), bisabolol oxide A (55.08%), bisabolol oxide B (4.35-18.93%) and bisabolone oxide A (63.85%).

As shown in the table below, German chamomile can be differentiated into four chemotypes based on the comparative percentage of its constituents. (35)

The content and composition of the essential oil are dependent on the developmental stage of the plant. For example, the quantity of α–bisabolol, α–bisabolol oxide A and B and bisabolone oxide A reached a maximum in full bloom, whereas the farnesene content decreased rapidly with the growth and development of the flower.

There can be a slight variation from one year to another in German chamomile because of the existence of different chemotypes. It is therefore important when sourcing German chamomile

Type A:	α–bisabolol oxide B > α–bisabolol oxide A > α–bisabolol
Type B:	α–bisabolol oxide A > α–bisabolol oxide B > α–bisabolol
Type C:	α–bisabolol > α–bisabolol oxide B > α–bisabolol oxide A
Type D:	α–bisabolol oxide B = α–bisabolol oxide A =α–bisabolol

The four principal chemotypes of German chamomile

essential oil for its anti-inflammatory and antispasmodic effects, that the chemotype which has the higher (-)-α-bisabolol content be sourced.

Blends well with Bergamot, carrot seed, clary sage, everlasting, geranium, lavender, patchouli, jasmine, neroli, rose, rosewood, sandalwood, yarrow, ylang-ylang.

Properties Analgesic, anti-allergenic, anti-inflammatory, antiphlogistic, antispasmodic, bactericidal, carminative, cicatrisant, cholagogue, emmenagogue, hepatic, sedative, stomachic, sudorific, vasoconstrictor, vermifuge, vulnerary.

Indications

Mind and spirit While Roman and German Chamomile are generally considered calming oils, I prefer to use Roman chamomile. See Roman chamomile description.

Body The essential oil of German chamomile receives its deep blue colour, sometimes called blue chamomile, from the presence of chamazulene. It has been traditionally known that it is the main active constituent which gives German chamomile its most important actions such as soothing, calming and anti-inflammatory.

The presence of both the lipophilic (principally the sesquiterpenes) and the hydrophilic (principally the flavonoids) greatly contribute to the anti-inflammatory action of chamomile extracts. The (-)-α-bisabolol promotes granulation and tissue regeneration. (36)

German chamomile is valuable in treating inflammation, whether internal or external. It can be used in hot compresses on boils, abscesses, infected cuts, splinters, etc.

The properties and uses of German chamomile often overlap with those of lavender. German chamomile can be used in massage or cold compresses for muscular pain, and for arthritic inflamed joints. It is also useful for treating sprains, inflamed tendons and swollen painful joints in bursitis.

Chamomile is a good remedy for urinary stones, and is indicated when there is inflammation of the pelvis or ureter due to the presence of stones.

Peter Holmes (37) suggests using German chamomile to stimulate and restore the liver and gall bladder. Indications would include, poor appetite, slow painful digestion and hypochondriac distention.

Dr Valnet (38) cites German chamomile oil as being useful as a stimulant of leucocytosis and being good for engorgement of the spleen. Menstrual pain and menopausal problems can be relieved by the use of compresses, massage and baths. The action of chamomile as a vasoconstrictor can help reduce the redness of the cheeks due to enlarged capillaries.

Essential oils which are rich in sesquiterpenes exhibit a cholagogic and choleretic activity (39). The essential oil of German chamomile also has liver regenerating properties (40).

Skin and hair German chamomile is valuable for many skin problems, especially where the skin is very sensitive, red and dry. Its most important use is in the treatment of allergies, eczema, psoriasis and all itchy, dry, flaky skin problems. The antiphlogistic effects of chamazulene have already been mentioned, however more recently it has been reported by Isaac (41) that other components of chamomile oil are responsible for the antiphlogistic and anti-inflammatory properties, such as α–bisabolol. German chamomile can be diluted in evening primrose or jojoba oil and used as a massage oil.

Precautions Non-toxic, non-irritant and non-sensitising.

Chamomile, Roman

Botanical name *Chamaemelum nobile.*

Family Asteraceae (Compositae).

Synonyms *Anthemis nobilis*, garden chamomile.

Place of origin Italy, France.

Other species Chamomile, Maroc *(Ormenis multicaulis* or *O.mixta* or *Anthemis mixta)* is native to north west Africa and southern Spain and is distantly related to German and Roman chamomile, although it does not resemble them physically. Also see discussion listed under German chamomile.

Description   A small perennial herb, up to 25 cm high, with a hairy stem. It has feathery pinnate leaves, daisy white flowers which are larger than those of German chamomile. The plant has an apple-like scent.

Characteristics   A pale yellow colour with a warm fruity herbaceous scent.

Part of plant used   Flower heads.

Method of extraction   Steam distillation.

History   Joseph Miller describes Roman chamomile as,

'a plant of many virtues, being stomachic, hepatic, nervine, emollient and carminative'.

He recommends it for colic, jaundice, urinary stones and in fomentations for inflammation and tumours. William Whitla describes it as an aromatic stimulant and stomachic bitter,

'improving the appetite and aiding digestion by increasing the vascularity of the mucous membrane. Its chief use is in atonic dyspepsia.'

He refers to the oil as a tonic, stomachic, and antispasmodic and mentions that it diminishes reflex excitability. Mrs Grieve refers to chamomile as a remedy for hysterical and nervous affections in women, and as an emmenagogue (42). She writes:

'It has a wonderfully soothing, sedative, and absolutely harmless effect.'

Chemical constituents   A typical chemical composition of Roman chamomile is reported as follows (43):

α–pinene (0.5-10.0%), camphene (0.-0.5%), β–pinene (0-10.0%), sabinene (0-10.%), myrcene (0.-0.5%), 1,8 cineole (0.5-25%), γ–terpinene (0.-0.5%), caryophyllene (0-10.0%), propyl angelate (0.5-10.0%), butyl angelate (0.5-10.0%)

Blends well with   Bergamot, clary sage, geranium, lavender, lemon, sweet marjarom, neroli, orange, rose absolute or otto, rosewood, sandalwood, ylang-ylang.

Properties   Analgesic, antineuralgic, antiphlogistic, antiseptic, antispasmodic, bactericidal, carminative, cholagogue, cicatrisant, digestive, emmenagogue, febrifuge, hepatic, nerve sedative, stomachic, sudorific, tonic, vermifuge, vulnerary.

Indications

Mind and spirit   Roman chamomile is generally used to treat psychological problems. Susanne Fischer-Rizzi suggests using Roman chamomile (44):

'When you are feeling moody and grumpy, reach for some chamomile. Roman chamomile is beneficial for people who are short tempered, self involved, overly sensitive or rarely satisfied.'

It is a traditional remedy for children and is recommended when they are feeling impatient, disagreeable, or tense. Teething pain, colic or flatulence may be the underlying causes. If this is the case you will find a 1% dilution of Roman chamomile oil in apricot kernel very useful as a massage oil over their cheeks or abdomen.

It is useful as a mild sedative for children, having a calming but not a depressing effect. Julia Lawless describes Roman chamomile as (45):

'having a profound calming effect on the emotional level, so it is helpful for people who tend to be hyperactive, workaholic, think too much and worry a lot.'

Body   Roman chamomile has anti-inflammatory and anti-spasmodic effects, though to a lesser degree than German chamomile. The more pleasing aroma of Roman chamomile, due to its high ester content, is more suitable for its effects as an inhalation.

Roman chamomile is a useful oil for women with irregular periods and PMS, ideally used in a bath or as a massage oil. For abdominal pain; gall bladder and throat infections, and for children suffering from colic, moist warm or hot compresses assist healing.

Using Roman chamomile as an inhalation helps combat emotional anxiety and tension associated with asthma, hayfever and other allergies.

Skin and hair   While German chamomile oil is preferred in skin care because of its chamazulene and bisabolol content, Roman chamomile also has anti-inflammatory properties.

Artifically induced skin abrasions responded favourably to the application of Roman chamomile - both in terms of reducing inflammation and accelerating healing (46).

Precautions   Non-toxic, non-irritant and non-sensitising.

However, contact dermatitis has been reported with topical applications of Roman chamomile (47). The risk of dermal reactions using Roman chamomile has been attributed to the sesquiterpene lactones. Caution is required with atopic individuals. It has been noted that chamomiles have been contaminated with other allergenic plants. This highlights the need for strict control when sourcing plant matter to make essential oils.

Cinnamon

Botanical name   *Cinnamomum zeylanicum.*

Family   Lauraceae.

Synonyms   *C. verum, Laurus cinnamomum.*

Place of origin   Indonesia, Sri Lanka.

Other species   Cinnamon from Madagascar is considered superior to the various species such as Saigon cinnamon (*C. loureirii*) and the Batavia cinnamon (*C. burmanii*).

Description   A tropical evergreen tree up to 15 metres high. When the trees are six to eight years old, the bark is removed in long strips and left to dry in the hot sun. These strips are rolled into tubes, the 'quills' familiar as the culinary spice.

Characteristics   The bark oil has a sweet, warm, spicy smell, while cinnamon leaf oil has a warm, spicy but rather harsh smell lacking the body and depth of cinnamon bark oil.

Part of plant used   Bark or leaf.

Method of extraction   Water or steam distillation.

History   A very old spice native to Sri Lanka, but now cultivated in other countries such as India, Seychelles and Mauritius. Most prescriptions in China have made use of cinnamon where it was used as a tranquilliser, tonic, stomachic and as being good for depression and a weak heart.

In Ayurvedic medicine it is the basis for the three aromatics, along with cardamom and bay leaves. These three help promote digestion.

The spice is mentioned in the Bible under the name of 'quesiah'. In Exodus, God told Moses to take myrrh, cinnamon, olive oil and bulrushes with him from Egypt. The ancient Egyptians were known to have used it to keep epidemics at bay, and in embalming.

The Arab traders, who kept its origins a secret, supplied the spice to the Greeks and Romans. The quest for the coveted cinnamon was pursued so enthusiastically that it was the principal incentive of the Portuguese in discovering the route around the Cape to India and Ceylon (now Sri Lanka). The Dutch, who took control of Ceylon in the mid-seventeenth century, monopolised the cinnamon trade for over 150 years.

In traditional Chinese medicine, cinnamon was seen as a cure-all and most recipes include cinnamon. It was used as a nerve tranquillizer and tonic, and considered good for depression and a weak heart.

Chemical constituents   A typical chemical composition of cinnamon leaf and bark oil is reported as follows (48):

Leaf: eugenol(80-96%), eugenol acetate (1%), cinnamic aldehyde(3%), benzyl benzoate (3%),

Bark: cinnamic aldehyde(40-50%), eugenol(4-10%), benzyl benzoate (1.0%), α-pinene (0.2%), 1,8-cineole (1.65%), linalool (2.3%), caryophyllene (1.35%).

Blends well with   Black pepper, clove, eucalyptus, frankincense, ginger, grapefruit, lavender, lemon, orange, rosemary, tangerine, thyme, tea tree.

Properties   Analgesic, antiseptic, antispasmodic, aphrodisiac, cardiac, carminative, emmenagogue, insecticide, stimulant, stomachic, tonic, vermifuge.

Indications

Mind and spirit   As an inhalation it is excellent for exhaustion, feelings of depression, fainting, debility and weakness.

Body   It is a very effective antiseptic, digestive and anti-rheumatic. Cinnamon oil is regarded as one of the strongest antiseptic oils. Valnet (49) found that a 1 part in 300 dilution of cinnamon in water will kill the typhus bacillus. It is therefore useful for preventing infectious and contagious diseases.

It calms spasms of the digestive tract, dyspepsia, colitis, flatulence, diarrhoea, nausea and vomiting and stimulates secretions of gastric juices. Its tonic effect on the whole body makes it useful to ease muscular spasm and painful rheumatic joints. Peter Holmes (50) suggests using cinnamon to prevent or resolve cold and flu, relieving aches and pains and low vitality.

Like ginger, cinnamon is recommended for any condition of cold, deficiency and congestion.

Skin and hair   Not recommended for skin care. Traditionally used in clearing warts.

Precautions   The leaf oil is relatively non-toxic. As eugenol is the major constituent of cinnamon leaf oil and clove, it should be assumed to have similar hazards to clove oil.

The bark oil is considered a dermal toxin, irritant and sensitiser. Cinnamon bark oil should never be used on the skin.

Citronella

Botanical name   *Cymbopogon nardus.*

Family   Poaceae (Gramineae).

Synonyms   *Andropogon nardus.*

Place of origin   Native to Sri Lanka.

Other species   An essential oil is produced from Java citronella (*C. winterianus*). This variety is cultivated in the tropics worldwide, especially in Java, Vietnam, Africa, Argentina and Central America.

Description   A tall, aromatic perennial grass.

Characteristics   A yellowy brown liquid with a fresh powerful, lemony scent. The Java oil is colourless to pale with a fresh, woody-sweet fragrance.

Part of plant used   Fresh, part dried or dried leaf.

Method of extraction   Steam distillation.

History   The leaves of citronella have been used for their medicinal and aromatic properties in many cultures, for fever, intestinal parasites, digestive and menstrual problems, and most commonly as an insect repellent.

Chemical constituents   A typical chemical composition of citronella (51) from Sri Lanka contains 55-65% acetylizable alcohols (geraniol) and 7-15% total aldehydes (citronellal), whereas the Java citronella oil contains approximately 85% alcohols and 15% aldehydes.

Blends well with   Bergamot, cajeput, cedarwood, eucalyptus, geranium, lavender, lemon, peppermint, rosemary, sage, tea tree, thyme.

Properties   Antiseptic, bactericidal, deodorant, diaphoretic, febrifuge, insecticide, tonic.

Indications

Mind and spirit   It has an uplifting effect and can help ease feelings of depression.

Body   Citronella is commonly used as an insect repellent. It may be used in a spray, diffused into the air or it may be applied to the skin in a massage oil. It can be used because of its antiseptic properties as an inhalation against colds, flu and minor infections. Its deodorant and stimulating properties always refresh sweaty tired feet, activating the whole body.

Skin and hair   Useful for combatting excessive perspiration and oily skin.

Precautions   Non-toxic, non-irritant, may cause dermatitis in some individuals.

Clary Sage

Botanical name   *Salvia sclarea.*

Family   Lamiaceae (Labiatae).

Synonyms   Muscatel sage.

Place of origin   France, Russia.

Other species   Closely related to garden sage (*S. officinalis*) and Spanish sage (*S. lavendulaefolia),* which are both used for the production of essential oil.

Description   A short biennial or perennial herb up to 1 metre high with large, hairy leaves, with small purple or blue flowers.

Characteristics   A fruity-floral-herbaceous, nutty and heavy fragrance.

Part of plant used   Flowering tops and foliage.

Method of extraction   Steam distillation.

History   The name is derived from the Latin word 'clarus' meaning 'clear', possibly because the herb was once used for clearing mucous from the eyes. Originally grown in southern Europe, it was planted in German vineyards. When introduced to England in the sixteenth century, it was sometimes substituted for hops in brewing beer. In the middle ages it was known as 'Oculus Christi' meaning 'Eye of Christ'.

Chemical constituents   A typical chemical composition of clary sage is reported as follows (52):
Linalool, (10-20%), linalyl acetate (60-70%), caryophyllene (1.5-2.5%), α−terpineol (0.5-2.5%), geraniol (trace-1.5%), neryl acetate (0.3-1.0), sclareol (0.5-2.0%), germacrene D (3.0-5.0%)

Blends well with   Bergamot, cedarwood, German and Roman chamomile, frankincense, geranium, jasmine, lavender, sweet marjoram, neroli, orange, rosewood, sandalwood, ylang-ylang.

Properties   Antidepressant, antispasmodic, deodorant, emmenagogue, hypotensive, nervine, sedative, tonic, uterine.

Indications

Mind and spirit   Clary sage is well known for its euphoric action. It is an extremely valuable oil for treating nervousness, weakness, fear, paranoia and depression. It helps reduce deep seated tension, yet remains stimulating, regenerative, and revitalising.

Clary sage is well known for its euphoric action on the consciousness which dispels depression, especially when arising from nervous burn-out (53). It acts on the thalamus and also helps to relieve anxiety states including those involving fear, paranoia and delusions. Holmes suggests that clary sage may be used to centre and ground scattered thinking, absent-mindedness and unrealistic ideas.

Patricia Davis (54) suggests using clary sage to bring us more closely in touch with dreamland, which can teach us so many spiritual lessons. Clary sage may be used to encourage vivid dreams, or it may be used to enhance dream recall. It may be used in an evening bath, in an oil burner or a drop on the pillow.

Susanne Fischer-Rizzi (55) recommends using clary sage for people involved in creative work, as it opens the path to the unknown, unusual, creative, and intuitive.

Body   Its antispasmodic and emmenagogue properties make it useful for helping with uterine problems such as easing pre menstrual syndrome, regulating scanty periods and easing painful cramps in the lower back. Also encourages labour, enabling the expectant mother to relax and eases post-natal depression.

A recent clinical study involving the use of essentials oils being used during labour found clary sage was beneficial for its analgesic effects, relaxing effects and its ability to accelerate labour. (56) Clary sage combines well with lavender, jasmine, neroli, and sandalwood during childbirth.

The oil is one of several that promotes oestrogen secretion. It is believed to act on the pituitary, thus having a harmonising effect in most menstrual disorders. It inhibits prolactin which tends to dry up breast milk. Clary sage is considered quite useful during menopause when symptoms such as hot flushes, dizziness, headaches, night sweats, palpitations and irritability are prominent.

Clary sage may also be useful for treating asthma as it both relaxes spasm of the bronchial tubes and helps with the anxiety and emotional tension often found in asthma sufferers.

Skin and hair   Ideally used in hair care, it may be used to clear greasy hair and dandruff by reducing excessive production of sebum.

Precautions   Non-toxic, non-irritant and non-sensitising. Not to be used during pregnancy.

Clove

Botanical name   *Eugenia caryophyllata.*

Family   Myrtaceae.

Synonyms   *Eugenia aromatica, E. caryophyllus, Syzygium aromaticum.*

Place of origin   Zanzibar, Madagascar, Java and Sri Lanka.

Description   A slender evergreen tree which grows up to 12 metres. At the start of the rainy season long buds appear with a rosy-pink corolla at the tip; as the corolla fades the calyx slowly turns deep red. The calyxes are beaten from the tree and, when dried, provide the cloves of commerce.

Characteristics   Strong, spicy and penetrating. The odour of the bud oil is considered to be softer and more floral.

Part of plant used   Bud/stem/leaf.

Method of extraction   Water distillation.

History   The Greeks called the tree 'caryophyllum' meaning 'leaf of walnut tree' and this derived through Arabic to 'girofle', part of the French name for the spice, clou de girofle. Clou is the French word for nail, derived from Latin clavus (the dried buds look like little nails).

Pliny praised cloves, as did the great Roman doctor Alexander Trallianus. St Hildegarde, in her book *Morborum Causae et Curae*, wrote that cloves were included in treatments for headaches, migraines, deafness after a cold, and dropsy. She advised that cloves would warm people feeling cold, and cool down those who felt hot. During the Renaissance, pomanders were made with cloves to keep epidemics and the plague at bay.

In Chinese medicine, cloves are considered a warming agent, good for hypertension. They are still used today as a stress-relieving agent for anxiety, tension, hysteria and insomnia.

Chemical constituents   A typical composition of the bud, stem and leaf oil can be differentiated as follows (57):

Compound	Clove Leaf	Clove Stem	Clove Bud
Eugenol	85-90%	87-92%	80-85%
Eugenyl acetate	0-10%	3-3.5%	8-12%
Isoeugenol	-	trace	-
Caryophyllene	10-15%	6-8%	6-10%
Isocaryophyllene	-	-	0-2.0%

Blends well with   Basil, black pepper, cajeput, cinnamon, ginger, lavender, spike lavender, lemon, Spanish marjoram, nutmeg, orange, peppermint, rosemary, thyme.

Properties   Analgesic, antiseptic, antispasmodic, carminative, stomachic, uterine.

Indications

Mind and spirit   A positive and stimulating effect on the mind, lifts depression and is recommended as an inhalation when feeling weak and lethargic.

Body   Clove is excellent as an antiseptic, because of the high proportion of eugenol. It may be used for the prevention of viral diseases. Being a carminative and antispasmodic it helps stimulate digestion, restores appetite and relieves flatulence.

The dental value of cloves is well known. Because of its minor anaesthetic effect, the oil has been traditionally used to relieve toothaches.

Recent studies have shown that clove oil and other essential oils commonly known to irritate the skin such as cinnamon and thyme triggered the release of anti-inflammatory substances, and inhibited the prostoglandins type 2 which are well known mediators of inflammatory processes (58).

Clove oil is beneficial for treating inflammatory conditions such as rheumatoid arthritis and other musculoskeletal conditions.

Skin and hair   Not used in skin care, except to treat infectious wounds, skin sores and leg ulcers.

Precautions   Clove oil can cause skin irritation. Clove bud oil is safer to use than clove leaf or clove steam oil due to its lower eugenol content. It should never be used in concentrations of higher than 1% when applied to the skin.

A near fatal ingestion of clove oil was recently reported involving a 2 year old boy who had drunk between 5-10 ml of clove oil from an open-mouthed bottle. (59)

Clove oil, when administered orally, is described as a hepatotoxin and an inhibitor of blood clotting. This is assumed to be due to the eugenol content. (60)

Cypress

Botanical name   *Cupressus sempervirens.*

Family   Cupressaceae.

Synonyms   Italian cypress, Mediterranean cypress.

Place of origin   France, Germany.

Other species   There are many species of cypress found throughout the world. Always use *Cupressus sempervirens* for aromatherapy purposes.

Description   A tall evergreen tree with slender branches and a statuesque conical shape. It bears small flowers and round brownish-grey cones or nuts.

Characteristics   Woody, slightly spicy yet clear and refreshing.

Part of plant used   Fresh leaves and cones.

Method of extraction   Distillation.

History   The word sempervirens means 'ever-living' and the ancient Greeks, Romans and Egyptians dedicated the tree to their gods of the underworld. The ancient Greeks dedicated the tree to Pluto, god of the underworld hence the use of the trees in cemeteries.

Hippocrates recommended cypress for severe cases of haemorrhoids with bleeding. Dioscorides and Galen recommended macerating the leaves in wine with a little myrrh for a fortnight. This was recommended for bladder infections and internal bleeding.

Culpeper says of cypress:

'The cones, or nuts, are mostly used, the leaves but seldom; they are accounted very drying and binding, good to stop fluxes of all kinds, as sitting of blood, diarrhoea, dysentery, the immoderate flux of the menses, involuntary miction; they prevent the bleeding of the gums, and fasten loose teeth: outwardly, they are used in styptic restringent fomentations and cataplasms.'

Chemical constituents   A typical chemical composition of cypress is reported as follows (61):

α–pinene (20.4%), camphene (3.6%), sabinene (2.8%), β–pinene (2.9%), δ-3-carene (21.5%), myrcene and α–terpinene (1.1%), terpinolene (6.3%), linalool (0.07%), bornyl acetate (0.3%), cedrol (5.35%), cadinene (1.7%).

Blends well with   Bergamot, clary sage, fennel, grapefruit, juniper, lavender, lemon, lime, orange, pine, rosemary, tangerine.

Properties   Antiseptic, antispasmodic, astringent, deodorant, diuretic, haemostatic, hepatic, styptic, sudorific, tonic, vasoconstrictor.

Indications

Mind and spirit   Cypress strengthens an overburdened nervous system and restores calm. Seems to have a soothing effect on anger, apparently cleansing the spirit and removing psychic blocks.

Susanne Fischer-Rizzi (62) suggests using cypress when one experiences uncontrollable crying spells. Cypress may be used to strengthen an overburdened nervous system and restores calm.

Patricia Davis (63) suggests using cypress at times of transition such as career changes, moving home and major spiritual decisions. Cypress also helps with painful transitions such as bereavement or the ending of a close relationship.

Body   Cypress oil can be used where there is excessive discharge of fluid. It has astringent and vaso-constrictor properties which are beneficial for circulatory problems such as varicose veins and haemorrhoids. For varicose veins it should be blended with lemon, wheatgerm oil and infused calendula oil and massaged lightly into the legs every day.

Dr Jean Valnet used cypress oil in hospital for coughs and bronchitis; a few drops of the oil under the patient's pillow stopped coughing. In France cough pastilles were once made using crushed cypress cones. It has antispasmodic properties, being useful for asthma, whooping cough, and all spasmodic coughing.

Cypress also has a regulating effect on the menstrual cycle. It stimulates oestrogen secretion, promoting and increasing the periods in conditions associated with dysmenorrhoea. It helps relieve painful periods and reduces abnormally heavy blood loss, particularly when it happens in the early stages of menopause.

Skin and hair   Cypress is both a deodorant and astringent and when used in a foot bath it will help to reduce excessive perspiration of the feet. For skin care cypress can be used for oily and over hydrated skin.

Precautions   Non-toxic, non-irritant and non-sensitising.

Eucalyptus Leaf Oils

Family   Myrtaceae.

Place of origin   Native to Australia.

Common species   There are over 700 species of eucalyptus, of which fewer than 20 have ever been exploited commercially, many of them outside Australia (64).

- *Eucalyptus globulus*, commonly known as blue gum, is used for the commercial production of eucalyptus oil. *Eucalyptus globulus* was introduced into Europe during the last century and grown mainly for the timber as mine props and paper pulp production.

- *Eucalyptus polybractea* (blue mallee) which is a small tree commercially grown and harvested for the essential oil. *E. polybractea* is a prime source of cineole-rich oils and is currently the major species used in commercial oil production in Australia. This species is ideally suited to mechanical harvesting.

- *Eucalyptus radiata* is a commercially grown tree and has a 1,8-cineole content of

around 75%. This oil, also known as 'narrow-leaved peppermint gum' is considered to be an ideal choice as the 1,8-cineole content is high enough to have the desired therapeutic effect, yet not too overpowering. This oil is often referred to by its trade name: '*Eucalyptus australiania*'.

- *Eucalyptus smithii*, commonly known as 'gully gum', 'white iron bark'; and also Smith's gum after H.G. Smith, Australia's foremost pioneer of eucalyptus essential oil. This species is widely grown in southern Africa where the leaves are harvested for oil production.

- *Eucalyptus citriodora*, commonly known as lemon scented eucalyptus is a tall evergreen tree with a smooth dimpled bark. The oil has a strong fresh citronella like odour with a sweet balsamic undertone.
  Eucalyptus citriodora appears to have bacteriostatic activity towards *Staphylococcus aureus* (65). This is due to the synergy between citronellol and citronellal present in the oil.

- *Eucalyptus dives,* commonly known as broad-leaved peppermint eucalyptus is a robust, medium-sized eucalyptus tree, with a short trunk, spreading branches and fibrous grey bark.
  There are two types of broad-leaved peppermint although they look identical. One is rich in cineol (*E. dives* var. *C.*) and one is rich in piperitone (*E. dives* var. *Type*). It is also similar to peppermint eucalyptus (*E. piperita*) and the grey or narrow-leaved peppermint (*E. radiata* var. *phellandra*).
  The piperitone rich oil with a fresh camphoraceous, spicy-mint odour is used in the manufacture of menthol (used in linaments and mouth washes).

Many eucalyptus oils have been redistilled and rectified. In reality much of the residue left behind from the rectification of the crude oils is rich in precious constituents such as the rare phenol australol. Even if the proportion of these constituents seems low, they work in synergy with the main components and should be retained in order for the essential oil to express its full healing potential.

Lassak cites work conducted by Penfold and Grant who noticed that the high boiling residues of eucalyptus oil extracted from the rectified essential oil exhibited a greater germicidal power than the refined oil. (72)

Characteristics   The scent of a crude *E. globulus* essential oil is similar to the crushed leaf, a camphorous odour with a woody sweet undertone. The scent of *E. radiata* essential oil is much lighter and fresher.

Once the nose has inhaled the genuine and crude essential oils of eucalyptus, it will turn down the rather vulgar smell of rectified eucalyptus oil which is more like the odour of pure 1,8-cineole.

Part of plant used   Fresh or partially dried leaves.

Method of extraction   Steam distillation.

History   The name comes from the Greek word 'eucalyptos', meaning 'well covered', because the flower buds are covered with a cup-like membrane which is thrown off as the flower expands.

The eucalyptus has long been a favourite home remedy in Australia, the white settlers learning of its properties from the aborigines. The aborigines used the burning leaves as fumigation for the relief of fever (66):

'heat went out of sick man and into fire'.

The pharmacist Joseph Bosisto, a Yorkshireman who migrated to Australia in 1848, began the first serious investigations of eucalyptus oil. Bosisto established himself by the 1860s as the first commercial producer of eucalyptus oils in Australia.

The Australian eucalyptus industry experienced its real boom during World War I. Eucalyptus oil was used for medicine, for a meningitis outbreak and the 1919 worldwide influenza epidemic. However by the 1930s eucalyptus oil was being produced from overseas plantations and this impacted heavily on Australian companies because of their higher production costs.

The eucalyptus oil industry in Australia reached its peak in the early post-war years when, in 1947, total production reached almost 1 000 tonnes of which 70% was exported. Since then the industry has declined. Today the world eucalyptus market is about 2 000 - 3 000 tonnes per annum of which about 5 - 10% is produced in Australia.

Early works on the antibacterial properties of the oil were published in Germany by doctors Cloez (1870), Faust and Homeyer (1874). They classified eucalyptus oil as being sudorific, a stimulant, anti-catarrhal, and astringent. It was prescribed for all respiratory system problems such as bronchitis, flu, asthma and coughs.

Chemical constituents   A typical chemical composition of various eucalyptus oils is reported as follows (67):

Eucalyptus globulus: α–pinene (10.66%), β–pinene (0.18%), α–phellandrene (0.09%), 1,8-cineole (69.10%), limonene (3.29%), terpinen-4-ol (0.22%), aromadendrene (1.63%), epiglobulol (0.80%), piperitone (0.1%), globulol (5.33%).

Eucalyptus radiata: α-pinene (15-21%), 1,8-cineole (57-71%), limonene (5.0%), p-cymene (0.3-1%).

Eucalyptus polybractea: α–pinene (0.90%), β–pinene (0.23%), 1,8-cineole (91.90%), limonene (1.10%), terpinen-4-ol (0.51%), globulol (0.05%).

Eucalyptus smithii: α–pinene (4.08%), β–pinene (0.11%), 1,8-cineole (80.54%), terpinen-4-ol (0.11%), globulol (2.36%).

Eucalyptus citriodora: Citronellal (56.3%), citronellol (7.8%),1,8-cineole (2.0%),γ–terpyl acetate (1.8%), citronellic acid (5.7%), citronellyl acetate (11.4%).

Eucalyptus dives: Piperitone (40-50%), phellandrene (20-30%), globulol/ viridoflorol (6%), 1,8-cineole (0.45%), limonene (0.3%), terpinen-4-ol (4.00%), p-cymene (3.36%).

Blends well with Aniseed, basil, cajeput, cedarwood, citronella, frankincense, ginger, hyssop, juniper, lavender, lemon, sweet and Spanish marjoram, myrtle, niaouli, pine, peppermint, rosemary, spearmint, tea tree, thyme.

Properties Analgesic, anti-bacterial, anti-inflammatory, anti-neuralgic, anti-rheumatic, antiseptic, antispasmodic, antiviral, astringent, balsamic, cicatrisant, decongestant, deodorant, depurative, diuretic, expectorant, febrifuge, hypoglycaemic, rubefacient, stimulant, vermifuge, vulnerary.

Indications

Mind and spirit Psychologically, eucalyptus oil serves as a refreshing and stimulating substance. It also assists concentration.

Body According to most medical references the active principal constituent of eucalyptus oil is 1,8-cineole. The medicinal properties of the oil are specified by minimum quantity of constituents which are defined in the British, United States and other pharmacopoeia and standards (eg Australian Standards 2113 and 2115 of 1977).

These specifications require eucalyptus oil to contain not less than 70% 1,8-cineole and be practically free of α- and β-phellandrene.

The expectorant activity of eucalyptus oil may be directly traced to the 1,8-cineole, which has the property of reducing the swelling of mucous membranes and of loosening phlegm, thus making breathing easier. Anecdotal evidence also indicates that eucalyptus oil supports the pancreas and lowers blood sugar. (68) (69)

In 1955 Atkinson and Brice (70) reported that:

> *'The genus Eucalyptus gave rather poor results against the bacteria Staph.'*

Dr Lyall Williams (71) also confirmed that the 1,8-cineole component of eucalyptus failed to show any zone of inhibition against all the microorganisms that he tested. Dr Lyall Williams' work is confirmed by comments made by Lassak (72) who states that:

> *'It was odd to note that many settlers did use eucalyptus oil as a reputed antiseptic, as most cineole rich essential oils exhibit relatively little bactericidal activity.'*

He suggests that the clean, crisp smell of eucalyptus oil resulted in easier and deeper breathing, and plenty of good clean air has always been associated in folk medicine with good health.

Traditionally eucalyptus is one of the most valuable oils for treating the respiratory system. According to Valnet the spraying of a 2% emulsion containing eucalyptus oil kills off 70% of local, airborne staphylococci (73). Eucalyptus oil influences the breathing process. It increases the oxygen supply to the body's cells. The essential oil is a traditional remedy for asthma, bronchitis, colds, flu, as well as sinus problems and throat infections.

According to Dr Daniel Penoel (74) 1,8-cineole-rich oils such as those of the eucalyptus species stimulate the immune system because they have an enhancing effect on gamma and beta globulins. They reduce the primary phase of the inflammatory reaction and therefore their effect is said to be immunomodulant.

The piperitone found in *Eucalyptus dives* is used for the manufacture of menthol (used in linaments). Dr Penoel (75) recommends not using the oil due to the high content of the neurotoxic ketone piperitone. However Julia Lawless (76) indicates that *Eucalyptus dives* is suitable for all respiratory conditions, muscular soreness, rheumatism, headaches and nervous exhaustion.

Skin and hair It is a good remedy for indolent wounds and ulcers, and should be used where there is any toxaemia or sepsis.

Precautions Non-toxic, non-irritant and non-sensitising. When taken internally eucalyptus oil is toxic.

There is a reported incident (77) where, for about the past five years, a man had been in the habit of swallowing five to ten drops of eucalyptus oil to keep colds at bay and to 'make him feel good'. He began to feel discomfort and pain in the region of the liver. After entering hospital for a check-up, he was informed him that he had been diagnosed with cirrhosis of the liver and that, unless he stopped drinking, his condition would further deteriorate. This man had never drunk alcohol. The apparent cause of his condition was the ingested eucalyptus which he had assumed would improve his health.

Everlasting

Botanical name   *Helichrysum angustifolium.*

Family   Asteraceae (Compositae).

Synonyms   Immortelle, helichrysum, St John's herb.

Place of origin   Native to the Mediterranean region, it is cultivated in Italy, the Balkans, Spain and France.

Other species   There are several other species such as *H. arenarium* commonly used by florists and *H. stoechas* which is also used to produce an absolute.

Description   A strongly aromatic herb. Grows up to 60cm high with brightly coloured daisy-like flowers.

Characteristics   An intense, rich, honey-like scent with a delicate tea-like undertone.

Part of plant used   Flowering tops.

Method of extraction   Steam distillation.

History   Immortelle has long been used medicinally. It was the chosen remedy for chronic ailments of the skin and lymphatic system. It has also been used in Europe for respiratory complaints such as asthma, chronic bronchitis and whooping cough; also used for headaches, migraine and liver ailments.

Chemical constituents   A typical chemical composition of everlasting is reported as follows (78):
α–pinene, camphene, β–pinene, myrcene, limonene, 1,8-cineole, linalool, terpinen-4-ol, neryl acetate, nerol, geraniol, eugenol, italidone and other β–diketones.

Blends well with   Bergamot, German chamomile, clary sage, frankincense, lavender, geranium, neroli, orange, rock rose, rose, rosewood, yarrow.

Properties   Anti-allergenic, anti-inflammatory, antimicrobial, antitussive, antiseptic, astringent, cholagogue, cicatrisant, diuretic, expectorant, fungicidal, hepatic, mucolytic, nervine.

Indications

Mind and spirit   Everlasting has a strong psychological effect, similar to vetiver and cypress. According to Susanne Fischer-Rizzi (79), its earthy fragrance may be beneficial for people who have lost contact with the earth, have become too cerebral, or acquired cold feet. Everlasting has a grounding effect without being heavy.

Fischer-Rizzi also suggests that everlasting, which loves growing in hot dry places, transfers the warmth the plant receives from the sun to the essential oil. This makes the oil ideal for people who feel cold or who may not have received warmth and affection as children.

Julia Lawless (80) suggests using everlasting to increase dream activity and awareness, and to stimulate the right side of the brain.

Body   The oil is ideal to use in lymphatic drainage massage, acting as a stimulant for the liver, gall bladder, kidneys and spleen - the organs responsible for detoxifying the body. For gall bladder inflammations, compresses of everlasting and rosemary are very effective. It can be used to help recovery from hepatitis and for treating headaches that originate from liver upsets.

A number of unusual compounds have been found in everlasting - sesquiterpenes which have anti-inflammatory and anti-allergenic properties and di-ketones, one being italidone (having 20 carbon atoms). Most ketones that are found in essential oils are of the 10 carbon atom size.

Italidone has been found to have strong mucolytic (mucous thinning), expectorant and cicatrisant properties.

Its mucolytic and expectorant properties coupled with its antispasmodic effects make it useful for sinus infections, bronchitis, spasmodic coughing and whooping cough. Everlasting can be used as an inhalation.

Its anti-inflammatory properties make it useful for treating rheumatoid arthritis, tendonitis and bursitis. It may also be used to treat prostatitis in men.

Skin and hair   For skin care, everlasting is very useful in combination with rock rose and lavender for chronic ailments of the skin involving the lymphatic system.

Everlasting has excellent cicatrisant properties, speeding cellular growth and assisting in wound healing of all types. It reduces old scar tissue, stretch marks and loosens adhesions after injuries. It has both anti-inflammatory and anti-allergenic properties, being useful for treating eczema and dermatitis.

Precautions   Non-toxic, non-irritant and non-sensitising.

Fennel

Botanical name   *Foeniculum vulgaris.*

Family   Umbelliferae.

Place of origin   Grows in Mediterranean countries.

Other species   Two types of fennel are known, sweet fennel (*F. vulgare.* var. *dulce*) and bitter fennel (*F. vulgare* var. *amara*).

Description   A biennial or perennial herb up to 2 metres high with feathery leaves and golden yellow flowers.

Characteristics   Sweet aniseed-like fragrance.

Part of plant used   Crushed seeds.

Method of extraction   Steam distillation.

History   A very popular plant with the ancient Chinese who used it as a cure for snake bite. A herb of ancient repute, believed to encourage longevity, courage and strength. Theophrastus and Pliny preferred it to anise, and Dioscorides and Hippocrates both said it promoted the flow of breast milk. Pliny valued it as an eye herb. The Romans valued it for its digestive properties. The Greeks believed fennel to be a slimming herb. As it is a diuretic there is some basis for this belief. Fennel has also been regarded as an appetite suppressant in traditional therapies. A seventeenth century herbalist, William Cole, wrote:

'Fennel is much used in drinks and broths for those that are grown fat, to abate their unwellness and cause them to grow more gaunt and lank.'

The seeds were carried by Roman soldiers on long marches, to chew when they did not have time to stop and have a meal. Christians also used fennel on fasting days.

Culpeper says of fennel:

'Fennel is good to break wind, provoke urine, ease pains of the stones and help break it... The seeds help to open obstructions of the liver, spleen and gall.'

Chemical constituents   A typical chemical composition of sweet fennel is reported as follows (81):
α–pinene (1.8-3.3%), myrcene (0.5-0.8%), fenchone (19.0-21.6%), trans-anethole (64.0-69.2%), methyl chavicol (3.9-6.5%), limonene and 1,8-cineole (1.2-1.7%), anisic aldehyde (0.1-0.3%).

Blends well with   Basil, clary sage, cypress, geranium, grapefruit, juniper, lavender, lemon, peppermint, rosemary, rose, sandalwood.

Properties   Antiseptic, antispasmodic, carminative, depurative, diuretic, emmenagogue, expectorant, galactagogue, laxative, stimulant, splenic, stomachic, vermifuge.

Indications

Mind and spirit   The oil is said to give strength and courage in adversity.

Body   According to traditional Chinese medicine and Galenic medicine (82) the main qualities of fennel are warming and drying. Since these qualities invigorate the stomach, spleen and intestines it is not surprising to find that fennel is one of the best choices as a digestive remedy, being used to relieve nausea, flatulence, indigestion, colic and hiccups.

Fennel is also a diuretic, and is recommended to assist in detoxifying the body. It may be used for the treatment of cellulite, when accumulations of toxic wastes and fluids in the subcutaneous fat produce a characteristic wrinkled appearance.

Fennel is traditionally used for treating gout and general bladder irritation due to high uric acid or stones.

Fennel is also known to have potent oestrogenic activity. According to Balacs (83) the oestrogenic potency of fennel may be due to the plant polymers of anethole, such as photoanethole and dianethole. This possibly explains its apparent usefulness in regulating the menstrual cycle. It may also be used at menopause in reducing the unpleasant symptoms caused by fluctuating hormonal levels, and stimulating the production of oestrogen by the adrenal glands after the ovaries have stopped functioning.

Oestrogen is needed to maintain muscle tone, elasticity of the skin and connective tissue, a healthy circulation and strong bones, so maintaining the supply can postpone the degenerative effects of ageing.

Like aniseed, fennel is also used for the lungs as an antispasmodic and expectorant. Fennel may be used in cold conditions and bronchitis as well as for whooping cough.

Skin and hair   It is often reputed to be useful in skincare for its ability to minimise the effects of wrinkles, this is possibly due to its oestrogenic properties. However care is needed as it may be considered sensitising to the skin tissue.

Precautions   Non-irritant, relatively non-toxic, can cause sensitisation in some individuals.

Due to trans-anethole's oestrogen-like action, it is advisable to avoid the use of fennel oil, until conclusive safety data is available, during breast feeding, oestrogen-dependent cancers, pregnancy and endometriosis. (84)

It should also be avoided by people suffering from epilepsy.

Fir Needle

Botanical name   *Abies alba.*

Family   Pinaceae.

Synonyms   White spruce, *A. pectinata.*

Place of origin   Native to the north European mountainous regions, cultivated in Switzerland, Poland, Germany, France, Russia and Canada.

Other species   Oils that are distilled from twigs and needles of various members of the coniferous families, *Abies, Larix, Picea, Pinus* and *Tsuga,* are all commonly called fir needle oil. It is therefore important to know the specific botanical name. There are many other members of the *Abies* family, notably the Canadian balsam *(A. balsamifera)* and the Siberian fir *(A. siberica).*

Description   A relatively small coniferous tree, with a regular pyramidal shape and silvery white bark, grown chiefly for timber and as Christmas trees.

Characteristics   A pleasing rich sweet balsamic odour.

Part of plant used   Needles and young twigs.

Method of extraction   Steam distillation.

History   The native American Indians used the resin for medicinal and religious purposes and it was introduced into Europe some time during the seventeenth century. It is used in shaving soaps, bath preparations, room sprays, deodorants, disinfectants and inhalations.

Chemical constituents   A typical chemical composition of fir is reported as follows (85): Santene (1.2-4.0%), tricylene (0.4-1.2%), α−pinene (4.7-9.4%), camphene (3.9-10.9%), β−pinene (21.4-44.3%), myrcene (1.0-2.5%), carene (7.3-35.6%), limonene (2.7-19.7%), phellandrene (2.7-5.8%), terpinolene (0.3-0.7%), borneol (0.1-0.6%), terpinen-4-ol (trace-0.2%), α−terpineol (0.1-0.4%), bornyl acetate (8.7-23%), piperitone (0-0.3%).

Blends well with   Basil, black pepper, cajeput, cedarwood, eucalyptus, frankincense, ginger, lavender, lemon, myrtle, niaouli, peppermint, pine, rosemary, rosewood, tea tree, thyme.

Properties   Analgesic, antiseptic, antitussive, deodorant, expectorant, rubefacient, stimulant, tonic.

Indications

Mind and spirit   It is useful as an inhalation for anxiety and stress. Considered useful for its grounding effect.

Body   It is ideal for respiratory difficulties. It has a beneficial effect on chest conditions especially obstructions of the bronchi such as mucus. Its warming effect is beneficial in massage blends for the relief of muscular aches and pain due to rheumatic or arthritic conditions.

Precautions　Non-toxic, non-irritant and non-sensitising.

Frankincense

Botanical name　*Boswellia carteri.*

Family　Burseraceae.

Synonyms　Olibanum.

Place of origin　The tree originates from the Middle East.

Description　A small shrub with abundant pinnate leaves and white or pale pink flowers. It yields a natural oleo gum resin which is collected by making incisions into the bark. At first, a milky-white liquid appears which then solidifies into amber or orange brown crystals of resin. It can be difficult to judge what quality of frankincense gum to use for essential oil production as there are many grades. The age, appearance, moisture level and olfactory characteristics determine the quality of the oil. The following grades are used to determine the quality of the resin:

- Grade 1: Oil from 'Tears' - most carefully selected, white, or yellow in colour

- ungraded: Oil from a mixture of yellow/white and reddish angulated masses with particles of bark and other foreign substances

- oil from dust and siftings.

Characteristics　A warm, woody, sweet balsamic, spicy fragrance with a hint of lemon.

Part of plant used　Resin.

Method of extraction　Steam distillation.

History　Frankincense has been used since ancient times in religious ceremonies and is still used in many churches today. It was very highly valued by many early cultures - thus one of the three gifts from the Magi to the infant Jesus.

Dioscorides mentions the therapeutic use of the gum to treat skin disorders, haemorrhages and pneumonia. Ambroise Pare, a sixteenth century surgeon, treated soldiers' wounds and noted that it stopped bleeding and helped scar tissue to form quickly.

Chemical constituents　A typical chemical composition of frankincense is reported as follows (86):
α–pinene (4.6%), camphene (1.1%), octanol (8.0%), linalool (2.5%), octyl acetate (52.0%), bornyl acetate (1.0%), incensole (2.4%), incensyl acetate (3.4%).

Blends well with　Basil, bergamot, black pepper, geranium, jasmine, lavender, lemon, myrrh, neroli, orange, patchouli, pine, rose, rosewood, sandalwood, vetiver, ylang-ylang.

Properties　Antiseptic, astringent, carminative, cicatrisant, cytophylactic, diuretic, emmenagogue, expectorant, sedative, tonic, uterine, vulnerary.

Indications

Mind and spirit　Frankincense slows down breathing and produces feelings of calm. This tends to bring about an elevating and soothing effect on the mind. Ideally used for meditation, it has been discovered that burning frankincense produces a psycho-active substance, trahydrocannabinole, which expands consciousness (87). Its comforting and refreshing action is helpful for anxious and obsessional states linked to the past.

Body　Like most other oils extracted from resins, frankincense is effective for respiratory catarrhal discharge and respiratory congestion. Used in inhalations, it may be helpful for asthma sufferers as it eases shortness of breath and increases the amplitude of the breath.

Its astringent properties may relieve uterine haemorrhages as well as heavy periods and generally acts as a tonic to the uterus.

Skin and hair　Its cytophylactic properties make it an ideal oil for mature, wrinkled skin in need of a lift. Its astringent properties may also help balance oily skin conditions.

Precautions　Non-toxic, non-irritant, non-sensitising.

Geranium

Botanical name   *Pelargonium graveolens.*

Family   Geraniaceae.

Synonyms   A common misnomer is *Pelargonium odorantissimum* or *P. odoratissimum.* This species has an apple aroma, grows about 20 cm tall as a creeping or cascading plant and therefore is not the pelargonium species grown for geranium oil production which is about 1 metre tall with a completely different leaf and oil.

Place of origin   Native to South Africa; widely cultivated in Spain, Reunion (Bourbon geranium), Morocco, Egypt and Italy. The Bourbon geranium has been considered to be the finest and most expensive oil, however in recent years the French government has allowed the Bourbon label to be used for oils derived from different countries.

Other species   There are over 700 varieties of cultivated geranium, many of which are grown for ornamental purposes. There are several oil producing species such as *P. odorantissimum* and *P. radens*, but *P. graveolens* is the main one commercially cultivated for its oil.

The most sought after geranium oil is from Bourbon, however this oil is often blended with other, less expensive geranium oils from other countries. Some people refer to the Bourbon geranium as rose geranium, because of its 'rosy' aroma. Most essential oils sold as rose geranium however are inexpensive geranium oils distilled over roses, or a blend of geranium and rose odorants.

Description   A perennial shrub up to 1 metre high with small pink flowers.

Characteristics   Sweet and heavy, a little like rose with a minty overtone.

Part of plant used   Leaves and flowers.

Method of extraction   Steam distillation.

History   There is little mention of geranium in the old manuscripts, although there is reference by Dioscorides to 'geranion', but it is believed to be a different plant.

Chemical constituents   A typical chemical composition of geranium is reported as follows (88):
α–pinene (0.18-0.39%), myrcene (0.21-0.4%), limonene (0.17-0.59%), menthone (0.74-2.11%), linalool (10.26-13.64%), geranyl acetate (0.34-4.38%), citronellol (20.89-27.74%), geraniol (14.36-17.43%), geranyl butyrate (0.58-1.14%).

Blends well with   Bay, basil, bergamot, carrot seed, cedarwood, citronella, clary sage, frankincense, grapefruit, jasmine, lavender, lemon, lime, neroli, orange, palmarosa, patchouli, petitgrain, rose, rosemary, rosewood, sandalwood, ylang-ylang.

Properties   Anti-depressant, antiseptic, astringent, cicatrisant, cytophylactic, diuretic, deodorant, haemostatic, styptic, tonic, vermifuge, vulnerary.

Indications

Mind and spirit   Geranium oil has a balancing effect on the nervous system. It relieves anxiety and depression and lifts the spirits. Because of its balancing action on the adrenal cortex, whose hormones are essentially of a regulatory, balancing nature, it is ideal for treating stress.

Body   Geranium is considered an ideal oil for maintaining homeostasis of the body. Its stimulating effect on the adrenal cortex has a regulatory affect on the hormonal system.

It is therefore useful for treating PMS and menopausal problems such as depression, lack of vaginal secretion and heavy periods. It is also a lymphatic stimulant which can help relieve congestion, fluid retention and swollen ankles.

The oil is a diuretic, and can be used for the treatment of jaundice, gall stones and is effective when general elimination is poor and the system is congested. The haemostatic properties of geranium restrain bleeding from the nose, mouth and internal organs.

Skin and hair   Useful for all skin conditions as it balances sebum, the fatty secretion in sebaceous glands and keeps the skin supple. Good for sluggish, congested and oily skins.

It has cicatrisant and antiseptic properties, making it an excellent remedy for burns, wounds and ulcers.

Precautions   Non-toxic, non-irritant and generally non-sensitising.

Ginger

Botanical name   *Zingiber officinalis.*

Family   Zingiberaceae.

Place of origin   China, Indonesia and the West Indies.

Other species   Another member of the same family is also known as ginger root or Chinese ginger.

Description   A perennial herb up to 1 metre high with thick, spreading, tuberous roots, which are very pungent.

Characteristics   Spicy, sharp, warm and pleasant with a hint of lemon and pepper.

Part of plant used   Roots.

Method of extraction   Steam distillation.

History   A spice highly esteemed through the ages for its therapeutic properties. The Chinese used it to break up phlegm and strengthen the heart. Dioscorides recommended it as a stomachic, to help a sluggish system and as a stimulant of the digestion. Ginger was used in the middle ages to counter the Black Death.

In Ayurvedic medicine ginger was considered a universal medicine, was used to preserve food and treat digestive problems and was also considered a physical and spiritual cleanser. Chinese sailors chewed ginger to prevent sea sickness and Chinese physicians prescribed it to treat arthritis and kidney problems.

Chemical constituents   A typical chemical composition of ginger is reported as follows (89):
α–pinene (trace-0.5%), camphene (0.1-2.1%), β–pinene (trace-2.0%), 1,8-cineole (4.1-11.2%), linalool (0.8-2.7%), borneol (0.5-2.2%),γ–terpineol (0.4-2.4%), nerol (0.1-2.8%), neral (8.1-27.4), geraniol (3.1-23.0%), geranial (12.7-35.8%), geranyl acetate (trace-29.4%), β–bisabolene (0.9-2.9%), zingiberene (1.8%-13.7%).

Blends well with   Atlas cedarwood, bay, black pepper, cajeput, cinnamon, clove, eucalyptus, frankincense, geranium, lemon, lime, myrtle, nutmeg, orange, rosemary, peppermint, tangerine, tea tree, thyme.

Properties   Analgesic, antiseptic, antispasmodic, bactericidal, carminative, cephalic, expectorant, febrifuge, laxative, rubefacient, stimulant, stomachic, sudorific, tonic.

Indications

Mind and spirit   Its warming effect makes it ideal when you are feeling emotionally cold and flat. It sharpens the senses and aids memory. Very stimulating and grounding oil.

Body   Ginger is well known as a warming stimulant and as an aid for digestive problems. It is an ideal remedy for treating nausea or vomiting, including travel sickness. Peter Holmes (90) describes ginger as:

> '...*warming and invigorating for the stomach and intestines, awakening the appetite and settling the stomach.*'

Holmes also suggests that ginger stimulates and warms the uterus, promoting menstruation and easing menstrual cramps.

It is useful for the treatment of colds, coughs and sore throats. It is indicated on the onset of cold or flu, especially if there are feelings of cold, chilliness and fatigue. It is recommended for catarrhal lung conditions.

A massage blend with ginger makes an effective warming massage oil for swellings caused by fluid retention or for rheumatism.

Skin and hair   Helpful in clearing bruises.

Precautions   Non-toxic, non-irritant, may cause sensitisation in some individuals.

Grapefruit

Botanical name   *Citrus paradisi.*

Family   Rutaceae.

Synonyms   *C. racemosa, C. maxima* var. *racemosa.*

Place of origin   Native to tropical Asia and the West Indies. Cultivated in California, Israel and Australia.

Other species   *C.paradisi* is a recent hybrid of *C.maxima* and *C.sinesis*.

Description   A cultivated tree, with glossy leaves and large yellow fruits.

Characteristics   A fresh, sweet and citrusy aroma.

Part of plant used   Fruit rind.

Method of extraction   Cold pressed.

History   The tree was first believed to have been cultivated in the West Indies some time in the eighteeth century. It was then known as 'Shaddock fruit' apparently after the sea captain who introduced the fruit to that part of the world.

Chemical constituents   A typical chemical composition of grapefruit is reported as follows (91):

α–pinene (0.2-1.6%), sabinene (0.7%), myrcene (1.4-2.1%), limonene (86-95%), geraniol (0.1-0.2%), linalool (0.3-0.4%), citronellal (0.14%), decyl acetate (0.15%), neryl acetate (0.2%), terpinen-4-ol (0.08%).

Blends well with   Basil, bergamot, cedarwood, carrot seed, citronella, fennel, frankincense, juniper, geranium, ginger, lavender, lime, orange, palmarosa, rosewood, rosemary, tangerine, ylang-ylang.

Properties   Antidepressant, antiseptic, depurative, diuretic, disinfectant, stimulant, tonic.

Indications

Mind and spirit   It has an overall uplifting and reviving effect making it valuable in states of stress, depression and nervous exhaustion.

Body   Grapefruit oil acts as a lymphatic stimulant and controls liquid processes. It is useful for treating water retention and its detoxifying and diuretic properties make it ideal for treating cellulite. It has a stimulating effect on the digestive system.

Skin and hair   Helpful in treating acne, congested and oily skin.

Precautions   Non-toxic, non-irritant, non-sensitising and non phototoxic.

Hyssop

Botanical name   *Hyssopus officinalis.*

Family   Lamiaceae (Labiatae).

Synonyms   Azob.

Place of origin   France, Spain and Southern Europe.

Other species   There are four main subspecies of hyssop, but *H. officinalis* is the main oil producing species.

Hyssopus officinalis var. *decumbens*, a chemotype of hyssop, produces an oil with very little or no pinocamphone or isopinocamphone.

Description   An attractive perennial, up to 60cm high with a woody stem and purplish blue flowers.

Characteristics   A pleasant aromatic, warm, sweet and penetrating aroma, reminiscent of sage, marjoram and lavender.

Part of plant used   Leaves and flowers.

Method of extraction   Steam distillation.

History   The name comes from the Greek word, hyssopus, itself derived from the Hebrew word ezob, meaning good scented herb. Both the flowers and leaves have been highly valued since antiquity for their therapeutic properties, and it was one of the bitter herbs mentioned in the Old Testament.

Hippocrates, Galen and Dioscorides favoured its bechic and pectoral properties. In pagan festivals, hyssop was sprayed on worshippers to purify them. The Romans used it medicinally and culinarily.

According to Culpeper:

'It is good to wash inflammations, and takes away the blue and black marks that come by strokes, bruises or falls...it is an excellent medicine for the quinsy, or swelling in the throat, to wash and gargle it... The hot vapours of the decoction taken by a funnel in the ears, eases the inflammation and singing noise of them... It is good for falling sickness [epilepsy], expectorates tough phlegm, and is effectual in all cold griefs, or diseases of the chest and lungs.'

Chemical constituents A typical chemical composition of hyssop is reported as follows (92):
α–pinene (0.74%), camphene (0.14%), β–pinene, sabinene (1.72%), myrcene (0.72%), limonene (0.68%), pinocamphone (42.66%), isopinocamphene (30.88%),γ–terpineol (1.00%), 1,8-cineole (0.64%), thujone (0.33%).

Blends well with Carrot seed, cajeput, clary sage, eucalyptus, fennel, lavender, lemon, myrtle, niaouli, orange, rosemary, tangerine, rosemary, tea tree, thyme.

Properties Antiseptic, astringent, antispasmodic, carminative, cicatrisant, digestive, emmenagogue, expectorant, febrifuge, hypertensive, nervine, sudorific, vermifuge, vulnerary.

Indications

Mind and spirit It enhances feelings of alertness and mental clarity. It also eases emotional pain by bringing deep feelings into focus.

Body Hyssop has a special affinity with the respiratory system. It liquefies mucus and relieves bronchial spasms. It is effective for treating colds, sore throats, influenza, bronchitis and asthma. As a hypertensive it has a regulatory effect on the circulation and helps raise low blood pressure.

It is a tonic to the digestive system and acts as a mild laxative, relieves stomach cramps, expels wind and has traditionally been used to eliminate worms.

Relieves menstrual problems associated with water retention during periods and is effective for treating amenorrhoea and leucorrhoea.

Skin and hair Has a healing effect on the skin by helping to form scars and dispersing bruises.

Precautions Non-irritant, non-sensitising; the oil is slightly toxic due to its pinocamphone content. Should be used sparingly and avoided by people suffering from high blood pressure, epilepsy, and during pregnancy.

The presence of terpene ketones such as pinocamphone and isopinocamphone in hyssop oil accounted for its toxicity which caused epileptic crises and cortical and muscular manifestations in laboratory rats (93).

As *Hyssopus officinalis* var. *decumbens* contains very little pinocamphone or isopinocamphone it is relatively safe to use.

Jasmine

Botanical name *Jasminum grandiflorum.*

Family Oleaceae (Jasminaceae).

Synonyms *Jasminum officinalis.*

Place of origin Jasmine orginates from Iran and northern India. It was not until around 1600 when jasmine was brought to Spain by the Moors that it made its first appearence in Europe. It is now commercially cultivated in France, Egypt, Morocco and Italy.

Other species From a botanical point of view, jasmine comes from *Jasminum grandiflorum*, however in order to make the plant more adaptable to different growing conditions, it is often grafted onto *J. officinalis.*

Description An evergreen shrub or vine with delicate, bright green leaves and star shaped very fragrant white flowers.

Characteristics Jasmine is the most exquisite of scents; the oil is a deep reddish-brown colour with a sweet, floral and exotic, slightly heady fragrance.

Part of plant used Flower.

Method of extraction Enfleurage/ solvent extraction.

History Known as the 'king of flowers', it has long been used in perfumery and therapeutically. In China the flowers are used to treat hepatitis, liver cirrhosis and dysentery.

Jasmine was imported from Persia to Europe in the seventeeth century. Grasse, a town in the south of France became the principal supplier of jasmine oil, but that region can no longer meet the high demand. Today huge plantations can be found in Morocco, Algeria and India.

According to Culpepper:

'Jessamine warms the womb and heals schirrhi therein and facilitates the birth. It is useful for coughs and difficulty in breathing.'

Chemical constituents   There are well over 100 constituents found in the oil. A typical chemical composition of jasmine is reported as follows (94):

Benzyl acetate (65%), linalool (15%), benzyl alcohol (5%), indole (2.5%), benzyl benzoate (3%),cis-jasmone (3%), geraniol (10%), methyl anthranilate (0.5%), and trace amounts of p.cresol, farnesol, cis-3-hexenyl benzoate, eugenol, nerol, ceosol, benzoic acid, benzaldehyde, γ−terpineol, nerolidol, isophytol, phytol and many others.

Blends well with   Bergamot, clary sage, frankincense, geranium, lavender, orange, mandarin, neroli, palmarosa, rose, rosewood, sandalwood, ylang-ylang.

Properties   Antidepressant, antiseptic, antispasmodic, aphrodisiac, cicatrisant, expectorant, galactagogue, parturient, sedative, uterine.

Indications

Mind and spirit   The essential oil of jasmine has a great influence on the emotions. Susanne Fischer-Rizzi (95) describes the powerful effects of this heavenly smelling essential oil:

> *'The fragrance diminishes fear, it is helpful in enhancing self confidence and defeating pessimism. No other oil is quite as capable of changing our mood so intensely, it offers little choice other than optimism.'*

Jasmine is especially helpful for emotional dilemmas, particularly when they involve relationships and sex. Existing problems seem easier to solve, because they usually result from unresolved emotional blocks.

According to Marcel Lavabre (96) jasmine is supremely sensual:

> *'Jasmine releases inhibition, liberates imagination and develops exhilarating playfulness.... It has the power to transcend physical love and fully release both male and female sexual energy.'*

Jasmine oil has aptly been called an antidepressant and is equal to melissa, basil and ylang-ylang in this respect.

Body   It is the most valued oil in childbirth. If it is used as a massage oil on the abdomen and lower back in the early stages of labour it will relieve the pain and strengthen the contractions. It helps with the expulsion of the placenta after delivery and aids post-natal recovery.

It is also known as a hormonal balancer and is effective in the treatment of post-natal depression. Can also be used to relieve spasms of the uterus, and soothes menstrual pain.

Skin and hair   It is particularly useful in skin care and is used to treat dry, aggravated skin. It is also used to treat dermatitis and eczema.

Precautions   Non-toxic, non-irritant and generally non-sensitising.

Juniper

Botanical name   *Juniperus communis.*

Family   Cupressaceae.

Place of origin   Native to northern hemisphere: Siberia, Scandinavia, Hungary, France, Italy, the Balkans and Canada.

Other species   In the Balkans an oil is produced from the fruits and twigs of *J. smerka*, less rich and sweet than that of *Juniperus communis*. Other species of juniper include *J oxycedrus* which produces cade oil and *J. sabina* which produces savin oil.

Description   An evergreen shrub or tree which grows up to 6 metres high. It has small flowers and little round berries, which are green in the first year, turning black in the second and third years.

Characteristics   Clear, refreshing and slightly woody.

Part of plant used   Berries; an inferior oil is obtained from the leaves and twigs.

Method of extraction   Steam distillation.

History   Juniper played a major medicinal role in many contagious diseases and was used to guard against the plague by fifteenth and sixteenth century herbalists. Juniper and rosemary twigs were burnt in French hospitals to clear the air and it was looked upon as a cure-all in Yugoslavia. Of course it is famous as an ingredient in gin.

According to Culpeper:

'It is a remedy for dropsy, brings down the terms, helps fits of the mother, expels the wind and strengthens the stomach. It provokes the urine and is good for gout and sciatica, and strengthens the limbs.'

Chemical constituents   A typical chemical composition of juniperberry is reported as follows (97): α–pinene (33.7%), camphene (0.5%), β–pinene (1.1%), sabinene (27.6%), myrcene (5.5%), α–phellandrene (1.3%), α–terpinene (1.9%), γ–terpinene (3.0%), 1,4-cineole (4%), β–phellandrene (1.3%), p-cymene (5.5%), terpinen-4-ol (4.0%), bornyl acetate (0.4%), cayophyllene (0.6%), and trace amounts of limonene, camphor, linalool, linalyl acetate, borneol and nerol.

Blends well with   Bergamot, cypress, fennel, frankincense, geranium, grapefruit, orange, lavender, lemongrass, lemon, lime, rosemary, sandalwood.

Properties   Antiseptic, antirheumatic, antispasmodic, astringent, carminative, depurative, rubefacient, stimulating, stomachic, sudorific, tonic, vulnerary.

Indications

Mind and spirit   Clears, stimulates and strengthens the nerves. It purifies the atmosphere, supporting the spirit in challenging situations.

According to Patricia Davis (98) juniper is great for clearing any negative energy, especially if this is through contact with other individuals with whom one doesn't feel any attunement. She also suggests using the oil for people who feel a sense of uncleanliness in relation to their own lives. This may be due to past actions that they now regret. Juniper oil should be used to help clear these feelings of uncleanliness from the most subtle layers of the aura.

Body   Regarded as one of the most effective detoxifiers and diuretics. It may be used to help eliminate uric acid making it useful for treating gout, arthritis and rheumatism. It is a valuable oil to use for the treatment of cellulite.

Juniper has a special affinity to the urino-genital tract, being the best choice for the treatment of cystitis and pyelitis. Use a douche or hip bath. Cystitis responds well to aromatherapy treatments, but if there is blood or pus in the urine, or fever, do not delay in obtaining medical help. Juniper will dramatically relieve retention of urine.

A study of juniper revealed that it acts by enhancing glomerular filtration and that increased amounts of potassium, sodium and chlorine are excreted. Helpful in relieving urine when the prostate gland is enlarged.

At the 24th International Symposium of Essential Oils, a paper was presented, indicating that juniper oil is not a kidney irritant. It was concluded that the reputation for juniper oil as a renal irritant may have come from the use of juniper oils containing high levels of α and β-pinene which are known irritants to the urinary tract. Higher levels of pinenes would result from co-distillation of needles, branches and unripe berries with ripe berries. It was decided that ripe juniperberries, and oil distilled only from the ripe berries, can be used safely in diuretic therapy. (99)

Juniper oil helps promote the menses and relieves painful menstrual cramps before onset and is beneficial for regulating periods.

Skin and hair   A tonic for oily and congested skins. Its detoxifying and antiseptic properties make it useful for treating acne, blocked pores, dermatitis, weeping eczema, psoriasis and inflammations.

Precautions   Sensitising, may be slightly irritating, non-toxic. Due to its possible nephrotoxic effect, it should not be used by those with kidney disease. Its use during pregnancy is not recommended.

Lavender

Botanical name   *Lavendula angustifolia.*

Family   Lamiaceae (Labiatae).

Synonyms   *Lavendula officinalis, L. vera.*

Place of origin   Indigenous to the Mediterranean region, now cultivated mainly in France, Spain, England and Tasmania.

Other species   There are many varieties of lavender; *Lavendula angustifolia* is divided into two subspecies - *L. fragrans* and *L. stoechas.* Cotton lavender *(Santolina chamaecyparissus)* and sea lavender *(Statice caroliniana)* belong to different botanical families. Lavandin *(Lavandula x intermedia)* is a hybrid plant developed by crossing true lavender with spike lavender.

Description An evergreen woody shrub, up to 1 metre tall, with pale green, narrow linear leaves and violet-blue flowers. The whole plant is highly aromatic.

Characteristics Floral, herbaceous, sweet scent with balsamic woody undertone.

Part of plant used Fresh flowering tops.

Method of extraction Steam distillation.

History Lavender has been used since ancient times as much for its perfume as for its medicinal properties. Romans added lavender to their bath water, hence the name derived from the word 'to wash', lavare. The ancients classified lavender as a stimulant, tonic, stomachic and carminative.

Herbalists regard lavender as the most useful and versatile essential oil for therapeutic purposes.

'This is called lavender. If this be sodden in water, give that water to drink to a man that hath the palsy, and it will heal him. It is hot and dry.'

Blanckes's Herbal.

'It is of especial use in pains of the head and brain which proceed from cold, apoplexy, falling sickness, the dropsy, or sluggish malady, cramps, convulsions, palsies, and often faintings. It strengthens the stomach, and frees the liver and spleen from obstructions, provokes women's courses'

Nicholas Culpeper.

Chemical constituents A typical chemical composition of lavender is reported as follows (100):
α−pinene (0.02-0.67%), limonene (0.02-0.68%), 1,8-cineole (0.01-0.21%), cis-ocimene (1.35-2.87%), trans-ocimene (0.86-1.36%), 3-octanone (1.75- 3.04%), camphor (0.54-0.89%), linalool (29.35-41.62%), linalyl acetate (46.71-53.80%), caryophyllene (2.64-5.05%),

terpinen-4-ol (0.03-4.16%), lavendulyl acetate (027-4.24%).

Blends well with Bay, bergamot, German and Roman chamomile, citronella, clary sage, geranium, jasmine, lemon, mandarin, orange, palmarosa, patchouli, pine, tangerine, thyme, rosemary, rosewood, ylang-ylang.

Properties Analgesic, anticonvulsive, antidepressant, antiphlogistic, antirheumatic, antiseptic, antispasmodic, antiviral, bactericide, carminative, cholagogue, cicatrisant, cordial, cytophylactic, decongestant, deodorant, diuretic, emmenagogue, hypotensive, nervine, rubifacient, sedative, sudorific, vulnerary.

Indications

Mind and spirit It is well known for its nervine - sedative properties, and is useful for treating a variety of nervous and psychological disorders including depression, insomnia, migraine, nervous tension, hysteria and paralysis. As a sedative - analgesic it is very good for headaches and migraines. Like geranium, lavender is considered normalising, hence its considerable versatility.

Lavender is useful to alleviate stress. Stress that becomes counterproductive on a physiological level involves either the sympathetic or parasympathetic nervous system. Sympathetic hyperfunctioning is triggered more by physical stress, while parasympathetic hyperfunctioning is caused more by emotional stress. Both types of stress will produce symptoms such as spasms, cramps, pain, irritability and mental distraction.

Lavender oil will inhibit both the sympathetic and parasympathetic nervous system functions. By selectively inhibiting either sympathetic or parasympathetic nervous excess, lavender can therefore assist responses to unproductive stress of any kind.

Peter Holmes (101) suggests using lavender in an acute crisis situation dominated by sudden, unpredictable and spontaneous change; for example, a family crisis, or stress associated with withdrawal symptoms. He states that lavender can promote personal renewal in every way by washing away past habits and opening us up to new possibilities. It will also help by producing inner acceptance of a painful situation, easing fear and creating the strength that allows us to move on.

Lavender has been the focus of many clinical trials and is being used in many hospital wards as a massage oil, being vaporised to help dispel anxiety, and as an alternative to using orthdox drugs to help patients sleep.

Body Without a doubt if one were to choose only a single essential oil to keep in the first aid kit, lavender would be the undisputed choice. Of all the essential oils lavender is undoubtedly the most versatile. Its antiseptic properties make it ideal to use for treating coughs, colds, catarrh, sinus, flu, as well as the treatment of wounds, ulcers, cystitis and catarrhal discharges.

According to Tisserand, (102) lavender inhibits mycobacterium tuberculosis, staphylococcus, gonococcus, Eberth's bacillus (typhoid) and Leoffler's bacillus (diptheria). Vaporised lavender will destroy pneumococcus and haemolytic streptococcus within 12 to 24 hours.

Being a good antispasmodic it can be used for the management of conditions such as asthma. Bronchitis also responds well to lavender used in massage and inhalations.

Lavender is helpful in the treatment of all types of pain. Headaches respond well to the application of lavender; a drop can be rubbed on the temples or a compress placed on the forehead and back of the neck to bring relief. In cases of muscular pain and rheumatism, lavender's antispasmodic, relaxant and analgesic properties are useful in a massage or bath oil.

Lavender has both a sedative and a tonic action on the heart. It will help lower blood pressure and ease nevous tension and palpitations, while it has a stimulating effect for someone with a weak heart, shortness of breath, fatigue upon exertion, cold extremities and depression.

As an emmenagogue lavender is good for scanty menstruation, and may be used for period pains. It is an excellent remedy for leucorrhoea, used in vaginal douches.

Because of its low toxicity it is considered, along with German and Roman chamomile, one of the safest essential oils to use with children. It is

of benefit for treating childhood infections, cuts, scratches etc.

Skin and hair Lavender is the essential oil most commonly associated with burns and healing of the skin. Its effectiveness in the treatment of burns has led to its use in burns units in European hospitals. It also has antiseptic and analgesic properties which will ease the pain of a burn and prevent infection. As it also has cytophylactic properties it will promote rapid healing and help reduce scarring.

Its anti-inflammatory and soothing properties have a balancing effect on the skin. It can also be used for the treatment of dermatitis, eczema, psoriasis, boils and acne. It may be used in general skin care for all types of skin. When using lavender for inflammatory conditions please use only low concentrations of less than 1%.

Lavender is also useful for the treatment of sunburn and sun stroke. It can be combined with peppermint in a 1% dilution and used as a massage oil. Finally it can be used as an insect repellent and may be used to treat insect bites - preventing the itching and scratching.

Precautions Non-irritant, non-toxic and non-sensitising.

Lavender, Spike

Botanical name *Lavendula spica.*

Family Lamiaceae (Labiatae).

Synonyms *L. latifolia,* aspic.

Place of origin A more robust plant than the true lavender and somewhat taller. It enjoys growing by the sea. The essential oil is commercially produced in Spain, Italy and France.

Other species There are several species of spike lavender. The French spike lavender is reputed to have a more delicate, aromatic scent than the Spanish variety.

A hybrid plant was developed by crossing true lavender *(L. angustifolia)* with spike lavender *(L.latifolia).* This plant is known as lavandin and is a much larger plant than true lavender.

Description   An aromatic evergreen shrub up to 1 metre high with lance-shaped leaves, broader and rougher than true lavender. The flowers are more compressed and of a dull grey-blue colour.

Characteristics   Similar to lavender though clearer and fresher.

Part of plant used   Fresh flowering tops.

Method of extraction   Steam distillation.

History   Culpeper recommends spike lavender for a variety of ailments including:

'Pains of the head and brain which proceed from cold, apoplexy, falling sickness, the dropsy, or sluggish malady, cramps, convulsions, palsies, and often in fainting'.

He also warned that the oil of spike is of a fierce and piercing quality, and ought to be used carefully, a few drops being sufficient for inward or outward maladies.

Spike lavender is listed in the British Herbal Pharmacopoeia, indicated for flatulent dyspepsia, colic, depressive headaches and the oil (topically) for rheumatic pain.

Chemical constituents   A typical chemical composition of spike lavender is reported as follows (103):
α–pinene (1.7%), camphene (0.5%), β–pinene (1.5%), myrcene (1.4%), 1,8-cineole (23.5%), p-cymene (0.6%), camphor (20.0%), linalool (32.4%), terpinen-4-ol (1.5%), borneol (4.6%), geraniol (1.8%).

Blends well with   Bergamot, black pepper, chamomile, eucalyptus, geranium, lemon, marjoram, orange, petitgrain, pine, rosemary, rosewood, sage.

Properties   Analgesic, antidepressant, antiseptic, antispasmodic, cholagogue, cicatrisant, cytophylactic, decongestant, diuretic, emmenagogue, insecticide, rubifacient, sudorific, vulnerary.

Indications

Mind and spirit   It helps clear a stuffy head making the senses calmer yet more alert.

Body   Spike lavender is particularly effective for treating respiratory complaints such as bronchitis and laryngitis. It eases breathing and clears the head, relieving headaches associated with catarrh. Its analgesic properties make it useful for reducing muscular and rheumatic pain promoting relaxation. It is useful in relieving painful insect bites and stings.

Spike lavender has been used for cases of bronchitis, chronic emphysema and asthma (104). The results indicated that it had a positive expectorant effect by acting on secretory motor cells and by dissolving sputum. It also has a detoxifying effect on bacteriotoxins. The article also discusses spike lavender's ability to reduce pain and swelling, and improve blood sedimentation and mobility.

Skin and hair   Spike lavender may be used as an insect repellent. May also be used in skincare as is lavender.

Precautions   Non-toxic, non-irritant and non-sensitising. Due to spike lavender's camphor content (approximately 20%) it may be advisable to avoid using it in cases of pregnancy and epilepsy.

Lemon

Botanical name   *Citrus limon.*

Family   Rutaceae.

Synonyms   *C. limonum.*

Place of origin   A small thorny evergreen tree, native to India now common in southern Europe, Florida and California.

Other species   There are about 47 varieties of lemon.

Description   A fresh and sharp citrus fragrance.

Characteristics   Fresh, sharp, sweet citrus smell.

Part of plant used   Peel of the fruit.

Method of extraction   Cold pressed.

History   The fruit became known in Europe in the middle ages, but it was known to the Greeks and Romans. The therapeutic value of lemons was recognised by the middle ages. Nicholas Lemery in his book on simple drugs in 1698 mentioned lemons as being digestives, as a blood cleanser, and as helping sweeten the breath after a heavy meal. Lemons reached the height of their fame when they were issued to counteract the effects of scurvy in the British Navy.

Chemical constituents A typical chemical composition of lemon is reported as follows (105):
α–pinene (1.8-3.6%), camphene (0-0.1%), β–pinene (6.1-15.0%), sabinene(1.5-4.6%) myrcene (1.0-2.1%), α–terpinene (0-0.5%), linalool (0-0.9%) β–bisabolene(0.56%), limonene (62.1-74.5%), trans–α–bergamotene (0.37%), nerol (0.04%), neral (0.76%).

Blends well with Bergamot, eucalyptus, fennel, frankincense, ginger, juniper, lavender, neroli, rose, rosemary, sandalwood, ylang-ylang.

Properties Anti-anaemic, antimicrobial, antirheumatic, antisclerotic, antiseptic, antispasmodic, astringent, bactericidal, carminative, cicatrisant, depurative, diaphoretic, diuretic, febrifuge, haemostatic, hypotensive, insecticidal, rubifacient, tonic, vermifuge.

Indications

Mind and spirit Refreshing and cooling when feeling hot and bothered. Research in Japan has found that lemon improves one's ability to concentrate. In one study it was found to reduce typing errors by 54%, when the essential oil was vaporised in the air. (106)

Other research into lemon essential oil found that it reduced health symptoms reported. According to Susanne Fischer-Rizzi lemon oil 'hums like a bumblebee' and lifts the spirits, especially during times of mental fatigue. It has been found to be useful for stimulating and clearing the mind and aids the decision making process.

Body Lemon oil is highly prized for its high antibacterial properties. Dr Jean Valnet (107) cites research which shows that the essential oil will kill Diphtheria bacilli in 20 minutes at a low dilution of 0.2%. Lemon oil is able to stimulate the action of the white blood corpuscles, the body's own defence. Lemon oil is also haemostatic.

It improves the functioning of the digestive system, counteracts acidity in the body and makes the stomach more alkaline. Other problems arising from too much acidity in the body give rise to painful symptoms, including rheumatism, gout and arthritis. Whenever the body does not rid itself effectively of uric acid, this forms crystals which cause pain and inflammation of the joints.

Lemon oil can be used in cases of toxaemia, such as rheumatism, arthritis, gout, high blood fat and cholesterol, general obesity, cellulite and abscesses, boils and carbuncles.

Lemon has a tonic effect on the circulatory system and is useful in treating varicose veins. It is helpful in cases of high blood pressure and can be used in preventative regimes against arteriosclerosis.

Skin and hair Being an astringent it has an effective cleansing effect on greasy skin. At the same time its antiseptic properties make it useful for treating cuts and boils.

Precautions Non-toxic, may cause dermal irritation or sensitisation reaction in some people. Phototoxic so avoid using on skin and then exposing to the sun.

Lemongrass

Botanical name *Cymbopogon citratus.*

Family Gramineae.

Synonyms *Andropogon citratus* also known as West Indian lemongrass; *Andropogon flexuosus* also known as East Indian lemongrass.

Place of origin Native to Asia, now cultivated mainly in the West Indies, Africa, and tropical Asia.

Other species There are several varieties of lemongrass of which the East Indian and the West Indian types are most common.

Description A fast growing, tall aromatic perennial grass up to 1.5 metres high.

Characteristics Strong, lemony and herbaceous.

Part of plant used Fresh and partially dried leaves.

Method of extraction Steam distillation.

History   Employed in traditional Indian medicine for infectious illness and fever; modern research in India shows that it also acts as a sedative on the central nervous system.

Chemical constituents   A typical chemical composition of lemongrass is reported as follows (108):

Constituent	C. flexuosus	C. citratus
myrcene	0.21%	8.2-19.2%
limonene	7.77%	trace
linalool	0.8-1.1%	-
citronellal	0.25%	0.1%
citral	79.1%	trace
geranyl acetate	0.85%	1.00%
nerol	0.33%	0.3-0.4%
geraniol	1.95%	0.5-0.4%
neral	-	25-28%
geranial	45.2-55.9%	-
borneol	0.1-0.4%	-

Blends well with   Basil, bergamot, cedarwood, geranium, lavender, lemon, niaouli, palmarosa, petitgrain, rosemary, tea tree.

Properties   Analgesic, antidepressant, antimicrobial, antipyretic, antiseptic, astringent, bactericidal, carminative, deodorant, febrifuge, fungicidal, galactagogue, insecticidal, nervine, sedative (nervous system), tonic.

Indications

Mind and spirit   Its invigorating properties stimulate, revive and energise, useful for treating symptoms of jet lag, clearing the head and relieving fatigue.

Buchbauer (109) investigated a number of inhaled essential oils. Lemongrass oil was found to amplify over-agitation induced by caffeine injection while lavender reduced the over-agitation. This finding is contrary to the reputed sedative effects of the inhaled odour of lemongrass.

Body   It is considered an excellent tonic for the body. It boosts the parasympathetic nervous system which assists recovery from illness, stimulating glandular secretions and the muscles for digestion. Could also be useful for colitis, indigestion and gastroenteritis.

Its strong antiseptic properties prevent the spread of contagious diseases. According to Dietrich Gumbel (110) lemongrass is the 'connective tissue oil'. It has an excellent effect for aching muscles, relieves pain making them more supple.

He suggests that:

> *'One should not miss the application of this oil in the after-care of sports accidents, sprains, inner effusions of blood, bruises and dislocations.'*

The analgesic action of myrcene, a constituent found in *Cymbopogon citratus*, but not in *Cymbopogon flexuosus*, has been confirmed (111).

Skin and hair   It has been used to tone the skin and is effective for open pores. While traditionally recommended to clear acne and balance oily skin conditions, I do not recommend its use for this purpose because it is known to be a dermal irritant.

Precautions   Non-toxic, possibly dermal irritant and/or sensitisation in some individuals, so use with care for skin applications.

Topically applied lemongrass oil has been found to be non-irritant or sensitising at dilutions of up to 3%, whereas isolated citral is a cause of major dermal irritation (112). It appears that other monoterpene constituents of lemongrass exert a quenching effect upon the irritant properties of citral.

Lime

Botanical name   *Citrus medica.*

Family   Rutaceae.

Synonyms   *C. medica* var. *acida, C. latifolia.*

Place of origin   Originally from Asia, the lime fruit is cultivated in many warm countries notably Italy, the West Indies and the Americas.

Other species   There are several species of lime such as the Italian lime *(C. limetta)* and the leech lime *(C. hystrix).*

Description   A small evergreen tree which produces a small bitter fruit similar to a lemon.

Characteristics   The cold expressed lime oil has a fresh, sweet, citrus peel odour. The steam distilled lime oil has a sweeter fresh fragrance reminiscent of lime beverages.

Part of plant used   Peel of the fruit.

Method of extraction   Cold expression of the peel of the unripe fruit and steam distillation of the whole ripe fruit.

History   Apparently introduced into Europe by the Moors and subsequently brought to America by the Spanish and Portuguese explorers around the sixteenth century. Ships bearing lime were called 'lime juicers' since the crews relied upon it to prevent scurvy - a dietary deficiency causing general weakness. Lime has since been a good source of Vitamin C.

Chemical constituents   A typical chemical composition of lime is reported as follows (113):
Cold pressed oil contains approximately: 74% monoterpene hydrocarbons [α–pinene (3%), β–pinene (18.2%), sabinene (3.2%), myrcene (1,2%), limonene (42.7%), γ–terpinene (7.4%), terpinolene (0.5%)]; 1.0% saturated aldehydes [octanal, nonanal, decanal, undecanal, dodecanal, tridecanal, tetradecanal, pentadecanal; trans-α– bergaptene (0.6%), caryophyllene (0.5%), β–bisabolene (1.0%); 6.2% citral- neral and geranial; 0.5% esters- neryl acetate and geranyl acetate] 0.6% monoterpene alcohols [α–terpineol (0.3%), and traces of linalool].

Distilled lime oil contains approximately: α–pinene (0.5-1.6%), β–pinene(0.4-9.0%), myrcene (0.5-1.4%), limonene (42.5-50.3%), terpinolene (3.6-9.3%), 1,8-cineole (0.25-3.0%), linalool (0.05-1.0%), borneol (0.3-0.5%) and traces of neryl acetate and geranyl acetate.

Blends well with   Bergamot, cedarwood, geranium, grapefruit, lavender, lemon, mandarin, neroli, nutmeg, orange, palmarosa, petitgrain, rose, rosemary, rosewood, tangerine, vetiver, ylang-ylang.

Properties   antiseptic, antiviral, astringent, bactericide, disinfectant, febrifuge, haemostatic, restorative, tonic.

Indications

Mind and spirit   Very refreshing and uplifting, ideal for fatigue and a tired mind. Very stimulating and activating especially where there is apathy, anxiety and depression.

Body   As with most citrus oils it is considered a digestive stimulant. It has disinfectant properties so it is useful for treating sore throats and influenza. The cold pressed lime oil also has detoxifying properties.

Skin and hair   Its astringent, toning and refreshing properties help clear oily congested skin.

Precautions   Non-toxic, non-irritant and non-sensitising. However the cold expressed oil is phototoxic.

Mandarin

Botanical name   *Citrus reticulata.*

Family   Rutaceae.

Synonyms   *C. nobilis, C. deliciosa, C. madurensis.*

Place of origin   Produced in Brazil, Spain, Italy and California.

Other species   While tangerine is from the same source, it differs as it is a hybrid of mandarin.

Description   Another member of the orange family, the mandarin is smaller and more spreading than the orange tree, with smaller leaves and fruits which are slightly flattened at both ends. The tangerine is larger than the mandarin and rounder, with a yellower skin, more like the original Chinese type.

Characteristics   Yellow, orange liquid with an intense sweet fresh citrus scent.

Part of plant used   Fruit peel.

Method of extraction   Cold pressed.

History   The name originates from the fruit which was a traditional gift to the mandarins of China. In France it has long been regarded as a safe children's remedy for indigestion and hiccups. It is also useful for the elderly since it helps strengthen the digestive function and the liver.

Chemical constituents   A typical chemical composition of mandarin is reported as follows (114):
α–thujone (0.76-0.96%), α–pinene (2.12-2.54%), camphene (0.02%) sabinene(0.24-0.29%), β–pinene (0.25-1.82%), myrcene(1.69-1.77%), limonene (67.92-74.00%), γ–terpinolene (16.78-21.02%), linalool (0.05-0.16%), citronellal (0.02-0.04%) terpineol-4-ol (0.02-0.06%), nerol (0.01-0.02%), geranial (0.03-0.06%).

Blends well with   Bergamot, German and Roman chamomile, black pepper, grapefruit, jasmine, lavender, lemon, lime, sweet marjoram, neroli, orange, palmarosa, petitgrain, rose, sandalwood, tangerine, ylang-ylang.

Properties   Antiseptic, antispasmodic, carminative, cholagogue, cytophylactic, depurative, digestive, diuretic, sedative, tonic.

Indications

Mind and spirit   Its refreshing aroma has an uplifting quality often used to eliminate depression and anxiety. According to Patricia Davis (115):

'Its delicate aroma breathes a message of happiness, especially to children or the child that is within each of us. It helps us to get in touch with that inner child.'

Body   Mandarin oil has similar properties to tangerine and orange oil - tonic, stomachic and a mild sedative for the nervous system. It has long been used for babies suffering from colic or hiccups. It has a tonic effect on the digestive system, helping to regulate metabolic processes and aids the secretion of bile and breaking down of fats. Also useful for calming the intestines and relieving flatulence.

Skin and hair   Often used in combination with neroli and wheatgerm oil to help prevent stretch marks during pregnancy.

Precautions   Non-toxic, non-irritant and non-sensitising.

Marjoram, Sweet

Botanical name   *Origanum marjorana.*

Family   Lamiaceae (Labiatae).

Synonyms   *Marjorana hortensis.*

Place of origin   Native to the Mediterranean region, Egypt and North Africa. Major oil producing countries are France, Tunisia and Egypt.

Other species   There is much confusion regarding the various species of marjoram. Should not be confused with Spanish marjoram *(Thymus mastichina)* which actually belongs to the thyme species or oregano *(Origanum vulgare)* which is used to produce oregano oil.

Description   A bushy perennial plant growing up to 60 cm high with a hairy stem, dark green oval leaves and small whitish flowers in clusters. The whole plant is strongly aromatic.

Characteristics   A warm, woody, spicy-camphoraceous odour.

Part of plant used   Dried, flowering herb.

Method of extraction   Steam distillation.

History   It was very popular with and a common medicinal plant amongst the ancient Greeks. The name originates from a Greek word meaning 'joy of the mountains'. It is a very useful herb which has been used for its soothing, fortifying and warming effects.

Nicholas Culpeper says of marjoram:

'Our common sweet marjoram is warming and comforting to cold diseases of the head, stomach, sinews (muscles) and other parts, taken inwardly or outwardly applied. The oil is very warm and comforting to the joints that are stiff, and the sinews that are hard, to mollify and supple them.'

Culpeper saw the warming effects as being useful for diseases related to coldness or spasm for almost any part of the body.

Chemical constituents   A typical chemical composition of sweet marjoram is reported as follows (116):
Sabinene (3.0%), α–terpinene (3.0%), γ–terpinene (7.3%), p-cymene (5.3%), terpinolene (2.0%), linalool (3.3%),

cis-sabinene hydrate (7.1%), linalyl acetate (7.4%), terpinen-4-ol (31.6%),γ–terpineol (8.3%).

Blends well with   Bergamot, cedarwood, chamomile, cypress, lavender, mandarin, orange, nutmeg, rosemary, rosewood, ylang-ylang.

Properties   Analgesic, anaphrodisiac, antiseptic, antispasmodic, antiviral, bactericidal, carminative, cephalic, cordial, diaphoretic, digestive, diuretic, emmenagogue, expectorant, fungicidal, hypotensive, laxative, nervine, sedative, stomachic, vasodilator, vulnerary.

Indications

Mind and spirit   Marjoram has a calming effect on the nervous system, relieves anxiety, and stress. It is effective for insomnia especially when there is high blood pressure. Marjoram may be considered a useful remedy for conditions originating from grief as it has a warming and comforting effect on the heart.

Sweet marjoram may be used by those suffering from grief or loneliness, but it should not be over-used since it can have a deadening effect on the emotions. This is probably why sweet marjoram is reputed to be an anaphrodisiac (diminishing the desire for sexual contact).

Body   Applied as a massage oil sweet marjoram is warming and analgesic, making it useful for muscular spasm, rheumatic pains, sprains and strains. It can be used as an inhalation or diluted in a massage oil for most respiratory problems.

Because marjoram stimulates and strengthens intestinal peristalsis it is a good digestive and carminative, relieving constipation, colic, flatulence, and spasmodic indigestion.

Its antispasmodic and emmenagogue properties are beneficial for treating delayed, scanty or painful periods. Used as a massage or hot compress over the lower abdomen, it will ease menstrual cramps.

Skin and hair   Its warming properties make it useful for treating chilblains and it helps disperse bruises.

Precautions   Non-toxic, non-irritant and non-sensitising. Not to be used during pregnancy.

Marjoram, Spanish

Botanical name   *Thymus mastichina.*

Family   Lamiaceae (Labiatae).

Synonyms   Commonly mistaken for oregano.

Place of origin   Spain.

Other species   Not to be confused with sweet marjoram *(Marjorana hortensis).*

Description   A perennial plant growing up to 60 cm high with a hairy stem, dark green oval leaves and small reddish-purple flowers. The whole plant is strongly aromatic.

Characteristics   Warm, penetrating and slightly eucalyptus type odour.

Part of plant used   Dried flowering herb.

Method of extraction   Steam distillation.

Chemical constituents   A typical chemical composition of Spanish marjoram is reported as follows (117):
α–pinene (2.6%). camphene (0.2%), β–pinene (2.0%), sabinene (1.1%), myrcene (0.2%), limonene (2.8%), 1,8-cineole (55.0%), p-cymene (1.3%), camphor (4.0%), linalool (11.1%), linalyl acetate (1.5%), bornyl acetate (0.2%), terpinen-4-ol (0.7%), aromadendrene (0.2%), borneol (0.9%), geranyl acetate (0.1%), geraniol (0.2%).

Blends well with   Bergamot, black pepper, cajeput, clary sage, eucalyptus, ginger, lavender, lemon, nutmeg, peppermint, rosemary, tea tree, thyme.

Properties   Analgesic, antiseptic, antispasmodic, bactericidal, carminative, diaphoretic, digestive, diuretic, expectorant, hypotensive, nervine, stomachic, vasodilator, vulnerary.

Indications   Considered to have similar properties to sweet marjoram so please refer to indications listed under sweet marjoram. Due to the higher 1,8-cineole content of Spanish marjoram, this oil is more effective used as an expectorant for respiratory tract infections and spasms.

Precautions　　Non-toxic, non-irritant and non-sensitising.

May Chang

Botanical name　　*Litsea cubeba.*

Family　　Lauraceae.

Synonyms　　*L. citrata*, tropical verbena. This essential oil has always been known in English by its botanical name 'Litsea cubeba'.

Place of origin　　Native to Asia, especially China. It is cultivated in Taiwan and Japan. China is the main producer of the essential oil.

Other species　　Despite its folk names, it is not related to lemon verbena. It belongs to the same family as the rosewood or cinnamon tree.

Description　　A small tropical tree with fragrant, lemongrass-scented leaves and flowers. The small fruits that it produces are similar to peppers, from which the name 'cubeba' is derived.

The essential oil is chemically similar to lemongrass, melissa and other oils rich in citral, and the therapeutic effects are similar to lemongrass. Its odour, however, is finer than lemongrass; it is more lemon like; closer to a true verbena oil, but at a fraction of the cost.

Characteristics　　A sweet citrus and fruity fragrance.

Part of plant used　　Fruit.

Method of extraction　　Steam distillation.

History　　In traditional Chinese medicine May chang is used to treat dysmenorrhoea that is relieved with heat or pressure, stomach aches, lower back pain, chills, headaches and muscular aches from external conditions.

May chang fruits are reputed to alleviate chronic asthma, as well as being a treatment for coronary heart disease and high blood pressure.

Chemical constituents　　A typical chemical composition of May chang is reported as follows (118):

α–pinene (0.87%), β–pinene (0.39%), myrcene (3.04%), limonene (8.38%), neral (33.80%), geranial (40.61%), nerol (1.09%), geraniol (1.58%), linalool (1.7%), linalyl acetate (1.65%), caryophyllene (0.51%).

Blends well with　　Basil, bergamot, geranium, ginger, jasmine, lavender, lemon, neroli, orange, petitgrain, rose, rosemary, rosewood, ylang-ylang.

Properties　　Antidepressant, antiseptic, astringent, carminative, cordial, galactagogue, hypotensive, insecticide, stimulant, tonic.

Indications

Mind and spirit　　Very uplifting and stimulating.

Body　　May chang is known as a tonic to the heart and respiratory system. Much research has been done in China in the field of heart disease prevention and cure using may chang.

May chang was tested in China against experimentally induced cardiac arrhythmias. It was compared with propranolol (a beta-blocker, antihypertensive and anti-angina drug). The test's results confirmed may chang's ability to reduce arrhythmias from 15 minutes to 6.5 minutes, while propranolol reduced the arrhythymia time from 15 minutes to 0.6 minutes (119).

May chang has also been used as a bronchodilator and may be helpful in cases of bronchitis and asthma.

Skin and hair　　It has a tonic and astringent effect on the skin making it useful for the treatment of acne and oily skin.

Precautions　　Non-toxic, non-irritant and possibly sensitising in some individuals.

Melissa

Botanical name　　*Melissa officinalis.*

Family　　Lamiaceae (Labiatae).

Synonyms　　Commonly called 'lemon balm' or 'balm'.

Place of origin　　A native to the Mediterranean but commonly found in most parts of Europe. Mainly cultivated in Hungary, Egypt, Italy and Ireland.

Other species　　Real melissa rarely finds its way into bottles labelled as such. Most companies sell a 'nature identical' which is a blend of reconstituted essential oils, mainly lemongrass and citronella.

Description A sweet-scented bushy herb which grows up to 90 cm high with serrated leaves and tiny white or pink flowers. The high price of melissa is due to the fact that approximately 3 tonnes of plant material is required to yield approximately 0.5 litres of oil.

Characteristics The scent is often described as being reminiscent of lemons, melissa has a uniquely warm and intensely radiant fragrance.

Part of plant used Leaves and flowering tops.

Method of extraction Steam distillation.

History Melissa comes from the Greek for 'honey bee'. The English herbalist Gerard described the herb as:

> *'comforteth the hart and driveth away sadnesse'*

and physician Paracelsus described it as the 'elixir of life'. Many herbalists praised the uplifting and antidepressant properties of melissa. Nicholas Culpeper wrote that it:

> *'causeth the mind and heart to be merry'.*

The plant gives its name to 'Carmelite Balm Water', a medieval panacea, consisting mainly of distilled melissa, made by the Carmelite monks. Carmelite Balm Water, which was composed of distillates of melissa (30 parts), lemon (30 parts), clove (15 parts), cinnamon (10 parts), coriander (5 parts), marjoram (3 parts) and angelica (3 parts), was recommended for hysterical disorders, digestive problems, palpitations, nervous headaches, neuralgia, and fainting. (120)

Chemical constituents A typical chemical composition of melissa is reported as follows (121): trans-ocimene (0.2%), cis-ocimene (0.1%), 3-octanone (0.6%), methyl hepenone (0.6%), cis-3-hexenol (0.1%), 3-octanol (0.1%), 1-octen-3-ol (1.3%), copaene (4.0%), citronellal (0.7%), linalool (0.4%), β-bourbonene (0.3%), caryophyllene (9.5%), α-humulene (0.2%), neral (24.1%), germacrene D (4.2%), geranial (37.2%), geranyl acetate (0.5%), d-cadinene (1.1%), γ-cadinene (1.0%), nerol (0.1%), geraniol (0.1%).

Blends well with Bergamot, cedarwood, geranium, jasmine, lavender, lemon, sweet marjoram, neroli, rose, ylang-ylang.

Properties Antidepressant, antispasmodic, bactericidal, carminative, cordial, diaphoretic, emmenagogue, febrifuge, hypotensive, nervine, sedative, stomachic, sudorific, tonic.

Indications

Mind and spirit Many herbalists have praised melissa's uplifting and antidepressant properties.

Susanne Fischer-Rizzi describes (122):

> *'The spirit of balm seems like a gift from heaven ... for overstimulation of our nervous system that causes stress, anxiety, insomnia, depression and lost inner direction.'*

Research studies have confirmed melissa's sedative properties. Wagner and Sprinkmeyer (123) found that sedation increased slightly between thirty and sixty minutes after application, and remained constant for two hours. The study also found that smaller doses (1mg/kg) were more effective than larger doses (3mg/kg).

Body Melissa is one of the few essential oils which has been confirmed as having great antiviral properties. Studies in Germany have also found melissa to possess antiviral properties against viruses associated with influenza, herpes, smallpox and mumps.

According to Dr Wabner, a combination of rose and melissa oils was effective in the management of *Herpes simplex* (cold sore infections) and *Herpes zoster* (Shingles). Dr Wabner suggests that adults apply the undiluted essential oil directly onto the blisters. The herpes often disappears within 24 hours. Care should be taken to apply the oil to the blisters only, not to the surrounding skin, to minimize irritation. (123)

Melissa may also be used to settle upset stomachs, being recommended for nausea and indigestion.

Skin and hair One of the problems with melissa is that there is a risk of allergic reaction or irritation due to the high aldehyde content. This is curious as melissa is often indicated by some aromatherapists in the management of allergic skin problems.

There is evidence that the allergic reaction is likely to occur from individual aldehydes rather than from the whole oil.

Precautions   Non-toxic, possibly sensitising and dermal irritant. Please ensure that pure melissa oil is used and not a 'nature identical' or reconstituted melissa oil.

Myrrh

Botanical name   *Commiphora myrrha.*

Family   Burseraceae.

Synonyms   *Balsamodendrom myrrha.*

Place of origin   Native to north east Africa and south west Asia, especially the Red Sea region (Somalia, Yemen and Ethiopia).

Other species   There are several species of myrrh: African or Somali myrrh (*C. molmol*) and Arabian or Yemen myrrh (*C. abyssinica*).

Description   The *Commiphora* species which yields myrrh are shrubs up to 10 metres high. The trunk exudes a natural oleoresin, a pale yellow liquid which hardens into reddish brown tears, known as myrrh. The native collectors make incisions in the bark of the tree to increase the yield.

Characteristics   The essential oil is a dark brown oily liquid with a warm, rich spicy balsamic odour.

Part of plant used   The crude oleoresin.

Method of extraction   Steam distillation.

History   Myrrh was well known to the ancients. It was an ingredient of incense used for religious ceremonies and fumigations by the ancient Egyptians. It was also an ingredient of the famous Egyptian perfume 'kyphi', and was an important ingredient in embalming. Because of its ability to preserve the flesh myrrh oil was used as a cosmetic ingredient. It was reputed to reduce wrinkles and preserve a youthful complexion. Egyptian women used myrrh in their facial preparations. It has a slightly cooling effect on the skin, and so would be especially useful in a hot dry climate.

Myrrh's therapeutic properties are frequently mentioned in the Old and New Testaments, the Koran, and in Greek and Roman texts. Joseph Miller is very informative regarding the properties of myrrh:

> '*Myrrh is of an opening, heating, drying nature, resists putrefaction, and is of great service in uterine disorders, opening any obstruction of the womb, procuring the menses, expediting the birth, and expelling the secundines. It is good likewise for old coughs and hoarseness, and the loss of voice, and is very useful against pestilential and infectious distempers, both taken inwardly, and flung upon burning coals and the fumes received. Outwardly applied it cures wounds and ulcers, and prevents gangreens and mortifications.*'

Chemical constituents   According to Guenther (124), the oil of myrrh was reported to contain α–pinene, cadinene, limonene, cuminaldehyde, eugenol, m-cresol, a tricyclic sesquiterpene hydrocarbon then known as heerabolene, acetic acid, formic acid, and some other unidentified sesquiterpenes and acids.

Blends well with   Frankincense, lavender, palmarosa, patchouli, rose, rosewood, sandalwood, tea tree, thyme.

Properties   Anticatarrhal, anti-inflammatory, antimicrobial, antiphlogistic, antiseptic, astringent, balsamic, carminative, cicatrisant, emmenagogue, expectorant, fungicidal, sedative, digestive and pulmonary stimulant, stomachic, tonic, uterine, vulnerary.

Indications

Mind and spirit   Myrrh is one of the most renowned incenses along with frankincense. Myrrh is thought to enhance spirituality and may be used either in an oil burner or inhaled directly. Use it as a meditation aid or before any healing session.

Myrrh is particularly valuable for people who feel stuck emotionally or spiritually and want to move forward in their lives.

Body   Myrrh prevents infection and putrefaction, clears toxins and promotes tissue repair.

Myrrh is an excellent expectorant and as such is of value in coughs, bronchitis, colds and any condition involving excessive thick mucus, not only expelling mucus but soothing mucous membranes.

only expelling mucus but soothing mucous membranes.

It generates warmth and stimulates the stomach, thus being a useful remedy for treating diarrhoea, flatulence, abdominal distension and poor appetite. Myrrh tincture can be used as a mouthwash or gargle for the treatment of mouth ulcers, inflammation of the mouth (stomatitis) and pyorrhoea.

Myrrh is a uterine stimulant and promotes menstruation thus relieving painful periods and may be used for assisting prolonged, difficult labour during childbirth.

Skin and hair   The efficacy of myrrh for the treatment of chronic wounds and ulcers is legendary. This is due to its antiseptic, astringent, anti-inflammatory and antiphlogistic properties. It is specially valuable for wounds that are slow to heal, and for weepy eczema and athlete's foot. Myrrh is ideal in skin creams for deep cracks on the heels and hands.

Precautions   Non-irritant, non-sensitising, possibly toxic in high concentrations. Not to be used in pregnancy as it is a uterine stimulant.

Myrtle

Botanical name   *Myrtus communis.*

Family   Myrtaceae.

Synonyms   Corsican pepper.

Place of origin   Native to North Africa, cultivated throughout the Mediterranean.

Other species   Part of the same family which includes eucalyptus and tea tree, and bayberry or wax myrtle *(Myrica cerifera)* and the Dutch myrtle or English Bog myrtle *(Myrica gale)* which are used in herbal medicine though their essential oils are said to be poisonous.

Description   A large bush or small tree with many tough but slender branches, a brownish red bark and small sharp pointed leaves. It has flowers followed by small black berries; both the leaves and flowers are very fragrant.

Characteristics   A pale yellow or orange liquid with a clear, fresh, camphoraceous, sweet herbaceous scent similar to eucalyptus.

Part of plant used   Leaves and twigs.

Method of extraction   Steam distillation.

History   The ancient Egyptians knew of the therapeutic properties of myrtle, macerating the leaves in wine to counter fever and infection. Theophrastus later confirmed its place in therapy. Dioscorides also prescribed a wine in which the leaves had been macerated: this fortified the stomach and was effective for pulmonary and bladder infections, and for those who were spitting blood.

In 1876, Dr Delious de Savignac recommended myrtle for bronchial infections, for problems of the genito-urinary system, and for haemorrhoids. (125)

Chemical constituents   A typical chemical composition of myrtle is reported as follows (126):

α-pinene (8.18%), β-pinene (0.19%), limonene (7.58%), 1,8-cineole (29.89%), α-terpinen-4-ol (0.22%), myrtenol (0.58%), geraniol (0.3%), linalyl acetate (0.53%), myrtenyl acetate (35.9%), carvacrol (0.6%).

Blends well with   Bergamot, clary sage, clove, hyssop, eucalyptus, ginger, lavender, peppermint, rosemary, spearmint, thyme, tea tree.

Properties   Anticatarrhal, antiseptic, astringent, balsamic, bactericidal, expectorant.

Indications

Mind and spirit   Uplifting and refreshing effect. Myrtle may also soothe feelings of anger, greed, envy or fear. Susanne Fischer-Rizzi (127) suggests using myrtle for people with addictions or self destructive behaviours:

'Myrtle is helpful for people whose body seems draped in a gray brown veil from smoking, drug abuse, or emotions like anger, greed, envy or fear. In such cases myrtle oil helps to cleanse the person's delicate inner being to dissolve disharmony.'

Body   Myrtle is antiseptic and bactericidal, particularly in pulmonary and urinary infections. It is used in chronic conditions of the lungs, where there is excessive bronchial catarrh. Because of its low irritant characteristics it is suitable for children's coughs and chest complaints.

For the treatment of haemorrhoids the oil has an astringent effect particularly when mixed with witch hazel and cypress oil.

Skin and hair   The oil has long been used in cosmetic preparations, such as facial toners to cleanse oily, infected skin and acne. Myrtle oil has antiseptic and deodorising properties.

Precautions   Non-toxic, non-irritant and non sensitizing.

Neroli

Botanical name   *Citrus aurantium* var. *amara*.

Family   Rutaceae.

Synonyms   Orange flower or blossom, neroli bigarade.

Place of origin   Italy, Morocco, Egypt, France.

Other species   There are two types of orange tree, the sweet orange *(Citrus sinensis)* and the bitter orange. Oil from orange blossoms is known as neroli oil, and is extracted from the white blossoms of the bitter orange. Sweet orange flowers also yield an essence but it is of an inferior quality.

Description   An evergreen tree up to 10 metres high with glossy leaves and fragrant white flowers.

Characteristics   A powerful but delicate bitter-sweet floral fragrance.

Part of plant used   Fresh flowers.

Method of extraction   Steam distillation.

History   Although oranges have been known since the first century, it wasn't until the late seventeenth century that neroli oil was discovered; it was named after Anna Maria de la Tremoille, Princess of Nerola. The oil's therapeutic properties were valued at this time by the people of Venice who used it against the plague and other fevers.

Chemical constituents   A typical chemical composition of neroli is reported as follows (128):
α–pinene, camphene, β–pinene, α–terpinene, nerol, neryl acetate, farnesol, geraniol, linalool, nerolidol, linalyl acetate, methyl anthranilate, and indole.

Blends well with   Bergamot, clary sage, German and Roman chamomile, frankincense, geranium, jasmine, lavender, lemon, lime, mandarin, orange, palmarosa, rose, rosemary, rosewood, sandalwood, tangerine, ylang-ylang.

Properties   Antidepressant, antiseptic, antispasmodic, bactericidal, carminative, cicatrisant, cordial, deodorant, digestive, stimulant.

Indications

Mind and spirit   Neroli is considered one of the most effective sedative and antidepressant essential oils. It is useful for treating depression and is used in a similar way to rescue remedy in Bach flower therapy. It may be used as a natural tranquilliser for anxiety, depression or shock. Susanne Fischer-Rizzi (129) describes the sweet scent of neroli as:

> *'reaches deep down into the soul to stabilise and regenerate. It provides relief and strength for long standing psychological tension, exhaustion, and seemingly hopeless situations.'*

It is particularly useful for insomnia, particularly when the sleeplessness arises from anxiety. It is best used in the bath before bedtime.

Body   Neroli is well known for its ability to relieve muscle spasm of the smooth muscles, especially that of the small intestines. It is extremely useful for chronic diarrhoea, especially when this arises from nervous tension.

A recent clinical trial in England involved the use of neroli oil and foot massage for cardiac surgery patients. The results of the trial confirmed neroli's antispasmodic properties. Neroli was effective in diminishing the amplitude of heart muscle contraction, thus benefiting people who suffer from palpitations or other types of cardiac spasm. (130)

Skin and hair   Neroli oil is suitable for all skin types. Since it does not irritate, it may be used for the care and treatment of sensitive skin and inflamed skin. The essential oil is also useful for the treatment of broken capillaries under the skin's surface. It is an excellent oil which stimulates cellular activity and growth.

Precautions Non-toxic, non-irritant and non-sensitising.

Niaouli

Botanical name *Melaleuca viridiflora.*

Family Myrtaceae.

Place of origin Native to Australia and New Caledonia.

Description An evergreen tree with a flexible trunk and spongy bark, pointed linear leaves and bearing spikes of sessile flowers.

Characteristics A colourless, pale yellow or greenish liquid with a sweet, fresh, camphoraceous odour.

Method of extraction Steam distillation.

Part of plant used Leaves and young twigs.

History Sometimes referred to by the French term 'Gomenol' though assigned its botanical name during Captain Cook's voyage to Australia. Like cajeput it did not appear in Europe until the seventeenth century.

Chemical constituents A typical chemical composition of niaouli is reported as follows (131):
1,8-cineole, γ-terpineol, limonene, α-phellandrene, α- and β-pinene, linalool and piperitone.

Blends well with Basil, cajeput, eucalyptus, fennel, juniper, lavender, lemon, lime, myrtle, orange, pine, rosemary, peppermint, tea tree, thyme.

Properties Analgesic, antirheumatic, antiseptic, bactericide, cicatrisant, decongestant, febrifuge, insecticide, stimulant, vermifuge, vulnerary.

Indications

Mind and spirit Generally stimulating and uplifting. Clears the head.

Body Niaouli is considered an excellent antiseptic for treating pulmonary infections such as bronchitis, catarrh and sinus. For respiratory problems it blends well with peppermint, eucalyptus, pine and myrtle. Also used to treat cystitis.

Skin and hair Aids healing and is antiseptic for treating acne, boils, ulcers, burns and cuts. Useful for washing infected wounds.

Precautions Non-toxic, non-irritant, non-sensitising.

Nutmeg

Botanical name *Myristica fragrans.*

Family Myristicaceae.

Synonyms *M. aromata, Nux moschata.*

Place of origin Native to the Moluccas; cultivated in Indonesia, Sri Lanka, and the West Indies.

Other species The essential oil of nutmeg from Indonesia and Sri Lanka is referred to as the 'East Indian' nutmeg and is considered superior, while Granada produces the 'West Indian' nutmeg oil.

Description An evergreen tree up to 20 metres high with greyish-brown smooth bark, dense foliage and small dull-yellow flowers. 'Mace' is the name given to the bright red shell and seed, which are together contained within the fleshy fruit.

Characteristics A pale yellow liquid with a sweet, warm spicy odour.

Part of plant used The dried nutmeg seed.

Method of extraction Steam or water distillation.

History Nutmeg and mace are widely used as domestic spices in the East and West. They have been used for centuries as a remedy for digestive and kidney problems. In Malaysia nutmeg is used during pregnancy to strengthen and tone the uterine muscles. Nutmeg is currently listed in the British Herbal Pharmacopoeia for flatulent dyspepsia, nausea, diarrhoea, dysentery, and topically for rheumatism.

In Indonesia, nutmeg has traditionally been used to alleviate stomach cramps, flatulence, vomiting, rheumatism, whooping cough and nervousness. Nutmeg is still used in Indonesia as a body oil to warm and invigorate the body and alleviate the symptoms of influenza.

Chemical constituents   A comparison in chemical composition of the East Indian and West Indian nutmeg oil is as follows (132):

Constituent	East Indian Nutmeg	West Indian Nutmeg
α–pinene	18.0-26.5%	10.6-13.2%
camphene	0.3-0.4%	0.2%
β–pinene	9.7-17.7%	7.8-12.1%
sabinene	15.4-36.3%	42.0-50.7%
myrcene	2.2-3.7%	2.5-3.4%
α–phellandrene	0.4-1.0%	0.4-0.7%
α–terpinene	0.8-4.0%	0.8-4.2%
limonene	2.7-3.6%	3.1-4.4%
1,8-cineole	1.5-3.2%	2.5-4.2%
γ–terpinene	1.3-6.8%	1.9-4.7%
linalool	0.2-0.9%	0.3-0.9%
terpinen-4-ol	2.0-10.9%	3.5-6.1%
safrole	0.6-3.2%	0.1-0.2%
methyl eugenol	trace-1.2%	0.1-0.2%
myristicin	3.3-13.5%	0.5-0.9%

Blends well with   Bay, black pepper, cajeput, clary sage, eucalyptus, geranium, ginger, lavender, lime, mandarin, orange, peppermint, petitgrain, rosemary, ylang-ylang and most spice oils.

Properties   Analgesic, antirheumatic, antiseptic, antispasmodic, carminative, digestive, emmenagogue, parturient, prostaglandin inhibiter, stimulant, tonic.

Indications

Mind and spirit   Invigorates and stimulates the mind. Nutmeg is known for its psychotropic effects.

Body   It is a tonic and is recommended as a stimulant and cardiac tonic. It is most useful as a digestive stimulant, helping people who cannot assimilate food. Also useful for the treatment of wind, nausea, chronic vomiting, and diarrhoea.

Bennett et al (133) investigated the effect of eugenol, a constituent of nutmeg oil, for the treatment of diarrhoea. Eugenol was found to inhibit prostaglandin synthesis, thus lowering intestinal fluid accumulation. Eugenol also showed anti-inflammatory activity confirming its benefits in treating inflammations associated with arthritis.

Nutmeg is traditionally used in South East Asia as a tonic for the reproductive system. It is used to regulate scanty periods and soothes pain. Because of its parturient property, it should not be used during pregnancy. It is an excellent oil to add to a massage oil because of its warming property for muscular aches and pains as well as rheumatism.

Skin and hair   Not recommended for skin care use.

Precautions   Nutmeg is generally non-toxic, non-irritant, and non-sensitising.

The psychotropic effects often associated with nutmeg are believed to be due to the myristicin and elemicin found in the nutmeg (134). It is possible that myristicin and elemicin are metabolised to TMA (3,4,5-trimethoxyamphetamine) or MMDA (3-methoxy-4,5-methylenedioxyamphetamine), both of which are hallucinogenic substances. (135)

However, closer investigation has revealed the following (136):

Component	Psychotropic effect
whole nutmeg	highly active
whole nutmeg less the essential oil	no activity
nutmeg oil	weakly active
myristicin on its own	no activity

It appears that the psychotropic properties are due not only to the myristicin and elemicin but to other constituents found in the nutmeg.

While ground nutmeg is moderately to strongly psychotropic when taken in high doses, the effect of the essential oil is very weak, and it appears that non-oral doses will not have any effect at all.

Orange, sweet

Botanical name   *Citrus sinensis.*

Family   Rutaceae.

Synonyms   *C. aurantium* var. *dulcis.*

Place of origin   The orange tree is a native of China and India and was brought to Europe in the seventeenth century. It is now cultivated in the Mediterranean region, Israel and the Americas.

Other species   There are numerous cultivated varieties of sweet orange, for example Jaffa, Navel and Valencia.

Description   An evergreen tree, smaller than the bitter variety, less hardy with fewer or no spines. The fruit has a sweet pulp and non-bitter membrane.

Characteristics   A zesty and refreshing citrus fragrance.

Part of plant used   Fresh ripe or almost ripe outer peel.

Method of extraction   Cold pressed.

History   Orange was first brought to Europe by the Arabs, probably in the first century. A very nutritious fruit, containing vitamins A, B and C. In Chinese medicine the dried sweet orange peel is used to treat coughs, colds, and anorexia.

Chemical constituents   A typical chemical composition of orange is reported as follows (137):
α–pinene (0.52%), sabinene (0.38%), myrcene (2.03%) limonene (95.79%), linalool, (0.28%), citronellal (0.04%), neral (0.04%), geranial (0.06%).

Blends well with   Bergamot, cinnamon, clary sage, clove, cypress, frankincense, geranium, jasmine, juniper, lavender, neroli, nutmeg, petitgrain, rose, rosewood, sandalwood, tangerine, ylang-ylang.

Properties   Antidepressant, antiseptic, antispasmodic, carminative, cholagogue, digestive, febrifuge, sedative, stimulant (digestive and lymphatic), stomachic, tonic.

Indications

Mind and spirit   The cheerful, sensuous and radiant nature of orange conveys warmth and happiness. It assists people to relax and unwind. Orange oil is described by Susanne Fischer-Rizzi as (138):

> *'parfum d'ambiance: Its influence on mood is positive and joyful; it harmonises feelings and awakens creativity.'*

It is an ideal oil to use at home or for use as an introduction to aromatherapy. Children love the smell of orange, it can be used to help them sleep.

Body   The properties of orange oil overlap to a large extent with those of neroli (obtained from orange blossoms). Orange oil appears to have a normalising effect on the peristaltic action of the intestines, it is recommended for the treatment of constipation and is helpful for treating chronic diarrhoea. It stimulates lymph fluids, which is helpful in treating swollen tissue. As a cholagogue it stimulates the gall bladder.

Skin and hair   The oil is beneficial and soothing to dry, irritated, or acne prone skin conditions.

Precautions   Generally non-toxic, non-irritant and non-sensitising.

Palmarosa

Botanical name   *Cymbopogon martinii.*

Family   Gramineae.

Synonyms   *Andropogon martinii*, East Indian geranium.

Place of origin   Originally from India, now cultivated in the Comoro Islands and Madagascar.

Other species   Lemongrass and citronella also belong to the same family. It is also closely related to gingergrass which is a different chemotype known as *C. martinii* var. *sofia.*

Description   A wild growing plant with long slender stems and terminal flowering tops, the grassy leaves are very fragrant.

Characteristics   A sweet, floral slightly dry fragrance with a hint of rose.

Part of plant used   Fresh or dried grass.

Method of extraction   Steam or water distillation.

History   Also known as 'Indian Geranium Oil' and often used to adulterate the more expensive rose.

Chemical constituents   A typical chemical composition of palmarosa is reported as follows (139):
myrcene (0.13-0.28%), linalool (2.26-3.91%), geraniol (76.3-82.8%), geranyl acetate (5.09-11.8%), dipentene, limonene (0.15-2.16%).

Blends well with   Bergamot, citronella, geranium, jasmine, lavender, lime, neroli, orange, petitgrain, rose, rosewood, sandalwood, ylang-ylang.

Properties   Antiseptic, bactericide, cytophylactic, febrifuge, hydrating.

Indications

Mind and spirit   It has a calming yet uplifting effect on emotions.

Body   Acts as a tonic to the digestive system and is said to have a beneficial effect on pathogens in the intestinal flora. Stimulates the appetite and may be helpful to people suffering from anorexia nervosa.

Skin and hair   Palmarosa has a hydrating effect on skin tissue and stimulates natural secretion of sebum. It is also used to stimulate cellular regeneration.

Precautions   Generally non-toxic, non-irritant and non-sensitising.

Patchouli

Botanical name   *Pogostemon patchouli.*

Family   Lamiaceae (Labiatae).

Synonyms   *P. patchouly.*

Place of origin   Malaysia, Indonesia, India and China.

Other species   Closely related to Java patchouli (*P. heyneanus*), which is also known

as false patchouli, occasionally used to produce an essential oil.

Description   A perennial bushy herb up to 1 metre tall with sturdy, hairy stem, large, fragrant, furry leaves with white flowers.

Characteristics   A strong earthy and exotic fragrance.

Part of plant used   Dried leaves, usually subjected to fermentation.

Method of extraction   After drying the leaves and young shoots in the sun, they are steam distilled.

History   The name patchouli is from India and has a long history of medicinal uses in India, China, Malaysia and Japan. It was a renowned antidote against insect and snake bites.

Dried patchouli leaves were placed amongst folds of Indian cashmere shawls in Victorian times to protect the merchandise from moths. Patchouli is a popular base fixative in many Oriental type perfumes.

Chemical constituents   A typical chemical composition of a patchouli oil from Indonesia is as follows (140):
β-patchoulene (2.9-3.8%), α-guaiene (13.1-15.2%), caryophyllene (3.3-3.9%), α-patchoulene (5.1-5.9%), seychellene (8.6-9.4%), α-bulnesene (14.7-16.8%), norpatchoulenol (0.5%), patchouli alcohol (32.0-33.1%), and pogostol.

Blends well with   Bergamot, black pepper, clary sage, frankincense, geranium, ginger, lavender, lemongrass, myrrh, neroli, rose, rosewood, sandalwood, ylang-ylang.

Properties   Antidepressant, antiphlogistic, antiseptic, aphrodisiac, astringent, cicatrisant, cytophylactic, deodorant, diuretic, febrifuge, fungicide, insecticide, sedative, tonic.

Indications

Mind and spirit   This is one of the oils that Rovesti found useful when dealing with anxiety and depression. Patricia Davis (141) suggests using patchouli:

'for dreamers and people who tend to neglect or feel detached from their bodies. This may be considered useful for people who are engaged

on a spiritual path and are placing an undue share of importance on their mental/psychic experiences, to the detriment of their physical wellbeing.'

Patchouli will help ground and integrate energy and keep us in touch with our physical selves.

Body   Patchouli's binding action is due to its strong astringent and cicatrisant properties. It also has diuretic properties which make it useful in the case of fluid retention and cellulite. It also has a significant deodorising effect.

Skin and hair   Patchouli is used as a tissue regenerator helping stimulate regrowth of skin cells and forming scar tissue. Assists healing rough, cracked skin, sores, and wounds. Also useful for treating acne, eczema, fungal infections and scalp disorders.

Precautions   Generally non-toxic, non-irritant and non-sensitising.

Peppermint

Botanical name   *Mentha piperita.*

Family   Lamiaceae (Labiatae).

Place of origin   USA, Tasmania.

Other species   There are several species of peppermint. Originally a cultivated hybrid of *M. aquatica.* A mint grown in Japan, called *Mentha arvensis*, has such a high menthol content that menthol crystals may appear on the surface of the leaves.

Description   A perennial herb up to 1 metre high with underground runners by which it is easily propagated.

Characteristics   Strongly piercing, refreshing, sharp, menthol fragrance.

Part of plant used   Leaves and flowering tops.

Method of extraction   Steam distillation.

History   Mint was mentioned in Egyptian herbals as a stomach soother. From the Middle East, mint spread to Greece and entered Greek mythology. It is from Greek mythology that the name Mentha is derived. Pluto, god of the dead, fell in love with Minthe, a beautiful nymph.

Pluto's goddess-wife Persephone became jealous and changed Minthe into a plant. Pluto could not bring Minthe back to life, but he gave her plant form a fragrant aroma. The plant's botanical name, Mentha, was derived from the name 'Minthe'.

Peppermint, the most common of mints, has always been valued for its therapeutic properties.

'These grateful aromatics are rapidly absorbed into the system, and behave as mild diffusible stimulants. Coming into contact with the gastric mucous membrane, they exercise at first a stimulating and afterwards a local sedative effect, dispelling nausea, and correcting uneasiness. By their local stimulating action on the bowel they correct the irregular painful sensations caused by accumulations of flatus, giving speedy relief, probably through reflex act by driving on the imprisoned gas. Often after a large dose, pain instantly disappears, and flatus is expelled, and this may be frequently observed in infants and feeble females.'

William Whitla.

Culpeper says of peppermint:

'It is useful for complaints of the stomach, such as wind and vomiting, for which there are few remedies of greater efficacy.'

Today many practitioners, doctors and scientists have confirmed the therapeutic values of peppermint as being stomachic, carminative and antispasmodic, a tonic and stimulant; as being good for nervous disorders, nervous vomiting, flatulence and colitis.

Peppermint is used in two medicinal products 'Mintec' and 'Colpermin' which are used for the treatment of irritable bowel syndrome. Both products contain peppermint oil in enterically coated capsules designed not to dissolve until they reach the large intestine.

Chemical constituents   A typical chemical composition of peppermint is reported as follows (142):
Menthol (40.0%), menthone (18.7%), 1,8-cineole (7.3%), methyl acetate (3.8%), methofuran (3.0%), isomenthone(2.5%), limonene (2.5%), β–pinene (1.8%), α–pinene (1.4%), germacrene-d (1.3%), trans-sabinene hydrate (1.0%), pulegone (0.8%).

Blends well with   Basil, bergamot, cajeput, cedarwood, cypress, eucalyptus, lemon, lime, mandarin, marjoram, niaouli, pine, rosemary, spearmint, thyme.

Properties   Analgesic, anaesthetic, antigalactagogue, antiphlogistic, antiseptic, antispasmodic, astringent, carminative, cephalic, cholagogue, cordial, decongestant, emmenagogue, expectorant, febrifuge, hepatic, nervine, stimulant, stomachic, sudorific, vaso-constrictor, vermifuge.

Indications

Mind and spirit   Peppermint oil helps people becomes clear headed and refreshes the spirits. It may be beneficial for people who are unable to concentrate or who have mental fatigue. Peppermint is one of the oils described as a cephalic, making it ideal to use in an oil burner, in the office, in conference rooms, or in situations in which clear thinking and mental stimulation are required.

Body   Because of its antiseptic and expectorant properties, the oil may be beneficial in the treatment of colds and flu. It is ideal to use for sinus congestion, infection, or inflammation, and for a congestive headache. For headaches and migraines related to digestive or hepatic problems it is an excellent remedy.

It is an ideal remedy for all digestive disorders including indigestion, colic, flatulence, stomach pains, diarrhoea. It is an effective remedy for nausea and vomiting and is good for relieving travel sickness. Peppermint stimulates the gall bladder and secretion of bile. Therefore, it has been used for gall bladder attacks and gallstones.

The antispasmodic properties of peppermint have been confirmed in clinical trials. In one trial peppermint oil was found to be beneficial in helping reduce colonic spasm during endoscopy (143).

In another trial patients who were experiencing difficulties with their colostomies were given oral doses of enteric-coated capsules containing peppermint. Peppermint had been chosen as it not only had an odour which would help mask the odour from the colostomy bag, but also because of its effect on the smooth muscle of the bowel. It reduced colonic pressure and prevented foaming, all of which helped to reduce post-operative colic and the frequency of bag change. (144)

According to Dietrich Gumbel (145) peppermint oil has a special connection to everything aqueous, to blood, to tissue fluid, lymph, spinal and cerebral fluid. It is used in massage to stimulate the lymph system and drainage of lymph fluids.

Peppermint is used in linaments for the relief of muscle pain, lumbago, bruises and contusions, joint pain and insect bites. The local anaesthetic action of peppermint oil is quite strong.

Skin and hair   Peppermint can be used to relieve any kind of skin irritation or itching, but should be used in a dilution of 1% or less or the irritation will be made worse. It may be used for skin redness due to inflammation, or acne; it cools by constricting the capillaries, and is a very refreshing skin tonic.

Precautions   Non-toxic, non-irritant (except in concentration), possibly sensitising due to menthol. Use in moderation.

Petitgrain

Botanical name   *Citrus aurantium* var. *amara*.

Family   Rutaceae.

Synonyms   *C. bigaradia*, petitgrain bigarade.

Place of origin   The best quality comes from France. Also produced in North Africa and Paraguay.

Other species   The petitgrain oils are obtained from the leaves of citrus trees. The most commonly available petitgrain oil is derived from the bitter-orange tree.

Description   The oil of petitgrain is produced from the leaves and twigs of the same tree that produces bitter orange oil and neroli oil.

Characteristics   A fresh floral citrus scent and a woody herbaceous undertone.

Part of plant used   Leaves and twigs.

Method of extraction   Steam distillation.

History   The name means 'little grains' as petitgrain was originally distilled from unripe fruit rather than the leaves. One of the classic ingredients of Eau de Cologne.

Chemical constituents   A typical chemical composition of petitgrain is reported as follows (146):
Geraniol (2.33%), linalool (27.95%), nerol (1.01%),γ–terpineol (7.55%), geranyl acetate (2.61%), linalyl acetate (44.29%), myrcene (5.36%), neryl acetate (0.55%),trans-ocimene (3.32%).

Paraguayan petitgrain oil has a lower ester and higher alcohol content than does petitgrain bigarade of French origin.

Blends well with   Bergamot, cedarwood, clary sage, geranium, lavender, lime, jasmine, neroli, orange, palmarosa, rosemary, rosewood, sandalwood, ylang-ylang.

Properties   Antidepressant, antispasmodic, deodorant, sedative.

Indications

Mind and spirit   Calms anger and panic. It is considered uplifting and refreshing. Similar in its action to neroli which is, however, considered to be more effective with serious states of depression.

Patricia Davis (147) suggests that while neroli activates the highest psychic or spiritual levels of the mind, petitgrain relates more to the conscious, intellectual aspect of the mind.

Body   Petitgrain has a sedative effect on the nervous system, its relaxing properties are useful for the treatment of rapid heartbeat or insomnia. It also has deodorising properties.

Skin and hair   A tonic effect on the skin and helpful for clearing up skin blemishes and pimples.

Precautions   Non-toxic, non-irritant, non sensitizing and non phototoxic.

Pine

Botanical name   *Pinus sylvestris.*

Family   Pinaceae.

Synonyms   Forest pine, Scotch pine, pine needle.

Place of origin   Northern Europe, North America.

Other species   Like the fir tree, there are numerous species of pine which yield an essential oil from their heartwood as well as from their twigs and needles.

Other species which produce pine oil include the eastern white pine (*P. strobus*) from the eastern USA and Canada, the dwarf pine (*P. mugo* var. *pumilio*) grown in central and southern Europe, and the black pine (*P. nigrum*) from Austria. Many varieties, such as the long leaf pine *(Pinus palustris),* are used to produce turpentine.

Description   A tall evergreen tree, up to 40 metres high with a flat crown. It has a reddish brown, deeply fissured bark.

Characteristics   A strong, dry-balsamic, turpentine like odour.

Part of the plant used   Needles.

Method of extraction   Steam distillation.

History   Hippocrates recommended pine for pulmonary problems and throat infections. In his book *Natural History*, Pliny described the therapeutic properties of pine in great detail, emphasising its use in all problems of the respiratory system.

Mrs Grieve's Modern Herbal indicates that pine's medicinal actions are rubefacient and diuretic and that it is a valuable remedy for bladder, kidney and rheumatic conditions, diseases of the mucous membrane and respiratory complaints.

Marguerite Maury considered it good for rheumatic conditions such as gout, and an effective diuretic as well as a treatment for pulmonary infections.

Chemical constituents   A typical chemical composition of *Pinus sylvestris* oil is reported as follows (148):

Borneol, bornyl acetate, α- and β-phallandrene, α- and β-pinene, 3-carene.

Blends well with   Cajeput, cedarwood, cinnamon, clove, cypress, eucalyptus, lavender, Spanish and sweet marjoram, myrtle, niaouli, peppermint, rosemary, thyme, tea tree.

Properties   Antimicrobial, antineuralgic, antirheumatic, antiseptic, antiviral, bactericidal, balsamic, cholagogue, deodorant, diuretic, expectorant, hypertensive, insecticidal, restorative, rubefacient, stimulant of the adrenal cortex, circulation and nervous system.

Indications

Mind and spirit   Used as an inhalation it is great for general debility and mental fatigue. Pine oil is cleansing and invigorating, promoting feelings of energy and wellbeing. Pine oil may be used in a vaporiser to clear a healing or meditation space, especially if the room is also used for other purposes.

Body   Pine's antiseptic and expectorant properties are helpful in cases of asthma, bronchitis, laryngitis and influenza.

Pine oil may be used to tonify the Yang and it is recommended for overcoming mental, physical and sexual fatigue, chills and poor appetite. It is used to stimulate the adrenals, both medulla and cortex.

It is effective in treating cystitis, hepatitis and prostate problems. Reduces inflammation of the gall-bladder and reduces gall stones. It stimulates the circulation and with its warming properties may relieve rheumatism, gout, sciatica and arthritis. Used in compresses when these conditions are very painful.

Skin and hair   Not traditionally used in skin care as it is sensitising for people with sensitive skin.

Precautions   Dwarf pine (*Pinus mugo.* var. *pumilio*) is considered a dermal irritant, a common sensitising agent. However it is very likely that all pine oils are dermal irritants if they are oxidised. Dwarf pine oil is not considered toxic but use in aromatherapy is not recommended.

Both longleaf pine *(Pinus palustris)* and Scotch pine *(Pinus sylvestris)* are considered non-toxic, non-irritants (except in high doses) but possibly sensitising, so it is best to avoid them in massage or in baths where allergic skin conditions exist.

Rock rose

Botanical name   *Cistus ladaniferus.*

Family   Cistaceae.

Synonyms   Cistus oil, labdanum.

Place of origin   Native to the Mediterranean mountainous regions and the Middle East. The oil is now mainly produced in Spain.

Other species   Rock rose is also obtained from other Cistus species, notably *C. incanus*, and other subspecies.

Description   A small shrub up to 3 metres high with lance shaped leaves. The extracted gum, a dark brown solid mass, is obtained by boiling the plant material in water.

Characteristics   The oil has a warm, sweet, dry-herbaceous musky scent. The absolute has a sweet herbaceous balsamic odour.

Part of plant used   The leaves and twigs of the plant.

Method of extraction   The absolute is extracted by solvent extraction and the essential oil is extracted by steam distillation of the crude gum.

History   The essential oil has been used since the middle ages in ointments to treat infected wounds and skin ulcers. The gum was used for catarrh, diarrhoea, dysentery and to promote menstruation. It was also used to treat 'scrofulous' conditions, with skin and soft tissue disturbances and swollen lymph glands.

Chemical constituents   A typical chemical composition of rock rose is reported as follows (149):
Camphene, sabinene, myrcene, phellandrene, limonene, cymene, cineole, borneol, nerol, geraniol, fenchone and many other constituents.

Blends well with   Bergamot, chamomile, clary sage, cypress, everlasting, juniper, lavender, orange, patchouli, pine, sandalwood, vetiver.

Properties   Antimicrobial, antiseptic, astringent, emmenagogue, expectorant, tonic.

Indications

Mind and spirit   Rock rose fragrance is warm, deep, spicy and soothing. Susanne Fischer-Rizzi (150) describes the essential oil as:

> 'conveys a warmth that deeply affects the soul. Rock rose is favoured for treating patients who feel cold, empty or numb after a traumatic event.'

Body   When rock rose is added to a massage oil, it is known to increase lymph drainage. For swollen lymph nodes in the neck, apply warm rock rose compresses. For abdominal disorders caused by cold, cystitis or painful menstrual cramps, a sitz bath with equal parts of rock rose and marjoram is helpful.

Skin and hair   The oil is excellent in skin care for treating infected and inflamed skin and swollen lymph glands. The oil has proven to be useful for treating chronic slow healing skin disorders, eczema, and psoriasis.

Precautions   Generally non-toxic, non-irritant and non-sensitising. Avoid during pregnancy.

Rose

Botanical name   The two major species of rose used for essential oil production are *Rosa damascena* and *Rosa centifolia*.

Family   Rosaceae.

Synonyms   *Rosa damascena* is commonly known as Bulgarian rose, Turkish rose or otto of rose. *Rosa centifolia* is known as rose maroc, French rose, attar of rose and rose absolute.

Place of origin   Although the rose has been highly esteemed since the dawn of history, the oil was not extracted until the sixteenth century.

The first preparation of rose water was by Avicenna in the tenth century. The first rose otto was made in Persia. Through the Turks, the manufacture of rose otto was introduced into Europe, by way of Asia Minor, where it has since been produced. It was introduced into Bulgaria, then part of the Turkish Empire.

The Bulgarian rose industry is confined to one special mountain district, having for its centre the town of Kazanlik. The rose bush seems to thrive best in sandy soil with good drainage, well exposed to the sun and protected from the cold winter winds.

Other species   There are over 10,000 types of cultivated rose. There are several subspecies of *R. centifolia*, depending on the country of origin. There are also many species of *R. damascena*.

Bulgaria also grows a white rose (*R. damascena* var. *alba*) or the musk rose (*R. muscatta*). Other therapeutic species are the red rose (*R. gallica*), and the tea rose (*R. indica*).

Description   The rose that is used for the production of oil is a hybrid between *R. centifolia,* a pink rose, and *R. gallica*, a dark red rose. This hybrid is known as rose de mai, grows to a height of 2.5 metres and produces an abundance of flowers with large pink or rosy purple petals.

Rosa damascena that is used to produce Bulgarian rose is a small prickly shrub 1-2 metres high, with very fragrant pink blooms.

Characteristics   The essential oil which is steam distilled from the fresh flower petals of *Rosa centifolia* or *Rosa damascena* is a pale yellow liquid with a deep, sweet, rosy-floral, tenacious odour.

When rose otto is cooled, it congeals to a translucent soft mass, which is again liquefied by the warmth of the hand. The congealing temperature is about 15°C.

The absolute is a reddish orange viscous liquid with a deep, rich, sweet, rosy-spicy, honeylike fragrance.

Part of plant used   Fresh flower petals.

Method of extraction   About 30 roses are required to make 1 drop of oil. Rose distillers do not obtain all their otto directly from the petals, but draw the greater part by treating the water.

For example, a still is charged with 10 kg of flowers and 50 litres of water. The first 10 litres of the distilled water is drawn and from this a very small quantity of green oil is obtained. The 40 remaining litres of water is redistilled several times. It is believed that 4,000 kg of flowers are required to yield 1 litre of rose otto, of which one-third is the green essence, coming from the first distillation, and the other two-thirds is yellow oil coming from the second and subsequent distillations.

Rose absolute is extracted by solvent extraction.

History   On studying ancient European and Oriental materia medica it is obvious that up until the middle ages rose oil was highly appreciated. In Chinese and Sanskrit manuscripts rose was highly praised. Li Shin-Chen tells us of a highly fragrant rose, *Rosa rugosa*, which is cultivated in China:

> *'Its nature is cooling, its taste is sweet with a slight bitterishness, and it acts on the spleen and liver, promoting the circulation of the blood. It is prescribed in the form of an extract for haematemesis, and the flowers are used in all diseases of the liver, to scatter abcesses, and in blood diseases generally... Essence of rose is made by distilling the flowers of Rosa rugosa. Its medicinal action is upon the liver, stomach, and blood. It drives away melancholy.'*

In both ancient art and literature the rose was the predominant flower symbol. Its blossom symbolises beauty, love, youth, perfection and immortality.

In ancient Persia rose water was regarded as a panacea. Rose petals, fruits, leaves and roots were used in traditional medicine of the ancient Chinese, Indians, Assyrians, Persians, Romans and Greeks. Generally it was thought that rose medicines had a cooling and soothing influence. It is interesting to note that the fields of application of rose oil in ancient medicine are almost identical with those of modern aromatherapy.

Rose oil and rose products were employed extensively in English medicine, notably by the well-known physician Nicholas Culpeper, who used rose oil as an anti-inflammatory agent.

Chemical constituents   Rose is one of the most complex essential oils known. It contains more than 300 chemical compounds, of which the greater part is still unidentified. The following table identifies 86% of the rose composition. The

remaining 14% of the volatile part of the oil represents about 300 substances.

A typical chemical composition of Bulgarian rose otto and French rose absolute is as follows (151):

Constituent	Bulgarian rose otto *R. damascena*	French rose absolute *R. centifolia*
(-)-citronellol	34-55%	18-22%
phenyl ethanol	1.5-3%	63%
geraniol & nerol	30-40%	10-15%
farnesol	0.2-2%	0.2-2%
stearpoten	16-22%	8%

with traces of the following constituents: nonanol, linalool, nonanal, phenylacetaldehyde, citral, carvone, citronellyl acetate, 2-phenylmethyl acetate, methyl eugenol, eugenol, rose oxide.

The comparision between the rose otto and rose absolute is clearly seen in the content of phenyl ethyl alcohol which is almost negligible in the rose otto. Phenyl ethyl alcohol is a water soluble constituent which is lost in the distillation process.

Blends well with   Bergamot, German and Roman chamomile, clary sage, frankincense, geranium, jasmine, lavender, melissa, neroli, patchouli, palmarosa, rosewood, sandalwood, ylang-ylang.

Properties   Antidepressant, antiphlogistic, antiseptic, antispasmodic, antiviral, aphrodisiac, astringent, bactericidal, choleretic, cicitrisant, depurative, emmenagogue, haemostatic, hepatic, laxative, sedative (nervous system), stomachic, tonic (heart, liver, stomach, uterus).

Indications

Mind and spirit   As Susanne Fischer-Rizzi (152) says:

> *'The rose, queen of flowers! Her fragrance, captured in the essential oil, is the most precious of all heavenly scents. It refreshes the soul; its fragrant poetry brings joy to the heart.'*

Rose oil has been assigned to the heart. The essential oil of rose has a deep psychological effect. Most aromatherapists agree that rose oil is effective in all levels of life, for the soul, spirit and body. It is harmonising, anti-depressive and helps make sorrow easier. It opens the heart and soothes feelings such as anger, fear and anxiety.

Peter Holmes suggests that rose oil addresses sexuality, self-nurturing and self-esteem. Rose oil is beneficial for dealing with behavioural problems, emotional stress and anxiety. He also suggests using rose for sadness, grief or disappointment. The scent is well known to give comfort in heartbreaks, emotional losses, broken trusts and violated feelings in general. (153)

Body   Modern scientific research has been able to confirm some of the medicinal properties of roses as applied by the ancient Indians and Chinese and later by Culpeper and his contemporaries. Marguerite Maury comments that rose oil has an astonishing effect on the female sexual organs as a purifying and regulating agent.

The essential oil is used extensively for gynaecological conditions such as regulating hormones, functional infertility, uterine bleeding, strengthening the uterus, regulating menstruation, and relieving menstrual cramps.

Rose oil has traditionally been used as a refrigerant, therefore it is often recommended for heat conditions that may involve the liver, gall bladder and heart. These may be manifested as general irritability, bleeding, fever, cholecystitis, biliary dyspepsia, headaches and gastro-enteritis.

Dietrich Wabner (154) cites work done by Kirov and Vankov who demonstrated that rose oil can reduce high blood pressure and arrhythmias. The same review also covered the spasmolytic effect of rose oil and its ability to act as a protective against gastrointestinal ulceration.

The combination of rose and melissa on *Herpes zoster* and *Herpes simplex* has also been confirmed. According to Wabner (154) a chemist at the Technical University of Munich, the oil should be applied pure without dilution, two or three times a day for several days.

Skin and hair   Rose oil has excellent emollient and hydrating properties which, accompanied by their stimulating and antiseptic qualities, makes it ideal for all skin care, especially for mature, dry or sensitive skin. Rose oil can be used in an almond oil and calendula base for the treatment of broken capillaries, redness and inflammation of the skin.

A by-product of rose oil distillation is rose water. This is the condensed steam that has extracted the essential oil. It contains trace amounts of the essential oil constituents. Rose water is used in skin care for its soothing and mildly astringent properties.

One of the components of rose oil, farnesol, is important in cosmetics because of its bacteriostatic and exceptional dermatophile properties. Farnesol appears in concentrations of 0.2-2% in rose oil and can be applied in deodorants in a concentration up to 0.3%.

Precautions   Non-toxic, non-irritant and non-sensitising.

Rosemary

Botanical name   *Rosmarinus officinalis.*

Family   Lamiaceae (Labiatae).

Synonyms   *R. coronarium.*

Place of origin   Originally from Asia, rosemary has become a familiar sight in the Mediterranean region and much of the essential oil comes from France, Spain or Tunisia.

Other species   *R. officinalis* is the type used for essential oil production.

Rosemary is another plant which has several chemotypes. Three principal chemotypes of *R. officinalis* can be found:

- camphor-borneol (Spain)
- 1,8-cineole (Tunisia)
- verbenone (France).

Description   A shrubby evergreen bush up to 2 metres high with silvery green, needle shaped leaves and pale blue flowers.

Characteristics   Strong, clear and penetrating, a refreshing and stimulating herbal fragrance.

Part of plant used   Flowering tops and leaves.

Method of extraction   Steam distillation.

History   Rosemary is probably one of the best known and most used of aromatic herbs. The ancient Egyptians favoured it, and traces of it have been found in the first dynasty tombs. To the Greeks and Romans it was considered a sacred plant. They believed rosemary symbolised love and death.

Rosemary has been used medicinally for centuries. Theophrastus and Dioscorides recommended it as a powerful remedy for stomach and liver problems; Hippocrates, the 'father of medicine' said rosemary should be cooked with vegetables to overcome liver and spleen disorders, and Galen prescribed it for jaundice.

Rosemary has long been known as a cephalic as can be seen from Nicholas Culpeper's description:

'The decoction of rosemary in wine, helps the cold distillations of rheums into the eyes, and other diseases of the head and brain, as the giddiness and swimmings therein, drowsiness or dulness, the dumb palsy, or loss of speech, the lethargy, the falling sickness, to be both drunk and the temples bathed therewith... It helps a weak memory and quickens the senses.'

Chemical constituents   A comparative major component composition of various Rosemary oils is shown in the table above (155).

Due to their different compositions, these oils can be applied for different purposes to achieve maximum efficiency. The camphor type rosemary (Spain) is best used for muscular aches and pains, while the 1,8-cineole type rosemary (Tunisia and France) is best used in connection with pulmonary congestion and to facilitate elimination from the liver and the kidneys. The verbenone rosemary is considered a safe non-irritant essential oil and is excellent for high quality skin care preparations.

Compound	Tunisian	Spanish	French
α–pinene	10.3-11.6%	19.1-26.9	10.4%
Borneol	2.8-4.2%	2.4-3.4%	3.1%
β–pinene	4.9-7.7%	4.3-7.7%	7.6%
camphor	9.9-12.5%	12.7-20.7%	-
Bornyl acetate	1.0-1.2%	0.4-1.6%	13.2%
Camphene	4.0-4.3%	7.0-9.9%	4.2%
1,8-cineole	40.1-44.45	17.0-25.1%	49.1%
Limonene	2.0-4.8%	2.9-4.9%	2.1%

Blends well with   Basil, bergamot, black pepper, cajeput, cedarwood, frankincense, geranium, ginger, grapefruit, lavender, lemongrass, lemon, lime, mandarin, myrtle, orange, peppermint, petitgrain, tangerine, tea tree, thyme.

Properties   Analgesic, antidepressant, astringent, carminative, cephalic, cholagogue, cordial, digestive, diuretic, emmenagogue, hepatic, hypertensive, nervine, rubefacient, stimulant, sudorific, tonic.

Indications

Mind and spirit   Rosemary is considered one of the best tonics for the central nervous system, strengthening mental clarity and awareness. Rosemary is an excellent brain stimulant and has a long history of improving memory. Inhale a few drops of this oil to feel the mental clarity that it promotes.

Body   Rosemary is a valuable oil for many respiratory problems, ranging from the common cold, catarrh and sinusitis, through to asthma. It is a good analgesic and may be used in massage, baths and compresses to relieve pain in rheumatism and arthritis or for tired, stiff and overworked muscles.

Since rosemary stimulates blood circulation, it is a good remedy for low blood pressure. It may be used to help relieve cold feet, tired or weak legs and circulatory problems of extremities.

Rosemary is considered an excellent tonic for the liver and gall bladder. It is used in the treatment of gall bladder infections, biliary colic and gall stones. Rosemary helps lower high blood sugar, and is also an aid for arteriosclerosis. As Patricia Davis (156) suggests:

'It strengthens the heart. It may be considered a middle aged executive's best friend.'

Skin and hair   Rosemary has traditionally been used in skin and hair care for hundreds of years. It is used in shampoos and hair treatments to help stimulate blood circulation to the scalp, thus being beneficial for promoting hair growth.

Precautions   Its highly stimulating action may not be suitable for people with epilepsy or high blood pressure. Generally non-toxic, non-irritant and non-sensitising. Avoid during pregnancy.

Rosewood

Botanical name   *Aniba rosaeodora.*

Family   Lauraceae.

Synonyms   Bois de rose.

Place of origin   Brazil.

Description   Medium sized tropical, evergreen tree with a reddish bark and heartwood.

Characteristics   Sweet, woody, floral and slightly spicy.

Part of plant used   Tree/wood.

Method of extraction   Steam distillation.

History   Rosewood has been introduced to aromatherapy only recently. The Brazilian essential oil output is vast and to prevent extinction of the trees, the government has enacted legislation requiring distilleries to plant a new tree for each one cut down.

Chemical constituents   A typical chemical composition of rosewood is reported as follows (157):

α–pinene, camphene, geraniol, neral, geranial, myrcene, limonene, 1,8-cineole, linalool, benzaldehyde, linalool oxides, α–terpineol.

Blends well with   Bergamot, cedarwood, frankincense, geranium, lavender, mandarin, neroli, orange, palmarosa, patchouli, petitgrain, rose, rosemary, sandalwood, vetiver, ylang-ylang.

Properties   Antidepressant, antiseptic, bactericide, cephalic, deodorant, insecticide, stimulant.

Indications

Mind and spirit   Its uplifting and enlivening properties have an overall balancing effect. Helpful when feeling weary and over-burdened with problems. Its cephalic properties may relieve headaches.

Patricia Davis (158) suggests using rosewood for meditation or in preparation of any spiritual healing. It has an overall calming effect without inducing any drowsiness.

Body   Rosewood oil does not have as wide a range of therapeutic properties as some of the better known oils, but it makes a useful addition to most massage oils and bath oils.

It is antibacterial and makes a good deodorant. Rosewood is currently been used in the manufacture of many skincare and bath products.

Skin and hair   Regarded as a cell stimulant and tissue regenerator which makes it useful for treating aged skin. It is also ideal for people with dry, sensitive and inflamed skin.

Precautions   Non-toxic, non-irritant and non-sensitising.

Sage

Botanical name   *Salvia officinalis.*

Family   Lamiaceae (Labiatae).

Synonyms   Garden sage, Dalmatian sage.

Place of origin   Balkans.

Other species   There are several species of sage, and essential oils are produced from Spanish sage *(S. lavendulaefolia)* and clary sage *(S. sclarea)* - see separate entries for both of these oils.

Description   An evergreen perennial herb up to 80 cm in height with a woody base, soft silver, oval leaves and a mass of blue or violet flowers.

Characteristics   Clear, herbal, camphorous and sharp.

Part of plant used   Dried leaves.

Method of extraction   Steam distillation.

History   Apart from its widespread use in cooking, sage has always been used in folk medicine in many countries in the form of herbal infusions, gargles, vinegars and poultices, particularly for mouth and throat infections, to heal wounds and clear headaches. It has often been described in old herbals as a mental stimulant. John Geralde says:

'Sage is singularly good for the head and brain, it quickeneth the senses and memory.'

Chemical constituents   A typical chemical composition of sage is reported as follows (159): α–pinene (1.7-5.9%), camphene (3.1-7.5%), β–pinene (0.3-1.6%), myrcene (0.5-0.8%), limonene (1.1-2.0%), 1,8-cineole (6.9-11.2%), α–thujone (17.0-21.6%), β–thujone (1.7-3.7%), camphor (23.1-27.3%), linalool (0.5-0.7%), bornyl acetate (1.1-2.8%), borneol (3.7-4.5%).

Blends well with   Bergamot, cajeput, clary sage, eucalyptus, geranium, ginger, lavender, myrtle, niaouli, orange, peppermint, pine, rose, rosemary, tea tree.

Properties   Anti-inflammatory, antibacterial, antiseptic, antispasmodic, astringent, digestive, diuretic, emmenagogue, febrifuge, hypertensive, laxative, stomachic, tonic.

Indications

Mind and spirit   In small doses it has a calming effect on the nerves by soothing the parasympathetic nervous system. It is indicated for tiredness, depression and grief.

Body   In spite of the undoubted value of sage I strongly recommend that sage be used by professional aromatherapists only. The oil has a high thujone content which can provoke epileptic fits or convulsions, and in larger amounts it is toxic to the central nervous system and is capable of inducing paralysis.

Its medicinal uses include being a digestive stimulant and it is indicated where there is loss of appetite. It also has a beneficial effect on the female reproductive system since it imitates the hormone oestrogen, thereby regulating the menstrual cycle. Also useful for treating menopausal problems, particularly sweating. It can be used for people with general debility (convalescence) and for people with low blood pressure because of its tonic effects. Used in massage oils it will help relieve the aches and pains of rheumatism.

Skin and hair   Dr Jean Valnet (160) recommends sage for the treatment of dermatitis, atonic wounds, sores, ulcers, and for insect bites.

Precautions   Due to its high levels of thujone, it may be an abortifacient so must be avoided during pregnancy. Avoid for people with epilepsy or high blood pressure. Use with extreme care in aromatherapy.

Sage, Spanish

Botanical name   *Salvia lavendulaefolia.*

Family   Lamiaceae (Labiatae).

Synonyms   Lavender-leaved sage.

Place of origin   Native to the mountain regions of Spain. It also grows in south west France and the Balkans. The oil is mainly produced in Spain.

Other species   A similar oil which is used for pharmaceutical purposes is produced in Turkey from a Greek variety, *S. triloba.*

Description   An evergreen shrub, similar to the garden sage but with narrower leaves and small purple flowers. The whole plant has a scent reminiscent of spike lavender.

Characteristics   A fresh-herbaceous, camphorous, slightly pinelike odour.

Part of plant used   Leaves.

Method of extraction   Steam distillation.

History   In Spain it is regarded as a 'cure-all'. Believed to promote longevity and protect against all types of infection.

Chemical constituents   A typical chemical composition of Spanish sage is reported as follows (161): myrcene (0.6%), limonene (1.5%), α–pinene (6.2%), β–pinene (6.1%), camphene (6.8%), tricyclene (0.5%), linalool (1.1%), linalyl acetate (1.5%), borneol (2.2%), bornyl acetate (2.8%), 1,8-cineole (29.0%), camphor (34.0%), caryophyllene (0.35%).

Blends well with Cedarwood, citronella, eucalyptus, juniper, clary sage, lavender, pine, rosemary.

Properties Anti-depressant, anti-inflammatory, antimicrobial, antiseptic, antispasmodic, astringent, carminative, deodorant, depurative, digestive, emmenagogue, expectorant, febrifuge, hypotensive, nervine, stimulant (hepatobiliary, adrenocortical glands, circulation), stomachic, tonic.

Indications

Mind and spirit It can be used for headaches, nervous exhaustion and stress related conditions.

Body As a massage oil it is used for arthritis, fluid retention, muscular aches and pain and poor circulation. Its antiseptic, antispasmodic and febrifuge properties make it useful as an inhalation and it should be considered for asthma, colds, coughs, fever and laryngitis. It is extremely valuable for the treatment of amenorrhoea and dysmenorrhoea. Its depurative and digestive properties mean that it can be used to treat jaundice and liver congestion.

Skin and hair It can be used to treat cuts, acne, dandruff, dermatitis, eczema, excessive sweating, gingivitis, gum infections and sores.

Precautions Relatively non-toxic, non-irritant and non-sensitising.

The composition of another Spanish sage essential oil (162) indicated that it contained 3% sabinyl acetate, which is a well known hazardous constituent with abortifacient effects. There are variations in the chemical composition of Spanish sage oils, and the variation in the sabinyl acetate content is due to the existence of chemotypes.

The combination of sabinyl acetate and the high percentage of camphor found in Spanish sage indicates that it would be advisable to avoid using Spanish sage during pregnancy or for sufferers of epilepsy.

Sandalwood

Botanical name *Santalum album.*

Family Santalaceae.

Synonyms East Indian sandalwood, Mysore sandalwood.

Place of origin Native of Asia. The region of Mysore, India exports the highest quality oil.

Other species The Australian sandalwood *(S. spicatum)* produces a very similar oil, but with a dry bitter top note. The West Indian sandalwood *(Amyris balsamifera)* is a poor substitute and bears no botanical relation to the East Indian sandalwood.

Description A small, evergreen, parasitic tree up to 9 metres high. The tree must be over 30 years old before it is ready for the production of sandalwood oil.

Characteristics Woody, sweet and exotic, subtle and lingering.

Part of plant used Timber, inner heartwood.

Method of extraction Steam or water distillation.

History Sandalwood has a long history. In ancient India it was widely used in religious ceremonies. It was also a specific for genito-urinary infections. In India and Egypt it was used as a perfume, and was an ingredient of many cosmetics.

While sandalwood is valued for its essential oil, the closely-grained, fine, pale yellow wood was often referred to as 'botanical ivory' as the wood is used for carved objects of high quality.

The spread of the use of sandalwood throughout Asia followed the spread of Buddhism. The use of powdered sandalwood as incense is an example of how sandalwood has always been considered the aromatic foundation of Buddhist practice.

Chemical constituents A typical chemical composition of sandalwood is reported as follows (163):

	Age of tree (Years)	
	10	**30**
oil percentage	0.9%	4.0%
santalols	74.6%	89.2%
santyl acetate	5.4%	3.5%
santalenes	4.9%	2.3%

The best quality sandalwood essential oil has a high santalol content and is manufactured from the heartwood of trees which are at least 30 years old. The Indian standard for Mysore sandalwood oil is that it contain a minimum of 90% santalols.

Blends well with Basil, bergamot, black pepper, cypress, atlas cedarwood, frankincense, geranium, jasmine, lavender, lemon, myrrh, neroli, orange, palmarosa, rose, vetiver, ylang-ylang.

Properties Antiphlogistic, antiseptic, antispasmodic, astringent, carminative, diuretic, emollient, expectorant, sedative, tonic.

Indications

Mind and spirit Sandalwood has a calming, harmonising effect helping to reduce tension and confusion. It is an ideal remedy to use for nervous depression, fear, stress, and a hectic daily lifestyle.

The yogis describe sandalwood oil as the fragrance of the 'subtle body', the centre of the highest insight and enlightenment. It has been assigned to the root chakra, seat of the fertility organs and sexuality. It has long been considered an aphrodisiac.

According to Susanne Fischer-Rizzi (164):

'Sandalwood oil aids people who want to make human contact and overcome isolation. Sandalwood helps them accept others with an open heart and diminish their egocentricity. Sandalwood oil fosters openness, warmth and understanding.'

Body Sandalwood oil has a pronounced action on the mucous membranes of the genito-urinary tract and the pulmonary tracts and is often used for chronic infections of these areas.

Not only is the oil recommended for treating catarrh, it will also relieve a dry cough. The oil also relieves intestinal spasm and inflammation and may be useful in colic and gastritis. It is also useful for the treatment of chronic and acute diarrhoea.

Skin and hair Sandalwood oil is very useful in skincare for dehydrated skin. It also relieves itching and inflammation of the skin. As a mild astringent it is also excellent to use in oily skin conditions.

Precautions Non-toxic, non-irritant and non-sensitising.

Spearmint

Botanical name *Mentha spicata.*

Family Lamiaceae (Labiatae).

Synonyms *M. viridis,* common spearmint.

Place of origin USA, Australia.

Other species There are several different types of spearmint, especially in the USA, such as the curly mint *(M. spicata* var. *crispa).*

Description A hardy branched perennial herb with bright green, lance-shaped leaves, quickly spreading underground runners.

Characteristics Similar to peppermint though slightly sweeter, fresher and less harsh.

Part of plant used Flowering tops and leaves.

Method of extraction Steam distillation.

History Spearmint was used as a tonic and scent by the ancient Greeks who used it in their bath water. The Romans introduced spearmint into Britain where it was used to stop milk from curdling. In medieval times it became a feature in oral hygiene and was used to heal sore gums and for whitening teeth.

Chemical constituents A typical chemical composition of spearmint is reported as follows (165):
α-pinene (0.7%), β-pinene (2.3%), carvone (63.3%), 1,8-cineole (0.8%), linalool (1.1%),

limonene (20.2%), myrcene, caryophyllene (0.3%), menthol (0.5%).

Blends well with   Aniseed, basil, cedarwood, cajeput, eucalyptus, lavender, lemon, lime, grapefruit, peppermint, rosemary.

Properties   Antiseptic, antispasmodic, carminative, cephalic, emmenagogue, insecticide, restorative, stimulant.

Indications

Mind and spirit   Stimulating and uplifting for the tired mind.

Body   Spearmint shares similar properties to peppermint. It has trace constituents of menthol so is less harsh on the skin. This makes spearmint my choice of oils for children with digestive problems, such as nausea, flatulence, constipation and diarrhoea.

It relaxes the stomach muscles, relieves hiccups and nausea. It is excellent to relieve the effects of travel sickness. Used as an inhalation it can be used to decongest sinus problems and it has an uplifting effect, reducing mental fatigue and depression.

Skin and hair   Spearmint may be used to relieve pruritus.

Precautions   Non-toxic, non-irritant and non-sensitising.

Tangerine

Botanical name   *Citrus reticulata blanco* var. 'tangerine'.

Family   Rutaceae.

Synonyms   *Citrus nobilis* var. *delicosa*.

Place of origin   A native of China, the oil is largely produced in USA and Sicily.

Other species   The botanical origin of the tangerine and mandarin are similar. Unfortunately for the lay person the name tangerine has been used as a general name for loose skinned citrus fruit varieties such as tangerines, mandarins and tangelos. The tangerine represents a lower stage in the horticultural development of the fruit. Tangerines do not have pips.

Description   Similar to the mandarin.

Characteristics   A sweet, light and tangy aroma. The tangerine has a slightly weaker and more subtle aroma than mandarin.

Part of plant used   Fruit peel.

Method of extraction   Cold expression.

History   Tangerine was introduced into USA from China via Europe.

Chemical constituents   A typical chemical composition of tangerine is reported as follows (166):
α–pinene (1.00%), myrcene (2.03%), limonene (91.23%), γ–terpinene (3.09%), and trace amounts of citronellal, linalool, neral, neryl acetate, geranyl acetate, geraniol, thymol and carvone.

Blends well with   Basil, bergamot, chamomile, clary sage, frankincense, geranium, grapefruit, ginger, lavender, lemon, lime, neroli, orange, rose, rosemary, ylang-ylang.

Properties   Antiseptic, antispasmodic, cytophylactic, depurative, sedative, stomachic, tonic.

Indications

Mind and spirit   It is a relaxant and is helpful in alleviating stress and tension due to its soothing action on the nervous system. It can be used in the same way that mandarin is used.

Body   Its medicinal properties are similar to that of mandarin and orange. It has a tonic effect on the digestive system, dealing with gastric complaints such as flatulence, diarrhoea, constipation. It is a popular addition to a massage oil during pregnancy, helping reduce stretch marks, reducing fluid retention and stimulating circulation.

Skin and hair   Can be used in massage oils for acne, congested oily skin and in the treatment of stretch marks.

Precautions   Non-toxic, non-irritant and non-sensitizing.

Tea Tree

Botanical name   *Melaleuca alternifolia.*

Family   Myrtaceae.

Synonyms   Ti-tree.

Place of origin   Australia.

Other species   Tea tree is a general name given to all members of the Melaleuca family.

Description   A small tree or shrub, with needle-like leaves.

Characteristics   Fresh and antiseptic, rather pungent.

Part of plant used   Leaves and twigs.

Method of extraction   Steam or water distillation.

History   The Australian aborigines have long recognised the virtues of tea tree. The following discussion is an extract from *The Medical Journal of Australia,* March 29, 1930 by E. Morris Humphrey, M.B., Ch. M., Honorary Surgeon, Royal North Shore Hospital of Sydney (167):

'An essential oil extracted from a variety of tea tree growing in profusion on the North coast of New South Wales was brought to my notice about twelve months ago. Analysis by Mr. W.R. Penfold, Curator and Economic Chemist of the Sydney Technological Museum, showed that it was non-toxic, non-irritating and eleven to thirteen times stronger than carbolic as a germicide (Rideal-Walker coefficient).

Dirty wounds, such as the result of street accidents, may be washed or syringed out with a 10% watery lotion, the solvent properties will loosen and bring away the dirt which is usually ground in, and the tissues will remain fresh and retain their natural colour. Dressings dipped in a 2.5% solution may then be applied, changed every twenty four hours and healing will readily take place.

The pus solvent properties led me to try the lotion for paronychia which is usually so disheartening and so frequently results in the loss of the nail or deformity. Here the results were excellent. Infections which resisted treatment of various kinds for months, were cured in less than a week. The fingers were dressed with lint soaked in 10% solution and changed every twenty four hours.

Twenty drops in a tumbler of warm water used as a gargle quickly clears up a sore throat in the early stages; it should be an excellent prophylactic for many infective conditions which gain entrance to the body through the naso-pharynx.'

Chemical constituents   The Australian Standard for tea tree oil (AS2782 - 1985) requires that the 1,8-cineole content shall not exceed 15% and the terpinen-4-ol content shall be at least 30%.

A typical chemical composition of tea tree is reported as follows (168):
α-pinene (2.1%), β-pinene (0.4%), sabinene (0.2%), myrcene (0.4%), α-phellandrene (0.8%), α-terpinene (7.1%), limonene (1.4%), 1,8-cineole (3.0%), γ-terpinene (15.7%), p-cymene (6.2%), terpinolene (3.4%), linalool (0.2%), terpinen-4-ol (45.4%), α-terpineol (5.3%).

Blends well with   Cajeput, cinnamon, clove, cypress, eucalyptus, geranium, ginger, juniper, lavender, lemon, mandarin, orange, peppermint, pine, rosemary, thyme.

Properties   Antimicrobial, antiseptic, bactericide, cicatrisant, expectorant, fungicide, insecticide, stimulant, sudorific.

Indications

Body   Tea tree has a very wide range of applications which are all dependent on two outstanding properties of tea tree:

1. This oil is active against all three categories of infectious organisms: bacteria, viruses and fungi.

2. It is a very effective immuno-stimulant, so when the body is threatened with any of these organisms, tea tree increases the body's ability to respond.

Tea tree oil has many beneficial uses and makes a marvellous addition to any first aid kit. Here are examples of some of the possible uses of tea tree:

- Dirty wounds may be washed out with a solution of tea tree oil.

- An ancient bush remedy for skin lesions or infected injuries is to liberally apply pure tea tree oil to the area and then dip a dressing in a 2.5% solution of oil in water, or pure oil, then bandage the wound. The dressing is changed every 24 hours. This is suitable for any wound, skin abrasion, minor burn or weeping ulcer.

- A 2.5% solution may be used to frequently swab fungicidal outbreaks such as paronychia (nail infection), athlete's foot (tinea), vaginitis, thrush and cradle cap.

- Ten drops in a tumbler of water may be used as a gargle to help clear throat infections, mouth ulcers or to eliminate bad breath.

- Used in a vaporiser the oil is an excellent inhalation for congested nasal passage and respiratory infections.

- For the treatment of thrush, tea tree may be diluted 1 part to 200 parts of water in a douche. Apply daily. After seven days noticeable improvement should have occurred. Discontinue if severe discomfort occurs.

- For muscular aches and pain use tea tree oil as a massage oil or add ten drops to a warm bath.

Skin and hair   In skin care tea tree can be used to treat infected rashes, and is very effective in combination with lavender for the treatment of pimples and acne. It can be used in a cleansing gel or in a 1% dilution in a light oil such as apricot kernel or jojoba oil. It is massaged into the face then wiped off.

Tea tree may be added to a shampoo, being effective for the control of dandruff. For head lice apply directly to the affected parts. Leave for half an hour before washing out. Repeat treatment for ten days at two day intervals. To relieve insect bites and stings dab on pure essential oil or apply a tea tree ointment.

Precautions   Non-toxic, non-irritant, possible sensitisation in some individuals.

Thyme

Botanical name   *Thymus vulgaris.*

Family   Lamiaceae (Labiatae).

Synonyms   Red thyme.

Place of origin   Native to Spain and the Mediterranean region.

Other species   The many species of thyme are derived from the original wild thyme (*Thymus serpyllum*), also called 'Mother-of-thyme', native to southern Europe. Another species often used to make red thyme oil is Spanish sauce thyme (*Thymus zygis*) an inexpensive thyme oil with a high thymol content (50-75%).

There seems to be no other aromatic plant which possesses such a diverse range of chemotypes as *Thymus vulgaris*. Researchers have found it difficult to categorise the oil botanically. There are at least six different chemotypes (169):

- thymol
- carvacrol
- linalool
- geraniol
- thuyan-4-ol
- α-terpinyl acetate.

The two most common chemotypes are thymol and carvacrol, which are extracted from *Thymus vulgaris* which grows close to the Mediterranean sea, at low altitude. At higher altitudes, the linalool chemotype is found. These three chemotypes are the most common.

The geraniol, thuyan-4-ol and α-terpinyl acetate chemotypes are rare and are found mixed with the the first three chemotypes.

Description   A perennial evergreen herb up to 45 cm high with a woody root and branched upright stem.

Characteristics   A rather sweet, warm and strongly herbal fragrance.

Part of plant used   Herb/flowers and leaves.

Method of extraction   Steam distillation.

History   Thyme was used by the Sumerians as long ago as 3,500 BC. The ancient Egyptians called it Tham, and used it for embalming. Hippocrates recommended infusions of the herb to be drunk at the end of banquets for digestive purposes. Pliny recommended it as a remedy for epilepsy; he said that the herb should be made into a mattress and that sleeping on it, the patient would be relaxed and calm.

The Romans used thyme to dispel melancholy and promote bravery; the soldiers would have a bath with thyme in it before going to battle, an idea that was still used at the time of the Crusades, when ladies would embroider sprigs of thyme on their knights' scarves before they went into battle. In the middle ages, St Hildegarde prescribed thyme for the plague, leprosy and body lice.

Culpeper says of thyme:

'A noble strengthener of the lungs, as notable a one as grows, nor is there a better remedy growing for hooping cough. It purgeth the body of phlegm and is an excellent remedy for shortness of breath ... An ointment made of it takes away hot swellings and warts, helps sciatica and dullness of sight and takes away any pains and hardness of the spleen; it is excellent for those that are troubled with gout.'

Lemery, a seventeenth century French physician and chemist used thyme as a brain fortifier, and a stimulant of the digestive system.

In 1719, Neumann isolated and discovered the thymol in thyme.

Thyme has been prescribed in cases of asthma, depression, and respiratory infections, and for chronic coughs. Thyme oil was used, along with clove and lemon essential oils, as a disinfectant in hospitals until World War I.

Chemical constituents   A typical chemical composition of *various thyme oils* is reported as shown in the table on this page (169).

Blends well with   Bergamot, cajeput, cedarwood, chamomile, eucalyptus, juniper, lavender, lemon, niaouli, mandarin, rosemary, tea tree.

Properties   Antirheumatic, antiseptic, antispasmodic, bactericide, cardiac, carminative, cicatrisant, diuretic, emmenagogue, expectorant, hypertensive, insecticide, stimulant, tonic, vermifuge.

Chemical constituent	*Thymus vulgaris*			*Thymus serpyllum*
	thymol chemotype	**carvacrol chemotype**	**linalool chemotype**	
α-thujene	4.6%	4.9%	0.26%	1.53%
α-pinene	0.75%	4.3%	0.3%	0.7%
camphene	0.3%	0.8%	0.27%	0.2%
β-pinene	0.34%	0.35%	-	0.17%
p-cymene	26%	33.9%	2.0%	25.0%
α-terpinene	24%	44.85%	0.28%	4.85%
linalool	4.2%	4.2%	77.5%	3.4%
borneol	0.65%	0.8%	0.2%	-
β-caryophyllene	3.55%	2.5%	2.8%	2.5%
thymol	34%	5.5%	2.2%	8.3%
carvacrol	4.7%	24.5%	trace	14.2%
geraniol	-	-	-	9.0%

The chemical constituents of several varieties of thyme

Indications

Mind and spirit   Strengthens the nerves and aids in concentration. Revives low spirits and combats exhaustion. According to Scott Cunningham (170), thyme has the effect of closing down the psychic mind in favour of the conscious, intellectual mind. This may be particularly beneficial for people who tend to be dreamy, detached or immersed in their spiritual life to the detriment of their physical wellbeing.

Thymus vulgaris C.T. linalool is also classified as a cephalic and cerebral stimulant. It may be used in cases of mental overwork. According to Philippe Mailhebiau (171) the oil is also used for regulating 'instinctive reactions' such as bulimia, anorexia, violence and fears.

Body   *Thymus vulgaris* C.T. thymol has excellent broncho-pulmonary and immuno-stimulant properties and is ideal for treating colds, coughs, sore throats, bronchitis, whooping cough and asthma. According to Valnet (172):

> *'an aqueous solution of 5% thyme kills typhus bacillus in 2 minutes. It can kill colon bacillus in 2-8 minutes, staphylococcus in 4-8 minutes and streptococcus and diphtheric bacillus in 4 minutes.'*

It is good for the circulatory system and helps raise low blood pressure. Its warming and analgesic properties make it ideal for treating rheumatism, gout, arthritis and sciatica. It is a digestive stimulant and helps with sluggish digestion.

Thymus vulgaris chemotype linalool is very different, from both an olfactory and a therapeutic perspective, from *Thymus vulgaris* chemotype thymol. The linalool chemotype has very few phenolic compounds and is considered ideal to use for children and is more of an immunostimulant than an antibacterial.

Due to its ester content it is also good for spasmodic, dry coughs especially if taken in conjunction with cypress.

Skin and hair   Because of its phenol content it should not be used for any skin care treatments.

Precautions   Thyme contains phenols which will irritate mucous membranes, cause dermal irritation and may cause sensitisation in some individuals. Use in moderation and in low dilution. Should not be used by anyone with high blood pressure.

Vetiver

Botanical name   *Vetiveria zizanoides.*

Family   Poaceae (Gramineae).

Synonyms   *Andropogon muricatus*, vetivert.

Place of origin   India, Java and Haiti.

Other species   Botanically related to lemongrass and citronella.

Description   A tall, tufted, perennial, scented grass, with a straight stem, long narrow leaves and an abundant complex of underground white roots.

Characteristics   Deep, smoky and earthy fragrance. Like the oils of patchouli and sandalwood, vetiver oil is a base note that is used as a valuable fixative for Fougere, Oriental and Chypre perfumes. Because of its potency it is best used in no more than one drop per 25 ml of carrier oil.

Part of plant used   Roots.

Method of extraction   Steam distillation.

History   The roots have been used in the East for their fine fragrance since antiquity. The root of vetiver is considered an emblem of vitality. In India and Sri Lanka the dried thin, wiry roots are woven into fans, screens and mats.

Chemical constituents   A typical chemical composition of vetiver is reported as follows (173): Benzoic acid, vetiverol, furfurol, α- and β-vetivone, vetivene, vetivenyl vetivenate.

Blends well with   Frankincense, geranium, grapefruit, jasmine, lemon, lavender, patchouli, rose, rosewood, sandalwood, ylang-ylang.

Properties   Antiseptic, nervine, sedative, tonic, vermifuge.

Indications

Mind and spirit   Vetiver is an interesting oil to use in aromatherapy. Some people can barely tolerate the smell while others are affected quite deeply by its aroma, which can be likened to the smell of a damp forest floor. Susanne Fischer-Rizzi (174) describes vetiver as:

> '*the scent of mother earth, mysteriously hidden in a deep, dark recess, drawing on the fullness of her life-giving force. This essential oil can be used for physical and emotional burnout resulting in total exhaustion.*'

Micheline Arcier (175) refers to it as the oil of tranquility and may be used as a protection against oversensitivity. The oil may be applied to the solar plexus to prevent becoming as Patricia Davis (176) calls it a 'psychic sponge'. To do this apply one drop of vetiver on the fingertips and gently massage it to the solar plexus in an anticlockwise direction.

The oil is considered a classic for physical, mental and emotional burnout which may result in total exhaustion. Holmes (177) suggests that vetiver's grounding and centring qualities will:

> '*mulch into the ground scattered ideas and abstract intellectual ideas into more practical earth-centered concepts.*'

On an emotional level, vetiver helps to soothe states of irritability, anger and hysteria. Neurotic behaviour and other behaviour that thrives on stress and tension will be pacified.

Body   It is often recommended for treating PMS caused by oestrogen or progesterone deficiency which tends to cause feelings of unworthiness and loss of purpose. The essential oil seems to have an effect on the hormone secretions of oestrogen and progesterone. This would make vetiver an appropriate choice during menopause when both these hormones need boosting.

Skin and hair   Vetiver is considered nourishing and moisturising to the skin and is recommended for dry, dehydrated or irritated skin. Vetiver's vulnerary and cicatrisant properties are utilised to prevent and reduce wrinkles, stretch marks during pregnancy, and to improve the tone of slack or tired-looking skin.

Precautions   Non-toxic, non-irritant and non-sensitising.

Yarrow

Botanical name   *Achillea millefolium.*

Family   Asteraceae (Compositae).

Synonyms   Milfoil, common yarrow.

Place of origin   Can be found growing in most temperate zones of the world. The oil is distilled in Germany, Hungary, and France.

Other species   A very extensive species. Other varieties include the Ligurian yarrow (*A. ligustica*) and the musk yarrow (*A. moschata*), which also produces an essential oil containing mainly cineol.

Description   A perennial herb with a simple stem up to 1 metre high, with fine dissected leaves giving a lacy appearance, bearing numerous pink-white, dense flower heads.

Characteristics   Slightly sweet, herbaceous and spicy. The blue oil obtained from yarrow possesses a characteristic aroma reminiscent of wormwood and German chamomile.

Part of plant used   Leaves and flowering heads.

Method of extraction   Steam distillation.

History   A plant of divination used as a charm in Scotland. Credited with powers to ward off evil spirits. Young maidens were also hopeful about its magical powers and placed it under their pillows to dream of true love. A myth goes that Achilles tended his soldiers' wounds with yarrow during the wars with Troy.

An age old herb used for a wide variety of complaints including fever and respiratory infections, digestive problems, nervous tension and externally for sores, rashes and wounds.

Chemical constituents   A typical chemical composition of yarrow is reported as follows (178):
Tricyclene (0.27%), α–pinene (9.41%), camphene (6.02%), β–pinene (7.13%), sabinene(12.35%), borneol acetate (2.10%) 1,8-cineole (9.59%),γ–terpinene (3.71%), limonene (1.71%), isoartemisia ketone (8.6%), borneol (2.55%), camphor (17.79%). Traces of chamazulene have also been identified: (this is not unexpected as the oil has a blue colour).

Blends well with   Bergamot, German and Roman chamomile, clary sage, juniper, lavender, lemon, neroli, pine, rosemary, vetiver.

Properties   Anti-inflammatory, antirheumatic, antiseptic, antispasmodic, astringent, carminative, cicatrisant, diaphoretic, digestive, expectorant, haemostatic, hypotensive, stomachic, tonic.

Indications

Mind and spirit   According to Susanne Fischer-Rizzi (179):

'the oil is helpful during times of major life changes (such as mid-life crisis, menopause, or other times of transition).'

She also suggests that yarrow strengthens intuitive energies and deepens our understanding of the earth's energies. This is beneficial to prevent an over emphasis on the purely intellectual while at the same time keeping our imagination in check.

Body   Yarrow is useful for gynaecological problems and is often used as a balancing remedy. It may be useful for the relief of irregular menstrual cycles and painful periods. The oil may be applied in a massage, compress or foot bath.

The oil is used for the treatment of varicose veins, rheumatic pain and neuralgia, in which it is best used as a compress or in a linament. For infections of the pelvic region, yarrow may be useful in a sitz bath, compress or poultice to aid ongoing therapy. For vaginal infections and irritations, make a douche by adding two to three drops of yarrow to warm water.

Skin and hair   Yarrow is used for treatment of wounds and open sores because of its astringent, antiseptic and anti-inflammatory properties. It may be applied as a compress or in a therapeutic bath. It is also excellent for the treatment of eczema and allergic skin reactions.

Precautions   Non-toxic, non-irritant, possibly sensitising in some people.

Ylang-ylang

Botanical name   *Cananga odorata.*

Family   Annonaceae (Compositae).

Synonyms   *Unona odorantissimum*, flower of flowers.

Place of origin   Philippines, Madagascar.

Other species   Closely related to cananga (*C. odorata* var. *macrophylla*). Cananga oil is produced in South East Asia. This essential oil finds extensive uses in less-expensive perfumes, soaps and a variety of other applications.

Description   A tall tropical tree which grows up to 20 metres high with large, tender, fragrant flowers, which are pink, mauve or yellow. The yellow flowers are considered best for extraction of essential oil.

Characteristics   Sweet, floral, exotic and heavy.

Part of plant used   Flower.

Method of extraction   The large, yellow flowers of *Cananga odorata* are subjected to fractional steam distillation to produce four grades of ylang-ylang oil known as ylang-ylang extra, first, second and third. A 'complete' ylang-ylang oil is also produced by combining ylang-ylang extra, 1st grade and 2nd grade.

In the production of ylang-ylang oils, the first portion of the distillate is collected over several hours and is called 'extra', and is considered the most superior and expensive grade, traditionally reserved for use in perfumery. The ylang-ylang oils grades 1 to 3 are then collected at increasing intervals of time, the distillation being stopped on each occasion and the oil removed.

History   In Indonesia, the flowers are spread on the bed of newly-weds on their wedding night. In the Molucca Islands, an ointment is made from ylang-ylang in coconut oil for cosmetic and hair care purposes. In the Victorian age, the oil was used in a popular hair treatment: macassar oil, due to its stimulating effect on the scalp and encouraging hair growth.

A French physician, Gal, investigated the therapeutic properties of ylang-ylang in 1873. At the turn of the century further work by chemists Garnier and Rechler found the oil useful for the treatment of malaria, typhus and other fevers. They recommended it as an antiseptic for intestinal infections, diarrhoea and flatulence. They also recognised its regulatory and calming effect on the heart.

Chemical constituents   A typical chemical composition of the various grades of ylang-ylang is reported as follows (180):

Constituents	Extra	1st grade	2nd grade	3rd grade
linalool	13.6	18.6	2.8	1.0
geranyl acetate	5.3	5.9	4.1	3.5
caryophyllene	1.7	6.0	7.5	9.0
p-cresyl methyl ether	16.5	7.6	1.8	0.5
methyl benzoate	8.7	6.4	2.3	1.0
benzyl acetate	25.1	17.4	7.0	3.7
benzyl benzoate	2.2	5.3	4.7	4.3
other sesquiterpenes	7.4	28.8	54.5	97.0

The operators of the stills producing ylang-ylang oils grade the different qualities by specific gravity and by odour, but, since there are no agreed standards, the quality of a given grade varies from one producer to the other, a fact that has to be considered when ylang-ylang is purchased.

The first fractions have the higher ester content, hence a more pleasant sweet floral odour, while the lower grades have an increase in the sesquiterpene content and a harsher oily odour character.

The traditional use of ylang-ylang in aromatherapy as a relaxant and anti-depressant indicates that the extra or grade 1 would be more suitable than the 3rd grade, as esters are chemical constituents which traditionally have such qualities.

Blends well with   Bergamot, grapefruit, geranium, jasmine, lavender, lemon, neroli, orange, patchouli, rose, rosewood, sandalwood, tangerine.

Properties   Antidepressant, antiseborrhoeic, antiseptic, aphrodisiac, hypotensive, nervine, sedative.

Indications

Mind and spirit   According to Susanne Fischer-Rizzi (181):

'The spirit of ylang-ylang usually fits the person naturally drawn to it. Upon inhaling ylang-ylang with its heavy seductive, sweet aroma one can imagine a fiery, temperamental, passionate and erotic person with an awesome radiance and confidence, never losing her balance. She would always dress in bright and colourful clothing and loves to wear jewellery.'

Therefore, we can use ylang-ylang for the woman who does not allow herself to live, who hides her femininity, dresses drably, and does not care what she looks like. She lacks self confidence, may be extremely frustrated, she appears nervous, depressed and tense.

Susanne Fischer-Rizzi (181) also suggests using ylang-ylang:

'for men allowing them to become less harsh towards themselves and others. It allows them to bring out their feminine side and arouses their understanding and intuition.'

Many men may reject the intense fragrance. If this is the case it should be blended with orange, bergamot, or sandalwood. Ylang-ylang has tension-relieving properties and it is particularly beneficial for nervous depression that is accompanied by severe tension.

Body   Ylang-ylang is particularly useful in reducing rapid breathing and rapid heart beat and its sedative properties are used to help lower high blood pressure. It is highly beneficial for treating PMS, which has manifested in some women with extreme mood swings that occur just before menstruation.

Skin and hair   It has a balancing effect on sebum making it effective on both oily and dry skin. Also use as a scalp oil to promote healthy hair.

Precautions   Excessive use may lead to headaches and nausea. Non-toxic, non-irritant, a few cases of sensitisation have been reported.

Chapter 13

Carrier Oils

As most holistic aromatherapy treatments involve massage it is important that carrier oils that are pure, unadulterated and naturally extracted are chosen:
- because they possess therapeutic properties
- because they enhance the absorption of essential oil into the skin
- because they are rich in fatty acids and other nutrients.

This chapter will discuss not only the important role that carrier oils play in aromatherapy, but also the nutritional benefits of cold pressed vegetable oils.

Introduction

Vegetable oils, which are the most familiar carrier oils used in aromatherapy, have many interesting properties and benefits not only in massage, but more importantly in the field of nutrition. Natural vegetable oils extracted from nuts and seeds have played an important role in many cultures as medicines, beauty treatments and food supplements.

In recent years, no single area of nutrition has changed more radically than the types of oils and fats consumed. In an attempt to combat heart disease, lose weight and become healthier there has been a movement away from high fat foods, an increased intake of low-cholesterol and fat free products and, in some cases, fatty foods have been avoided altogether. However, the trend towards a fat free diet, which often means excluding oils as well, may pose a risk to overall health and wellbeing.

A balanced diet is one that contains the correct amount of nutrients needed by the body to function effectively and includes fats, proteins, carbohydrates, vitamins and minerals.

By cutting out certain fats such as the unrefined oils, people run the risk of deficiency in vital nutrients found in oils such as essential fatty acids, which can lead to significant health problems. It is not the quantity but the type and quality of the fat or oil that is fundamental to optimum health.

Fatty acids

All edible oils and fats are classified as lipids, and are largely composed of fatty acids which, in turn, are composed of two parts, one fatty and the other acid. Linked, they are appropriately named: fatty acid. The fatty acids are the major building blocks of fat in the human body and in food and are important sources of energy for the body. They are also major structural components of the membranes which surround subcellular organelles and are therefore important in the building and maintenance of healthy cells.

A fatty acid molecule contains a non-polar, fatty and water-insoluble carbon chain of variable length, made entirely of carbon and hydrogen atoms, ending in a methyl ($-CH_3$) group. The other end of the molecule is a weak organic acid called a carboxyl ($-COOH$) group. The diagram below shows the structure of a fatty acid.

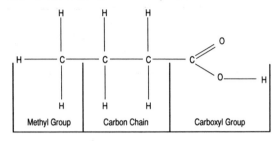

Basic structure of a fatty acid

Fatty acids may be saturated or unsaturated. To determine whether a fatty acid is saturated or unsaturated check the number of double bonds that occur in its structure. These double bonds result in fewer hydrogen atoms in the molecule. Fewer hydrogen atoms in the structure means less saturated. Since there can be many double bonds, or only a few, in a long chain fatty acid, the terms *mono-unsaturated* (one double bond), and

Saturated Fatty Acids

Mono-unsaturated Fatty Acids

Polyunsaturated Fatty Acids

Examples of saturated, mono-unsaturated and polyunsaturated fatty acids

polyunsaturated (two or more bonds) have come into general use.

Function of fatty acids

Fatty acids containing fewer than 16 carbon atoms, and all saturated fatty acids are oxidised in the body to produce energy, calories and heat. The shorter the length of the carbon chain of the saturated fatty acid, the more readily it oxidises and the easier it is to digest. This is important for people who suffer from a weak or diseased liver. Since one of the important functions of the liver is to metabolise fats, symptoms of liver malfunction are: difficulty in digesting fatty foods, and a feeling of tiredness or heaviness after eating a fat-rich meal. Shorter chain fatty acids are less demanding on the liver and are preferable in diets of people with liver disorders.

Unsaturated fatty acids can be lengthened or more double bonds inserted and the highly unsaturated molecules which result are used for special functions in the most active tissues such as brains, sense organs, adrenal glands and sexual organs. Some unsaturated fatty acids can be partially oxidised, and in this process, which is enzyme controlled, the fatty acids are changed into prostaglandins, which regulate many functions of all tissues in a hormone like way.

Saturated fatty acids

Saturated fatty acids have no double bonds. Each carbon atom is linked to hydrogen atoms by single bonds. Saturated fatty acids are mostly of animal origin such as red meat and dairy produce and are easy to identify as they tend to be solid at room temperature (eg lard, butter or cheese). The longer the carbon chain in a saturated fatty acid, the higher its melting point and the harder it is.

Short chain saturated fatty acids with up to ten carbon atoms are found in butter, milk fat and in coconut oil. The human body uses saturated fatty acids up to 14 carbons in length primarily as:

- a source of energy for the body to burn
- an insulator to keep your body warm.

The three most common saturated fats in food are myristic, palmitic and stearic acids. These longer chained saturated fatty acids appear to be

Name of Fatty Acid	Number of Carbon Atoms	Melting Point °C
butyric	4	-8
caproic	6	03
caprylic	8	17
capric	10	32
lauric	12	44
myristic	14	54
palmitic	16	63
stearic	18	70
arachidic	20	75
behenic	22	80
lignoceric	24	84

Chain length, structural formula and melting point of saturated fatty acids.

the most potent elevators of cholesterol and low-density lipoproteins (LDL) that encourage deposits in the arteries and raise the risk of heart attacks and thrombosis.

This is a problem in cardiovascular disease and other diseases of fatty degeneration, which plague those populations whose diet is high in beef and dairy foods (1).

Unsaturated fatty acids

Unsaturated fatty acids differ from the simpler saturated fatty acid in only one respect. They contain one or more double bonds between carbon atoms in their fatty carbon chain. Physically, they are liquid at room temperature.

The mono-unsaturated fatty acid, oleic acid, is found abundantly in olive oil, while polyunsaturated fatty acids are found in a number of vegetable oils, including safflower seed, sunflower seed, sesame, soybean, wheatgerm and corn. Indeed, polyunsaturated fatty acids are characteristic of vegetable oils, with the notable exceptions of palm and coconut oils, which are high in saturated fat.

Examples of polyunsaturated fatty acids are linoleic, linolenic and arachidonic acids. These

Chain length and structural formula of some saturated fatty acids

fatty acids are collectively known as the 'essential fatty acids', because they are essential for life.

None of these are produced by the body, although linolenic and arachidonic acids may be synthesised from other nutrients. Linoleic acid, however, must be obtained from diet. By eliminating all fats and oils from daily intake, people run the risk of precipitating deficiency disease.

Oleic acid is the most important mono-unsaturated acid in nutrition. It is found in olive oil, almond oil, and many other seed oils, in the membranes of plant and animal cell structures, and in the fat deposits of most land animals. It is not an essential fatty acid as the body can make its own, however it is a valuable addition to the diet. In excess it can interfere with the metabolism of essential fatty acids.

Essential fatty acids

The most important fatty acids in human nutrition and health are two acids with 18 carbon links:

- linoleic acid
- linolenic acid.

Linoleic acid and the omega 6 family

Linoleic acid can be metabolised to produce two useful fatty acids: gamma-linolenic acid (GLA), and dihomogamma-linolenic acid (DGLA). These are obviously names which the chemists have had fun with, so for our purposes they will be called GLA and DGLA. Collectively these are called the omega 6 fatty acids because of their structures.

Linoleic acid is the main omega 6 polyunsaturated fatty acid found in most cold pressed vegetable oils. A deficiency of linoleic acid can lead to disorders such as eczema-like skin eruptions, loss of hair, liver degeneration, excessive sweating with thirst, susceptibility to infections, poor wound healing, sterility in males, miscarriage in females, arthritis, heat and circulatory problems, and growth retardation. (2)

GLA has a few natural sources, in particular evening primrose oil and borage seed oil. This fatty acid is vital and has been very successful in the treatment of premenstrual syndrome, atopic eczema, psoriasis, heart and vascular disease, rheumatoid arthritis and multiple sclerosis. (3)

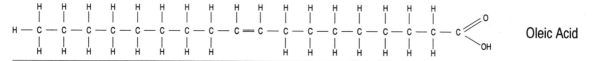

Chain length and structural formula of a mono-unsaturated fatty acid

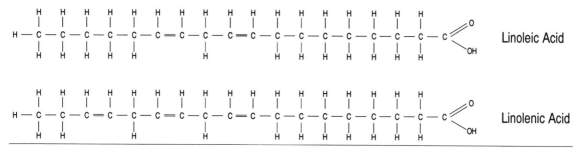

Chain length and structural formula of essential fatty acids

Linolenic acid and the omega 3 family

Linolenic acid, otherwise known as alpha linolenic acid, is found in high concentrations in vegetable oils such as linseed and canola, and in the oils from cold water fish such as salmon, sardines, mackerel and tuna. When it is metabolised in the body, linolenic acid forms a number of members of the omega 3 fatty acid family, with the most important ones being eicosapentaenoic acid (EPA), and docosahexanoic acid (DHA).

A deficiency of linolenic acid is known to cause a variety of disorders including retardation of growth, muscular weakness, lack of co-ordination. tingling of arms and legs, disturbances of vision and behavioural changes. The omega 3 fatty acids do not have the broad spread of actions of the omega 6 fatty acids. Their effect is on the cardio-vascular system.

Research into the omega-3 fats has shown that they can (4):

- prevent blood clots

- prevent dangerous abnormalities in heart rhythm which are a common feature in sudden heart attack

- reduce the levels of triglycerides in the blood

- stop certain cells sticking to the walls of the arteries

- prevent some inflammatory reactions in the body such as rheumatoid arthritis

- help lower blood pressure

- provide immunity to certain diseases.

Since these are many of the causes of heart disease in Western countries, it is not surprising that the use of the omega 3 family has increased greatly around the world, for prevention of heart disease alone. An adult requires about 5gm of each essential fatty acid each day. A deficiency may

Polyunsaturates		
Omega-6		Omega-3
High Linoleic	GLA Oils	High Linolenic
Corn Cotton Soya Safflower Sunflower	Borage Evening primrose	Linseed Fish Oils Menhaden Salmon Mackerel Tuna Anchovy

Food sources of polyunsaturated fatty acids

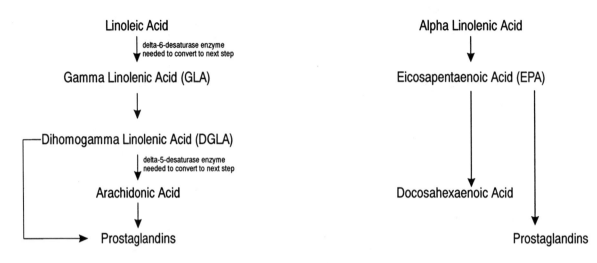

Essential fatty acid metabolism

result in rough or dry skin, dull hair, or abnormal nails. Polyunsaturated fatty acids are also important because of the role they play in reducing fatty deposits within the body. This leads us to a consideration of dietary cholesterol and its link with atherosclerosis and coronary heart disease.

Toxic fatty acids

Several natural oils contain toxic fatty acids, and are not good oils for human consumption. Cotton seed oil contains from 0.6-1.2% of a cyclopropene fatty acid with 19 carbon atoms, which has toxic effects on the liver and gall bladder. This fatty acid also slows down sexual maturity on a biochemical level, and destroys the desaturase enzymes which are responsible for metabolising the unsaturated fatty acids. It also enhances the ability of alfatoxins to cause cancer. (5)

Cotton seed oil has been known to have a very high content of pesticide residue. Cotton farmers are known to severely over-spray their crops in order to keep cotton pests under control. Refining removes part of the toxic fatty acids and pesticides, however cotton seed oil is not recommended for human or animal consumption.

Rape seed oil (canola) contains erucic acid, a 22 carbon chain fatty acid. Until 1974 rapeseed oil produced in Canada contained up to 40% erucic acid. In response to government concerns over the results of rat studies which showed erucic acid causes fatty degeneration of the heart, kidneys, adrenals and thyroid, geneticists have bred new varieties of rape seed with a lower content of erucic acid. According to some government standards, less than 5% erucic acid content in canola oil is permissible. (6)

However when researchers did the same test with rats, but using sunflower seed oil (which contains no erucic acid), the rats ended up with the same condition. As it turned out, rats do not metabolise fats and oils well as their normal diet consists of low-fat vegetables and grains!

It seems that the millions of dollars spent in developing new varieties of rapeseed was a waste of money and effort because of an error made in the interpretation of research results from animal tests.

In China and India, millions of people use high erucic acid mustard oil and rapeseed unrefined oil as a staple part of their diets without developing the problems that the laboratory rats developed with rapeseed oil.

Even more disturbing is the fact that erucic acid has beneficial effects. Lorenzo's oil, a preparation of 20% erucic acid and 80% oleic acid, has been used to treat a rare, fatal degenerative genetic condition known as adrenoleukodystrophy (ALD), in which a buildup of very long-chain fatty acids (C22 to C28) destroys the myelin in the brain. Erucic acid has been found to normalise these fatty acids, although it does not reverse damage already done to nerves and myelin (7).

The story of Lorenzo Odone and his parents' fight to get erucic acid treatment for their son has been captured in the highly moving film *Lorenzo's Oil*.

Another toxic fatty acid is the hydroxy fatty acid ricinoleic acid which makes up 80% of the fatty acid content of castor oil. This fatty acid stimulates the secretion of fluids in the intestine and for this reason is used as a purgative in medicine. Apart from causing very powerful intestinal contractions, castor oil has no harmful effects. (8)

Cholesterol

The fat called 'cholesterol' is generally considered a 'baddie' in nutritional terms, however this is somewhat over-simplifying matters. As usual, it is a case of maintaining the right balance. The body uses cholesterol as a component of the membranes surrounding every living cell. Its function is to ensure that the fats we need to transport can be moved around in the largely water-based fluids such as blood and lymph. Cholesterol also helps maintain healthy nerve fibres and is needed for the manufacture of hormones. Because cholesterol is so important the liver is able to manufacture the body's requirements.

There is no other substance as widely publicised by the medical profession. It has become a powerful marketing gimmick for vegetable oil and margarine manufacturers who advertise their products as 'cholesterol free'. The problem cholesterol causes is not entirely due to the substance itself. The unwanted build up of cholesterol is simply a symptom of the body's not being able to process its blood fats correctly, and this is dependent on the type of oils in the diet. It is necessary to understand how fats are transported in the body and the role cholesterol plays.

Fats are insoluble in water, and to be transported by the blood they have to be modified. They bind with proteins (which are usually soluble in water) to form lipoproteins, and these in turn fall into two categories:

- low density lipoproteins (LDL), which are the main carriers of cholesterol in the blood and transport cholesterol to the tissues

- high density lipoproteins (HDL), which transport cholesterol away from the tissues to the liver, where it can then be excreted in bile.

This means that it is the amount of LDL cholesterol that we should be concerned about, since it is these fatty deposits that will settle inside the wall of the arteries. As the arteries become increasingly clogged there is less room for the blood flow, thus we have a condition called atherosclerosis.

The importance of cold pressed oils is that they are high in polyunsaturated fatty acids, which help to reduce the risk of atherosclerosis. Saturated fats in the diet, on the other hand, are more likely to cause the formation of blood clots which in due course can lead to a heart attack. The essential fatty acids have a vital function of reducing the adhesiveness of fatty deposits on the lining of the arterial wall. The prostaglandins which are formed from the essential fatty acids also help to control the clustering of platelets in the blood.

How we produce cholesterol

One of the causes of high cholesterol levels is a high intake of saturated fats. These fats are broken down in the liver to ketoacids which are normally used for energy production in the muscle cells. For this, the ketoacids need the breakdown products of the sugar metabolism (glycolysis). If you have an habitually raised adrenalin level or insensitivity to insulin (eg diabetes), these sugar metabolites are in short supply, which can cause ketoacids to accumulate. In addition, a deficiency of chromium will also interfere with the fat metabolism. The liver now attempts to get rid of the ketoacids by converting them to surplus cholesterol.

Another factor responsible for cholesterol overproduction in the body is the overconsumption of sugar. When sugar is ingested, the blood insulin level is raised. A key enzyme of cholesterol synthesis is actually

Hydrogenation

regulated by insulin. This means that a higher sugar intake generates a higher insulin level and with this higher fat and cholesterol levels. It can be seen that a diet high in fat and sugar is the main cause of a raised cholesterol level, while the cholesterol content of food ingested has repeatedly shown little impact on body cholesterol levels.

A direct connection has also been shown to exist with oxy-cholesterol. If cholesterol in food is heated, especially with access to air, then it is oxidised to oxy-cholesterol. Animal experiments with high intakes of either cholesterol or oxy-cholesterol have shown atherogenic degeneration only with the latter, not with cholesterol itself. This implies that the main contributing factor to the high rate of heart disease is the habit of overly heating, and in particular frying, meats, eggs and milk products.

Modified oils

An effective way to destroy the nutritional value (essential fatty acids) in a natural vegetable oil is to hydrogenate the oil. In this process, oils which contain unsaturated fatty acids in their natural state, (all cis-) are reacted at a high temperature (120° - 210°C) and under pressure with hydrogen gas in the presence of a metal catalyst, usually nickel, platinum or copper for up to eight hours.

Once the process is complete all the double bonds in the oil are saturated with hydrogen. As a result the oil now has no essential fatty acid activity. Such oils are now considered very useful for commercial purposes, as they have a long shelf life, and when heated will not produce toxic byproducts. Oils such as coconut and palm oil which are often hydrogenated (these oils are over 90% saturated to begin with) are ideal to use in

products such as chocolate which needs to be hard enough so that it does not melt except in very hot weather and yet will melt in the mouth.

In partial hydrogenation the process of hydrogenation is not brought to completion and a product containing many intermediate substances is formed. Double bonds turn from cis- to trans-configuration, and double bonds may shift, producing conjugated fatty acids.

cis-configuration

trans-configuration

Cis- and trans- configurations of fatty acids

The simple change that occurs in the shape from cis- to trans- has significant effects on the physical properties and therefore, the functions of the molecules. Trans- molecules are more stable than cis- molecules, however in terms of its biological activity, the trans- configuration can fit into only half of the enzyme and membrane structures, which can only identify the cis-configurations. Thus not only can't the trans-configurations do the job of the cis-configurations, but they also block out the cis-forms.

Partial hydrogenation is used to make margarines and shortenings. Consequently there are high percentages of trans-fatty acids and other altered fat substances which are known to be detrimental to health because they interfere with normal biochemical processes, and many others have not been adequately studied to know what their effects on health might be.

216

Two statements summarise my opinion on hydrogenated oils and their by-products such as margarine.

The first statement, made by Brisson (9), Professor of Nutrition at Laval University in Quebec, says that:

'it would be practically impossible to predict with accuracy either the nature or the content of these new molecules....there is a world of chemistry that alters profoundly the composition and physicochemical properties of natural oils.'

Herbert Dutton (10), one of America's most knowledgeable oil chemists says:

'If the hydrogenation process had been discovered today, it probably could not be adopted by the oil industry.'

He continues,

'... the basis of such comment lies in the recent awareness of our prior ignorance concerning the complexity of isomers formed during hydrogenation and their metabolic and physiological fate.'

The way in which oils are used in cooking will affect the fatty acid profile of the oil. Heating oils to temperatures of 160°C or higher produces many toxic substances including trans-fatty acids.

Frying and deep-frying are two of the most popular methods of fast food preparation, but foods prepared by these methods are damaging to health because the heat modifies and damages the fatty acids in the vegetable oils used. Many toxic substances are produced during the heating and some have not even been identified.

Besides producing atherosclerosis, the oils after use in frying and deep-frying can impair cell respiration and other cell functions, inhibit immune functions, and lead to cancer.

My advice is simply to not use fresh cold pressed, unrefined, EFA-rich seed oils for frying. If frying or deep frying, use oils which contain the lowest amount of EFAs and use sulphur-rich garlic and onions to minimise free-radical damage.

According to Udo Erasmus the oils and fats which are least damaged by high temperatures include (11):

- butter
- tropical fats such as coconut oil
- high oleic sunflower oil
- high oleic safflower oil
- sesame seed oil
- canola oil
- olive oil.

How are vegetable oils extracted?

In most modern oil pressing factories many things happen to the seeds and the natural oil that it contains before the oil is actually extracted. This section summarises these processes.

Cooking

The seeds are initially mechanically cleaned, crushed and cooked for up to 2 hours at varying temperatures depending on the seed being used. An average temperature used is 120°C. This process makes the next step easier by destroying the cells which contain the oil.

Unrefined oil production stage

Expeller pressing

The crushed seeds are pressed in an expeller press, which is a continually rotating spiral shaped augur which moves the seed forward and pushes the seed against a metal press head. The pressure generated in the head of an expeller press reaches several tonnes per square centimetre. The turning augur further crushes the seed and creates friction in the seed mass, which produces heat in the press head. Both the heat and pressure force the oil out of the seed and the oil runs out through slots or holes in the side of the press head, while the oil cake, the solid remainder of the seed mash, is pushed out through slits at the end of the press head. This pressing process usually takes a few minutes at temperatures around 85°C.

The oil is then filtered and bottled and sold as 'cold pressed oil'. Most commercial manufacturers will then treat this 'unrefined oil'

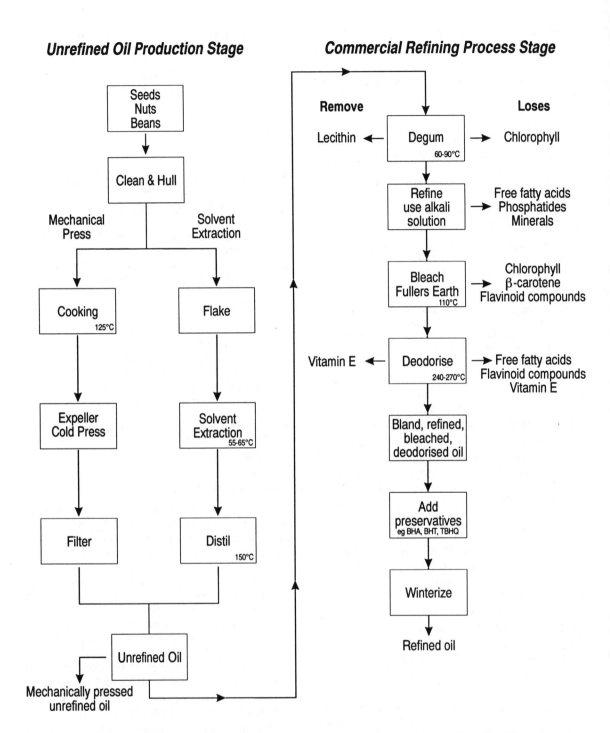

Schematic of the steps involved in the processing of vegetable oils (1)

by several processes such as degumming, refining, bleaching and deodorising.

Solvent extraction

An alternative method of removing the oil from the seed is to extract the oil from the seed meal with a solvent such as hexane. This same method is often used to get the last oil remaining in the oil cake after expeller pressing, and thus increase the yield of the oil from the seed. Once the oil-solvent mixture has been separated from the seed meal, the solvent is evaporated at a temperature of about 150°C. This oil is now ready to be treated by the processes described below.

Commercial refining process stage

Degumming

In this process, gums (protein-like compounds), and complex carbohydrates called polysaccharides are taken out of the oil. Lecithin, well known for its health benefits, is also isolated and sold separately (at twice the price). Degumming is carried out at 60°C, with water and phosphoric acid. Degumming also removes chlorophyll, calcium, magnesium, iron, and copper from the oil.

Refining

In this process the oil is mixed with sodium hydroxide (caustic soda) and sodium carbonate. This removes free fatty acids from the oil. Free fatty acids form soap with sodium hydroxide, and the soap then dissolves in the watery part of the mixture. Phospholipids, protein-like substances, and minerals are also further removed in this process. The refining temperature is around 75°C. At this stage the oil still contains pigments.

Bleaching

Acid treated clays and Fuller's Earth are used to remove the pigments of chlorophyll and beta-carotene and the remaining traces of soap. Bleaching takes place at 110°C. During bleaching, toxic peroxides and conjugated fatty acids are formed from the essential fatty acids present in the oil.

Deodorisation

This involves steam distillation under pressure and exclusion of air to remove aromatic oils, more free fatty acids, pungent odours and unpleasant tastes, which are not present in the natural oil in the seed before the processing began. Deodorisation takes place at the high temperature of 240°C to 270°C for 30 to 60 minutes.

The peroxides produced in the refining step are removed. Vitamin E, phytosterols and some pesticide residues and toxins are also removed by deodorisation. The oil is finally odourless, tasteless and cannot be distinguished from oils derived from other sources which have been similarly treated. Believe it or not this oil can still be sold as 'cold pressed', because no external heat was applied during the pressing of the oil.

Preservative and winterisation stage

Before distributing the refined oil to the supermarkets, several antioxidants will be added to them. These may include butylated hydroxytoluene (BHT), butylated hydroxyanisole (BHA), propyl gallate, tertiary butylhydroquinone (TBHQ) or citric acid, to replace the natural antioxidants beta-carotene and vitamin E which were destroyed in the refining process. Defoamers may also be added, and the oil is bottled and sold.

Winterisation is the process whereby an oil is cooled and filtered again to prevent it from developing turbidity when it is cooled in the refrigerator.

What are cold pressed oils?

The term 'cold pressed' implies that no heat is used in extracting the oil. It really means that no external heat has been applied to the seed while it is being pressed. During pressing the temperature reached by the oil press rarely exceeds 100°C. In some countries it is illegal to call an oil 'cold pressed' if the highest temperature which the oil has reached in the entire process, from seed to oil, exceeds 50°C.

Why should vegetable oils be extracted without heat? The higher temperatures break down and destroy many of the nutritive qualities of the vegetable oil. Many of the unsaturated fatty acids contained in the oil thus begin to change their molecular arrangement from the natural cis-configuration to the unnatural trans- configuration (which is a toxic substance) once the temperature begins to exceed 160°C. Therefore the heat produced during pressing normally does not damage the oil.

Commonly used vegetable oils

The seeds of most plants contain oil, which serve as the high energy starter for the seedling. Just like the chicken's egg the plant seed has to contain enough energy to sprout a whole plant. The tougher the environmental conditions, the more oil the seed needs to store. The colder the climate, the more of the unsaturated fatty acids it contains in its oil to increase its metabolic rate. For this reason, the amounts of the various fatty acids contained in the oil from different seeds varies greatly. The amount of oil found in the different seeds varies from 4% for corn oil to over 70% for pecans.

Sweet almond oil

Botanical name: *Prunus amygdalus*

The almond tree is a native of the Middle East. There are two varieties of tree, the sweet almond *(dulcis)* and bitter almond *(amara)*. It is the sweet almond that is widely used, as the bitter almond contains traces of amygdalin that can be hydrolysed or distilled to produce the deadly hydrocyanic acid (cyanide).

The earliest use of almond oil dates back to the Romans who used it extensively in skincare preparations. Almond oil was a favourite beautifier throughout Europe, and in Britain the sixteenth century herbalist John Gerald wrote:

> '*Almond oil makes smoothe thye hands and face of delicate persons and cleanseth the skin of spots and pimples.*'

It stores reasonably well, protects and nourishes the skin, and is ideal for chapped or irritated skin. Almond oil is highly nutritious and has been shown to be twice as effective as the better known olive oil in the reduction of cholesterol. According to clinical trials published,

participants' cholesterol levels dropped by an average of 11%. (12)

A typical analysis of sweet almond oil is:

Fatty Acid	Name	Percentage
C14	Myristic	0.1
C16	Palmitic	6.6
C16:1	Palmitoleic	0.5
C17	Heptadecenoic	0.1
C17:1	9-Heptadecenoic	0.1
C18	Stearic	1.3
C18:1	Oleic	64.6
C18:2	Linoleic	26.3
C18:3	Linolenic	0.2
C20	Arachidic	0.1
C20:1	Eicosenoic	0.1

Apricot kernel oil

Botanical name: *Prunus armeniaca*

Apricot kernel oil is a good source of polyunsaturated fatty acids. It has a wonderful light texture making it very easily absorbed by the skin. The light texture of this oil makes it especially suitable for facial massage blends. It is good for the treatment of mature, dry, sensitive or inflamed skins.

A typical analysis of apricot kernel oil is:

Fatty Acid	Name	Percentage
C16	Palmitic	4.9
C16:1	Palmitoleic	0.9
C17	Heptadecenoic	-
C17:1	9-Heptadecenoic	0.1
C18	Stearic	1.0
C18:1	Oleic	62.0
C18:2	Linoleic	30.6
C18:3	Linolenic	0.2
C20	Arachidic	0.1
C20:1	Eicosenoic	0.1

Avocado oil

Botanical name: *Persea americana*

The avocado tree was first found growing in South American swamp lands where it was nicknamed 'alligator pear'. Technically, avocados are a fruit because they have a stone.

The oil is extracted from the flesh which contains up to 30% pure oil - a figure rivalled only by olive and palm fruit. Crude avocado oil is produced by mechanical pressing on hydraulic presses, followed by centrifugal extraction.

The oil is rich in many nutrients including Vitamin A and D, lecithin and potassium. It is also rich in chlorophyll, the reason for its dazzling green colour. Although the oil is mono-unsaturated, it is not as stable as olive oil at high temperatures, so is not suitable for cooking.

Avocado oil can be used to soothe the skin, being useful for conditions such as nappy rash and eczema. It has moisturising properties and is ideal for dry, mature skin and assists in the treatment of climate-damaged, parched, undernourished or aging skin.

A typical analysis of avocado oil is:

Fatty Acid	Name	Percentage
C16	Palmitic	12.0-16.0
C16:1	Palmitoleic	4.3-6.8
C18	Stearic	2.0
C18:1	Oleic	60.0-72.0
C18:2	Linoleic	8.0-15.03
C18:3	Linolenic	2.0

Canola oil

Botanical name: *Brassica napus*

Also known as Rapeseed oil, this oil has been extensively used in commercial food preparation. The rape plant belongs to the cabbage family and grows 1.5 to 1.8 metres high with vivid yellow flowers. Rape is a versatile crop. The seeds contain 35-40% pure oil, and the young leaves can be served as a vegetable. Because of its rather unfortunate name the Canadians decided to register the name Canola for the oil produced from the rapeseed.

Canola oil has the highest percentage of unsaturated fats of any oil. It contains over 90% mono- and polyunsaturates and is a light oil with very little flavour. It is unstable at high temperatures and will produce more toxic effluents when cooked.

A typical analysis of canola oil is:

Fatty Acid	Name	Percentage
C16	Palmitic	3.0-4.5
C16:1	Palmitoleic	0.2-0.3
C18	Stearic	1.3-1.7
C18:1	Oleic	56.0-62.0
C18:2	Linoleic	19-24
C18:3	Linolenic	8.2-13.0
C22:1	Erucic	0.2-1.8

Evening primrose oil

Botanical name: *Oenothera biennis*

The evening primrose is a tall, spiky plant that blooms only in the evening, hence its common name. The North American Indian medicine men were the first to recognise its potential as a healing agent and used to brew the seed pods to make an infusion for healing wounds.

Evening primrose oil is rich in fatty acids, one in particular, gamma linolenic acid (GLA). The gamma linolenic acid found in evening primrose oil is biologically important as it affects much of the enzyme activity in the body. Every process that takes place in the body, including the production of prostaglandins, is triggered by the action of various enzymes. These hormone like substances are responsible for:

- lowering blood pressure
- inhibiting thrombosis
- inhibiting cholesterol
- inhibiting inflammation
- inhibiting platelet aggregation

- regulating oestrogen, progestogen, and prolactin in the luteal phase of the menstrual cycle.

Prostaglandins are the end result of a chemical chain reaction which starts with essential fatty acids- notably linoleic acid which is found in cold pressed oils. The diagram on this page shows the synthesis of prostaglandins from linoleic acid.

A prostaglandin imbalance or deficiency results in a wide range of disorders such as poor skin conditions, eczema type lesions, reproductive problems, problems of the circulatory system, increased susceptibility to infection, poor wound healing and many other cellular and enzymatic disorders.

Linoleic acid is converted into gamma-linolenic acid, the substance found in evening primrose oil, and then to dihomogamma-linolenic acid and then to arachidonic acid. The latter two are present in all cell structures and are the precursors of prostaglandins. It is assumed that this conversion process is efficiently dealt with in the body.

Research shows that the following factors inhibit the production of GLA: (13)

- a diet rich in saturated fats
- a diet rich in processed vegetable oils
- consumption of alcohol
- diabetes
- aging process
- a lack of zinc, magnesium and vitamin B in the diet - all of which are necessary for GLA formation
- viral infections, radiation, cancer
- stress.

This is where evening primrose oil steps in. It has been found that the GLA from this oil is a more efficient precursor of arachidonic acid than the linoleic acid found in sunflower seed oil.

GLA is essential to the formation of a number of compounds, the most important being PGE1 which:

- prevents thrombosis
- lowers blood pressure

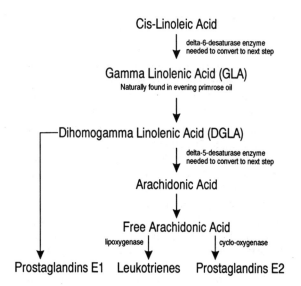

Prostaglandin synthesis from the linoleic family

- opens blood vessels and relieves angina pain
- slows down the production of cholesterol
- enables insulin to work more effectively
- prevents inflammation and controls arthritis.

Rheumatoid arthritis, inflammatory bowel disease, ulcerative colitis, Crohn's disease as well as eczema, multiple sclerosis and other diseases involving inflammation and immunity are all affected by prostaglandin levels. They all have a common feature: excessive production of Class 2 prostaglandins (PGE2).

The elevated level of Class 2 prostaglandins is believed to be a major contributor to local inflammation and it now appears to be linked with lack of adequate amounts of PGE1. If this is correct, aspirins and other steroid medications often given for rheumatoid arthritis are not the answer as they inhibit the biosynthesis of prostaglandins. Instead the PGE1 levels should be adjusted through nutritional sources such as evening primrose oil.

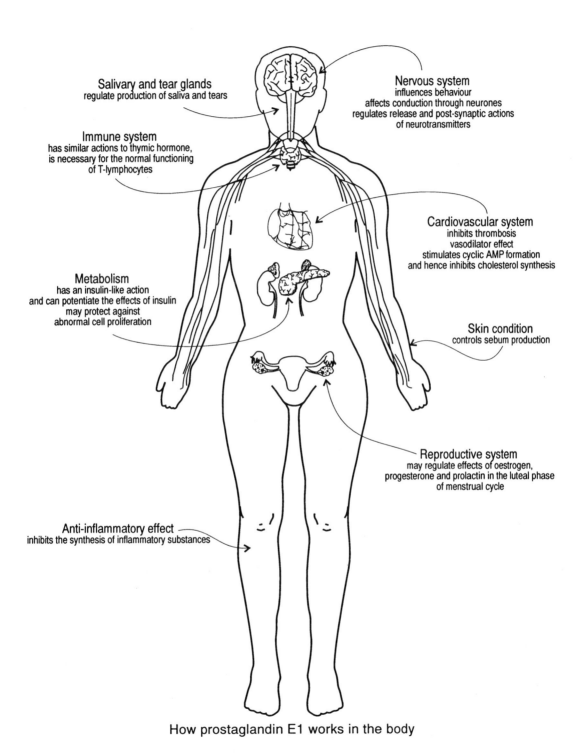

How prostaglandin E1 works in the body

Evening primrose oil can be used externally as a massage oil and has been found to be effective for the treatment of eczema and psoriasis, pre-menstrual syndrome, rheumatoid arthritis and weight reduction.

A typical analysis of evening primrose oil is:

Fatty Acid	Name	Percentage
C16:1	Palmitoleic	6.1
C18:1	Oleic	1.9
C20:0	Arachidic	0.3
C22:0	Behenic	0.1
C18:1w9	Oleic	6.3
C18:1w7	Oleic	0.6
C20:1w9	Eicosenoic	0.2
C22:1w9	Erucic	-
C24:1w9	Tetracosenoic	-
C18:2w6	Linoleic	65.0-73.9
C18:3w6	Gamma linolenic	8.5-11.5
C18:3w3	Alpha linolenic	0.2

Joboba oil

Botanical name: *Simmondsia chinensis*

The jojoba plant was first recorded by British botanist H. F. Link in 1822, when he landed at Baja California in northern Mexico and observed the wild shrub in its natural state. Link named the plant *Simmondsia chinensis*, after a fellow British botanist and explorer, T.W. Simmonds.

It was not until the early 1970s when the U.S. Government banned whaling, that active research began in the production of jojoba oil as a substitute for sperm whale oil. Jojoba oil (pronounced ho-ho-ba) is unique because the oil is not composed of fat but of liquid wax.

In scientific terms, waxes are esters of long-chain fatty acids with long-chain monohydroxyl alcohols, whereas fats are esters of long-chain fatty acids with glycerine. Being composed of mostly wax esters means that there is little likelihood of the oil's deteriorating.

Jojoba oil is ideal for use in cosmetics because of its molecular stability and its natural moisturising and healing properties. Jojoba's resistance to oxidation means that it does not require additional chemical preservatives. It is suitable for all skin types, whether dry, oily or sensitive.

When applied to the scalp as a treatment, jojoba oil acts to regulate and remove the sebum. Research indicates that jojoba oil is beneficial in the treatment of certain dry scalp and skin problems such as psoriasis and eczema. The oil is an excellent emollient for the skin, rendering it soft and smooth.

A typical fatty acid profile of jojoba oil is:

Fatty Acid	Name	Percentage
C16:0	Palmitic	1.5
C16:1	Palmitoleic	0.4
C18:0	Stearic	10.1
C18:1	Oleic	13.9
C18:2	Linoleic	0.3
C18:3	Linolenic	0.2
C19:0	Nonadecenoic	trace
C20:0	Arachidic	0.1
C20:1	Eicosenoic	71.2
C22:0	Behenic	0.2
C22:1	Erucic	11.2
C24:0	Lignoceric	0.1
C24:1	Nervonic	0.9

Linseed oil

Botanical name: *Linum usitatissimum*

Linseed oil takes its name from the Latin for 'most useful' and is extracted from the flax plant. Flax is an annual crop with rich blue flowers and tiny brownish seeds. There are several varieties, each with a different use. The long stemmed variety is grown for its lengthy fibres that are woven into linen, while the seeds of the short stemmed varieties are commonly used for oil production.

The use of linseed oil can be traced back to Hippocrates who recorded that it was a useful treatment for stomach and skin disorders. Linseed is valued by herbalists for its mucilage properties, meaning it contains a slimy material that is not absorbed but passes straight through the body.

Linseeds are very effective and gentle bulking agents and can be used as laxatives when swallowed whole with plenty of water. The mucins and water binding substances in linseed work by increasing the volume of the stool. This then presses against the intestinal walls and triggers the peristalsis movement. In addition, the mucins form a protective and gliding film which covers the sensitive mucous membranes. This can be useful for healing intestinal wall irritations. Linseeds can be crushed and used as a poultice to draw out excess fluid from body tissues.

Linseed oil contains mainly omega-3 fatty acids which are normally found in fish oils and is therefore recommended for vegetarians who prefer not to take fish oils. One of the drawbacks of linseed oil is that it needs to be used fresh as it turns rancid much faster than other oils, so it needs to be kept in a refrigerator and a tightly sealed amber bottle.

A typical fatty acid profile of linseed oil is:

Fatty Acid	Name	Percentage
C16	Palmitic	5.5
C16:1	Palmitoleic	-
C18	Stearic	3.5
C18:1	Oleic	19.1
C18:2	Linoleic	15.3
C18:3	Linolenic	56.6

Macadamia oil

Botanical name: *Macadamia integrifolia* or *M. ternifolia*

Macadamia oil is high in palmitoleic acid, a mono-unsaturated fatty acid not commonly found in many other oils. Palmitoleic acid is also found in sebum, thus macadamia oil has been often recommended for older skin which starts to dry as the sebum production diminishes. It is a highly nourishing and emollient oil recommended for dry and mature skin.

A typical fatty acid profile of macadamia oil is:

Fatty Acid	Name	Percentage
C14	Myristic	0.6-1.6
C16	Palmitic	7.0-11.0
C16:1	Palmitoleic	18.0-25.0
C18	Stearic	2.0-4.0
C18:1	Oleic	55.0-62.0
C18:2	Linoleic	1.0-4.0
C20	Arachidic	2.0-4.0
C20.1	Eicosenoic	2.0-4.0

Olive oil

Botanical name: *Olea europaea*

The olive is traditionally regarded as a symbol of peace. The ancient Greeks wore garlands of olive leaves in their hair as they prayed for peace. Even in the modern political setting, an olive branch within a dove's beak is the accepted symbol of peace.

The best oil comes from the fruit which is nearly fully ripe, and hand picked. The oil itself comes from the pulp, not the kernel, and mills crush the fruit gently so that the stone does not fracture. The oil is separated by a centrifugal process, and filtered for purity. This is true 'virgin olive oil', but there are various grades of virgin oil, which are graded according to the aroma and degree of acidity.

Olive oil is amongst the heavier oils, which enables it to be used in soaps and cosmetics. Many people find olive oil a little heavy for massage but it may be blended with less viscous vegetable oils for this purpose.

A typical analysis of olive oil is:

Fatty Acid	Name	Percentage
C16	Palmitic	11.0
C16:1	Palmitoleic	1.2
C18	Stearic	2.7
C18:1	Oleic	75.5
C18:2	Linoleic	8.0
C18:3	Linolenic	0.7

Pumpkin seed oil

Botanical name: *Curcurbita pepo*

The seeds from the commonly cultivated pumpkin, *Curcurbita pepo*, produce an oil with a pleasant nutty aroma and very high in protein, zinc and polyunsaturated fats.

It is prescribed for the treatment of urinary tract infections. 5 to 10 drops should be taken orally three times a day for four weeks. Taken orally as described above, pumpkin seed oil also aids in maintaining the health of the lungs and mucous membranes giving relief to symptoms of catarrh.

A typical fatty acid profile of pumpkin seed oil is:

Fatty Acid	Name	Percentage
C16:0	Palmitic	10.6
C18:0	Stearic	6.1
C18:1w9	Oleic	41.4
C18:2w6	Linoleic	39.7
C18:3w3	Alpha Linolenic	0.4
C20:0	Arachidic	0.5
C20:1	Eicos-11-enoic	0.2
C22:1	Erucic	0.2

Rosehip oil

Botanical name: *Rosa rubiginosa*

Rosehip oil is produced in Chile and has recently become a popular oil, particularly in regenerative skin care. The oil is usually obtained by solvent extraction.

It is extracted from the seeds of a rose bush which grows wild in the southern Andes. Extensive clinical work conducted in South America claims that the oil is extremely beneficial in tissue regeneration for conditions such as burns, facial wrinkles, and treatment of scars following surgery.

The oil has been used successfully to reduce wrinkles and signs of premature aging. It also helps to counter the drying effects of the sun which are usually noticed by the fine wrinkles or 'crows feet' around the eyes and mouth. The oil was also used to attentuate scars (both surgical and accidental), by reducing the redness or hyperpigmentation, reducing the formation of keloid scar tissue formed and loosening up fibrous cords. (14)

It is believed that these important functions in the regeneration and repair of skin tissue are due to the amazingly high level of both linoleic (47.4%) and linolenic (33.0%) fatty acids.

Safflower oil

Botanical name: *Carthamus tinctorius*

Safflower, also known as American saffron, belongs to the sunflower family. The oil is extracted from the seeds of the plant and has a bland, slightly nutty flavour. Among the natural vegetable oils it is one of the least expensive and it usually has a high percentage of unsaturated fatty acids.

Unfortunately, safflower oil becomes rancid if not stored in a refrigerator and it is not suitable for deep frying because its nutritional properties are unstable at high temperatures.

A typical analysis of safflower oil is:

Fatty Acid	Name	Percentage
C16	Palmitic	6.0-7.5
C16:1	Palmitoleic	trace - 0.1
C18	Stearic	2.0-2.5
C18:1	Oleic	11.0-13.5
C18:2	Linoleic	76.0-80.0
C18:3	Linolenic	trace - 0.1

Sesame seed oil

Botanical name: *Sesamum indicum*

Sesame, also known as benne, is one of the oldest herbs grown specifically for its seeds. The Chinese cultivated sesame some 5,000 years ago, the Egyptians ground it to produce flour, and Roman soldiers mixed sesame seeds with honey to give them extra strength for their long arduous military campaigns.

The sesame oil can be extracted from raw seeds, or seeds which have been roasted prior to being pressed. The latter oil is dark and smoky red and is often used in Chinese cooking. The natural oil is light in colour and slightly nutty to taste. Sesame seed oil is comparatively stable and does not turn rancid on contact with the air.

The oil is also high in Vitamin E, B complex vitamins, and the minerals calcium, magnesium and phosphorus. It is a good source of vegetable protein and comparatively rich in lecithin. Because it is high in calcium, sesame seed oil is not acid forming and is therefore a good laxative for those suffering from stomach disorders. The oil can be used in skin care as a natural moisturiser.

A typical fatty acid profile of sesame seed oil is:

Fatty Acid	Name	Percentage
C16	Palmitic	5.5-9.5
C16:1	Palmitoleic	-
C18	Stearic	4.0-6.0
C18:1	Oleic	33.5-46.0
C18:2	Linoleic	41.0-51.0
C18:3	Linolenic	trace-1.0 max

Soyabean oil

Botanical name: *Glycine max*

Soyabean oil comes from the soya plant which belongs to the pea or legume family. It can be traced back 5,000 years to its first recorded cultivation in mainland China. The oil is extracted from the smooth egg-shaped beans which have an oil content of approximately 20%.

Cold pressed soyabean oil is the second best natural source of vitamin E found in cold pressed vegetable oils (87 mg per 100 ml). It contains more lecithin than any other vegetable oil. The oil is comparatively high in unsaturated fatty acids. It can be used in massage, being suitable for all skin types.

A typical analysis of soyabean oil is:

Fatty Acid	Name	Percentage
C16	Palmitic	10.4
C16:1	Palmitoleic	0.1
C18	Stearic	4.1
C18:1	Oleic	23.9
C18:2	Linoleic	53.5
C18:3	Linolenic	6.8

Sunflower oil

Botanical name: *Helianthus annuus*

Sunflowers were prized by the South American Indians who ground the seeds of the flower in a mortar and pestle to make meal. Sunflower seeds contain vitamins A, D, B-complex and E and are also rich in minerals such as calcium, zinc, potassium, iron and phosphorus.

The oil from the seeds of sunflower resembles that of safflower, to which it is related. Sunflower is an inexpensive oil to use for massage and may be blended with other cold pressed oils.

A typical analysis of sunflower oil is:

Fatty Acid	Name	Percentage
C16	Palmitic	6.4
C16:1	Palmitoleic	0.1
C18	Stearic	4.2
C18:1	Oleic	14.2
C18:2	Linoleic	73.5
C18:3	Linolenic	0.2

Wheatgerm oil

Botanical name: *Triticum durum* or *T. aestivum*

Wheat is the most widely cultivated cereal grain in the world and is derived from a hybrid wild wheat that grew in the Middle East 10,000 years ago. Most varieties of cultivated wheat belong to two basic types: *Triticum durum* and *Triticum aestivum*. The latter is used to produce bread, while *Triticum durum* is a harder type of wheat used to make semolina, spaghetti and other forms of pasta.

Wheat grain consists of three parts: the bran, or outer husk, representing 12% of the grain by weight; the germ (about 3%) and the starchy endosperm (about 85%). Milling of white flower separates the wheatgerm altogether. Unfortunately it is the wheatgerm that contains 25% of the protein and a vast array of vitamins and minerals.

Wheatgerm oil is extracted by warm pressing or solvent extraction from the 'germ' of wheat. It is an extremely valuable source of vitamin E (190 mg per 100 gm) and essential fatty acids. Because of its vitamin E content it is a natural anti-oxidant and is well protected from the elements, such as light and heat, that usually break down vegetable oils. It promotes the formation of skin cells, improves blood circulation, and helps relieve symptoms of dermatitis.

Its anti-oxidant properties help to remove cholesterol deposits from the arteries and are thus of vital importance in combating heart disease.

A typical fatty acid profile of wheatgerm oil is:

Fatty acid	Name	Percentage
C14:0	Myristic	less than 0.1
C16:0	Palmitic	15.77
C16:1	Palmitoleic	0.2
C18:0	Stearic	1.02
C18:1	Oleic	19.15
C18:2	Linoleic	53.9
C18:3	Linolenic	7.07
C20:0	Arachidic	0.19
C20:1	Ecisadenoic	1.54
C20.2	Eicosadinoic	0.14
C22:0	Behenic	0.13
C24:0	Lignoceric	0.4
C24:1	Nervonic	less than 0.1

Macerated oils

Macerated oils include arnica, calendula, carrot, and hypericum oils, but almost any plant can be macerated.

To make your own macerated oil place freshly harvested herbs loosely in a transparent, wide-mouthed glass jar and add a cold pressed vegetable oil such as sweet almond or apricot kernel to cover. Seal the jar so that it is air tight and leave it for four to eight weeks, shaking vigorously once a day. At the end of the period, the oil is drained and filtered and is ready to use as a macerated oil. Store the oil in a dark bottle.

Arnica

Botanical name: *Arnica montana*

The herb arnica grows almost exclusively in the high mountainous regions of Northern Europe. The German folk name for arnica literally means 'mountain well-being'. The flowering heads of the plant are used for the preparation of either a macerated oil or a tincture of arnica and the root stock is usually employed for homoepathic preparations.

Arnica oil or the tincture should be used for external applications only. The main application is for the external treatment of all types of injuries in which the skin is not broken, such as bruises, strained muscles, tendons, contusions, haemorrhages and swellings, incuding bone fractures. Arnica may be used as a compress and if applied immediately or as soon as possible it has astonishing healing qualities.

Calendula

Botanical name: *Calendula officinalis*

Calendula should not be confused with tagetes which is also known as marigold.

Calendula has anti-inflammatory properties and vulnerary properties, making it useful for stubborn wounds, ulcers, bed sores, varicose veins and bruises. It is effective in treating skin problems such as rashes and in particular, chapped and cracked skin, and makes an excellent base oil for treating eczema.

Calendula oil has also been used for treating venous complaints. In case of all venous inflammation the ointment should be lightly applied, preferably blended with cypress and lemon essential oils. When applied consistently, calendula oil decreases the symptoms of varicose veins and veinous congestion by inhibiting inflammation, toning tissue and promoting enhanced blood supply to tissue.

Calendula is a native of the Mediterranean region and the whole flower blossom, not the petals alone, is employed for medicinal purposes. The flower's bright yellow-to-orange colour is due to the high carotenoid content, a substance of great importance to calendula's skin regenerative properties. The carotenoid compounds are only soluble in fats.

The wound healing properties of calendula have been documented in many studies and it was found that a combination of lipophilic extracts (oil extracts) and hydrophilic extracts (containing flavonoids and saponins) promoted healing and skin repair and had anti-inflammatory properties (15).

Carrot

Botanical name: *Daucus carota* subsp. *sativus*

Carrot oil is manufactured by using a carrot root extract macerated in a vegetable oil. Carrot oil is rich in beta carotene, vitamins B, C, D, and E. It is useful as a skin rejuvenator and is recommended for dry and aging skin types.

Hypericum

Botanical name: *Hypericum perforatum*

Hypericum perforatum is commonly known as St John's Wort, named after John the Baptist, possibly because it blooms on the anniversary of John the Baptist's birthday. The red sap in the stems, leaves and flower is supposed to represent the blood of John the Baptist and the herb is supposed to show its red spots on 29th August, the day that John the Baptist was beheaded.

St John's Wort is not a native to Australia, however since its introduction into Australia in the 1800s it has been declared a noxious weed due to the effects produced on grazing cattle. (16)

Hypericin is believed to be the principal active constituent of the plant. Hypericin is contained in the viscid oily substance in the glands on the leaves, petals and stems of the plant. Studies recently completed evaluated the hypericin concentration in various parts of the plant. The lowest is in the main stem (120ppm), leaves (290-380ppm) and flowers and buds (2150 ppm). (17)

Hypericin is known as a psychotropic activator of neuronal metabolism. This possibly accounts for its antidepressant and mood lifting properties. (18)

Recent studies have shown that hypericin is a potent anti-viral drug, especially against enveloped viruses. Studies have confirmed hypericin's activity against the AIDS viruses in laboratory tests. (19)

The oil is used topically for mild burns, bruises, haemorrhoids, varicose veins, wounds, sores and ulcers. It has also been indicated for nerve pain such as neuralgia, sciatica and for some rheumatic pain.

The oil is easily prepared by crushing the flowers and covering them in a fixed oil such as sweet almond oil, and then placing it in the sun for approximately three weeks. Press and strain. The oil which is bright red, can be used externally for massage purposes to treat many of the conditions indicated previously.

There is one possible side effect that is associated with hypericin. It increases photosensitivity so it should not be used before going into the sun.

Chapter 14

Hazardous Essential Oils

This chapter includes detailed information on some of the hazardous essential oils, which are not recommended for use in aromatherapy practice or need to be used with extreme caution by qualified aromatherapy practitioners only.

Introduction

Essential oils have been used for centuries and the toxicology of the majority of essential oils is well documented. Some 10 to 15% of all essential oils are hazardous in some way, and the purpose of this chapter is to discuss the hazards of this group of oils.

From the data presented on the hazardous essential oils the following points need to be considered:

- The majority of essential oils were toxic only if the oils were ingested.

- When essential oil poisoning did occur, resulting in death, the amount of oil taken was considerably higher than the normal therapeutic dosages.

- Undesirable side effects are caused by diliberate abuse or by gross overdosing.

- Toxicity testing of essential oils is mainly done for perfumes and cosmetic products.

- Many of the plants from which toxic essential oils are derived are still used safely in herbal medicine.

Ajowan

Botanical name   *Trachyspermum copticum.*

Family   Apiaceae (Umbelliferae).

Part of plant used   Seeds.

Major constituents   A typical chemical composition of ajowan oil is reported as follows (2): α–pinene (0.63%), β–pinene (1.56%), camphene (0.63%), limonene (2.25%), γ–terpinene (20.35%), p-cymene (23.78%), thymol (48.5%), carvacrol (6.8%).

Hazards   Dermal and mucous membrane irritant.

Contra-indications   Information regarding the safety of ajowan is scarce, its composition is similar to that of thyme oil and similar hazards (eg dermal irritant) may be assumed.

Comments

It has been extensively used in the pharmaceutical industry for the isolation of thymol. However since the introduction of synthetic thymol, ajowan has ceased to be an important source of thymol as it was not economic to remove natural thymol from the oil. The seeds are used extensively in curry powders and as a general remedy for intestinal problems in India.

Almond, bitter

Botanical name   *Prunus amygdalus* var. amara.

Family   Rosaceae.

Part of plant used   Kernels.

Major constituents   A typical chemical composition of bitter almond oil is: benzaldehyde (95%), hydrocyanic acid also known as prussic acid (3%).

Hazards   Toxin.

Contra-indications   Should not be used in therapy.

Comments

The bitter almond tree is widely cultivated in Spain, Turkey, Morocco, Algeria, Tunisia and Egypt. A fixed oil is produced by separating the kernels from their shells and then crushing them in a press. The crushed kernels yield about 30% of a fixed oil similar to sweet almond oil. The powdered cake left after pressing is then macerated in water to split the naturally occurring glycoside, amygdalin by enzymatic action, and then distilled to yield 1% of the essential oil of bitter almond.

Human ingestion of 7.5 ml has resulted in death (1). Prussic acid, known as cyanide, is the main chemical constituent of bitter almond oil, and is a well-known poison. It is not present in the nuts in their natural state. Bitter almond oil is used in flavouring after the prussic acid has been removed by alkali washing and rectification. It is used as 'almond essence' or as food flavours. The oil is now being replaced by synthetic benzaldehyde in food flavouring.

Boldo

Botanical name   *Peumus boldus.*

Family   Monimiaceae.

Part of plant used   Dried leaves.

Major constituents   A typical chemical composition of boldo oil is reported as follows (3): α-pinene (4.0%), β-pinene (0.8%), camphene (0.6%), limonene (1.6%), γ-terpinene (1.0%), p-cymene (28.6%), ascaridole (16.1%), 1,8-cineole (16.0%), linalool (9.1%).

Hazards   Toxin.

Contra-indications   Extremely toxic, should not be used in aromatherapy.

Comments

The essential oil of boldo is steam distilled from the leaves of the boldo tree which grows wild in South America, particularly in Chile.

Boldo oil's toxicity is due to ascaridole. In animal tests convulsions were produced by doses as low as 0.07g/kg. (4) The oil has powerful therapeutic effects, however it is considered harmful to the human organism even when used in very small doses.

In herbal medicine the dried leaves are used for genito-urinary inflammation, gallstones, liver and gall bladder pain, cystitis and rheumatism. The dried leaves are currently listed in the British Herbal Pharmacopoeia as a specific for cholelithiasis.

Buchu

Botanical name   *Agothosma betulina* or *Agathosma crenulata.*

Family   Rutaceae.

Part of plant used   Leaves.

Major constituents   There are two varieties of buchu: *Agathosma crenulata* and *Agathosma betulina.*

A typical chemical composition of *Agothosma betulina* oil is reported as follows (5): the essential oil contains sulphurated terpenoid ketones, including 8-mercapto-p. menthane-3-one, 8-acetylthio-p.menthone- 3-one.

A typical chemical composition of *Agathosma crenulata* oil is reported as follows (5): d-pulegone (50%), iso-pulegone (10%), diosphenol (1%), 4-diosphenol (1%), iso-menthone (22%), menthone (6%).

Hazards   Toxin.

Contra-indications   *Agathosma crenulata* oil is considered toxic because of the pulegone content. Should not be used in aromatherapy.

It is recommended that both types of buchu be avoided in aromatherapy.

Comments

Buchu, which is the local South African name given to the plant, provides us with the oil of commerce. The oil has an exceptionally pungent phenolic-blackcurrant, semi-sweet, medicinal aroma due to its content of diosphenol.

The leaves are used in herbal medicine for infections of the urinary tract such as cystitis, urethritis and prostatitis. It is currently listed in the British Herbal Pharmacopoeia 1983.

Calamus

Botanical name   *Acorus calamus* var. *angustatus.*

Family   Araceae.

Part of plant used   Roots.

Major constituents   A typical chemical composition of European calamus oil is reported as follows (6): acorenone (8.0%), β-gurjunene (6.7%), isoshyobunone (6.2%), β-asarone (5.2%), calamendiol (3.8%), α-selinene (3.8%), α-calacorene (3.5%), calamusenone (3.2%), camphone (3.2%), shyobunone (2.6%)

Hazards   Toxin, carcinogenic and hepatotoxic.

Contra-indications   Should not be used in aromatherapy.

Comments

Calamus, also known as sweet flag, is a perennial, semi-aquatic, marshy plant native to northern Europe and Asia. The oil is extracted by steam distillation of either the fresh root or the unpeeled dried root. The oil has a warm, spicy odour, reminiscent of a sweet forest.

The properties of the herb are mainly due to the essential oil constituents, found mainly in the root. The root was considered highly valued for its use in treating nervous complaints, vertigo, headaches and dysentery. It is listed in the British Herbal Pharmacopoeia, for acute and chronic dyspepsia, gastritis, intestinal colic, anorexia and gastric ulcer.

However the essential oil contains a carcinogenic constituent asorone. Fed to rats at 0.05-0.5% in a daily diet, calamus oil caused malignant tumours to develop in the duodenum after 59 weeks. Asorone is also responsible for the oral toxicity of the oil. Oral toxicity signs in rats included severe tremors from 30 minutes to 2 hours after ingesting the oil. Convulsions and severe liver and kidney damage occurred, but test animals surviving for 3 days recovered completely from any liver or kidney damage. (7)

Camphor

Botanical name   *Cinnamomun camphora.*

Family   Lauraceae.

Part of plant used   Crude camphor is collected from the trees in crystalline form. The essential oil is produced by steam distillation from the wood, root stumps and branches and then rectified under vacuum and filter pressed to produce three fractions, known as white, brown and yellow camphor.

Major constituents   The chemistry of camphor is very complex and continues to maintain biochemical intrigue. There are five main chemotypes:

- camphor
- cineole
- safrol
- linalool
- sesquiterpene.

A typical analysis of the *Cinnamomum camphora* subsp. *eucamphor* was reported as follows (8): α–pinene (3.76%), camphene (1.64%), β–pinene (1.26%), sabinene (1.47%), phellandrene (0.17%), limonene (2.71%), 1,8-cineole (4.75%), γ–terpinene (0.24%), p-cymene (0.14%), terpinolene (0.3%), furfural (0.16%), camphor (51.5%), linalool (0.68%), bornyl acetate (0.02%), terpinen-4-ol (0.57%), caryophyllene (1.49%), borneol (0.02%), piperitone (2.41%), geraniol (0.63%), safrole (13.4%), cinnamaldehyde (0.08%), methyl cinnamate (0.08%), eugenol (0.12%).

The yellow and brown fractions have a very high safrole content (yellow: 10-20%; brown: 80%).

Hazards   Brown and yellow camphor are toxic and carcinogenic. White camphor does not contain safrole however it is considered a convulsant and neurotoxin.

Contra-indications   Should not be used in aromatherapy.

Comments

White camphor has a long standing traditional use in the treatment of infectious disease. In addition to its valuable use for respiratory diseases, it was also used for heart failure. However in its crude form it is poisonous, and has been removed from the British Herbal Pharmacopoeia.

The symptoms of camphor oil poisoning by ingestion include nausea, vomiting, colic, headaches, dizziness, delirium, muscle twitching, epileptiform convulsions, depression of the central nervous system and coma. Death from respiratory failure is rare though fatalities in children have been recorded from ingesting 1 g of camphor oil. (9)

A 77 year old man who ingested 60 ml of camphorated oil developed vomiting and convulsions. He recovered following treatment by haemodialysis with 8 litres of soya oil for 4.5 hours to remove the camphor from his system. (10)

Another incident reported in the British Medical Journal involves a man who attempted suicide by ingestion of 150ml of camphorated oil. He suffered peripheral circulatory shock, severe dehydration due to vomiting, and three attacks of severe and prolonged grand mal epilepsy. He recovered after intensive supportive treatment. The dosage was believed to be one of the highest to be followed by survival. (11)

Camphorated oil is prepared with 20% camphor in any fixed oil.

Cassia

Botanical name   *Cinnamomum cassia.*

Family   Lauraceae.

Part of plant used   Bark, leaves and twigs.

Major constituents   A typical chemical composition of cassia is reported as follows (12): cinnamic aldehyde (87%), cinnamyl acetate (0.08%), benzaldehyde (4.73%), linalool (0.13%), chavicol (0.33%).

Hazards   Dermal irritant and sensitiser, mucous membrane irritant.

Contra-indications   As the essential oil is such a strong skin sensitiser and irritant it should never be used on the skin.

Comments

The dried herb is used extensively as a spice. It is used in much the same way as cinnamon, mainly for digestive complaints such as flatulence, dyspepsia, colic, diarrhoea and nausea. The powdered bark is listed in the British Herbal Pharmacopoeia as a specific for flatulent dyspepsia or colic with nausea.

Cinnamon Bark

Botanical name   *Cinnamomum zeylanicum.*

Family   Lauraceae.

Part of plant used   The dried inner bark of young trees.

Major constituents   A typical chemical composition of cinnamon bark oil is reported as follows (13): cinnamic aldehyde(40-50%), eugenol(4-10%), benzyl benzoate (1.0%), α-pinene (0.2%), 1,8-cineole (1.65%), linalool (2.3%), caryophyllene (1.35%)

Hazards   Dermal irritant and sensitiser, mucous membrane irritant.

Contra-indications   As the essential oil is such a strong skin sensitiser and irritant it should never be used on the skin.

Comments

Cinnamon bark is highly sensitising and undiluted will cause severe irritation to the skin. Tested at 4% and 8% respectively, cinnamon bark produced 20 sensitisation reactions from two groups of 25 volunteers each. (14)

The IFRA recommends that cinnamon bark oil be limited to 1%. This recommendation was based on the RIFM test results showing an absence of sensitisation reaction at this concentration.

Clove

Botanical name   *Eugenia caryophyllata.*

Family   Myrtaceae.

Part of plant used   Dried flower bud, or leaf or stem.

Major constituents   A typical composition of the bud, stem and leaf oil can be differentiated as follows (15):

Compound	Clove leaf	Clove stem	Clove bud
eugenol	85-90%	87-92%	80-85%
eugenyl acetate	0-10%	3-3.5%	8-12%
isoeugenol	-	trace	-
caryophyllene	10-15%	6-8%	6-10%
isocaryophyllene	-	-	0-2.0%

Hazards   Dermal irritant, hepatotoxic, mucous membrane irritant.

Contra-indications   Should not be used on the skin, except in dilutions of 1% or less and used with caution.

Comments

Of the three types of clove oil commercially available (bud, stem and leaf oils), clove leaf oil is produced in the largest volumes and has the highest content of eugenol. Clove bud is slightly less toxic than clove stem oil, and clove leaf oil seems significantly more toxic than either clove bud or stem oils (16).

A case was recently reported of a near fatal ingestion of clove oil (17). A two year old boy drank between 5 to 10 ml of clove oil from an open-necked bottle. One hour after ingestion the boy was drowsy and distressed and almost unconscious. Within three hours he was in a deep coma, had a high acidosis and a very low blood glucose level. The child remained unconcious for three days and showed signs of disseminated intravascular coagulopathy with concurrent liver failure. After three days of treatment with heparin, plasma, fibrinogen, antithrombin III, protein C and factor VII, the patient began to recover, but only after continuing deterioration in liver function and signs of raised intracranial pressure.

Costus

Botanical name   *Saussurea lappa.*

Family   Asteraceae (Compositae).

Part of plant used   Dried roots.

Major constituents   The essential oil of costus root is predominantly made up of costus lactones (18): costuslactones (50%), costunolide (50%), cyclocostuniolide, alantolactone, iso-alantolactone, dihydrobehdrocostus lactone.

Hazards   Dermal sensitiser.

Contra-indications   Should not be used in aromatherapy.

Comments

The root has long been used in India and China for digestive complaints, respiratory conditions and for infections such as cholera and typhoid. The essential oil is also suggested for nervous exhaustion and stress related conditions.

The essential oil contains certain sesquiterpene lactones having a sensitisation potential. Tested on 25 volunteers at 4%, costus produced sensitisation reaction in all 25 test volunteers, extremely severe in 8 of them. (19)

Elecampane

Botanical name   *Inula helenium.*

Family   Asteraceae (Compositae).

Part of plant used   Dried roots.

Major constituents   A typical chemical composition of elecampane is: alantolactone, iso-alantolactone, dihydroiso-alantolactone, alantic acid, azulene.

Hazards   Dermal sensitiser.

Contra-indications   Should not be used on the skin. The essential oil contains certain sesquiterpene lactones with an α-methylene butyrolactone structure which causes dermal sensitisation.

Comments

It has been used as a herb of ancient medicinal repute in both Western and Eastern herbalism, mainly in the form of a tea for respiratory conditions such as asthma, bronchitis and whooping cough, disorders of the digestion, intestines and gall bladder.

Pliny said of elecampane:

'Let no day pass without eating some root of inula, considered to help digestion and cause mirth.'

and Culpeper said,

'The fresh roots of elecampane preserved with sugar are very effectual to warm a cold windy stomach and stitches in the side, caused by spleen and to relieve cough, shortness of breath and wheezing in the lungs.'

It is listed in the British Herbal Pharmacopoeia as a specific for irritating coughs or bronchitis.

Horseradish

Botanical name   *Cochlearia armoracia.*

Family   Brassicaceae (Cruciferae).

Part of plant used   Roots.

Major constituents   A typical chemical composition of horseradish oil is reported as follows (20): allyl isothiocyanate (44.3-55.7%), phenyl ethyl isothiocyanate (38.4-51.3%).

Hazards   Toxin, dermal irritant, mucous membrane irritant.

Contra-indications   This is one of the most hazardous of all essential oils. It should never be used in aromatherapy.

Comments

The essential oil is chemically similar to mustard, except that the allyl isothiocyanate content is around 99% in mustard. Both essential oils have a similar irritating effect to the eyes, nose, mucous membranes and the skin.

The main medicinal uses of horseradish root as a herb are as a stimulant, rubefacient, diuretic and antiseptic. Culpeper said of horseradish,

'If bruised and applied to a part grieved with sciatica, gout, joint-ache or hard swellings of the spleen and liver, it doth wonderfully help them all.'

If eaten at frequent intervals during the day at meals, horseradish root is said to be most efficacious in getting rid of persistent cough following influenza. (21)

Mugwort

Botanical name   *Artemisia vulgaris.*

Family   Asteraceae (Compositae).

Part of plant used   Leaves and flowering tops.

Major constituents   A typical chemical composition of mugwort oil is reported as follows (22): α–thujone (36-82%), β–thujone (6-16%) 1,8-cineole (2.0%), camphene (2.6%), camphone (15%).

Hazards   Toxin, neurotoxin and abortifacient.

Contra-indications   Should not be used at all in aromatherapy.

Comments

In has traditionally been used in Europe as a protective charm against evil and danger. It was used as a womb tonic, for painful or delayed menstruation and as a treatment for hysteria and epilepsy. It was used to expel worms, control fever and as a digestive remedy.

Gerarde said of mugwort:

'Mugwort cureth the shakings of the joynts inclining to palsie.'

and Culpeper directs that the tops of the plants are used fresh, and says:

'A very slight infusion is excellent for all disorders of the stomach, preventing sickness after meals and creates an appetite.'

In Chinese medicine the dried herb is compressed to make moxa. The herb is currently listed in the British Herbal Pharmacopoeia as a specific for amenorrhoea and dysmenorrhoea. The herb is used both in herbal and homoeopathic medicine as a remedy for convulsive fits.

Mustard

Botanical name   *Brassica nigra.*

Family   Cruciferae.

Part of plant used   Black mustard seeds.

Major Constituent   Not less than 92% allyl isothiocyanate.

Hazards   Toxin, dermal irritant, mucous membrane irritant.

Contra-indications   This is one of the most hazardous of all essential oils. It should never be used in aromatherapy.

Comments

Grieve (23) describes mustard as an irritant, stimulant, diuretic and emetic. Mustard seeds are used in the form of poultices for external application near the seat of inward inflammation, chiefly in pneumonia, bronchitis and other diseases of the respiratory system. It relieves congestion of various organs by drawing the blood to the surface, as in head affections, and is beneficial in the alleviation of neuralgia and other pains and spasms.

The essential oil is not present in the fresh seed, or the powder, and so preparations made from these do not contain Allyl isothiocyanate. The essential oil is only formed when the mustard seeds come in contact with water. A glycoside, located in certain cells, is decomposed by hydrolysis under the influence of an enzyme, and forms the essential oil, which is then distilled.

White mustard seeds do not contain any essential oil, nor do they produce any of the conditions described above. Mustard oil is used extensively in the pickle and canning industries.

Mustard oil when inhaled produces extremely unpleasant sensations in the occipital regions of the head and causes an inflammation of the conjunctiva of the eyes and the mucous membranes of the respiratory system. The strongest effect is caused by applying mustard oil to the skin which provokes a burning sensation even when used in a weak concentration.

Oregano

Botanical name   *Origanum vulgare.*

Family   Lamiaceae (Labiatae).

Part of plant used   Dried flowering herb.

Major constituents   A typical chemical composition of mugwort oil is reported as follows (24): carvacrol (14%), thymol (12%), p-cymene (3%),cis-ocimene (13.5%), caryophyllene (9.2%), linalool (3%).

Hazards   Dermal irritant, mucous membrane irritant.

Contra-indications   Should not be used on the skin.

Comments

There are several species of oregano used for producing essential oils. The main species is *O. vulgare*; other species include Italian oregano *(O. gracile)*, Greek oregano *(O. heracleoticum)*, Turkish oregano *(O.smyrneaum)*, Syrian oregano *(O.maru)* and Moroccan oregano *(O. virens)*. The plant called Spanish oregano *(Thymus capitatus)* is actually a species of thyme, similar to Spanish marjoram *(Thymus mastichina)*.

Parsleyseed

Botanical name   *Petroselinum sativum.*

Family   Apiaceae (Umbelliferae).

Part of plant used   Seeds.

Major constituents   A typical chemical composition of parsley seed oil is reported as follows (25):

Three distinct chemotypes of parsley seed oil exist. They are:

myristicin chemotype
myristicin 49-77%
2,3,4,5-tetramethoxyallylbenzene 1-23%
apiol 0-3.%

apiol chemotype
myristicin 9-30%
2,3,4,5-tetramethoxyallylbenzene trace-6%
apiol 58-80%

2,3,4,5-tetramethoxyallylbenzene chemotype
myristicin 26-37%
2,3,4,5-tetramethoxyallylbenzene 52-57%
apiol 0 - trace.

Hazards   Abortifacient, hepatotoxic.

Contra-indications   Avoid during pregnancy.

Comments

The essential oil of parsley seed, because of its depurative property, is traditionally used in aromatherapy for the treatment of arthritis, cellulite and accumulation of toxins. It is also an emmenagogue and is recommended for the treatment of amenorrhoea, dysmenorrhoea and as an aid during childbirth.

However the apiol content of the essential oil contributes to the oil's use as an abortifacient (26). Parsley seed oil, therefore, is a high risk oil and its use is not recommended during pregnancy.

There are recorded cases of fatal poisoning from ingestion of as little as 1gm of apiol (26). Common signs of apiol poisoning are fever, severe abdominal pain, vaginal bleeding, vomiting and diarrhoea.

Parsley seed oil contains myristicin which is believed to contribute to the psychotropic effects of nutmeg oil. However the myristicin appears to have no such effect in parsley seed oil.

Pennyroyal

Botanical name   *Mentha pulegium.*

Family   Lamiaceae (Labiatae).

Part of plant used   Fresh herb.

Major constituents   A typical chemical composition of pennyroyal oil is reported as follows (27): pulegone (52-63.5%), menthone

(0.5-30.8%%), iso-menthone (5.2-19.8%), neomenthone (3%).

Hazards   Toxin, abortifacient.

Contra-indications   Should not be used in aromatherapy.

Comments

The herb has a long traditional use as a carminative, diaphoretic, stimulant and emmenagogue. The herb and oil were traditionally used to strengthen the nerves, being valuable in hysteric disorders, nervous exhaustion and externally applied for neuralgia. The oil warms and comforts the stomach and relieves nausea, vomiting and flatulence. It promotes the flow of bile, and is recommended for jaundice caused by bile duct blockage. Pennyroyal also has a deserved reputation as an insect repellent.

Pennyroyal essential oil has been found to produce acute liver and lung damage. Its toxicity is due to the pulegone, isopulegone and menthofuran. In 1897, the Lancet reported a case of a 23 year-old woman who had taken a tablespoonful of pennyroyal in an attempt to bring on menstruation, which had been absent for six months. She suffered from acute gastritis, but recovered fully. (28)

Another case was reported in the Lancet in 1955. It does not specify the dosage taken, but the effects were abortion, vaginal bleeding, haemolytic anaemia (destruction of the red blood cells) and acute destruction of the kidney tubules, which resulted in death following a massive ureal leakage into the blood. (29)

A case involving pennyroyal was also recorded in 1979 in the Journal of the American Osteopathic Association. The woman, who took 15ml of pennyroyal to induce menstruation, suffered CNS depression, vomiting and fluid on the lungs. She was treated by gastric lavage, activated charcoal, milk of magnesia and acetylcysteine, which is a liver protector. This resulted in rapid improvement and discharge from hospital after 96 hours. (30)

Botanist Dr Walter Lewis cites a case of a Colorado woman who took one ounce of pennyroyal oil,

'Within two hours she vomited blood, bled from the vagina and eyes and by the third day her liver was damaged. On the sixth day, she sank into a deep coma and died on the seventh day.' (31)

Another plant called American pennyroyal *(Hedeoma pulegeoides)* also produces an essential oil very rich in pulegone at 62-82%.

The pennyroyal herb is currently listed in the British Herbal Pharmacopoeia for flatulent dyspepsia, intestinal colic, the common cold, delayed menstruation and gout.

Rue

Botanical name   *Ruta graveolens.*

Family   Rutaceae.

Part of plant used   Fresh herb.

Major constituents   A typical chemical composition of rue oil is reported as follows (32): 2-nonanone (18%), 2-nonyl acetate (11%), 2-undecanone (30%), 2-butanone (3%), psoralen (1.28%), bergaptene and xanthotoxin (7.24%).

Hazards   Toxin, skin and mucous membrane irritant, abortifacient, phototoxic and neurotoxic.

Contra-indications   Rue should not be used at all in aromatherapy. When applied to the skin rue oil may produce a burning sensation, erythema (redness) and vesication (blisters).

Comments

The oil is considered toxic and ingestion of large amounts of rue oil has been known to produce epigastric pain, nausea, vomiting, confusion, convulsions and death. It may harm the mucous membranes and irritate the skin, producing erythema and vesication after frequent dermal contact. (33)

According to an IFRA report (34), rue was found to be extremely phototoxic. This is not surprising when we consider the high percentage of the phototoxic constituent, bergaptene.

As a herb, rue was a favoured remedy of the ancients as an antidote to poison. Gerard said of rue:

'If a man be annointed with the juice of rue the poison of wolf's bane, mushrooms or toadstooles, the biting of serpents, stinging of

scorpians, spiders, bees, hornets and wasps will not hurt him.'

Culpeper recommends it for sciatica and pains in the joints. Externally, rue is an active irritant, being employed as a rubifacient. If the fresh leaves are bruised and applied the leaves will ease severe pain of sciatica.

In many cultures it was believed to protect against evil. It was also used for disorders in the head, nerves and womb, convulsions and hysteric fits, colic, weakness of the stomach and bowels. It resisted poison and cured venomous bites. It is currently listed in the British Herbal Pharmacopoeia for atonic amenorrhoea.

Sassafras

Botanical name   *Sassafras albidum.*

Family   Lauraceae.

Part of plant used   Dried root bark.

Major constituents   A typical chemical composition of sassafras oil is reported as follows (35): safrole (80-90%), 5-methoxy-eugenol, asarone, coniferaldehyde, camphone and traces of menthone, thujone, anethole, apiol, elemicin, myristicin and eugenol.

Hazards   Carcinogenic.

Contra-indications   Should not be used in aromatherapy.

Comments

A few drops of sassafras oil has been considered lethal and records exist in the USA of a male adult who died following the ingestion of a teaspoon of sassafras oil. The symptoms of poisoning were those of CNS depression, vomiting and nausea (36). Large doses of sassafras oil cause fatty changes in the liver and kidneys. The use of sassafras oil may lead to accumulation in the body of safrole which is considered a hepatocarcinogen (37).

Sassafras has traditionally been used for treating high blood pressure, rheumatism, arthritis, gout, menstrual and kidney problems and for skin problems. The herb is listed in 1983 British Herbal Pharmacopoeia for head lice, cutaneous eruptions, rheumatic pains and gout.

The carcinogenicity of sassafras oil is due to its content of safrole. Currently essential oils containing asarone have been banned by the FDA. (38) It is reported to be carcinogenic in rats producing malignancy of the connective tissues, blood and lymphatic cells.

Sassafras was traditionally used in the food flavouring industry for preparations such as toothpastes, mouthwashes and in flavouring sarsaparilla root beer.

Savin

Botanical name   *Juniperus sabina.*

Family   Coniferae (Cupressaceae).

Part of plant used   Twigs and leaves.

Major constituents   A typical chemical composition of savin is reported as follows (39): sabinyl acetate (37.5-38%), sabinene (26-30%), α–pinene (2.2-6.8%), limonene (0.6-1.2%), terpinene-4-ol (2.0-3.2%), α–cadinene (1.5-4.5%).

Hazards   Toxin, dermal irritant, abortifacient.

Contra-indications   Should not be used at all in aromatherapy.

Comments

The principal constituents sabinene, sabinol and sabinyl acetate, are responsible for the toxic effects of this oil. Savin is an irritant when administered internally or locally. It is a powerful emmenagogue and serious and fatal cases of poisoning have resulted from its attempted use as an abortifacient (40). The odour is very unpleasant; the taste bitter and repulsive. The oil is banned from sale to the public in many countries due to its toxic effects.

Savory (winter & summer)

Botanical name   *Satureja hortensis* (summer)
Satureja montana (winter).

Family   Lamiaceae (Labiatae).

Part of plant used   The whole dried herb.

Major constituents   A typical chemical composition of winter savory oil is reported as follows (41): carvacrol (60-75%), thymol (1.0-5.0%), p-cymene (10-20%), γ-terpineol (2.0-10.0%), 1,8-cineole (3.8%), borneol (12.5%), α-terpineol 2.5%).

Hazards   Dermal irritant, mucous membrane irritant.

Contra-indications   Should only be used with great care. Not to be used during pregnancy.

Comments

There are two main species of savory used for producing essential oils; they are the winter or garden savory *(Satureja montana)* and the summer or mountain savory *(Satureja hortensis)*. The chemical composition and odour of the two savory oils are very similar, summer savory being harsher than winter savory oil.

Traditionally the herb was used as a tea for digestive complaints, menstrual problems and respiratory conditions such as asthma, catarrh and sore throat. Applied externally the fresh leaves bring instant relief from insect bites, bee and wasp stings.

Tansy

Botanical Name   *Tanacetum vulgare.*

Family   Asteraceae (Compositae).

Part of plant used   Whole herb.

Major constituents   A typical chemical composition of tansy oil is reported as follows (42): thujone (66-81%), isopinocamphone, camphor, borneol, camphone, artemisone, piperitone.

Hazards   Toxin, abortifacient, neurotoxin.

Contra-indications   Should not be used at all in aromatherapy. Tansy oil, like other essential oils containing high doses of thujone, is a poison which causes convulsions and epileptic-like attacks.

Comments

Signs of tansy oil poisoning due to its thujone content include vomiting, gastro-enteritis, flushing, cramps, loss of consciousness, rapid breathing, irregular heart beat, rigid pupils, uterine bleeding and hepatitis. Death results from circulatory and respiratory arrest and organ degeneration. (43)

Traditionally used to expel worms, to treat colds and fever, to prevent possible miscarriage and to ease dyspepsia and cramping pains. Externally, the crushed leaves were used as a remedy for scabies, bruises, sprains and rheumatism. The herb is listed in the 1983 British Herbal Pharmacopoeia for the treatment of round or thread worm infestation in children and topically applied for scabies.

Thuja

Botanical Name   *Thuja occidentalis.*

Family   Cupressaceae.

Part of plant used   Fresh leaves and twigs.

Major constituents   A typical chemical composition of thuja oil is reported as follows (44): α-thujone (60.0%), β-thujone (9.5%), α-pinene (1.3%), camphene (1.2%), d-sabinene (1.8%), fenchone (14%), camphone (2.0%), terpinen-4-ol (1.2%) and bornyl acetate (2.3%).

Hazards   Toxin, neurotoxin, abortifacient.

Contra-indications   Should not be used at all in aromatherapy. In pregnancy may cause abortion by reflex uterine contractions.

Comments

The herbal infusion of the twigs may produce abortion by reflex action on the uterus from severe gastro-intestinal irritation. Because of the presence of thujone the essence is toxic in large doses and constitutes a neurotoxin which can lead to spasms, epileptiform convulsions, diarrhoea, and gastro-enteritis.

Thuja twigs are listed in the 1983 British Herbal Pharmacopoeia for bronchial catarrh, enuresis, cystitis, psoriasis, amenorrhoea and rheumatism. Topically applied it is used for the treatment of warts.

Wintergreen

Botanical name   *Gaultheria procumbens.*

Family   Ericaceae.

Part of plant used   Leaf.

Major constituents   A typical chemical composition of wintergreen oil is reported as follows (45): methyl salicylate (98%), gaultherilene.

Hazards   Toxin.

Contra-indications   Should be avoided in aromatherapy, both internally and externally.

Comment

Wintergreen is listed in the 1983 British Herbal Pharmacopoeia for rheumatoid arthritis, lumbago and sciatica. True wintergreen is virtually identical with sweet birch oil, and with methyl salicylate, the principal constituent of both these essential oils. Methyl salicylate has been incorporated into linaments and ointments for muscular skeletal problems.

Wintergreen was tested at 85% dilution for 48 hours on 27 volunteers and did not produce any irritation or sensitisation reactions. However other tests have shown that methyl salicylate can be a moderate irritant at a concentration as low as 1%. Urticaria occurred on several occasions in a patient sensitive to asprin following exposure to a linament. (46)

Ingestion of relatively small amounts of methyl salicylate may result in fatal poisoning. Signs of poisoning include nausea, vomiting, acidosis, pulmonary oedema, pneumonia and convulsions. The lethal dose for children may be as little as 4 ml. A ten year old boy suffered from severe metabolic acidosis after ingesting approximately 10 ml of methyl salicylate. Many cases of methyl salicylate poisoning have been reported with 50-60% death rate. (47)

Wormseed

Botanical name   *Chenopodium ambrosioides.*

Family   Chenopodiacae.

Part of plant used   The whole plant including fruit.

Major constituents   A typical chemical composition of wormseed oil is reported as follows (48): ascaridole (60-80%), cymene, limonene, terpinene, myrcene.

Hazards   Toxin, neurotoxin.

Contra-indications   Should not be used at all in aromatherapy.

Comments

Wormseed was traditionally used for the expulsion of round worms and hookworms. However, it is toxic to the liver and kidneys and has been replaced by less toxic drugs.

The essence is toxic even at small doses due to its depressive action on the heart. Several cases of fatal human poisoning by wormseed have been reported. Toxic effects include irritation of the digestive tract, provoking nausea and vomiting, leading to vertigo, ataxia, deafness, and visual difficulties, circulatory collapse due to vasomotor paralysis and sometimes pulmonary oedema. (49)

Four drops of wormseed oil in a steam inhalation led to an unpleasant sensation of vertigo in the frontal part of the cranium, and caused moderate irritation of the nasal mucous membrane. The vertigo persisted for one hour. (50)

The ascaridole in wormseed oil is an unstable compound and may cause the essential oil to explode when treated with organic acids. (51)

Wormwood

Botanical name   *Artemisia absinthium.*

Family   Asteraceae (Compositae).

Part of plant used   Leaves and flowering tops.

Major constituents   A typical chemical composition of wormwood oil is reported as follows (52): α–thujone (2.76%), β–thujone (46.44%), sabinene (2.7%), myrcene (1%), trans-sabinol 3.2%, trans-sabinyl acetate and linalyl acetate (27.78%) and geranyl propionate (1.4%).

Hazards   Toxin, neurotoxin, abortifacient.

Contra-indications   Should not be used in aromatherapy.

Comments

Artemisia absinthium herb is listed in the 1983 British Herbal Pharmacopoeia for nematode infestation, anorexia and atonic dyspepsia.

Wormwood was used in the liqueur absinthe. Prolonged consumption of this drink became known as 'absinthism'. The symptoms included auditory and visual hallucinations, hyperexcitability, intellectual enfeeblement and addiction. Many people believe it was absinthe that finally drove the unstable and psychotic painter Vincent van Gogh to suicide. (53)

It is believed that thujone and delta-9-tetrahydrocannabinol, the most active ingredient in cannabis, interact with a common receptor in the CNS and thus have similar effects (54).

Thujone, the major constituent, is a convulsant and neurotoxin. In 1915 the French banned the production of a drink called absinthe which contained wormwood, due to its narcotic and habit forming properties.

243

UNIT IV

PRACTICAL MATTERS

Unit IV outlines the knowledge and skills required for the
practice of aromatherapy.
The chapters:
• explain the requirements for professional practice
• explain the importance of a consultation before a treatment
• describe the skills necessary to select the appropriate
essential oils
• outline the aromatherapy massage treatment

Unit IV includes the following chapters:

Chapter 15 Requirements for Professional Practice

Chapter 16 The Consultation

Chapter 17 Guidelines to Prescribing

Chapter 18 Methods of Application

Chapter 19 The Aromatherapy Massage

Chapter 15

Requirements for Professional Practice

Aromatherapy is a health service which utilises holistic procedures such as the use of essential oils in massage for the improvement of the client's wellbeing. The aromatherapist has an ethical responsibility to the public and to individual clients to maintain a high level of professionalism. This chapter outlines the duties and responsibilities of the professional aromatherapist.

Introduction

In health care, practitioners of different modalities are able to perform duties as prescribed by their occupation and their level of training.

Many occupations and professions have National or State regulatory and training boards to develop and upgrade professional standards and to regulate licensing procedures. However, at the time of publication, no State in Australia has adopted licensing procedures to regulate the practice of aromatherapy. Regardless of this, it is important for aromatherapists to practice within professional boundaries.

Professionalism

According to the Oxford dictionary professionalism means:

'Belonging to a profession, following occupation as a means of livelihood; maintaining a proper standard, not amateurish.'

While there may be many definitions of 'professional' they all have the same basic message: A person who is focussed on and committed to a given profession, who is not seeking personal gain by jumping on the latest bandwagon.

Aromatherapy is now recognised by many members of the community as a therapy that can offer genuine assistance to the health industry as a whole. There is often a general perception that therapists involved in the natural therapy industry belong at the bottom of the paramedical hierarchy. Natural therapists are often accused by the medical fraternity of using unproven and unscientific practices.

Unfortunately there is a lack of control over training standards. This means that someone can set up practice after having done a 'mickey mouse' training course and that inadequately trained people can set themselves up as practitioners.

This often has a negative influence on the therapist with a genuine commitment to the profession. Professional aromatherapists should be proud of their accomplishments and skills and be actively promoting their standing as professional practitioners. Professional aromatherapists can, directly or indirectly, help:

- save taxpayer's money through the promotion and practice of preventative medicine

- reduce degenerative and iatrogenic diseases

- treat or manage many so-called incurable diseases that have defied the medical system with all its millions of dollars of research, latest technology and hospitals

- introduce the benefits of aromatherapy into hospitals for patient care.

The role of the aromatherapist

It is important for an aromatherapist to be well trained and to have the required technical knowledge. Aromatherapists require dedication and commitment and must believe in what they are doing. Most importantly they must be aware that they are in a profession dealing with people and so being sympathetic and caring is important.

As soon as the client arrives at the clinic, it is important for the aromatherapist to concentrate completely on the needs of the client in order to correctly assess the situation and to decide which is the best treatment. Imagine the aromatherapist's thoughts being projected onto a screen for the client to see.

It is the duty of an aromatherapist as a professional to give the client, and the public in general, the best possible treatment and accurate information. This also means that aromatherapists should be bringing to the attention of the community issues such as:

- therapists' credentials and qualifications

- the safe use and application of essential oils

- the contraindications and the quality of the essential oils

- the restorative benefits of the aromatherapy treatments.

Aromatherapists need to able to explain to the client how the treatment works. A few clear explanations can often help. The therapist also needs to have a wider understanding of the other natural therapies available, in order to be able to advise and to refer the client in the right direction when necessary. Most importantly the aromatherapist must have the wisdom to recognise when medical advice should be sought. Aromatherapists are not doctors and to gain the respect of medical practitioners, must show professionalism by staying within the limits of the speciality.

Belonging to a professional organisation is very important for all practitioners who see themselves as professionals. It is important also to abide by that organisation's code of practice. For example, the International Federation of Aromatherapists (IFA) does not endorse the ingestion of essential oils unless the practising aromatherapist has medical qualifications or holds an insurance policy which specifically covers the ingestion of essential oils.

Professional ethics

Ethics are standards of acceptable and professional behaviour by which a person or business operates. A code of professional ethics will provide the aromatherapist with clear guidelines so that the high standards of the profession of aromatherapy will be maintained. The code should include:

1. Treat all clients with the same fairness and courtesy.

2. Provide the highest quality care for those seeking professional services.

3. The consultation and all communication with the client must be confidential.

4. The aromatherapist should perform only those services for which qualifications are held and should refer to appropriate practitioner when indicated.

5. Respect and cooperate with other ethical health care providers to promote health and wellbeing.

6. Be honest in all advertising of services providing such advertising does not bring discredit on the profession of aromatherapy.

7. Know and obey all relevant rules, laws and regulations of your local town, council, state and country.

8. Do not discriminate against colleagues or clients.

9. A therapist will not deliberately mislead a client seeking advice.

10. The clinic must be clean, neat and professionally presented to reflect the profession of aromatherapy. Remember that people judge the profession by first impressions of individual practitioners and their clinic.

11. Maintain physical, mental and emotional wellbeing.

12. All practitioners should maintain active participation in professional associations and should pursue continuing education and training.

13. A professional dress code is essential.

Counselling skills

As an aromatherapist you will be providing your client with a comfortable, safe and nurturing environment. This environment facilitates your client's level of trust in you. As the clients relax into this environment they will frequently disclose issues in their lives other than those you have been asked to treat, such as difficulties in sexual relationships or sexual abuse.

While a knowledge of psychology is of great help, it is important to realise our limitations. You need to be caring and understanding, and you need to listen to your client's problems, but it is unwise to become emotionally involved. Effective caring means:

*   going through rough patches with the client, but allowing them to stand on their own two feet

*   taking off your own shoes before putting yourself in theirs

- being sensitive and avoiding the 'she'll be right mate' attitude
- being human and allowing them to be human
- being non-judgemental
- being ready to listen to their story and being patient.

An aromatherapy practitioner without formal counselling qualifications may easily get drawn into the role of a counsellor. As a professional it is important that, when necessary, you refer your client to other practitioners who will be able to offer the necessary advice and care.

What do you do when you find your client is revealing personal problems to you? For example, someone tells you how hurt they are. Your response could be 'I can see how you would be hurt'. Avoid questions that require a yes or no answer as this closes the conversation. Offer an open inquiry such as 'How do you feel?'.

At this initial stage the client has an undefined sense of difficulty. Once the client knows what the problem is they may decide to see a counsellor. Some people may choose to hold onto their problem if the problem is too threatening. The person would have to give up what gives them sympathy, martyrdom, a reason not to, or something to talk about. They will not want your help and will give you a million reasons why your suggestions will not work. Other people will want to resolve their problems. They still need a supportive environment to express their problems and difficulties but the last thing this person needs is to be constantly reminded of the painful situation by hearing 'Oh, how terrible' or 'You poor thing'.

The client does not need a practitioner ghoulishly poring over every detail such as 'What did you do then?', or, 'What happened next?'. This might be harmful in the sense that you may prevent the client from seeing the problem as it really is and perhaps what part they play in it. The person at this stage needs to know how to use their defence mechanisms and needs to be able to continue in their life so that they can develop strategies to find a solution and initiate healing.

Without specific training it is very difficult to know what sort of person your client is. You can

actually prevent a person from moving on to health, therefore the damage you can inadvertently do is extensive. Apart from your skill as an aromatherapist, the most precious gift you can give your client is listening, attentive ears and the honesty to refer if necessary!

Personal hygiene and health

To inspire trust and confidence in the client the therapist should project a professional appearance at all times. This means maintaining personal health and grooming practices that are essential for the protection of the therapist and the client. An aromatherapist's personal hygiene and health habits should include the following:

- Health and personal hygiene should be such as to cause no danger to a client.
- The aromatherapist should be well groomed and wear appropriate clothing.
- Therapists must not eat, drink or smoke while at practice.
- The hands must be clean. Finger nails should be clean and filed so that they never come into contact with the client's skin.
- Ensure that time is set aside for relaxation and physical fitness.
- Eat a well-balanced and nutritious diet.
- Be aware of good posture when walking, standing, sitting and at work. Poor posture such as slouching contributes to fatigue and foot problems and places strain on the back and neck.

Setting up a clinic

The facilities in which an aromatherapist works should reflect a professional appearance yet at the same time be comfortable and relaxing. The image of the place of business is very important as it makes an impression on clients.

There are many options available for an aromatherapist to establish a practice:

- private practice from home

- private office or clinic

- another facility such as fitness club, resort, health professional's office or salon.

Regardless of the location of the business, the set-up of the therapist's clinic should reflect the professional services that the therapist is offering. The following guidelines are recommended for any aromatherapists setting up clinics and expecting to conduct themselves in a professional manner:

- Lighting in the room should not be harsh and glaring. Avoid direct overhead lighting or any light that can shine directly into the client's eyes. Reflective or soft, natural light is preferred.

- You must be aware of all the local authority's safety by-laws in connection with setting up a clinic.

- The atmosphere in the treatment room should be professional yet harmonious and warm, and should provide a genuine retreat from the hustle and bustle of the real world.

- Eliminate all possible distracting noise with the exception of some soothing music. Music is optional; some practitioners feel it distracts the client and prevents inward focussing and obtaining a full experience of what is happening to the body. The use of an answering machine will ensure that the telephone does not cause any interruptions which can destroy the concentrated mood you want to create.

- It is advisable to have a wash basin with hot and cold water nearby

- Maintaining good records is important for continuity of professional client care.

- The size of a treatment room needs to be approximately 3 metres wide by 4 metres long. This will allow enough space for all equipment, as well as enough space to move about the massage table.

- The temperature of the clinic room should be comfortable enough so that the client does not feel cold or hot.

- The room should be well ventilated.

Equipment and products

Equipment and products should be checked regularly to ensure they are in proper condition and that sufficient quantity is on hand. Each room should have the appropriate furnishings and equipment for treatments to be given. All supplies must be kept in a clean and sanitised condition.

A professional massage table is essential. It should provide a firm, comfortable base, as well as a cushioned opening where the face can rest comfortably when the client is lying on the stomach. The height of the table is important; it should reach the flat of the hand when the arms are down at the side fully extended. This height enables the application of appropriate pressure without any strain. Leaning over a table can be hard on the back.

The following is a checklist of equipment and supplies generally needed. You may add your own suggestions to this list.

essential oils and carrier oils
massage table
empty, clean, amber-glass bottles
blank labels
glass measuring cylinders
ointment or cream base
glass jars
eye droppers
a supply and linen cabinet
desk and chairs
sheets, blankets and towels
pillows
clothes hangers
small table or trolley
wall charts
bathroom scales
foot basin
alcohol or other sterilising agents
cotton for facial cleansing
facial tissues

Sanitary and safety practices

The aromatherapist has a duty to protect his or her own health as well as the health of the client. A practitioner's hands may pick up bacteria from the client's skin, therefore it is important to clean the hands thoroughly before and after a treatment to prevent bacteria spreading. Hygiene and safety are of utmost importance. Some guidelines follow:

- All furniture must be kept clean and disinfected at all times.

- Supplies such as blankets, towels and sheets should be clean and fresh for each client.

- Linen and towels should be washed in hot water and soap. Chlorine bleach may be used for its germicidal benefits.

- Clean linen should be stored in closed cabinets.

- An adequately-stocked first aid kit should be kept on the premises.

- Make sure first aid skills are maintained and upgraded as necessary.

- The clinic should be well ventilated and kept at a comfortable temperature.

- Check to make sure clients are not sensitive or allergic to any essential oils or products used.

- Use proper procedures in dealing with illness and injury. Refer to proper medical authorities when conditions indicate.

- Ensure that all supplies (essential oils, massage oils, lotions etc.) are stored in sealed containers.

Chapter 16

The Consultation

This chapter explains the importance of the consultation before an aromatherapy treatment. During the consultation, clients should give relevant information about themselves and why they are seeking the services of the aromatherapist. The aromatherapist should inform clients about the services provided. Chapter 16 will also explain why it is important to keep records and how to prepare a case study.

Introduction

The purpose of the consultation is to gather and exchange information. A consultation should consist of:

- introduction to the client
- explaining the procedure and policies
- the assessment
- a treatment plan.

Keep the consultation relaxed yet ensure that it is directed towards pertinent information. The first consultation is usually the most extensive, as it is the first time the therapist and client meet, and the therapist needs to record details of the client's medical history, family history, social history and present health status. It is also the time for the therapist and client to clarify their intentions and expectations for the aromatherapy treatment and to agree on some goals. The therapist will need to explain to the client what can be expected from an aromatherapy treatment.

Subsequent sessions with the client will not require detailed consultations, however each should begin with a short question and answer period to determine any changes in conditions or course of treatment since the previous session.

Introduction to the client

Begin by introducing yourself to the client. Ensure there are no distractions present, and if the client's friends or relatives are present they should be courteously asked to leave. If this is required, make sure they are given an estimate of when they should return.

The impressions made in the first minutes of contact will often determine the response of both the practitioner and client. Joseph Sapira suggests that: (1)

'As the physician is evaluating the patient, the patient is evaluating the physician.'

Explaining procedures and policies

During the first appointment, aromatherapists should clearly explain the aromatherapy procedure, the expected benefits of an aromatherapy treatment and the requirements of a consultation as well as policies such as payment of fees and the procedures for missed or late appointments, so that awkward situations are avoided.

There is no set manner in which these policies should be presented, but it is preferable that they be in writing. They may be displayed in the reception area of your clinic or they may be on a printed form.

Assessment

It is necessary to find out why the client is seeking an aromatherapy treatment, the client's expectations and any existing condition which may benefit from the aromatherapy treatment. In order to do this, questions, which may be written or verbal, must be asked.

If written forms are used, the aromatherapist should review the form after completion. Ask questions to clarify the written answers and to gain more specific information about the client's condition and reason for coming. To determine what aromatherapy procedure to perform on the client, the aromatherapist must correctly assess the client's condition. The assessment usually involves:

- inquiring
- physical examination.

A thorough assessment will expose any contraindication for aromatherapy. When an assessment has been completed, the aromatherapist should have a clearer understanding of the client's condition and will be better able to develop a treatment strategy.

Some problems that may be encountered during the consultation include:

The client who denies the relevance of psychological factors

Some people will deny psychological factors or simply not see their relevance. The client is paying for the therapist's services so is entitled to accept or reject any diagnosis made at any level. A client-rejected connection made between life events and illnesses should not be reiterated by the therapist in a contentious manner.

The demanding client

Some clients pressure the practitioner with an insistent demand for rapid treatment and assessment. In this case the therapist should advise the client that until a complete consultation and assessment is done, it will not be possible to determine the treatment strategy.

The therapist should be honest in their appraisal and clearly state the importance of the treatment and the need for the cooperation of the client for the condition to improve.

The uncooperative client

It is the therapist's duty to determine whether or not a client is following the treatment plan. If they are not, then it is the therapist's duty to determine if the client is having difficulties with the treatment plan, or if they are being uncooperative.

If they are uncooperative a number of strategies may be employed:

- Acknowledge that it takes time, dedication and commitment to follow a treatment plan, or to make lifestyle modifications. For example, if the prescribed lifestyle changes have been too great, then it is best to set goals that are achievable. It is difficult to change, overnight, ingrained patterns of thought that have existed for years, sometimes a lifetime. Therefore change should be implemented slowly without self punishment or deprivation.

- Share the decision making with the client. Describe the treatment strategy to the client and allow them to make choices as to the options that have been proposed.

One thing that the therapist must remember is that they cannot take responsibility for their client's health. It is the client who must be willing to take responsibility for their own health.

A client who begins to cry

If the client begins to cry, this is a sign that the interview was successful in eliciting emotion-laden material, and in a manner that permitted the client to express it. Give the client a tissue, and permit them to finish crying. Do not leave the client alone while in this state.

The professional client

A client who tells the therapist a long list of ailments diagnosed by medical doctors, acupuncturists, herbalists, naturopaths, chiropractors and even knows what *Readers Digest* has stated about the complaints, has spent a lot of money for little relief. Before proceeding further, such a client may want to know if you can help, at what cost, and your opinion on the other modalities. The therapist should explain the need for a detailed history and examination before an assessment can be made.

This person is possibly a 'professional client' as indicated by all of the prior consultations in so many different modalities. (A professional client is someone who looks too eagerly for illness and personal problems, who doesn't really want to get better but makes out they do - some will try out different therapists just to prove how hopeless their case really is.)

Many people could benefit from lifestyle and dietary changes and although they know this, choose to continue with their current habits and are prepared to accept responsibility for their decision. These clients may view the condition that they are suffering from as less of a problem than changing some other aspects of their lives. Dr John Harrison states that:

'Those clients who do not get what they need from me will seek out another therapist. It is the cornerstone of my thinking about why so many patients accept bad and ineffective treatment from doctors that people choose the doctor and the treatment they want, that is, they choose for

themselves what seems a bad and ineffective treatment.'

Many diseases help one maintain a belief system about oneself, others and the world which, although damaging in some way, effectively mask deep-seated and fundamental fears. Becoming ill may spare the trauma of examining those aspects of ourselves we have chosen to suppress. When a therapist attempts to instruct a client on the true nature of the disorder, the client may become scared and may resist or redefine the information. If the therapist persists, then the client will often seek alternative advice.

All the diet, homoeopathy, acupuncture, chiropractic, herbalism and naturopathy or any other healing art will not significantly contribute to the wellbeing of the client without regard for the psychology of the client. All of these healing modalities can contribute to the wellbeing of clients who are in the process of working through their reasons for giving themselves the disorder.

Inquiring

A detailed case record will ensure that the aromatherapist has all the necessary information to provide the correct treatment. The following information may be used as a guideline to developing your own consultation form.

A. Identification data

Name, age, sex, marital status, occupation, religion, work address, home address, telephone number.

B. Main complaint

The main complaint is a statement in the client's own words of their present condition. In order to analyse the condition, it must be fully described in all its dimensions. The following parameters might be used:

- time
- quantity
- location
- aggravating factors
- alleviating factors
- quality.

Other questions that should be asked include:

- What do you think is your problem?
- What do you want to do about it?
- What has been happening in your life recently?

C. Family History

Record the age and health (or death and cause of death where applicable) of parents, siblings and children. Is there a history of any of the following conditions in the family: diabetes, high blood pressure, stroke, heart problems, cancers, tumours, arthritis, gout, alcoholism, epilepsy, glaucoma, blindness, deafness, kidney problems, bladder problems, migraines, asthma, breathing problems, allergies, skin problems, stomach problems, bowel problems, gall bladder problems, liver problems, genetic or inherited diseases, other unusual diseases.

D. Past medical history

1. General health: Ask the client to rate their own health, eg excellent, good, fair or poor
2. Serious illnesses. Ask the client if they have ever had chicken pox, measles, rheumatic fever, polio, herpes, pneumonia, diverticulitis, hernia, haemorrhoids, tension/anxiety problems, depression.
3. Injuries: Ask the client if they have ever had broken bones, lacerations, or other injuries.
4. Operations: Ask the client to list surgical procedures they have undergone.
5. Medications: Ask the client to list current medication (also include any nutritional or naturopathic supplements).

E. Diet

Brief breakdown of daily meals, special diets, alcoholic beverages, coffee, teas, bowel movement.

F. Review of systems

The main symptoms referrable to each system are reviewed. Information that belongs with the present illness will frequently be obtained and should be recorded here. Repetitions are to be avoided by referring to the preceding sections that contain the same information.

1. Skin.: Texture, colour, sweating pattern, bleeding, bruising, eruptions, pimples, eczema, cracked skin, boils or itching.

2. Lymph nodes: enlargement, pain, sinuses, drainage.

3. Head: headaches, injury, fainting, seizures.

4. Respiratory: asthma, oppressed breathing, acute or chronic bronchitis, cough, expectoration, hayfever, sinus, allergies, smoking.

5. Cardiovascular: amount and type of exercise, angina, chronic heart disease, sluggish circulation, palpitations, oedema, hypertension, varicose veins.

6. Gastrointestinal: appetite, nausea, vomiting, constipation, diarrhoea, unusual stool colour or consistency, abdominal pain, food intolerances.

7. Endocrine: impotence, sterility, menstrual history (age at onset, cycle, duration, amount, dysmenorrhoea, amenorrhoea, menorrhagia, date of last period, premenstrual syndrome, number of pregnancies, obstetric complications, age of menopause, hot flushes, post menopausal bleeding).

8. Urinary: passing urine, frequency, pain, colour, foul smelling.

9. Musculoskeletal: Pain, swelling, stiffness, limitation of motion of joints, fractures, serious sprains.

10. Neuropsychiatric: headaches, convulsions, loss of consciousness, paralysis, weakness, involuntary movements.

11. Predominant moods: anxiety, depression, sleep pattern, memory, thought content, attitude (towards friends, associates, family, disease).

G. Social history

Record nativity, occupation, marital status, client's emotional relationship to parents throughout life. Marital history should contain age, health, occupation, education of partner and number of children. Describe the extended family group. Who do they live with at home? Learn exactly what the client does in their occupation with particular attention to the degree of emotional tension or health hazard. Are there any debts or economic problems that may influence convalescence? How much do they participate in the civic, social, religious and political activities

of their particular economic and social group? Find out in detail how the client spends their day, what hobbies, how they relax, how the family responds to an illness.

Physical examination

The physical examination will vary according to your skills as a practitioner. A physical examination should include the following:

* the general appearance
* facial features and expressions
* identifying the skin type and the general health of the skin
* defining the muscle tone
* the quality of the body tissue
* the condition of the lymphatic system.

The client's expressions are an outward manifestation of vital functions, the eyes, facial colour, facial signs, appearance and physical shape of the client.

Hostility, fear, sadness and joy are usually reflected in the voice. There is a certain detectable resonance to a happy person's voice. There is a wide range of vocal abilities in a happy person, reflecting the person's ability to express how they are feeling at the time.

A person who suppresses their anger usually speaks with their mouth partially closed, for fear of exposing their anger. When sadness predominates, the voice will be weak and often breathless. When someone is afraid, the speech will be shallow and rapid, with little expansion of the chest. Often these people will hunch their shoulders to hide their chest from view, as the heart is considered vulnerable.

Developing a treatment plan

The treatment plan is an outline the aromatherapist can follow to determine the most appropriate aromatherapy treatment to be prescribed for the client. Using the information provided in Chapter 17 the treatment plan will determine:

- the essential oils to be selected
- duration and frequency of the treatment
- the dosage to be used
- how the essential oils will be applied.

The treatment strategy may involve several sessions, but every session will have to be assessed individually and should have a treatment plan. The treatment plan should be discussed with the client so that he or she can be actively involved in the therapy process. Clients who actively participate in the therapy generally respond to the treatment faster, and tend to follow through for a more lasting remedy.

When discussing assessment findings and treatment strategies with a client, use terminology that the client can understand. Some clients will be more interested than others. Be clear in describing assessment findings and give enough information to inform clients without saturating them with unnecessary technicalities.

Client files

The client file is the record that the aromatherapist uses to document the work that has been done with the client. It is important to keep files updated to ensure the aromatherapist has access to current information regarding the client. Suggested information that should be included on the client file is:

- identification data
- medical history
- treatment plan and recorded notes
- financial and billing information.

Keeping accurate records is a tedious but essential part of a professional operation. All data should be recorded with each treatment, including accurate records of the client's responses to the treatment. This will permit the therapist to render more effective treatments and to achieve better results.

The file should always be reviewed before a client comes in for a return visit. This will assist the therapist in planning the session and becoming familiar with the client. There is nothing worse than a practitioner who relies on memory and forgets important factors about a client from one session to the next. This is a sure way to lose trust with the client which is so necessary in a therapeutic relationship.

The therapist should never discuss or give out personal details about the clients. All records should be kept in a secure place. A practitioner should not divulge information about a client's personal details without the consent of the client.

Case history

The case history is the complete story the therapist composes to help understand the client's condition. The purpose of writing a case history is to present a summary of the:

- client assessment
- details of the treatment and client's response to the treatment
- an evaluation of the treatment
- any future recommendations.

Education of the client

Once the aggravating factors of the illness are understood by the therapist, this understanding can be transmitted to the client who can then take the necessary steps to avoid or reduce these factors.

Treatment and education combine to relieve the disharmony. In some simple situations, treatment alone is sufficent; in others, the disharmony may be redressed solely by the remedial actions of the client. Generally, both the treatment and remedial measures carried out by the client are required to achieve lasting improvement. This is especially true of complex chronic deficiency disharmonies. Unless the client is given a clear understanding of the origins of the illness, and is shown what remedial procedures to adopt, the disharmony may drag on indefinitely, although being partly relieved by the treatment. Therefore the appropriate actions of clients to help themselves can greatly reduce their suffering and their need for treatments.

There are two main aspects of client education.

- The first is concerned with the identification of the originating factors of the illness, and then with prescribing the appropriate remedial measures to these factors.

- The second is concerned with helping clients at a more personal level. To help people to help themselves it is first necessary to help them understand themselves, then accept themselves, and yet also to determine to change themselves.

This is the basis of client education.

Many origins of disease are not physical factors, but disharmonious patterns of thought and emotion. Changing these ingrained patterns of disharmony is the most important and the most difficult part of client education, since people are distinctly reluctant to change their personalities. The regulation of these deeply embedded patterns of feeling and belief is the core of client education. Since some individuals may have difficulty in changing, progress must be gradual and only at a rate within the capacity of the client. The three main components to the basic formula of change are:

- understanding

- motivation

- discipline.

Understanding

Clients must first understand, as thoroughly as it is appropriate, the pattern of their disharmony in the context of the pattern of their lives. They need to know which aspects of their behaviour or constitution became the originating factors of their illness. In this way they can understand which of their patterns of thought, emotion and behaviour need to be modified, and thus which preventative and remedial measures are appropriate.

Motivation

Understanding alone is not enough. There must be the motivation to put the understanding into practice. This can only be done with motivation from within the client. The therapist may act as a catalyst, but cannot supply motivation to a person who altogether lacks it.

Discipline

Momentary enthusiasm, temporary motivation, is useless. Changing ingrained patterns of thought and emotion is the work of a lifetime. Discipline is the steady application of understanding and motivation over long periods of time, despite setbacks and discouragements. This is the only way that lasting change can be effective. Discipline does not mean sudden, harsh bursts of self punishment and deprivations; it is the slow, steady, gentle implementation of change.

Chapter 17

Guidelines to Prescribing

The combination of the complexity of the essential oils and real clinical practice (which is never as simple as the textbooks describe) can make it difficult to determine the most appropriate aromatherapy treatment to prescribe for the client. This chapter provides the necessary guidelines to assist the aromatherapist in prescribing the most appropriate treatment.

Introduction

A number of factors need to be considered when prescribing essential oils in aromatherapy:

- essential oil selection
- duration and frequency of treatment
- the dosage used
- how the essential oils are used
- essential oil blending.

All of these factors will influence the therapeutic effect and outcome, and the aim of the aromatherapist is to find the right combination of prescribing factors for each condition being treated. As with anything, experience will prove to be the best teacher, and the guidelines should not be seen as hard and fast rules. From both a theoretical and practical perspective it is usually impossible to take all factors into account.

Essential oil selection

The effectiveness of correct selection of essential oils is based on the accuracy of the differential diagnosis. Such a diagnosis includes an assessment of the nature, location, origin, aetiology and progression of a disease condtion. When the various parameters of a conditon are assessed, the essential oils can be selected according to their therapeutic properties.

Since there are so many essential oils to choose from, how does one decide which essential oils should be selected? The essential oils should be selected using the following guidelines:

- the physiological condition
- the psychological condition
- the practical availability of the essential oils.

The physiological condition

To select the essential oils according to the physiological condition it is necessary to determine whether the condition is:

- chronic or acute
- internal or external

- empty or full
- cold or hot

as well as knowing what:

- other presenting symptoms exist.

Once the type of condition present has been determined it is possible to outline the treatment method and the essential oils to be chosen. This may involve the use of essential oils with the following actions:

- eliminating
- restoring or tonifying
- regulating or harmonising
- treating symptoms.

Eliminating

The conditions that are treated by 'eliminants' are full or excess conditions. These conditions are usually characterised by stagnation and obstructions. This may come in many forms, usually in the form of undesirable substances such as:

- mucous
- faeces
- urine
- menstrual blood
- other toxins.

Therefore essential oils which promote elimination work on expelling injurious waste matter. These essential oils may have properties such as:

- diaphoretics (promoting sweating, thus assisting the excretory functions of the skin)
- expectorants (promoting expulsion of mucous, thus assisting the respiratory system)
- diuretics (promoting urination, thus assisting the excretory functions of the kidneys)
- laxatives (promoting bowel movement, thus assisting the excretory functions of the large intestine)

- hepatic (enhancing liver function, thus assisting the liver's detoxifying function)

- emmenagogues (promoting menstruation, thus assisting in the elimination of menstrual blood) The treatment of amenorrhoea with menstrual retention may involve specific factors such as emotional shock, going off and on the contraceptive pill, ovarian tumours or cysts, menopause, hormone imbalances and pregnancy. These factors should be addressed if necessary.

All of the above properties will help promote detoxification for the treatment of general toxaemia.

Restoring or tonifying

The conditions that are treated by restoring and tonifying essential oils are termed deficient or empty conditions. A deficiency consists of the absence of some positive function or structural element ant this must be replenished or restored.

Therefore essential oils which restore are those which are normally classified as:

- astringents, cardiac, cephalics, cordials, digestives, hepatics, nervines, rubefacients, stimulants, stomachics and uterines.

Regulating and harmonising

Regulating and harmonising essential oils keep check of natural physiological responses such as fever, inflammation and nervous tension that have become excessively chronic and are counterproductive to healing. The effect is qualitative rather than quantitative, meaning that they simply create a harmony where there is a qualitative imbalance. These essential oils may be typified by the following properties:

- anti-inflammatory, febrifuges, hormone regulators, hypotensives, hypertensives.

Symptom treatment

It may also be necessary to choose essential oils according to their symptomatic properties, irrespective of the underlying condition. Treating a distressing symptom is equally important in aromatherapy, because it assists the body in rebalancing the disharmony. In most cases the use of essential oils for symptomatic treatment will not suppress symptoms in the same way as pharmaceutical drugs.

Some of the more common classifications of essential oils according to their symptomatic actions include:

- relief of pain (analgesics, antispasmodics, rubefacients)

- promoting tissue repair (cytophylactics, cicatrisants)

- enhancing the mind and spirit (antidepressants, cephalics, relaxants, sedatives)

- stimulating immunity (immunostimulants)

- restraining infection (antibacterial, antimicrobial, antifungal, antiviral)

- enhancing and assisting pregnancy and childbirth (uterine tonics, parturients).

The psychological condition

The treatment of the physiological conditions alone will not be sufficient to restore total balance. A holistic approach may include identification and treatment of the disease but it does not focus exclusively on the physiological conditions. The holistic assumption is that the body knows how to heal itself, and that many symptoms are often an opportunity for one to examine one's life, to reconsider values and habits, to re-evaluate personality and relationship, to expand awareness and to change. It was Doctor Bach who said (1):

'As long as our souls and personalities are in harmony, all is joy and peace, happiness and health. It is when our personalities are led astray from the path laid down by the soul, either by our worldly desires or the persuasion of others that conflict arises. This conflict is the root cause of disease and unhappiness.'

In addressing the psychological condition, the olfactory aspect of the essential oil is often important. In seminars I will often pass around unlabelled bottles of essential oils. I then ask the students to make the following observations:

- What memory associations do you have with the essential oil?

- What emotional response do you have to the essential oil?

- Use intuition to describe the essential oil.

- Identify the character of the essential oil.

Memory associations

It is almost impossible to accurately assess an individual's reaction to a particular fragrance for its therapeutic purpose. The memory and emotional responses are often so varied. Specific odour memories are personal, and will vary from one individual to another and the memories are often incredibly strong. It has been demonstrated that the long-term memory of odour is stronger than the long-term visual memory association (2).

It is interesting to note that the limbic system plays a significant role in selecting and transmitting information between the short- and long-term memories. Selection of and transmission to these two memories, is performed via corresponding associated regions of the limbic system that receive their information from the olfactory stimuli. It is therefore understandable why the perception of fragrances can often be connected with a recollection of specific experiences, or why, when we recall or experience odours associated with our childhood we simultaneously perceive our past emotions and experiences. When considering the role of memory associations the following factors need to be considered:

- age and childhood memories

- cultural background and learned fragrance needs.

Unlike taste, there are no innate perceptions of bad or unpleasant odours. Only substances that overly irritate the infant's nasal mucous membrane are perceived as being unpleasant or painful. What is in later life assessed as being an unpleasant or pleasant odour is a result of the learning experiences of socialisation.

For example, many people today associate patchouli with an alternative/ hippy lifestyle. This life-style association is of course influenced by the abundant use of patchouli in the late 60s and early 70s. The lifestyle of a person, which includes attitudes and ideas, can also be strongly influenced by intellectual factors.

The smell of frankincense is often associated with religious ceremonies by many Christian religons, because of its regular use in church. Western culture has usually associated rose with love, sexuality and compassion. Constance Classen discusses how the association with roses varied throughout history and different cultures (3).

'The Romans were so fond of roses that one Roman emperor, Heliogabulus, once suffocated his guests by showering them with an overabundace of roses... Roses were believed to relieve headaches... Not only was rose considered a pleasant luxury, but essential to health and wellbeing... However early Christian church leaders banned roses because of their association with 'Roman idolatry', and their assumed tendency to lead to sensualism.'

Emotional response

For a person to be drawn towards a particular fragrance it may correspond to the emotional needs of that person. However, it had been considered in the past that the preference for various fragrances was made on an irrational basis and could not be explained on the basis of specific factors (4). Others such as Jellinek (5) are of the opinion that external characteristics, such as hair and eye colour are decisive factors. Jellinek also proposed a classification of odour types and their

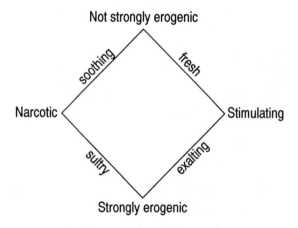

Jellinek's scheme of odour types and
psycho-therapeutic effects

associated psycho-therapeutic effects as shown in the diagram opposite.

In an attempt to relate personality type to different fragrances, Mensing & Beck (6) conducted a survey of 270 perfume users. There was a choice of four different perfume types:

- fresh
- floral powdery
- oriental
- woody-resinous.

They were asked to choose from one of the perfume types and complete a questionnaire and two colour charts to determine their personality and emotional mood. The data revealed that extroverts displayed a significant tendency towards fresh. stimulating odours, while introverts tended to prefer oriental, spicy fragrances. Emotionally stable people showed no statistical significance in favour of any particular fragrance, but emotionally ambivalent persons tended to choose the floral-powderey type of odours.

Tisserand proposes that essential oils may be used to influence emotion and mood in four different ways (7):

- to evoke positive feelings
- to counter negative feelings
- to influence our own mood
- to influence the mood of others.

Intuition

The best teacher will be the essential oils and your intuition. To develop your intuition, use the essential oils regularly, have them beside your desk when you study them. Pour a drop out and look at it, smell it, allow yourself to be receptive to the nature and personality of the oil. You may often find that your experience may not be the same as mine or that of other aromatherapists.

People are often automatically drawn to the essential oil which is most suitable for them.

As Stoddart explains:

For a scent or perfume to fulfil its function to the maximum extent it is important that it is tailored to the wearer's natural odorant signature; few people can get away with

wearing the equivalent of a 'sloppy joe' pullover odour. (8)

To develop your intuition and fully appreciate and experience the healing power of the essential oils, we often need to look beyond the little brown bottle.

Every time you use an oil, having a clear picture of the plant or flower, will help develop your intuitive understanding of the oil. When you consider the plant from which the oil was obtained, you might ask yourself:

- What does the colour of the plant tell me?
- What part of the plant yields the essential oil?
- What is the shape of the plant?
- What is the shape of the leaves, flowers, etc., and what can these aspects tell me about its energies?
- What is the habitat of the plant?

The character of the essential oils

When Doctor Edward Bach developed the Bach flower remedies in the 1930s, the psychological and emotional characteristics of the individual were central to the remedy being chosen. The remedy chosen by a therapist or by the individual, considers not only the condition, but other things such as relationships and feelings. For example, larch will be recommended for lack of confidence while heather is selected for persons always concerned about themselves.

Dr Bach believed that each person's personality and nature could be matched with a particular remedy, which will be taken for a short-term or long-term basis to deal with the passing problem.

As an example Susanne Fischer-Rizzi (9) discusses the nature of ylang-ylang, emphasising the need to not only treat the symptoms but the role which the clients play in their own disharmony:

'The spirit of ylang-ylang usually fits that person who is naturally drawn to the oil. She is much like the title character Carmen, from George Bizet's opera - fiery, temperamental, passionate and erotic. Although her emotions are deeply felt, she never loses her balance. Aware of her own fascinating radiance, she is

capable of casting magical spells. Her wardrobe is bright and colourful and she loves to wear jewellery.'

According to Fischer-Rizzi, the second type of client who uses ylang-ylang as a healing remedy is:

'... this second woman often does not allow herself to live, who hides her femininity, dresses drably, and does not trust her intuitive powers. Extremely frustrated, she appears nervous, depressed, and tense. This may often cause hormonal problems, such as PMT and irregular or painful periods.'

This very nature of ylang-ylang may also be utilised to help dominating masculine men bring out their feminine side, to awaken their understanding and intuition. The intense feminine quality of ylang-ylang may be seen to threaten their masculinity. If this is the case blending the ylang-ylang with sandalwood, bergamot or orange will help disguise the fragrance of ylang-ylang.

Another good example is vetiver oil. Some people can barely tolerate this oil, while others adore it. The oil is distilled from the roots of a grass. The heavy, earthy, musty rare fragrance of vetiver gives us an indication that it is a source of vitality and regeneration. The fact that the roots reach deeply into the ground and are strong and hardy, that the plant can survive periods of drought and is used to protect against soil erosion also indicates that it connects us to earth's energy. As Fischer-Rizzi explains (10):

'Vetiver is ideal for treating severe nervousness, exhaustion, or anorexia. It is valuable for exhausted people whose diminished energy reservc makes them vulnerable under stress.'

According to Phillipe Mailhebiau (11), a French aromatherapist who has drawn up aromatic characterologies for many essential oils:

'The idea of a characterology seems natural when one applies oneself to objectivising the psychosensory effect of essences by defining the personalities corresponding to them....'

He suggests that it is a search for affinities between the essential oil and the patient. It makes it possible to better understand the personality of the patient, which cannot be dissociated from the aetiology of the illness. An aromatherapy treatment that is based on the character of the essential oil will be more suited to restore a patient's 'terrain'.

The practical availability of the essential oil

This needs no further elaboration. If a particular essential oil that is required is not available, then by turning to Appendix Three, Therapeutic Cross Reference, a substitute oil which has similar properties may be found.

Duration and frequency

The length of time in hours, days, weeks or months for which treatments should be administered can vary a great deal. The main considerations are to:

- treat the constitution of the individual
- rebalance the condition of disharmony
- relieve symptoms.

If the essential oils are used as preventative measures, extended or regular treatments are necessary. If the treatment is for symptomatic relief (not suppression), short-term use is enough.

If the condition is chronic or degenerative such as M.S. or rheumatoid arthritis, the treatment might be ongoing and permanent. With acute conditions, short-term treatments may be sufficient. Please note that the imbalance which occurs from acute symptoms often needs further attention and longer-term treatments. Systemic conditions, such as those usually underlying skin eruptions, for example, are more likely to take longer to treat than purely local conditions such as injury or local infection.

Dosage

One of the aspects that makes aromatherapy so intriguing is the range of principles involved. At one end of the spectrum the essential oils are being used for their pharmacological action, similar to allopathic medicine, yet under the assumption that the whole natural extract is best suited to induce true healing.

At the other end of the spectrum is the psychotherapeutic use of the essential oils, where the scent is considered the most important agent to bring about healing. Research into olfactory perception indicates that only a few molecules are needed to have a substantial effect, such as the recalling of memories and associations.

According to Schnaubelt (12) the effects caused by olfactory triggering mechanisms in aromatherapy work in the same concentration ranges as low homoeopathic potencies.

The question of how much essential oil is needed to achieve the desired effect is important in aromatherapy. The size of most essential oil constituents, their volatile and lipophilic natures mean that the essential oils have the ability to penetrate human tissue.

Many natural substances have been found to have a certain effect at one concentration and the opposite effect at another concentration. Robert Tisserand (13), for example states that:

'... patchouli oil seems to be one of those oils that is stimulating in small doses, and sedative at larger doses. Its yang effect is most pronounced on the nervous system; it seems to be a very strong nerve stimulant, reminiscent of ginseng..... The effect of sedation or stimulation not only depends on the dose but also on the state of the individual.'

Peter Holmes (14) also gives an example of this using lavender:

'Lavender can exert a cooling or a warming effect on the body. This would depend on the dosage of lavender used and the type of condition being treated. A person with a hot and acute condition- typified by congestion, inflammation or fever, dilutions of one percent or less are recommended. This will have a cooling, anti-inflammatory effect.
On the other hand someone with a cold and chronic condition, characterised by chills, fatigue, cold extremities - a higher dosage of lavender may be used to generate warmth and activity, both local and systemic.'

Therefore lavender can cool and sedate or warm up and stimulate, depending on the dosage used.

Many studies have demonstrated that the inhalation of essential oils for their expectorant effect is most effective when the essential oils were present in concentrations so low that they could barely be detected by smell. Increases in the concentration of essential oils in the inhaled air reduced the expectorant effect.

Aldehydes such as citral and citronellal have been described as having sedative properties, however this is dependent once again on the dosage used. Used at concentration levels of 1mg/kg of body weight, citral was found to have good sedative properties, however it is well known that indiscriminate use of lemongrass oil which has high levels of citral can produce strong irritation. (15)

The question of accumulation of essential oils in the body also needs to be addressed. Because of their 'high mobility', essential oils are quickly eliminated from the body. In a study essential oils were inhaled as they evaporated from a hot water bath. The concentrations of different terpenoid compounds in the blood serum were measured and were found, after 15 minutes of inhalation, to reach levels that could be considered therapeutically active. It was also found that after 3-4 hours practically all of the essential oil constituents were eliminated. (16)

It is usually advisable to use essential oils in small dosages. Test this yourself by using half the amount of essential oil you are currently using for a certain problem. I am sure you will be surprised to find that the observed effectiveness of the remedy will not be diminished.

How the essential oils are used

Applying the essential oils correctly is one of the most important things if the full benefit of their properties is to be obtained. It is obvious that, in many cases, while applying the essential oils by one method such as massage, the essential oils will also be inhaled, so there will be not only a physiological effect but also an olfactory/ limbic/ hormonal/ emotional response.

One of the benefits of aromatherapy is the ease with which it can be administered and the fact that the essential oils can be administered in so many different ways as listed below:

- massage
- inhalation
- bath
- compresses
- douches
- ointments
- creams and lotions.

Blending

Blending is an important aspect of aromatherapy. It allows one to prescribe the most appropriate essential oils in an aromatherapy treatment. Blending is the creative aspect of aromatherapy and it requires a balance of practice and intuition.

Essential oils are dynamic remedies because they are 'synergistic', meaning that they work together in harmony. Essential oils generally work better when mixed together with other essential oils.

When essential oils are blended, it is always worth keeping the fragrance in mind. It is more pleasing to use a remedy that has a pleasant odour for the individual concerned. Some essential oil fragrances can be quite incompatible.

Some basic hints before you blend are:

- Do not blend more than three to four essential oils in the one blend until you have gained enough experience.
- Check the properties of the essential oils and ensure that they are suitable for your client's condition.
- Ensure that your client does not have any allergies to the essential oils that you have selected.
- Ensure that your client does not have unpleasant memory associations with the essential oils that you have selected.
- Ensure that the environment in which you are working is free of other odours, and that the temperature in the room is stable.

- As John Steele mentioned at a workshop I attended; 'Learn to listen through your nose'. He suggests that it is important for the person blending to be 'empty and receptive' as one would be during meditation.

The following guidelines will be of assistance in preparing balanced and satisfying blends.

- enhancing
- classical blending techniques
- balancing.

Enhancing

When essential oils are blended, a certain effect, eg a calming, uplifting antiseptic effect, can be enhanced by blending the most suitable essential oils.

This concept is referred to as synergy. For example, bergamot may be blended with a variety of oils, each time enhancing a particular aspect of the bergamot:

Bergamot and tea tree:	antiseptic properties; acne, oily skin, cystitis
Bergamot and lavender:	relaxing properties; anxiety, stress
Bergamot and rosemary:	stimulating properties; exhaustion, fatigue
Bergamot and jasmine:	sensuous qualities; depression, aphrodisiac

Classical blending techniques

In the nineteenth century a Frenchman, Piesse, developed a method of classifying odours according to the notes in a musical scale. He transposed the idea of musical harmony into the realm of fragrances where the notes corresponding to each scent formed perfectly balanced chords or harmonics when they were combined.

The practice of classifying essential oils and perfume ingredients into top notes, middle notes and base notes still forms the basis of creating a well-balanced perfume and these principles may be applied to aromatherapy. A good perfume composition should harmoniously balance essential oils in these three categories.

A combination of orange and sandalwood, for example, can be very fresh and fruity at first, becoming more woody and balsamic later.

Top notes

Top notes are sharp, penetrating, highly volatile and the fastest acting. Top notes will hit you first in a blend. They do not last very long, but they are very important in a blend as they give you the first impression of the blend. Top notes are usually uplifting and refreshing.

Typical top notes are: all citrus oils (such as bergamot, neroli, lemon, lime, orange, lemongrass), peppermint, thyme, cinnamon and clove. While most citrus top notes can be used liberally in a blend the spice oils should be used in very small amounts.

Middle notes

Middle notes give body to blends; they smooth the sharp edges. They include oils such as geranium, lavender, rosewood, rosemary and marjoram. They are warm, round and soft. They primarily affect functions of the body, eg digestion and the general metabolism of the body.

Base notes

Base notes, also known as fixatives, deepen the blend and draw it into the skin, giving it permanence. Typical base notes are sandalwood, patchouli, myrrh, frankincense, cedarwood and vetiver. When smelled from the bottle, base notes may appear faint, but when applied to the skin, they strongly react and release their power, which lasts for several hours. Base notes have a sedative and relaxing effect. They are deep, intense and profound.

Base notes slow down the evaporation of the more volatile essential oils, making their fragrance last longer.

Carles, a perfumer of high repute, suggests the following ratio of top, middle and base notes in a typical perfume blend. (17)

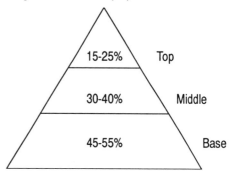

The division into top, middle and base notes is of course arbitrary depending on the essential oils used.

Carles seems to overemphasise the importance of the base notes, when he wrote that they

'...will serve to determine the chief characteristic of the perfume, for their scent will last for hours on end and will be eventually responsible for the success of the perfume.'

Balancing

Perfumers have developed analytical techniques for determining the odour intensity. The odour intensities presented below are obtained from Appell (18) and are rated on a scale from 1 to 10. Often the odour intensity may be used as a guide to blending. The key to balance is to achieve olfactory equilibrium which occurs when two or more essential oils are in a mixture and no single essential oil dominates the odour of the blend.

For example: if making a blend of everlasting and lavender, the respective odour intensities are 7 and 5. This means that the everlasting odour is stronger than that of lavender. As a result, mixing one drop of everlasting and one drop of lavender does not produce a fragrance representing both essential oils. Everlasting would dominate. To create a blend which can be perceived as a balanced combination of both essential oils it may be necessary to mix one drop of everlasting to three drops of lavender (or even more). While the figures given for the odour intensity do not give an exact mixing ratio, they do make it easier to find the right proportions.

Lavabre (19) has developed his own classifications:

- equalisers
- modifiers
- enhancers.

He says that in working with fragrances any classification is bound to be highly subjective.

Blend equalisers

Blend equalisers are those essential oils that will smooth out the sharp edges in a blend. They will balance the blend and allow it to flow harmoniously. Lavabre cites the following essential oils as being equalisers: rosewood, Spanish marjoram, orange and tangerine. Fir and pine are ideal to use with cineole-rich essential oils.

The main purpose of the blend equaliser is to hold the blend together but it has little effect on the blend's distinctive personality.

Blend modifiers

Blend modifiers will give the blend a lift and contribute to its distinctive personality. If the blend is rather flat and uninteresting, adding a drop of a modifier may improve it. Blend modifiers include essential oils such as clove, cinnamon, peppermint, German chamomile, cistus and vetiver. They should be used sparingly as they have the ability to greatly affect the overall fragrance of the blend even when used in very small amounts.

Blend enhancers

These essential oils have a pleasant fragrance and slightly modify the blend without overpowering it. Blend enhancers include essential oils such as bergamot, cedarwood, geranium, clary sage, lavender, lemon, lime, may chang, palmarosa, sandalwood, spruce, jasmine, neroli, rose otto and myrrh.

angelica root	9	frankincense	7	patchouli	7
aniseed	7	ginger	7	pepper, black	7
basil	7	juniper	5	peppermint	7
bergamot	5	lavender	5	petitgrain	5
cedarwood	6	lavender, spike	6	pine	5
cinnamon	7	lemon	5	rose absolute	8
citronella	6	lemongrass	6	rose otto	7
clary sage	5	mandarin	5	rosemary	6
clove bud	8	myrrh	7	rosewood	5
eucalyptus	8	neroli	5	sage, Dalmatian	6
everlasting	7	nutmeg	7	sandalwood	7
fennel	6	orange	5	thyme, red	7

The odour intensity of commonly-used essential oils according to Appell (18)

Chapter 18

Methods of Administration

One of the benefits of aromatherapy is the ease with which it can be administered and the fact that the essential oils can be administered in so many different ways. This chapter discusses the different methods available for the application of essential oils.

Introduction

Applying the essential oils correctly is important if the full benefit of their properties is to be obtained. It is obvious that, in many cases, while applying the essential oils by one method such as massage, the essential oils will also be inhaled, so there will be not only a physiological effect but also a psychological response.

One of the benefits of aromatherapy is the ease with which it can be administered and the fact that the essential oils can be administered in so many different ways as listed below:

- massage
- inhalation
- bath
- compresses
- douches
- ointments
- creams and lotions
- internal use of oils.

Massage

Several studies have confirmed that essential oils are easily absorbed into the body upon application to the skin. One of the studies involved massaging lavender essential oil diluted in peanut oil over the stomach for ten minutes. Five minutes after the massage ended, traces of linalool and linalyl acetate were detected in the blood, increasing to give peak blood levels after 20 minutes. After 90 minutes most of the lavender oil had been removed from the blood. It was concluded that the effects of lavender oil after massage were due to absorption through the skin and inhalation of the oil. (1)

Aromatherapy massage uses gentle, relaxing techniques, and utilises the various energy systems of the body. The percussive techniques of Swedish massage or deep tissue work are not suitable for aromatherapy because they are too intense and stimulating when used with essential oils. Essential oils can be used very effectively in

reflexology, different oils being chosen to correspond with different areas of the foot.

It is not recommended to apply pure essential oils to the skin. They should always be diluted in a suitable carrier oil. For a typical aromatherapy massage place 15 to 30 drops of essential oil into 50 ml of carrier oil. This corresponds to a 1 to 3% dilution of the essential oil.

The carrier oil chosen should be a cold pressed vegetable oil such as sweet almond, apricot kernel, avocado, soybean, safflower or jojoba. Do not use mineral oils as this will impede the absorption of essential oils into the body. Adding 5% or less of wheatgerm oil to the massage oil will keep it from oxidising.

Conditions that respond to massage are:

circulatory problems, digestive problems, fluid retention, headaches, insomnia, menstrual problems, musculoskeletal disorders and nervous tension.

Benefits of Massage

- increases metabolism
- speeds up healing process
- relaxes muscles
- enhances removal of metabolic wastes
- improves circulation of blood and lymph
- relieves mental and physical fatigue
- reduces pain
- reduces tension and anxiety
- calming to the nervous system
- muscles and joints become more supple
- improves skin tone.

Inhalation

Inhalation of essential oils works predominantly on the mind via the olfactory/ limbic/ hormonal/ emotional response. This may help overcome problems such as depression, stress or over tiredness and any other emotional dilemma that may be encountered.

Giovanni Gatti and Renato Cayola (2) explored the effect of various essential oils used in the treatment of anxiety and depression. The experiments were conducted by inhaling the essential oils using a face mask with a cotton wool pad impregnated with an essential oil or an aromatic solution which was sprayed into the air. The results indicated that scents exerted an almost immediate influence on the emotions, in contrast to oral administration, where the essential oils were slowly absorbed via the digestive system.

Buchbauer (3) believes that the only effective way of administering essential oils is via inhalation.

'Aromatherapy applied in the correct way by inhalation only (where the resultant plasma concentrations of aroma compounds are 100 - to 10,000 smaller) leads to the desired effect.'

Marguerite Maury (4) describes the effect of fragrance on the psychic and mental state of an individual:

'Powers of perception become clearer and more acute, and there is a feeling of having, to a certain extent, outstripped events. They are seen more objectively and therefore in truer perspective.'

The use of essential oils as an inhalation for the treatment of respiratory conditions such as a congested nose, headache, sore throat and coughs is a common and effective practice (5). Bardeau (6) found that essential oils that were vaporised were able to kill 90% of airborne microbes within three hours. The oils that were most effective when vaporised included clove, lavender, lemon, marjoram, mint, niaouli, pine, rosemary and thyme.

One of the simplest methods to inhale the essential oil is to place about ten drops on a paper towel or handkerchief and regularly inhale. Another possibility is to place ten drops of essential oil into boiling water and breathe the vapours emitted. The most effective method of using the essential oils as inhalations is by using an oil burner or vaporiser.

Conditions that respond to inhalations are:

tension, headaches, respiratory problems, colds, sore throat, blocked sinuses and cough.

Benefits of Inhalation

- treats respiratory tract problems
- treats throat infections
- eliminates catarrhal conditions
- relieves mental and physical fatigue
- reduces tension and anxiety
- calms the nervous system.

Bath

One of the most common enjoyable methods of using the essential oils is in the bath. This is a very effective method because the oil can act in two ways: by absorption into the skin, and by inhalation, since the warm water causes evaporation of the essential oil.

Although the main method of application in holistic aromatherapy is massage, baths can be an excellent way of using essential oils for a client who cannot be massaged.

Foot and hand baths

For foot and hand baths, place five drops of an essential oil into a bowl of lukewarm water. After soaking the hands or feet for 10-15 minutes, wrap them in a dry towel.

Conditions that respond to hand and foot baths are:

arthritis, dermatitis, rheumatism, varicose veins and dry skin.

Full bath

For a full bath in a bath tub, I recommend the use of a dispersing bath oil. Add 3ml of essential oil to 100ml of dispersing bath oil. Dispersing bath oil is a naturally-derived substance which allows the water and essential oil to form an emulsion. Then add 10ml of bath oil to the tub of water and soak for 15 minutes.

Conditions that respond to body baths are:

circulatory problems, fluid retention, headaches, insomnia, menstrual problems, muscular disorders and nervous tension.

Be cautious when using citrus oils such as lemon or spice oils such as cinnamon and peppermint, because they can easily 'burn' the skin. A prickly sensation may be felt, or a rash may occur. If this happens the bath should be vacated immediately, the oil washed off and a vegetable oil such as jojoba should be applied to soothe the irritated skin.

Sitz bath

Sitz baths are also known as hip baths. A bowl or normal bath may be used, filled with enough water to cover the hips up to the waist only. Add 5 drops of essential oil to each litre of water and mix well. A sitz bath is very effective for treating urinary, genital and lower digestive conditions.

A cold hip bath which should last for one to three minutes only is stimulating, decongesting and is ideal for treating blood congestion. Cold hip baths are great for treating copious menstruation or inter-menstrual bleeding. They can also prevent colds, flu, and promote sound sleep.

A hot hip bath for about 15 minutes at 26°C will stimulate, relax, warm and relieve pain. It is typically used for gynaecological conditions such as delayed or painful periods, for lumbar pain, urinary ailments, gout, haemorrhoids and constipation.

Benefits of Baths

- relieve mental and physical fatigue
- reduce tension and anxiety
- calm the nervous system
- enhance removal of metabolic wastes
- clear heat, fever and inflammation
- improve circulation of blood and lymph
- reduce pain and inflammation.

Compresses

A compress is simply water and essential oils or herbs applied externally to the body with a cloth. A compress can be hot or cold, depending on the condition. A hot compress should be as hot as tolerable and a cold compress should have ice cubes in the water.

Hot compress

Hot compresses are used to reduce muscular or rheumatic pain, to draw out boils or splinters, and to relieve menstrual cramps and toothaches.

Cold compress

Cold compresses are used for treating sprains, swelling, headaches and to reduce fever. Cold compresses may also be used to relieve tiredness due to overwork or stress when in good health. Placed on the feet, legs or hands a cold compress is very reviving. The cold water compress is definitely more stimulating and decongesting than the cold foot bath.

Warm and cold compresses

Alternating warm and cold compresses may be used to help speed healing in pulled muscles, sprained ligaments and bruises. The normal dilution of essential oils in a compress solution is ten drops in 200 ml of water. Dip an un-medicated gauze, cloth or cotton wool into it and wring out the compress so that it does not drip and then cover the area being treated with the compress. Place a plastic wrap over the compress and then a towel or blanket on top. Leave the compress on for two to four hours. A cold compress should always be kept moist.

Benefits of Compresses

- relieve lymphatic and fluid congestion
- clear heat, fever and inflammation
- improve circulation and reduce pain
- relieve tiredness.

Douches

A douche is a vaginal wash using essential oils diluted in water. This method can be very helpful in the treatment of mucous lining in catarrhal or infectious conditions associated with the urinary tract or genital area, such as pruritus, cystitis or thrush. Add five to ten drops of essential oil to one litre of warm water and shake the mixture well. Add one tablespoon of cider vinegar to help maintain the pH balance. This mixture can be used in a sitz bath, bidet or in an enema or douche pot, which can be bought from some chemists.

The best position for applying a douche is lying on the back (to avoid spreading infection to the womb), and the douche should be retained for 10-20 minutes. Douches should be applied every day for up to a week when the symptoms are acute and once a month for maintenance. It should be kept in mind that douching should not be done on a regular basis as it disrupts the normal, healthy bacterial balance.

Benefits of Douches

- treat infectious conditions associated with the urinary tract or genital area.

Ointments

An ointment is an oil or fat extraction applied to the skin by rubbing. It is often called a 'salve' or 'unguent'. It has topical protective, healing, soothing, moistening and cooling properties and provides a long-term effect when continuously applied. Some examples of the preparation and application of ointments are:

- For treatment of boils, sores, infected cuts, fungal skin infections or inflamed skin conditions, a soothing and antiseptic ointment can be made from tea tree oil and infused calendula oil.

- The rubefacient and analgesic properties of black pepper, ginger, cinnamon, and peppermint can be used in an ointment to treat arthritis and sports injuries. Use before an event to keep the muscles warm and prevent injuries.

- To moisten, soothe and protect dry, irritative skin conditions such as eczema, dry chapped skin or lips use infused calendula oil, infused carrot oil, myrrh and German chamomile in an ointment.

For an ointment base, various types of fat or a vegetable oil blend with beeswax or lanolin may be used. Lanolin may be used alone as an ointment base. The essential oil dilution should vary according to the condition (1-5% dilution).

Benefits of Ointments

- protect and heal
- soothe and moisturise
- enhance long-term effects of essential oils
- relieve pain.

Creams and lotions

A cream is a light oil preparation emulsified in water. While similar to ointments, creams have the advantage of penetrating faster and they do not have the same clogging effect on the skin. Creams and lotions may be used to treat most skin conditions or any condition where a massage oil might be considered.

A lotion is simply a thinner, more liquid cream, diluted with water. Creams and lotions have the advantage of being able to be applied to the skin at any time of the day without the worry of the base oils staining clothing.

A simple recipe for making a cream base is as follows:

emulsifying wax	20 gm
coconut oil	20 ml
almond oil	40 ml
purified water	90 ml .

Melt the wax in a bain-marie and beat in the oils. Bring the water to the same temperature in a separate bowl. Remove both bowls from the heat and slowly stir the water into the wax mixture.

Continue beating until the mixture cools. Add 1-5% essential oil to the preparation and store in a jar.

Benefits of Creams and Lotions

- protect and heal
- soothe and moisturise
- ideal for skin care preparations
- penetrate quickly
- non-greasy feeling on the skin.

Internal use of essential oils

This is often an area of much controversy. The French medical practitioners often use essential oils internally, in much the same way as a doctor would prescribe the use of antibiotics. The essential oils are carefully prepared medications, usually in capsule form, and are formulated to be safe for ingestion.

Many people recommend the taking of essential oils in tea, water, honey or sugar. I do not recommended this practice. There is a real possibility of irritating the stomach lining if the oils are used incorrectly or in excessive amounts. The International Federation of Aromatherapists does not recommend that essential oils be taken internally unless under the supervision of a medical doctor who is also qualified in clinical aromatherapy as practised in France. In conclusion I agree with Madame Maury, a well known French aromatherapist and herself a biochemist:

'the responsibility for administering them internally could not be carried out except by a competent doctor.' (7)

Chapter 19

The Aromatherapy Massage

Aromatherapy works on the body as a whole, having a great influence not only on mood, but also on the treatment of many physical ailments. This chapter describes the aromatherapy massage technique and the expected benefits of the treatment.

Introduction

Massage is a healing art. It is the manipulation of the soft tissues of the body. It can be used to enhance relaxation, to relieve aches and pains, to encourage blood circulation or to assist lymph flow. As well as its undoubted physical benefits, massage also enhances a more optimistic outlook on life. It generally has a sedative effect, but it can be uplifting. Massage is also excellent for toning the skin, helping to regulate the secretion of the sebaceous glands and helping in the elimination of toxins.

Before I describe the aromatherapy massage technique in detail I will describe the benefits of the main massage techniques used in the aromatherapy massage.

Swedish massage

Swedish massage was developed early in the nineteenth century, by Professor Ling, of Sweden. He made a detailed scientific study of massage, thus laying down the foundations for what is now taught and practised as 'Swedish massage'.

Swedish massage is familiar to most people. It usually starts with long, slow, gentle strokes, referred to as effleurage, over the back and body. The smooth flowing effleurage techniques of Swedish massage are used extensively in all aromatherapy massage techniques.

Smoother but deeper kneading movements will follow, warming the muscles to do deeper work. Kneading is useful for aching muscles. Muscles begin to ache when chemical by-products from physical activity (mainly lactic acid) begin to build in the tissues. This usually happens when the muscles are being used beyond their normal capacity, and the blood and lymph cannot eliminate the lactic acid quickly enough from the area. Massage, especially kneading, stimulates the circulation and helps to disperse the lactic acid. At this point aromatherapy massage leaves Swedish massage and its more vigorous hacking and pounding movements.

While it is an excellent form of physical massage, Swedish massage does not usually take into account the mental and emotional state of the receiver. Other movements used in Swedish massage include petrissage, which is a deeper massage using the thumbs.

Neuromuscular massage

Neuro-muscular techniques are the backbone of the aromatherapy massage technique explained in this manual. The system evolved over the past 40 years from the original work of the late Stanley Leif (1). As a trained chiropractor and osteopath he studied the work of a practitioner of Hindu manipulation, Dewanchand Varma, who was practising in Paris. Varma used a system called 'Pranotherapy' and in his book *The Human Machine and its Forces* he states:

We have discovered that the circulation of the nervous currents slows down occasionally because of the obstruction caused by adhesions; the muscle fibres harden and the nervous currents can no longer pass through them.

The overall effect of this massage is the restoration of the balance of the autonomic nervous system.

According to Maria Ebner who speaks extensively of the connection between body tissue and the autonomic nervous system (2):

(a) Pathological conditions of organs cause reflexly pathological symptoms of the skin and the connective tissue element of the body surface, in the muscles, blood vessels and nerves, probably also in the bones if they depend for their innervation on the same segmental nerve supply;

(b) Pathological conditions of the tissues of the body surface including the skin and its connective tissue element of the body surface, in the muscles, blood vessels and nerves, probably also in the bones will eventually cause pathological dysfunction of organs within the same segmental nerve supply;

(c) Therapeutic agents applied to the surface tissues of the segment will influence beneficially the pathological condition of the affected organs within the segment.

Ebner's comments helped lay the foundation of the aromatherapy massage and also confirm the benefit of using essential oils on specific areas of the body to treat specific conditions.

Lymphatic massage

Lymphatic problems can be relieved by using specific lymphatic drainage massage techniques. Aromatherapy massage techniques developed by Maury and Arcier incorporate many lymphatic drainage movements.

The best known system of lymphatic massage was developed by Dr. Emil Vodder. Dr Vodder developed a system of movements which drained the lymph nodes and relieved the symptoms. He spent 40 years developing a system of lymphatic drainage massage which is now taught all over Europe.

You need to be aware of the contraindications of lymphatic massage and must observe them rigidly. Lymphatic massage should not be done on anyone who has active cancer, heart problems, thrombosis, phlebitis, high blood pressure, varicose veins, pregnancy, any acute inflammation or infection, or any other severe medical problem. Do not use these techniques on anyone who has recently undergone chemotherapy, since the toxins filtered by the liver for elimination will be released into the bloodstream and make the person feel very ill.

Acupressure massage and shiatsu

The word shiatsu comes from the Japanese word 'Shi', finger, and 'atsu', pressure. Like acupressure, it is based on the Chinese medical system that holds that the energy of the body 'Qi' in Chinese and 'Ki' in Japanese, circulates from the internal organs to the periphery of the body and returns again through the channels also known as meridians. There are six channels of yin energy and six channels of yang energy. In Oriental medicine the qualities of yin and yang are distinguished as follows:

- Yin energy is quiet, deep, passive and nourishing.
- Yang energy is active, purposeful, aggressive and functionally protective of the body.

It will be important to diagnose the imbalance between the yin and yang energy, and treat appropriately along these channels of energy. Along these channels the Qi may surface to the exterior of the body at specific points. By applying pressure at these points the Qi may be stimulated or sedated according to the body's requirements.

Reflexology

The most therapeutically effective massage of the feet is reflexology. Reflex points on the feet relate to every organ and gland in the body. Placed side by side, the soles of our feet reflect a map of our whole body. Applying pressure on the reflex points has been shown to have various effects:

- definite physiological changes eg decreased blood sugar levels
- a deep and long lasting sense of relaxation and well-being
- reduction in pain
- improved circulation
- a balanced energy flow in the meridians.

Research has indicated that reflexology can have powerful therapeutic effects on conditions such as asthma, premenstrual tension and chronic constipation.

Through the feet, the autonomic nervous system, the lymphatic system, the circulation and the energy meridians are all affected. This makes reflexology a uniquely holistic therapy which can be ideally combined with aromatherapy.

Polarity therapy

Some aromatherapy techniques use polarity therapy which is based on Dr. Randolph Stone's work. The human body is a living being, emitting an electromagnetic energy field of many different frequencies, which must be in balance to maintain good health. Each part of the body has either a positive or negative charge, and polarity therapy is the use of the therapist's own electromagnetic field to rebalance that of the client.

The autonomic nervous system

To understand the full benefits of the aromatherapy massage an understanding of the autonomic nervous system that regulates the activity of the smooth muscles, cardiac muscles and the glands is necessary.

The autonomic pathways consist of two neurons. One extends from the central nervous system to a ganglion. The other extends directly from the ganglion to the effector (muscle or gland). The ganglions are known as the cervical ganglia, thoracic ganglia, lumbar ganglia, and the sacral ganglia. From these ganglia pass nerve fibres which group themselves to form plexuses. From these plexuses, nerves radiate to supply the different organs in the thoracic, abdominal and pelvic cavities. These are responsible for controlling the processes which take place within the body but not under conscious control.

During the aromatherapy massage you will be using techniques to stimulate the ganglia (reflex points). These techniques often have a profound effect on the body. Most people who experience an aromatherapy massage who have also received different styles of massage comment on the gentleness of the technique, but are absolutely amazed at the way that they feel energised, if they were suffering from lethargy, or how relaxed they feel and how well they sleep. These responses are due to the effect that the aromatherapy massage has on the autonomic nervous system.

It is interesting to note that there is a similarity between the location of the ganglia and the position of the Chinese acupuncture points found along the bladder channel which runs bilaterally to the spine. The acupuncture points along the back are referred to as 'back shu' points or 'associated' points. Each associated point indicates a disharmony in that meridian, and in its associated organ or function. These points are similar to the location of the chain of ganglia situated on either side of the vertebral column from the base of the skull to the coccyx.

Aromatherapy massage guidelines

Before giving a massage the following advice will help you:

- Ensure that your nails are short.

- Try not to break contact unnecessarily from your client's body. A break in contact mid-flow can almost feel disconcerting to the recipient. Of course, breaks when you have reached a natural pause in the sequence are okay.

- Slow movements calm while brisk movements stimulate.

- Work with your whole body, rather than just your hands and arms. For example, when applying pressure, lean into the stroke, using your body weight rather than overworking your arms and wrists.

- If you forget what to do next, use simple effleurage techniques until you remember. It is far better to improvise than to stop mid-flow.

- Be totally relaxed and confident, otherwise your client will sense your nervousness.

- The timing of the aromatherapy massage is approximately 45 minutes to one hour.

Aromatherapy massage contraindications

There are a few times when aromatherapy treatment is not advisable or should be used with caution. Contraindications include the following conditions:

Do not massage if:

- the client has recently consumed alcohol

- the client has just had a large meal.

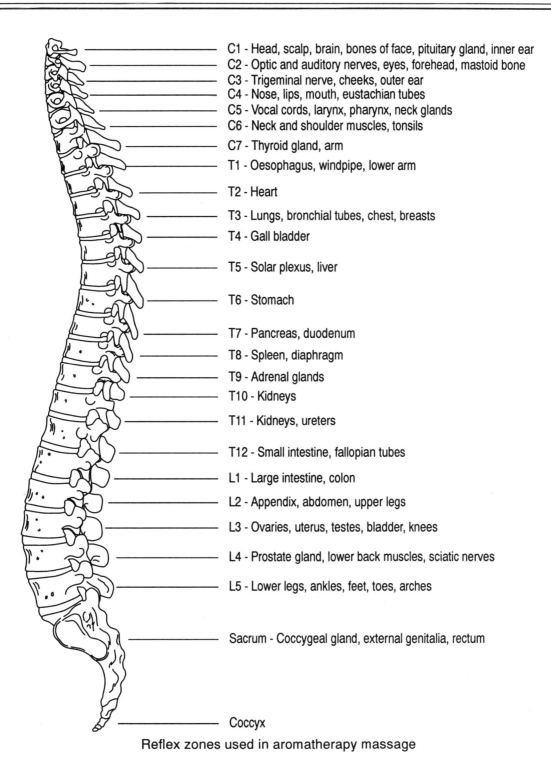

C1 - Head, scalp, brain, bones of face, pituitary gland, inner ear
C2 - Optic and auditory nerves, eyes, forehead, mastoid bone
C3 - Trigeminal nerve, cheeks, outer ear
C4 - Nose, lips, mouth, eustachian tubes
C5 - Vocal cords, larynx, pharynx, neck glands
C6 - Neck and shoulder muscles, tonsils
C7 - Thyroid gland, arm

T1 - Oesophagus, windpipe, lower arm

T2 - Heart

T3 - Lungs, bronchial tubes, chest, breasts

T4 - Gall bladder

T5 - Solar plexus, liver

T6 - Stomach

T7 - Pancreas, duodenum

T8 - Spleen, diaphragm

T9 - Adrenal glands

T10 - Kidneys

T11 - Kidneys, ureters

T12 - Small intestine, fallopian tubes

L1 - Large intestine, colon

L2 - Appendix, abdomen, upper legs

L3 - Ovaries, uterus, testes, bladder, knees

L4 - Prostate gland, lower back muscles, sciatic nerves

L5 - Lower legs, ankles, feet, toes, arches

Sacrum - Coccygeal gland, external genitalia, rectum

Coccyx

Reflex zones used in aromatherapy massage

Post operative states

Always seek permission of your client's general practitioner before massaging following any form of recent major surgery.

Heart conditions

If the client has a history of heart attacks, angina or strokes use only gentle massage that will help the circulation.

Cancer

Unless advised by a doctor, massage should not be used if a client has been diagnosed as having cancer. However, if permission has been obtained from your client's doctor, massage can be extremely beneficial.

Varicose veins

Treat with care and massage extremely lightly with upward stokes only (towards the heart). Massage above the area first.

Infectious diseases

Do not massage any topical infectious disease, but instead use essential oil compresses, which are useful for treatment of broken skin, wounds, inflammations and bedsores, etc. For respiratory infections such as sore throat or chest infections, chest massages are very helpful.

Inflamed joints

With conditions such as gout or rheumatoid arthritis, massaging directly over the area will be extremely painful, therefore compresses or baths are recommended. Massaging the joint above the affected area can be very beneficial to improve circulation.

A doctor's written consent should first be obtained before treating any of the above conditions. The wisest recommendation I can give is, if in doubt, **DON'T!**

Recent fractures and large areas of scar tissue

Do not massage a recent fracture or large area of scar tissue for at least two months. Use only gentle massage techniques to apply the aromatherapy oil blend to aid scar healing and minimize scarring.

Aromatherapy massage

Aromatherapy massage uses various holistic principles, but works mainly on the nervous system. As already explained, by applying pressure to the nerve ganglia along the spine, the aromatherapy massage works on the autonomic nervous system, having an instant regulating effect.

I am privileged to have trained with Micheline Arcier, who has developed this aromatherapy massage technique. The technique I will be describing is referred to as the 'Micheline Arcier Aromatherapy Massage'. I have not altered her sequence and have found it best to follow the exact sequence without alteration.

The actual massage should take only 45 minutes. Extending the duration of the massage is not recommended, as too much stimulation may neutralise the results. These are the main massage movements used. The massage movements are usually repeated five times.

1. Attunement

This technique relaxes your client and establishes contact. It is done with dry hands. Cup your left hand around the base of the occipital bone and keep it there as you do the following:

- Right hand flat on 5th thoracic for 20 seconds, then lift hand.
- Right hand flat on 10th thoracic for 20 seconds, then lift hand.
- Right hand flat on 2nd and 3rd lumbar for 20 seconds, lift hand.
- Right hand on iliac crest pushing gently towards feet, right side first then on the left side, lift hand.
- Leave left hand still on the occipital bone for 20 seconds, then slowly release.

2. Massaging the base of the cranium

- With dry hands start to massage the base of the cranium and the back of the neck.

- Then hold the right side of the head with the left hand and with the right thumb start to apply pressure on the left side of the cranium under the occipital bone. When the centre part is reached, invert the position, but this time using the middle finger to apply pressure on the right side of the cranium. This alleviates muscle contraction and fluid infiltrations.

Repeat these movements five times, more if there is tension. Due to tension and congestion some people are very tender in this area, so go gently at first, increasing the pressure if your client can tolerate it.

- Slide fingers up along cranium and then sweep your fingers over the top of the head and through the hair starting at the base of the skull. Carry the motion all the way to the ends of the hair, giving your hand a little flick at the end of each sweep. This stimulates the cranial nerves, releases the energy flow from the body and neutralises negative electrical charges from the body. Repeat this movement 5 times.

3. Applying the oil

Apply the prescribed oil all over the back with sweeping effleurage movements. Repeat a few times until the oil is well spread and the client starts to relax. Effleurage can be done throughout the treatment between steps to give continuity to the treatment.

4. Stimulation of nerve ganglia along the spine

The two thumbs are used, alternately pressing, releasing, sliding. Each side of the spine must be done alternately three times, starting at the coccygeal area, working all the way up the spine to the neck. Do not press on the spinal bone. Follow by a similar, deep sliding movement.

These movements stimulate the chain of ganglia that make up the sympathetic nervous system.

5. Decongesting the back tissue

The tissue on the back often becomes tight and congested with tension and fatigue. You are going to relieve this tension by picking up the skin between your hands. Begin just above the buttocks and continue all over the back up to the neck and top of the shoulders. Scoop up the skin going as deeply as possible. This movement also speeds up blood and lymph flow.

6. Liberation of nerve influx

Beginning at the base of the client's spine, poise finger tips of both hands at the edge of the spinal column pointing towards the table, and slide them over the back and down the massage table. This movement should be continued up the back to the shoulder, then repeated on the left side. You should be standing on the left side, so you will find that your thumbs now move over the body and down the table before the fingers. Repeat on both sides of the back, from bottom to top, three times.

7. The hips and buttocks

These movements can relieve problems associated with the uterus, bladder and sexual organs. When working on women this area often feels tender, and these techniques should break up much congestion. People with sciatic pain will also benefit.

- Effleurage hip and buttocks area
- Circular movement with thumbs from coccygeal to the hip bone
- Deep thumb sliding movement along ganglia from coccygeal to iliac crest, repeat fanning outward over the buttock area
- Apply pressure with the middle finger to the hip plexus for a count of four, and then rest flat of hand over the area to soothe. The hip plexus is collocated with GB 30,

and is located posterior and inferior to the head of the greater trochanter, in the major gluteal depression. The depression is very obvious when the buttocks are tensed. This point will help relieve pain in the lower hip region, pain and weakness in the lower extremities and will help the energy circulate around the body.

These movements speed up circulation and improve lymphatic drainage and relieve any congestive state.

8. Massaging the kidney area

Effleurage over kidney area.

9. Arms and hands

If your client's arms are not lying straight out, lift them onto the couch.

- Sliding movement from the coccygeal lumbar area to shoulder lymph points. Apply pressure with thumbs.

- Slide down arms, pressure on inside of elbows, inside of wrists and palm of hands, slide off hands.

These acupressure points affect lymph circulation and metabolism (shoulder point), lung and heart function (inside of elbows), and the kidneys and adrenal glands (hands).

10. Relaxing tension in the neck and shoulder area

Massage shoulders and neck. Finish by sliding along cranium to top of head.

11. Leg massage

Apply the oil using effleurage movements.

- Standing at the end of the table, place your entire hand on the sole of each foot, your left hand on the left foot, your right hand on the right foot. Hold your hands on your client's feet for at least ten seconds.

This movement uses polarity therapy, which utilises the magnetic field of the person to calm and stimulate. In this position you are charging the body with two poles of the same polarity. By using the flat of your hands the effect is calming and energising.

- Curve your hands around your client's ankles and hold for two seconds.

- Then run your two flat hands up to the back of the knees. The pressure should be firm, unless there is fluid retention. In this case always press lightly. Pause with the hands on the popliteal crease and apply pressure to acupressure point Bl 40 for two seconds.

- Now continue to run your hands on up the legs and then sliding back down the lateral aspect of the thighs from the trochanter to just above the knee, applying firm pressure.

- Circular and sliding movements with the thumbs on the sole of the feet. Slide up to the ankles, circular movements around ankles, slide up and rest hands on the popliteal crease for two seconds. Now slide up to just below the buttocks and, with the thumbs, press the lymphatic points. These lymphatic points are collocated with Bl 36 at the midpoint of the gluteal fold between the femoral biceps and the semitendinosus muscles and is used for the treatment of pain in the lumbar, sacral, gluteal and femoral regions.

Repeat leg movements three times and finish by resting hands on the soles of the feet.

12. Front

You are now ready to commence working on the head. neck and chest.

- Turn the client onto the back, continuing to drape with towels.

- The therapist should now wash his/her hands.

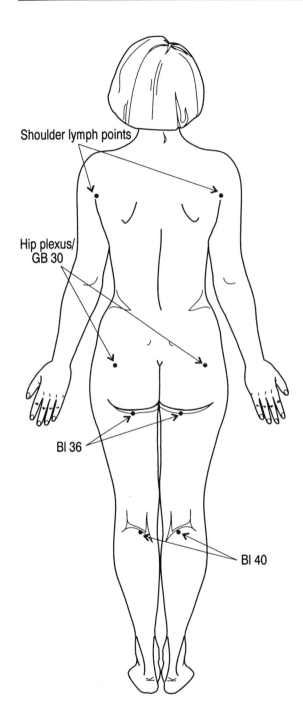

Shoulder lymph points

Hip plexus/
GB 30

BI 36

BI 40

Location of pressure points used in
aromatherapy massage

13. Pressing the head with your thumbs

- With dry hands, begin pressing the forehead with your thumbs. Put one thumb on top of the other to enhance the pressure, and press at 1 cm intervals, starting from the centre of the top of the forehead, then moving over the top of the head to the back of the head.

This movement affects the governor vessel meridian, and stimulates the endocrine system because of its stimulating effect on the pituitary gland.

14. Stimulating the scalp

- With your fingers spread, firmly massage the scalp all over. Actually move the scalp, don't let your fingers slide around on the hair.

This loosens the scalp, bringing nourishing blood flow to the hair follicles, and stimulating nerve endings that relieve tension to the head.

15. Magnetic cleansing

- Rake your fingers through the hair, starting at the scalp. Pull through to the very tips of the hair, giving your hands a flick as you reach the ends.

This cleansing action draws out negative magnetic charges from the head and the hair. Repeat six times.

16. Applying oil to the face and upper body

Apply a small amount of face oil into the palm of your hand, and apply it to the face, working both hands in unison on each side of the face, over the nose and chin, and carefully around the eyes.

17. Massaging the forehead

- With your two thumbs facing each other, start above the eyebrows in the centre of the forehead and press in a straight line out to the hairline on the side of the head, pressing at 2 cm intervals, and moving up until you reach the hairline at the forehead. Pressure is decreased when on the temples.

- Deep pressure is applied to the corrugator muscle, which is a small muscle on each side of the root of the nose, sliding up to the hairline. This will help release tension and soothes the frowning muscle.

- Complete by a soothing almost hypnotic movement, sliding the hands alternately over the forehead. The centre of your palm should make the most contact with the head.

18. Circling the eyes

- With either your second or middle fingers, circle the eyes, starting from the inside corner of the eyebrows and moving out and around below the eyes. Exert more pressure over the brow, and very light pressure over the eyelid.

Do not drag the skin tissue when performing this technique. This movement calms and revives the eyes and improves blood circulation.

19. Pinching the eyebrows

The corrugator muscle is lifted up and pressure applied inside the bone near the eye to relieve eye strain and sinus problems.

20. Decongesting the nose

- Using the fingers of both hands, make circles on each side of the base of the nose, working up the bridge. Then slide your fingers over the forehead to the hairline.

Be sure that you don't press too hard on the side of the nose as this may obstruct breathing. This technique decongests the nose.

21. Decongesting the sinuses

- Spread your fingers over the cheeks on each side of the nose. With firm pressure

'rake' over the cheek towards the ear. This helps drain the sinuses and benefits the lymph capillaries that run horizontally across the face into the submaxillary lymph glands in the jawbone under the ear.

- Just under the cheekbone at the nostrils, where the acupuncture point called 'colon 20' is located, press firmly, holding for ten seconds, then completing by sweeping fingers out towards the ear.

22. Liberating the lymph in the lower face

- Spreading your fingers of each hand over the upper lip and chin, rake outwards to the ear.

This encourages lymph flow into the nodes at the sides of the lower jaw, called the mandibular lymph nodes.

23. Stimulating the chin and jaw area

- Massage contours of the face with fingers placed under the jaw bone, and thumbs

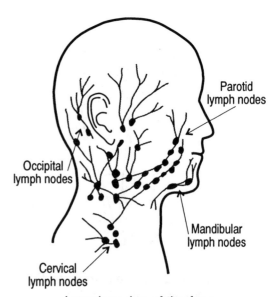

Lymph nodes of the face

working in a circular movement, from the chin to the end of the mandible.

24. Toning the neck

- Holding your left hand under the neck, slide your right hand around the front of the neck, working from left to right.

- Now change hands, placing the right hand underneath the neck, and sliding with the left.

You should use a flat hand and make sure you are using enough oil so that you don't pull the skin. This improves the skin tone of the neck.

25. Stimulating the neuro-lymphatic reflex points

- Begin this movement by sliding your hands to the base of the neck over the clavicle down to just above the breast; hold your hands about four inches apart. Hold for two seconds.

- Sweep your hands over the top of the shoulders and press them down, holding for ten seconds.

- Run your hands all the way up the sides of the neck and out through the hair.

As you move down the chest you are passing over lymph nodes, lymph vessels and nerves that affect the heart, liver, thyroid and lungs. If your client objects to oil in the hair, you can discontinue the movement at the hairline. Repeat the entire process three times.

26. Massaging the shoulders

- Slip your hands under your client's shoulders and massage with circular movements of the fingers, on the trapezius muscle in the shoulder area, to help relieve tension in the upper back and shoulders.

- A deep petrissage movement on the shoulders helps to relax muscles and release tension.

- Cup your fingers against the occipital bone slightly stretch the neck.

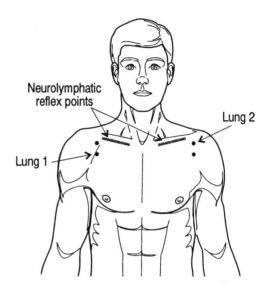

Neurolymphatic reflex points

Lung 1

Lung 2

- Hands cupped under the back of the neck, lift and vibrate. Do not lift the head from the massage table.

27. Stimulating the neuro-lymphatic reflex point below the clavicle

- Sliding from the neck down to the midpoints under the clavicle, press with your first two fingers for two seconds, using both hands.

- Massage below the clavicle working your way out to the shoulders, up the side of the neck and head and off through the hair.

You are stimulating the lung acupuncture points as well as the neurolymphatic reflex point in the area.

28. Calming and reviving the diaphragm

- Apply oil to the abdomen.

- Keeping your left hand on the client's arm inscribe a counterclockwise movement with the flat of your hand around the solar plexus, make the circular movements at least six times, moving slowly and concentrating on putting your body energy into the treatment.

- Then liberate the diaphragm by sliding hands down the ribs. If the client complains of deep pain stop the movement. If there is a lot of tension ask the client to do a few abdominal breathing exercises.

29. Massaging the feet

- Apply oil to the feet and legs using effleurage movements.
- Then with wrists tilted inwards, grasp the tops of the feet with your fingers, the thumbs on the heels.
- Now slide up the feet with your thumbs from the heel to the big toe. Repeat this movement, working towards the centre of the heel.
- When you cannot go any further in this position, move the hands to the outside of the feet and, grasping the tops of the feet with the fingers, work the thumbs up the heel to the little toe. Repeat this movement working towards the centre of the feet.

30. Stimulating the lymph in the feet.

- Hold the soles of the feet with your fingers. At the same time, stroke between the toes in the direction of the ankle with your thumbs.

This encourages the lymph that flows down to the toes to start its upward journey to the nodes in the knees.

31. Massaging the legs

- Sliding your hands from the feet to the ankles, massage them with a circular motion.
- Then slide your hands up to the knee and rest them for two seconds. The popliteal lymph nodes that drain the bottom of the legs are located in the front of the knees,

so by sliding up the leg and resting your warm hands on the knees you are encouraging lymph to travel into these nodes.

- From the knees slide up towards the groin and press in with your thumbs to stimulate the inguinal lymph nodes there. These nodes are located in the inguinal groove, level with the upper border of the symphysis pubis. This movement should be done with great care as the area is often tender and sensitive.

32. End of the treatment

End the aromatherapy treatment by placing the flats of your hands on the soles of your client's feet. This is always done at the end of the treatment to rebalance the flow of energy. Remember to wash your hands when the treatment is completed and shake them to release any negative magnetism.

UNIT V

CLINICAL INDEX

Unit V provides the knowledge and skills for the treatment of a wide range of conditions. Each condition is listed with a description of cause and symptoms and is followed by the recommended treatment - the essential oils used, their application, as well as suggestions with regards to diet, herbs, acupressure and additional therapies.

Unit V includes the following chapters:

Chapter 20 Circulatory system

Chapter 21 Respiratory system

Chapter 22 Musculoskeletal system

Chapter 23 Reproductive system

Chapter 24 Integumentary system

Chapter 25 Nervous system

Chapter 26 Lymphatic system

Chapter 27 Immune system

Chapter 28 Digestive system

Chapter 29 Aromatherapy skin care

Chapter 20

Circulatory System

This chapter summarises an holistic approach to the treatment of many common ailments and conditions associated with the circulatory system.
Not only have the aromatherapy procedures for each condition been outlined, but details have also been included on other forms of treatment such as diet, herbs, acupressure and exercise.

Conditions discussed in this chapter include:

Chilblains
Hypertension
Oedema
Palpitations
Varicose veins

Introduction

The circulatory system is made up of the heart, arteries, arterioles, capillaries, venules, veins and the blood. The basic function of the circulatory system is to ensure that blood reaches all parts of the body. Every cell must receive nourishment which is provided by the blood. The circulatory system also ensures that waste products of the cells (carbon dioxide, urea, lactic acid, etc.) are carried to the kidneys, intestines, lungs and skin where they are excreted.

Diseases of the circulatory system account for two thirds of all deaths in our western society. Many circulatory problems require professional medical diagnosis and treatment, however aromatherapy, as with other forms of natural therapy can play a vital role in the prevention of circulatory diseases.

Much evidence shows that lifestyle is a contributing factor to the disease process. Risk factors such as cigarette smoking, excess intake of salt, saturated fats and refined processed foods, alcohol, lack of exercise can all potentiate the disease process.

Biochemical risk factors such as high cholesterol and triglycerides, reduced high density lipo-proteins (HDL) levels, decreased levels of plasma copper, excessive zinc intakes, high blood sugar, pesticide residue in fatty tissues, increased blood viscosity and high blood pressure can also significantly influence circulatory problems.

The vitality and tone of the circulatory system are fundamental to life and to the integration of all the parts of the body. If there is weakness or congestion present, it will have profound effects on the tissues and organs involved. The blood may be healthy but if the supply of blood to the organs is not adequate, there will be problems. If the blood supply to the brain is obstructed brain death will occur in about six minutes.

Similarly, if waste materials produced in the metabolic process are not removed, damage to tissues will result. From this we may conclude that any disease focused in an organ may have its roots in an insufficiency of the circulatory system, either because the organ is not being properly supplied with blood, or because the waste it produces is not being adequately removed.

General considerations

Prevention is far better than having to resort to curing a disease that has developed. There are four specific factors relating to the circulatory system that apply to everybody:

- exercise
- diet
- tobacco and alcohol
- stress.

Exercise

Exercise is vital for a healthy circulatory system. This is the only way to ensure that the heart and blood vessels are effectively used, but it also reduces both stress and the risk of circulatory disease. The exercise program should, of course, be carefully designed, taking into account the patient's needs and circulatory condition.

Diet

The most important dietary factors that will reduce the risk of heart disease are:

- Reduce the consumption of dietary fat to 20% of total calories.
- Increase intake of fish oils or cold pressed polyunsaturated oils.
- Reduce the intake of salt to less than 2 to 3 gm per day.
- Avoid all tea , coffee, cocoa, and excessive sugar.
- Increase dietary fibre by eating raw fruit and vegetables.
- Reduce alcohol intake.
- Reduce weight if necessary.
- Eat more garlic, onion and ginger.

Tobacco and alcohol

Anyone with concerns for their health should stop smoking and keep the intake of alcohol to a minimal amount.

Statistics have shown that smokers have a 70% higher rate of death from circulatory disease. Smoking has been positively associated with increased sugar, alcohol and caffeine consumption (1). Cigarette smokers are also known to have higher concentrations of lead and cadmium and lower concentrations of ascorbic acid than nonsmokers (2).

Stress

There is a correlation between the level of stress in your life and the occurrence of health problems, particularly in the circulatory system. 'Stress' is a relative concept. It would be more appropriate to consider the individual's ability to deal with stress in his/her life rather than to look at stress itself.

Essential oils can play a vital role in assisting us to deal with stress, but it is far better and more realistic to go to the underlying cause within us and change that. Relaxation therapy, counselling, meditation, yoga and biofeedback techniques all have much to offer. 'Dis-ease' can be prevented by bringing ease into one's life. Psychological and spiritual harmony will create the inner environment for bodily harmony.

Aromatherapy considerations

Many circulatory and most cardiac problems require professional diagnosis and treatment, but aromatherapy in combination with simple preventative recommendations can prevent the deterioration of the circulatory and cardiovascular system.

Aromatherapy has been found to be extremely valuable in the care of post operative coronary heart disease patients. Stevenson (3), a qualified aromatherapist and nurse, found that neroli oil reduced discomfort and side effects of patients who had recently undergone cardiac surgery.

Neroli oil was chosen because of its abilities in calming the nervous system, helping insomnia, relieving anxiety, calming palpitations and being a cordial or heart tonic. Neroli's antispasmodic effect works particularly well on diminishing the amplitude of heart muscle contraction, thus benefiting people who suffer from palpitations or other types of cardiac spasm.

Studies in China have confirmed may chang's anti-arrhythmic properties. May chang and propranolol (a commonly prescribed beta-blocker) were tested against barium chloride-induced arrhythmias. The essential oil was given at the same dose as the drug. May chang reduced the time the arrhythmia persisted from 15 minutes to 6.5 minutes, while propranolol reduced the arrhythmia time to 0.6 minutes. (4)

Research in Belgium has identified eugenol and isoeugenol as the ingredients in nutmeg oil responsible for anti-platelet activity (5).

The following list of properties indicates how essential oils may be used to help prevent and treat some of the more common problems associated with the cardiovascular system.

Nervines

Anxiety and stress can lead to cardiovascular problems. The use of relaxing nervines such as *lavender, neroli* and *Roman chamomile* should be considered to reduce stress and anxiety.

Hypotensives

For reducing high blood pressure *lavender, sweet marjoram, may chang* and *ylang-ylang* are excellent essential oils.

Hypertensives

Hypertensives are used for poor circulation, chilblains, listlessness and low blood pressure. Essential oils such as *rosemary, thyme, peppermint* and *eucalyptus* are often used.

Circulatory tonics and astringents

Essential oils such as *cypress, geranium, yarrow,* and *lemon* are useful for treating swellings, inflammations and varicose veins.

Rubefacients

Oils such as *black pepper, sweet* and *Spanish marjoram, rosemary* and *ginger* stimulate circulation locally to the area which they are applied. Rubifacient oils cause the capillaries to dilate, increasing the blood flow, which speeds up the healing process.

While aromatherapy has much to offer in the treatment of circulatory problems, it must be emphasised that any serious heart problem should be treated under medical observation. The most common symptoms resulting from heart disease are fatigue, chest pain, palpitations and oedema. However, because any of these symptoms may be due to non-cardiac disorders, the proper interpretation of their significance depends upon correct diagnostic studies.

Associated conditions

Some of the serious conditions that affect the heart, blood vessels and blood include: coronary heart disease (heart attack and angina), blood clotting, peripheral vascular disease, strokes and high blood fat levels. It is not in the scope of this book to cover these conditions mentioned as diet and lifestyle modification are often more appropriate.

Chilblains

Useful Oils

Black pepper, cinnamon, clove, ginger, lemon, nutmeg, rosemary, Spanish and sweet marjoram, thyme

Clinical features

These are reddish blue discolourations of the skin, accompanied by swelling, which affect parts of the body which are exposed to cold, particularly toes, fingers, and the back of legs. Children are particularly prone to chilblains on their feet in winter. Poor circulation of the blood is a contributory factor.

Aromatherapy treatment

If the chilblains are unbroken, essential oils classified as rubefacients will help to stimulate the local circulation. The most effective essential oils are black pepper, ginger, nutmeg and Spanish marjoram.

Massage the affected area with a massage oil containing a 3% dilution of any of these oils. This will reduce pain and itching and help to disperse the chilblains. Massage and baths with essential oils of lemon and rosemary are also recommended.

Other treatments

- In the long term, the circulation needs to be improved. Garlic, and food containing high levels of vitamins C and E will help.

- Keeping the extremities warm is a practical and obvious step to take, since prevention of chilblains is much easier than cure.

Hypertension

Useful Oils

Bergamot, Roman chamomile, frankincense, lavender, lemon, juniper, sweet marjoram, may chang, melissa, neroli, rose, ylang-ylang

It is perfectly normal for the systolic blood pressure to increase on exertion or during emotional stress, but in a healthy body it will return to normal quite quickly. Blood pressure is a parameter which reflects the circulating blood volume, peripheral vascular resistance, efficiency of the heart as a pump, viscosity of the blood and elasticity of the arterial walls. Thus a change in any of these parameters will result in blood pressure changes.

The blood pressure reaches its highest point during systole and its lowest point during diastole. The blood pressure of a healthy young adult is approximately 120mm Hg (column of mercury) during systole and 80mm Hg in diastole. By convention, this is expressed as 120/80.

Clinical features

The criteria for the diagnosis of hypertension are arbitrary, because the arterial pressure rises with age and varies from one occasion of measurement to another. Most authorities consider hypertension to be present when the diastolic pressure consistently exceeds 100mm Hg in a person more than 60 years of age or 90mm Hg in a person less than 50 years of age.

Hypertension is an important preventable cause of cardiovascular disease. Studies have shown that without treatment, hypertension greatly increases the incidence of cardiac failure, coronary heart disease with angina pectoris and myocardial infarction, and renal failure. Arteriosclerosis and atherosclerosis are common precursors of hypertension. Because the arteries become obstructed with cholesterol plaque, circulation of blood through the vessels becomes difficult.

When the arteries become hardened and constricted, the blood is forced through narrower passageways. As a result the blood pressure becomes elevated. Hypertension is often asymptomatic. Advanced warning signs include persistant morning headaches, sweating, rapid pulse, shortness of breath, swollen ankles and fingers, recurrent nose bleeds, dizziness and vision disturbances.

Aetiology

High blood pressure can be divided into two categories: one of known origin, (renal, adrenal tumour types) referred to as secondary hypertension and the other of unknown origin referred to as essential hypertension.

92-94% of all diagnosed hypertension is essential hypertension (6). It is believed that the following factors are responsible for essential hypertension:

- genetic factors
- hyper-reaction to stressor agents, such as cold and emotion
- psychogenic factors (This disorder is prevalent in civilised communities and particularly in people under stress.)
- dietary factors (A low sodium diet will reduce hypertension.).

22% of all secondary hypertension is due to kidney disease. The kidneys secrete a large amount of a hormone called renin. The function of renin is to constrict the arterial walls, and in doing so, raise the pressure of the vessels. Many kidney diseases such as pyelitis, nephritis or polycystic kidneys increase the possibility of hypertension.

Aromatherapy treatment

Essential oils that dilate the peripheral blood vessels increasing the total volume of blood in the system and oils that help the kidneys to eliminate more water, reducing the fluid retained in the system can help lower blood pressure, although it will be critical to alter diet and lifestyle as well.

The following massage blend may be useful:

ylang-ylang	5 drops
lavender	20 drops
sweet marjoram	5 drops
cold pressed vegetable oil	50 ml.

These essential oils are known for their hypotensive properties and have a calming and relaxing effect. Massage has been shown to effectively reduce high blood pressure, and if massage is given regularly, the treatment is even more effective.

While the above oils assist in lowering high blood pressure, a selection of sedative, antidepressant and uplifting oils may also be used. Roman chamomile, bergamot, neroli, rose and frankincense are some of those that can be used. Detoxifying essential oils such as juniper and lemon can also be beneficial.

CAUTION

These essential oils are contra-indicated for hypertension: hyssop, rosemary, sage, thyme.

Other treatments

- Check blood cholesterol and blood sugar as these are usually elevated in hypertension. If elevated treat accordingly.

- Stress reduction techniques have been shown to have some value in lowering blood pressure.

- A salt free diet is essential to lowering blood pressure. Lowering salt intake is not good enough; eliminate all salt from the diet. Excessive consumption of dietary sodium chloride, coupled with diminished dietary potassium, induces an increase in extracellular fluid volume and an impairment of the blood pressure regulating mechanisms. This results in hypertension in susceptible individuals.

- Increase intake of calcium-rich foods. Calcium deficiency has been linked to high blood pressure.

- A high fibre diet and supplemental fibre are recommended. Oat bran is a good source of fibre. Eat plenty of fruit and vegetables.

- Avoid foods such as aged cheeses and processed meats. The diet must be low in fats. Avoid animal fats.

- Garlic, onions and ginger should be used in cooking often. Garlic has been shown to decrease the systolic pressure by 20-30mm Hg and the diastolic by 10-20mm Hg. (7)

- Keep body weight down. Regular moderate exercise is important to maintain proper circulation.

- Increasing the amount of cold pressed polyunsaturated vegetable oils which are an excellent source of linoleic acid has a profound hypotensive action (8). This is due to normalisation of the E series prostaglandins which are known to be decreased in hypertensive patients.

- Hawthorn berries have long been in use in Europe as a cardiovascular agent (9). Their healing properties are attributed to:

  - improvement of metabolic processes within the myocardium resulting in improvement in functional heart activity

  - improved coronary blood supply by dilation of coronary vessels

  - elimination of some forms of rhythm disturbances.

Oedema

Useful Oils
Carrot seed, cypress, fennel, grapefruit, juniper berry, geranium, mandarin, orange, rosemary, tangerine, sage

Clinical features

Fluid retention usually causes swelling of the feet and ankles and is made worse by standing and by hot weather. Being stationary for a long time, such as on a prolonged journey, may produce ankle swelling. More generalised fluid retention may result in swelling of the fingers, with tightness of rings on the fingers and puffiness of the upper and lower eyelids and face.

Aetiology

There are many possible causes, the most serious one being some form of kidney disease. Pregnancy, oral contraceptives, premenstrual tension, allergic reaction, standing or sitting for too long, and injury to the body can all cause the body to retain fluid.

Aromatherapy treatment

Massage is useful for reducing fluid retention of the legs and ankles that has occurred after prolonged standing. Massage the legs with long, upward strokes always moving away from the ankle.

Any essential oil which has diuretic properties may be added to a massage oil. The following blend is an example:

cypress	10 drops
juniper berry	20 drops
geranium	10 drops
grapefruit	20 drops
apricot kernel	100 ml.

The legs are one part of the body where self massage is possible, so a blend of these oils can be taken home and used daily, between aromatherapy treatments.

Citrus oils such as lemon, lime, grapefruit, tangerine, mandarin and orange are all lymphatic stimulants and help reduce water retention. All the above oils may be used in a bath.

Fluid retention is often caused by an accumulation of toxic wastes in the body, as in the case of cellulite. Detoxifying oils such as carrot seed, fennel, juniper and lemon can be helpful in such cases.

Other treatments

- Stop adding salt to food; salt helps retain fluid in the body.

- Cut right down on refined carbohydrates, such as sucrose-containing foods, honey and glucose. All these foods require a considerable amount of water to be metabolised. Often just cutting these foods out will alone increase the urine output.

- Food allergies produce significant fluid retention. Wheat, other grains and milk are particularly common culprits.

- Persistent fluid retention can be caused by heart problems which will require medical treatment.

- The following herbs may be helpful: dandelion root or leaves, juniper berries, celery seed extract, parsley and burdock root. These herbs have diuretic properties.

Palpitations

Useful Oils
Neroli, lavender, may chang, melissa, rose, ylang-ylang

Clinical features

Consciousness of rapid, forceful or irregular heart beat is the most common complaint referable to the heart. Awareness of these changes varies from person to person. Some may be supersensitive to these changes, others totally oblivious to any heart irregularity. Palpitations may be associated with exercise or emotion and with chest pain and shortness of breath.

Aetiology

Usually quite normal after exercise, or when stressed and frightened, or when stimulants such as caffeine or nicotine have been taken. Palpitations may, however, be the symptom of some underlying heart disorder, and if recurrent, should be checked by a doctor.

Aromatherapy treatment

As an emergency procedure simply inhale some essential oil such as neroli, lavender, rose or ylang-ylang directly from the bottle. A person who is subject to frequent palpitations would benefit from regular massage with any one of the above oils.

Other treatments

- Avoid coffee, tea, cola drinks, chocolate, alcohol and smoking.

- During an 'attack', dip the hands and arms up to the elbow in cold water for at least 10 seconds.

- Acupressure points Heart 7 and Pericardium 6 are traditionally used to relieve anxiety, nervous tension and palpitations..

- Reduce anxiety state through meditation or relaxation techniques.

- Stop smoking.

- Increase consumption of potassium, magnesium and calcium-rich foods.

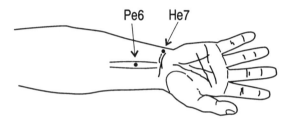

Location of acupressure points used to treat palpitations.

Varicose veins

Useful Oils
Calendula infused oil, cypress, lemon, geranium, juniper, rosemary, wheatgerm oil

Clinical features

Varicose veins are abnormally enlarged, swollen veins that usually occur in the legs. They are the result of a weakness of the valves inside the veins that allow the blood to flow back to the heart. If the valves do not work properly, blood accumulates in the veins, stretching them and causing varicosities. These prominent, blue, bulging veins are often accompanied by dull, nagging aches and pains. Swelling, sore legs, leg cramps and feelings of heaviness in the legs are also characteristics of varicose veins.

About 50% of middle-aged adults have varicose veins. The subcutaneous veins of the legs are commonly affected, due to the tremendous strain that standing has on the veins. When an individual stands for long periods of time, the pressure exerted against the vein can increase up to ten times. Hence individuals whose occupation requires long periods of standing are at greatest risk of developing varicose veins.

Generally, varicose veins are not considered harmful if the involved vein is near the surface. These veins are however, cosmetically unappealing. Although significant symptoms are not common, the legs may feel heavy, tight and tired.

A more serious form of varicose vein involves obstruction and valve defects of the deeper veins of the leg. This type of varicose vein can lead to problems such as thrombophlebitis, pulmonary embolism, myocardial infarction and stroke.

Aetiology

Several theories exist to explain the cause of varicose veins:

- genetic weakness of the veins or venous valves
- excessive venous pressure due to a low-fibre induced increase in straining during defecation
- lack of exercise, obesity, pregnancy and anything that reduces the circulation in the legs
- poor posture such as sitting cross-legged or standing upright all day long.

Aromatherapy treatment

Aromatherapy aims to improve the general tone of the veins. Peter Holmes (10) refers to cypress as a true venous blood decongestant as well as an astringent and recommends its use for the treatment of venous blood stagnation such as varicose veins, haemorrhoids and phlebitis. It should be used in a massage oil.

The massage should be very light and should never be done over the area affected by the veins. Massage the legs everyday with an oil consisting of:

calendula infused oil	50 ml
wheatgerm vegetable oil	50 ml
cypress essential oil	1 ml
lemon essential oil	2 ml.

Work up the legs from the feet towards the heart. It may take months to produce any improvement in the varicose veins, and as in any chronic situation, prolonged treatment is required. It is therefore important to vary the essential oils used from time to time. Alternate cypress and lemon for lavender, juniper, geranium or rosemary. Daily application is needed. These essential oils may also be used in a bath or blended in a clay lotion compress.

Other treatments

Therapeutic considerations in the treatment of varicose veins include the implementation of:

- modifying dietary factors
- increasing bulking agents
- physical methods
- botanical medicines.

These could be implemented by prescribing the following treatments:

- Vitamin C aids circulation and reduces tendency to blood clotting. Up to 3,000 mg daily is recommended.
- Regulate the diet carefully. The diet should be low in fat and refined carbohydrates and contain plenty of fresh fruit and vegetables. Avoid processed and refined foods.
- Flavonoid-rich berries, such as hawthorn berries, cherries, blueberries and blackberries are beneficial in the prevention and treatment of varicose veins since they increase the integrity of the walls of the veins (11). Consumption of these berries or their extracts is indicated for individuals with varicose veins.
- Make sure the diet contains adequate fibre to avoid constipation. A high fibre diet is the most important component in the treatment and prevention of varicose veins (and haemorrhoids). A diet rich in vegetables, fruits, legumes and grains promotes peristalsis. Fibre will attract water, forming a gelatinous mass which keeps the faeces soft, bulky, and easy to pass. The effect of a high fibre diet is less straining during defecation.
- Avoid standing as much as possible and lie with the feet higher than the heart.

- Do not sit cross-legged as the blood flow will be inhibited.

- Individuals with varicose veins have a decreased ability to break down fibrin. The result is that fibrin is deposited in the tissues near the varicose veins (12). The skin becomes hard and lumpy due to the presence of fibrin and fat. Herbs such as ginger, cayenne, garlic and onion all increase fibrin breakdown. Liberal consumption of these spices in foods is recommended for individuals with varicose veins and other disorders of the cardiovascular system.

- Wear loose clothing that does not restrict blood flow.

- Gentle exercise such as yoga and swimming is beneficial. Walking and gentle stretching exercises are suitable, but jogging, skipping, aerobics and other exercises which involve repeated impact can do more harm than good.

Chapter 21

Respiratory System

This chapter summarises an holistic approach to the treatment of many common ailments and conditions associated with the respiratory system.
Not only have the aromatherapy procedures for each condition been outlined, but details have also been included on other forms of treatment such as diet, herbs, acupressure and exercise.

Conditions discussed in this chapter include:

Asthma
Bronchitis
Catarrh
Coughs
Hayfever
Sinusitis
Sore throat
Tonsillitis

Introduction

Human life depends on the ability to utilise oxygen and to eliminate carbon dioxide. Respiration is defined as the exchange of oxygen and carbon dioxide between the atmosphere and the cells of the body. The respiratory system consists of the nasal passage, the larynx, the pharynx, the trachea, and the lungs which consist of the bronchial tubes, bronchioles and the alveoli sacs.

In order to understand the origin of many conditions associated with the respiratory system it is important to have a basic understanding of the functions of the respiratory system organs.

The lungs are an extremely efficient unit allowing gas exchange between air and fluid, made up of a vast network of fine blood capillaries surrounded by air whose movement is powered by an efficient bellows unit, the diaphragm.

What happens when we inhale air which is contaminated with dust, smoke and other pollutants? Sucking all this junk into a closed moist sponge (the lungs) would inevitably mean that a lot of rubbish will get trapped inside. Fortunately a number of ingenious systems ensure that the air we breathe is cleaned.

As the inhaled air is sent spiralling in a vortex down the bronchial tubes, the centrifugal forces ensure that most particles in air (eg dust) get thrown to the bronchial walls. A sticky mucous secretion traps the particles like flypaper. This film of mucus is supported on a bed of cilia, which are involved in a phased series of contractions, always upwards, which give the effect of repeated waves rising up the airways, carrying the impregnated mucus with them. This usually emerges at the throat as phlegm or sputum. This upward elimination is technically referred to as the 'mucociliary escalator'.

The air that reaches the fine alveoli in the lungs, where it meets the capillaries, is usually clean. However if there are impurities that are too fine or too copious to be trapped in the mucociliary escalator, then wandering phagocytes, powerful upheavals of the diaphragm, or coughing are required to remove them.

Therefore the cough, which is clearly an attempt at removal, is the body's natural response and is the back-up to the mucociliary escalator. Orthodox treatment often suppresses natural body reactions such as coughing.

The mucociliary escalator can fail because there may be:

- insufficient mucus
- too much mucus.

In the first instance, often seen in allergic and asthmatic conditions and in dry, irritating coughs, the mucus is too sticky to flow adequately. If the problem is prolonged, congestion may occur and chronic bronchitis can result.

In the second instance, otherwise known as a catarrhal condition, excessive mucus overloads the ciliary mechanism, leading to congestion. Opportunistic infection can easily occur and bronchitis and other lung infections may result.

With this in mind let us now develop an holistic approach to the treatment of respiratory problems.

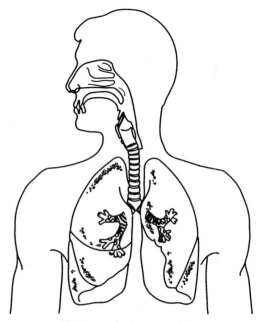

The respiratory system

General considerations

As with all disease, the best prophylactic is a correct lifestyle. Diet, exercise and quality of life all have a profound influence on the health of the lungs. To ensure healthy lungs, the inner environment must be in harmony, but the outer environment must be free from pollutants. Air contaminated with chemicals and particles, gases and smoke, should be avoided, which brings us to tobacco. Smoking places a wall of tar and ash between the individual and the world. This can lead to an impressive host of problems such as bronchitis or cancer, without taking into consideration the effects of diminished oxygen supply to the rest of the body.

There are other specific dangers to avoid. In the case of infections the simplest solution would be to avoid contact with the pathogens. However this is socially impossible, so we need to maintain our natural defences at their peak.

In the treatment of respiratory disease, diet and lifestyle are of paramount importance. Aromatherapy may assist by accelerating the healing process, by toning debilitating tissues, encouraging proper elimination of toxins and by relieving symptoms until the underlying causes have been dealt with. Treatment should follow holistic principles.

The following dietary and lifestyle measures should be considered essential for long term cure:

- restructuring the diet, including the acid/alkaline balance of the diet in favour of alkaline-forming foods

- reduction or elimination of refined sugar and refined wheat products

- reduction or elimination of salt, sugar, tea, coffee and alcohol

- reduction or elimination of suspected allergens, eg yeast, gluten, artificial food additives, and dairy products (Make sure that there is a corresponding supplementation of foods high in calcium.)

- restructuring the diet around whole grains, nuts, seeds, vegetables and fruits

- a high intake of foods high in vitamin C

- regular exercise, fresh air and correct breathing

- no smoking!

Aromatherapy considerations

Extensive research and clinical trials have proven that essential oils are very effective for treating respiratory problems. The best method of application of the oils is inhalations, chest and back massage, compresses, diffusers and oil burners.

Many of the essential oils used in treating respiratory problems come from trees: leaves, resins and woods. One school of thought suggests using the leaf oils for acute and short term problems of the respiratory system, and the wood and resin oils for more chronic conditions. Generally the wood and resin oils tend to be more drying and soothing, while the leaf oils are more stimulating and active in fighting pulmonary bacteria.

According to Dietrich Gumbel (1) the leaves of the plant have a direct affinity to the function of the lungs, since they are the respiratory organs for the plants, and indirectly for the earth itself.

The therapeutic properties of essential oils which have a particular affinity for the respiratory system are:

Antiseptics or antibacterial

Valnet (2) describes the antiseptic effect of vaporising essential oils in killing airborne bacteria and micro-organisms. Most essential oils are antiseptic to some extent, but the following are of particular value for the treatment of flu, colds, sore throats, tonsillitis and other infections: *thyme, eucalyptus, sage, pine, hyssop var. decumbens, cajeput, niaouli, tea tree* and *lemon*.

Antispasmodics

These essential oils have the effect of calming spasms in smooth muscle tissue and are used for the treatment of asthma, dry cough and whooping cough. Essential oils such as *cedarwood, cajeput, clary sage, cypress, eucalyptus, hyssop var. decumbens, sandalwood* and *thyme* can be used.

Expectorants

An expectorant promotes the ejection of phlegm by coughing or spitting. According to Boyd (3) an expectorant may be pharmacologically defined as a substance which increases the output of demulcent respiratory fluid. Expectorants are also used to alleviate coughing by:

- assisting the removal of a substance causing the cough reflex
- providing a more demulcent respiratory tract fluid.

Essential oils such as *aniseed, cajeput, fennel, everlasting, eucalyptus, frankincense, hyssop var. decumbens, spike lavender, myrrh, myrtle, pine, sandalwood* and *thyme* can be used.

Immunostimulants

Essential oils can support and strengthen the immune response in two ways; by directly inhibiting the threatening micro-organisms or by stimulating the immune system. A number of oils such as *cajeput, eucalyptus, lavender, lemon, rosemary* and *tea tree* act against a wide variety of bacteria and viruses while at the same time increasing the immune response.

Associated conditions

Asthma

Useful Oils
Aniseed, atlas cedarwood, cajeput, clary sage, Roman chamomile, cypress, fennel, frankincense, everlasting, eucalyptus radiata, hyssop var. decumbens, lavender, pinus sylvestris, spike lavender, lemon, mandarin, myrtle, peppermint, petitgrain, rosemary.

Clinical features

Asthma is the reversible narrowing of small air tubes (bronchioles), by inflammation of the mucous membranes or contraction of the muscular walls of the diaphragm. Difficulty in breathing, tightness in the chest, prolonged expiration phase, wheezing and coughing caused by excessive mucus are common symptoms.

General considerations

Asthma has typically been divided into two categories; extrinsic and intrinsic. Extrinsic or atopic asthma is generally considered an immunologically mediated condition with a characteristic increase in serum IgE. This is closely linked with the presence of eczema, hayfever, urticaria and migraine in the patient, or in his or her close relatives. People with this kind of family history are called atopic. If both parents have had a history of atopy then the chances of the child being affected are 50%; if one parent is affected the chance is 30%; and if neither parent is affected, the chance is approximately 12%.

Childhood asthma is often preceded for several months or even years by episodic coughing which later develops into a wheezy bronchitis and eventually into asthma. Such children often have a history of slow recovery from upper respiratory tract viral infections. It is interesting to note that asthma is particularly uncommon in certain tribal communities such as the Eskimos, some North American Indians and Highlanders from New Guinea. Environmental and/or dietary factors may also be important.

Intrinsic or nonatopic asthma is associated with a bronchial reaction that is not due to antigen-antibody stimulation, but rather to such factors as chemicals, cold air, exercise, infection, agents that activate the complementary pathway, and emotional upset.

Approximately 50% of asthmatics are nonatopic type, and in these it appears that reflex stimulation of the parasympathetic nervous system in susceptible individuals is the major mechanism. These patients do not demonstrate elevated IgE antibodies in their serum, and the history does not suggest hypersensitivity to specific allergens.

Aetiology

- inhaled allergens (Commonly inhaled allergens include the house dust mite; animal dander, and irritant gases including cigarette smoke.)

- ingested allergens: foods; drugs, eg aspirin; food additives; yeasts and moulds on food

- infecting organisms, either due to the infection itself or an allergy to the organism

- temperature change and changes in the weather - especially cold air

- lack of exercise and fresh air

- emotional stress, eg bereavement

- hormones

- certain chemicals in the workplace.

Signs and symptoms

The major symptoms of asthma are: cough, breathlessness, audible wheeze. Respiratory distress may be mild or severe. As a general rule, severe distress occurs only when the airway obstruction is gross. In exceptional circumstances, such as acetyl-salicyclic acid ingestion in an aspirin-sensitive patient, life threatening asthma may develop within minutes. More commonly such severe symptoms develop gradually over many hours or days.

General treatment plan

Treatment of severe asthma attacks must be promptly administered by a doctor. The following preventative practices may reduce the frequency and severity of the asthma:

- Determine and balance the underlying metabolic defect that causes the excessive inflammatory response.

- Find the allergens, and develop a lifestyle, diet and environment that will allow the allergens to be avoided.

- Prepare an effective treatment for the bronchoconstriction of the acute attack.

- Reduce mucus, reduce infections and use decongestants.

Aromatherapy treatment

Given the wide number of contributing factors the aromatherapist's approach will need to be flexible and varied according to the immediate circumstances of the asthma sufferer. During a crisis, inhaling essential oils that have antispasmodic properties will provide relief. This can be done by simply inhaling the essential oils from the bottle, or placing a few drops on a tissue or handkerchief.

The best-suited essential oils with antispasmodic properties which may be incorporated into gentle relaxing massage or used in a diffuser for inhalation include lavender, clary sage, Roman chamomile, cypress, petitgrain and mandarin.

Do not use steam inhalation as the heat from the steam will increase any inflammation of the mucous membranes and make the congestion even worse. Moisture however, is helpful and a humidifier with a few drops of essential oil added is a good idea. Between attacks the entire thoracic area, back and chest, should be massaged, with particular emphasis on techniques which open out the chest and shoulders.

The selection of essential oils is dependent upon:

- whether an infection is present

- whether emotional factors are involved

- whether an allergic response is involved.

Asthma precipitated by infection (cold, flu, bronchitis, etc.) with loose, copious mucus secretions is best treated with oils such as cajeput, *Eucalyptus radiata*, myrtle, lemon and spike lavender.

Asthma with viscid tenacious mucus is best treated using essential oils with expectorant properties such as aniseed, fennel, hyssop var. decumbens, rosemary and peppermint.

Asthma is sometimes representative of the psychosomatic illnesses present in industrial Western societies (4). The psychosomatic effect was observed with asthma patients who suffered allergies to cats. It was in many cases sufficient only to show the afflicted person a photograph of a cat in order to precipitate a crisis. Usually asthma patients are people who convey messages asking for love and attention. The typical personality of an asthma sufferer demonstrates extreme sensitivity with poor self-esteem. Typically, asthma sufferers have difficulty creating boundaries between themselves and others.

For asthma sufferers with allergies essential oils such as everlasting, lavender and Roman chamomile are recommended. Another oil which has been found to be useful is frankincense. Not only is it used as an expectorant to treat the congestion, but it is also known to slow and deepen the breathing which is considered useful as a preventative measure in asthma.

Other treatments

- Check for food sensitivities and avoid exposure to foods found to precipitate an asthma attack. Double-blind food challenges in children have shown that immediate onset sensitivities are usually due to (in decreasing order of frequency) eggs, fish, shellfish, nuts and peanuts. Delayed onset is triggered by milk, chocolate, wheat, citrus fruit and food colourings particularly tartrazine. (5)

- Vitamin B12 appears to be especially effective in sulphite-sensitive individuals. (6)

- Avoid all food colourings, if sensitive to aspirin, particularly tartrazine which gives the yellow colour to margarine. (7)

- Practise allergen avoidance as efficiently as possible, ie, keeping bedding/bedroom as dust free as possible, avoiding feather pillows, eiderdown, quilts etc. Wash linen in 1% tannic acid solution.

- Avoid drinking cold fluids.

- Reduce exposure to cigarette smoke, pollutants, cold winds and air conditioning ducts.

- Keep ambient temperature in the bedroom at a comfortable level of warmth to try to prevent airway cooling during the night. Avoid wide open windows in winter as warm humid conditions have been clearly shown to prevent asthma provoked by airway cooling.

- Garlic should be taken on a regular basis as it stimulates the immune system and also inhibits lipoxygenase and cyclo-oxygenase which generate inflammatory mediators from mast cells. (8)

- Asthma will respond well to herbs, but it is impossible to give a prescription that is appropriate in all cases as the various factors involved must be identified. Expectorant herbs such as liquorice and aniseed will help to eliminate excessive production of mucus while spasmodic asthma may be relieved by using cramp bark, skullcap and peppermint.

- Supplement the diet with essential fatty acids (GLA, EPA) or take linseed oil, one tablespoon per day, and cod liver oil, one teaspoon per day.

- Improve immunity by supplementing with anti-oxidant nutrients, zinc and vitamin B6.

- Relaxation and breathing exercises should be performed every day.

- Corticosteroids are still the allopathic drugs of choice for asthma, although the precise mode of action has not been totally elucidated
  Glycyrrhizin, the glycoside found in liquorice root, has a steroid-like activity and has long been used as an anti-inflammatory and anti-allergenic agent (9). Liquorice root is also an expectorant, a useful action to help alleviate asthma.

- Acupressure is particularly helpful in cases of acute asthmatic attack. It probably won't make the symptoms disappear but it will definitely alleviate them. Use of acupressure points Lung 1 and Kidney 27 will help to relieve chest congestion and asthma.

- According to Louise Hay (10), asthma is caused by 'smother love' and an inability to breathe for one's self. She states that an asthmatic feels as though he/she doesn't have the right to breathe. The asthmatic takes on guilt feelings for whatever seems wrong in his/her environment.

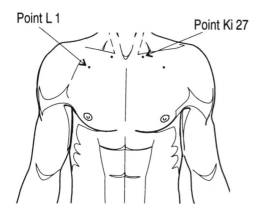

Point L 1

Point Ki 27

Location of acupressure points used to treat asthma

Bronchitis

Useful Oils

Aniseed, basil, bay, cajeput, cypress, atlas and virginian cedarwood, everlasting, eucalyptus, frankincense, ginger, hyssop var. decumbens, spike lavender, myrrh, niaouli, rosemary, peppermint, sandalwood, thyme.

Clinical features

Bronchitis is the inflammation or obstruction of the bronchi or the breathing tubes that lead to the lungs. The inflammation is followed by coughing and expectoration, fever, back and chest pain, sore throat and breathing difficulties.

Acute bronchitis typically follows upper respiratory tract infections such as influenza and often leads to pneumonia. Acute bronchitis is common in viral infections and, in a healthy adult, is rarely serious, but in infants and small children, respiratory obstruction may be severe and life threatening.

Chronic bronchitis results from frequent irritation of the lungs, but is not an infection.

Allergies may be the cause of chronic bronchitis. Cigarette smoking appears to be a common factor and very commonly there is coexisting emphysema.

Aetiology

- diet, especially high dairy intake
- improper treatment of the common cold, or flu
- lowered resistance, chest weakness, frequent colds
- smoking
- allergies
- poor digestive function.

General treatment plan

Eliminate the intake of impurities in the diet. It is imperative that the client be aware of the impact of diet on the respiratory condition. The client should lower the intake of fats, dairy foods, proteins of animal origin and sugars.

Acute bronchitis: According to Weiss (11) acute inflammatory conditions should be primarily treated with mucilaginous agents. These act as demulcents (soothing agents). Expectorant agents should only be used for chronic bronchitis. Careful differentiation of the condition will bring rapid relief to the patient and shorten the illness.

Bed rest is advisable and smoking should be prohibited. Sufficient fluids should be provided to prevent dehydration. Steam inhalations are useful to relieve cough.

Chronic bronchitis: the possibility that bronchitis is secondary to some serious underlying disease must always be kept in mind. Sources of possible irritants such as smoking, allergenic agents, or fumes should be avoided. A change of climate to a dry, temperate area may sometimes be warranted.

In patients with chronic respiratory insufficiency, the treatment strategy should include:

- anti-infectious essential oils
- essential oils to prevent degeneration
- immunostimulant essential oils
- soothing and healing the inflamed bronchial mucosa

- using expectorants to facilitate the removal of sputum from the bronchi and trachea

- relaxing bronchial spasms.

Aromatherapy treatment

Aromatherapy aims at combating the infection, reducing the fever, easing the cough and expelling mucus. In the first stages when the coughing is dry and painful, steam inhalations with eucalyptus radiata, spike lavender, cedarwood or frankincense will give a great deal of relief. These essential oils are used for their antispasmodic and expectorant properties. In the later stages of acute bronchitis, it is very important to clear all the mucus from the lungs and any essential oil such as hyssop var. decumbens, aniseed, basil, cajeput, eucalyptus, myrrh, or thyme may be used .

A person suffering from acute bronchitis needs to be kept warm and rested, preferably in bed. It is important to avoid anything which may aggravate the cough such as smoke, and very dry air. Make sure that there is sufficient humidity in the room, by using a humidifier or by simply using a large bowl of hot water and adding 10 drops of eucalyptus oil.

Essential oils such as bay and parsley seed oil may be used to ensure the tissue structure integrity of the lungs.

Most adults recover from bronchitis without complications, given the above care and treatment. However the elderly and frail, babies and young children and people with heart conditions or a history of lung infections, are at a much greater risk and must always be treated under properly qualified supervision.

Other treatments

- Balch (12) suggests a daily dosage of 3,000-10,000 mg of vitamin C plus bioflavonoids.

- The following herbs are recommended for acute bronchitis: echinacea, liquorice root, white horehound, marshmallow, thyme and ginger.

- The following herbs are recommended for chronic bronchitis: sundew, liquorice root, echinacea, ginger and golden seal.

- Add moisture to the air. Drink plenty of fluids.

- Chronic bronchitis sufferers should stop smoking.

Catarrh

Useful Oils
Aniseed, cajeput, atlas and virginian cedarwood, eucalyptus, everlasting, fennel, frankincense, ginger, hyssop var. decumbens, lavender, lemon, sweet marjoram, myrtle, peppermint, pine, rosemary, sandalwood, thyme, tea tree.

Clinical features

Common to many respiratory problems, catarrh is seen in holistic medicine as being a vicarious elimination mechanism. There is either faulty elimination by the usual organs responsible for detoxification, or an excessive intake of environmental and dietary toxins. The body will seek to restore its internal harmony by using the mucous membranes to expel these waste products/toxins.

Aetiology

Catarrh as a medical condition does not really exist, although the term is used extensively to explain the thick mucus that is expelled from the nose or coughed up from the throat.

The most common causes are asthma, colds, flu, hayfever, bronchitis, sinusitis and rhinitis. Many of these conditions are dealt with under separate headings.

General treatment plan

In addition to general dietary and lifestyle factors, long term treatment of catarrhal problems will involve the use of depurative or detoxifying essential oil remedies, particularly those that encourage drainage of the lymphatics, those that promote elimination of acid metabolites - diuretics, and those that stimulate the immune system.

Aromatherapy Treatment

Many essential oils are decongestants and expectorants - helping to clear out the chest and lungs - and therefore can help catarrh considerably. For the immediate relief of congestion, a steam inhalation with any of the following essential oils is excellent: aniseed, cajeput, cedarwood, eucalyptus, frankincense, ginger, hyssop var. decumbens, lavender, myrtle, peppermint, pine, rosemary, thyme or tea tree. The preparation of a massage oil for the upper back, chest and shoulders using any of the above essential oils will also be of assistance.

For catarrh caused by pollens and other irritants, anti-allergenic essential oils such as everlasting, lavender or German or Roman chamomile are the best choices. Massage of the face, with particular attention to the sinus area around the nose will help to drain away excessive mucus.

Other treatments

- Diet plays a part in many cases of catarrh. Dairy products and wheat are known to provoke catarrh in many people, and they should be avoided for a period by anybody who suffers catarrh frequently.

- See also asthma, bronchitis, hayfever, or sinusitis.

Coughs

Refer to asthma and bronchitis.

Hayfever

Useful Oils
Cajeput, German chamomile, eucalyptus, lavender, myrtle, peppermint, pine, rosemary, thyme, tea tree.

Clinical features

The symptoms of hayfever are: sneezing, runny nose, swelling of nasal mucosa, itching of the eyes, watery eyes, hypersecretion of mucus, headaches. These symptoms may be secondary to acute colds or flu, or hayfever.

Aetiology

Common antigens that precipitate symptoms in susceptible individuals are house dust, animal dander, fungus spores, feathers, powders, insecticides and many grass pollens. Sinusitis may also develop in these individuals due to bacterial infection that becomes associated with impaired drainage of the nasal mucosa. Symptoms of this condition are local pain and tenderness of the overlying facial skin, headaches and possibly fever.

General considerations

- avoiding or reducing exposure to the offending antigen

- reducing sensitivity by building integrity of mucosa and reducing inflammatory response

- improving immunity

- making dietary changes including low acid diet, reduction of dairy products etc.

Aromatherapy treatment

Essential oils that assist in the treatment of hayfever have expectorant, anti-inflammatory, astringent, antimicrobial and immunostimulant, restorative and tonic properties.

Any of the oils that relieve the symptoms of the common cold such as eucalyptus, spike lavender and pine may be used in inhalations to help reduce the sneezing and runny nose. If there are allergies present use German chamomile.

Other treatments

- A good diet can help hayfever sufferers overcome the tiredness and depression the disease can cause. A diet rich in raw vegetables and fresh fruit which contain vitamin C is recommended. Such a diet will also prevent constipation which many hayfever sufferers experience, and which may also contribute to the disease.

- Avoid milk and dairy products. These encourage the formation of catarrh and mucus in the alimentary tract.

- Pollen granules and garlic capsules are also considered useful.

- Louise Hay suggests that hay fever is caused by emotional congestion and a belief in persecution. (13)

Sinusitis

Useful Oils
Cajeput, eucalyptus, spike lavender, lavender, lemon, myrtle, niaouli, peppermint, pine, thyme, tea tree.

Clinical features

Sinusitis is an inflammation of the nasal sinuses that accompanies upper respiratory infection. More than 50% of all cases of sinusitis are caused by bacteria. The sinuses affected by this infection include those above the eyes, inside each cheekbone, behind the bridge of the nose and in the upper nose.

Symptoms of sinusitis include headache, earache, toothache, facial pain, cranial pressure, loss of sense of smell, tenderness over the forehead and cheekbones, and occasionally a high fever. Sometimes sinusitis produces a swollen face followed by a stuffy nose and thick discharge of mucus. If the mucus is clear after a week you probably do not have an infection. If mucus is greenish or yellowish, you do. If the mucus is clear without a cold, you probably have allergies.

Aetiology

Acute sinusitis is frequently caused by colds or bacterial and viral infections of the nose, throat and upper respiratory tract and can be extremely painful with headaches so severe that it is impossible to move the head without pain. Chronic sinusitis problems which give rise to dull pain in the forehead may be caused by small growths in the nose or injury to nasal bones.

Aromatherapy treatment

The use of essential oils at the onset of a cold can often prevent the infection from spreading to the sinuses. Essential oils such as tea tree, eucalyptus, cajeput, niaouli and thyme are effective bactericidals, while steam inhalations using essential oils such as cajeput, eucalyptus, spike lavender, lavender, lemon, niaouli,

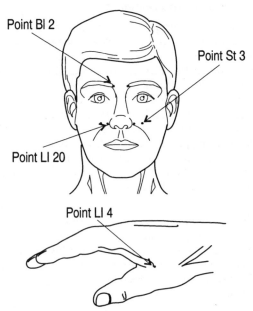

Acupressure points used to treat sinus problems

peppermint and pine relieve sinusitis. Eucalyptus, pine and peppermint help clear the stuffiness.

Special techniques for facial massage can be used to encourage the drainage of mucus from the nose and sinuses. These techniques may be too uncomfortable to perform during a severe attack. Massage may be introduced after a day or two, or whenever a steam inhalation has reduced the congestion enough for massage to be tolerable.

Other treatments

- Herbs that are considered effective for relieving the symptoms of sinusitis include fenugreek, elder flowers, eyebright, golden seal, marshmallow, and echinacea.

- Garlic is a valuable immune stimulant and natural antibiotic that keeps infection in check.

- Bee pollen increases immunity and speeds healing so a small daily supplement of bee pollen is recommended.

- A diet of 75% raw foods is recommended (14).

- Do not eat dairy foods because they increase mucus formation. Soured dairy products such as yoghurt and cottage cheese, however, do not.

- Vitamin C should be taken to increase immunity against infection and reduce mucus.

- Vitamin A increases the health of epithelial tissue lining of the sinuses.

- The throat may be affected by problems originating in the lungs, the nose, or the sinuses. A sore throat may take the form of tonsillitis, pharyngitis, or laryngitis.

- Acupuncture and acupressure are very effective therapies for sinusitis and can be used alongside aromatherapy. The acupressure points commonly suggested for the treatment of sinuses are LI 4 and Bl 2. Bl 2 is located at the bridge of the nose and is helpful for frontal headaches and sinus conditions, while LI 20 and St 3, on the face, are the best points for dealing with the maxillary sinuses located in the cheek area.

- Dr John Harrison (15) suggests that sinusitis is linked to poor bowel function and that constipation of the bowel reflects mental constipation, mostly in inflexible individuals, and often indicates a reluctance to cry.

Sore throat

Useful Oils
Cajeput, frankincense, lavender, lemon, niaouli, sandalwood, tea tree, thyme.

Clinical features

A sore throat can be caused by anything that irritates the sensitive mucous membranes at the back of the throat.

Aetiology

Some irritants include viral and bacterial infections, allergic reactions, dust, smoke, fumes, extremely hot foods and drinks, tooth or gum infections, and abrasions. Chronic coughing and excessive loud talking also irritate the throat. Typically, a sore throat is an extension of the common cold, tonsillitis, sinusitis, or a viral infection. An acute sore throat should run its course within a few weeks.

Aromatherapy treatment

Steam inhalations using essential oils of lavender, tea tree, niaouli, and cajeput will ease the discomfort. A gentle massage to the throat and chest area with a massage oil containing frankincense, lavender and sandalwood can be used. Any of these oils used in an oil burner will help especially if used at night before going to bed.

Other treatments

- Add five drops of tea tree oil to a glass of warm water, mix well and gargle at least two to three times a day. Continue until the condition has cleared up.

- An infusion of equal parts sage and thyme herbs has an antiseptic/astringent action and may be gargled three or more times a day.

- Vitamin C and bioflavonoids can be used to improve immunity and vitamin A can be used to increase the resistance of epithelial tissue.

- Honey and lemon juice is good for alleviating sore throats.

- The following herbs can be used to alleviate a sore throat:

  - to stimulate immunity or act as demulcents: echinacea, golden seal and slippery elm powder

  - infused liquorice root combined with honey has demulcent and expectorant properties

  - marshmallow tea will soothe a sore throat.

- Refer also to sinusitis and tonsillitis.

Tonsillitis

Useful Oils
Eucalyptus, lemon, tea tree, thyme.

Clinical features

Tonsillitis is an inflammation of the tonsils, the glands of lymph tissue located on either side of the entrance to the throat. Symptoms of tonsillitis include soreness, redness, pain and inflammation of the tonsils, difficulty in swallowing, hoarseness and coughing. Other possible symptoms are headaches, earache, fever and chills, nausea and vomiting, nasal obstruction and discharge, and enlarged lymph nodes throughout the body. People of any age can be afflicted with inflammation of the tonsils.

Aetiology

The inflammation is typically caused by viruses and other bacteria, often streptococcal organisms, which are present when the body's resistance is lowered. Tonsillitis can be caused by improper diet which is high in carbohydrates and low in protein and other nutrients. Repeated bouts of tonsillitis indicate a weak state of resistance, making it difficult to cure.

Aromatherapy treatment

Steam inhalations at frequent intervals will relieve the pain and help combat the infection. Not only are thyme, lemon and eucalyptus the best antiseptic essential oils to use, but they also have a local anaesthetic effect which will relieve the discomfort.

Other treatments

- Chamomile, echinacea, sage and thyme are excellent herbs to use for the treatment of tonsillitis.

- Use a warm salt-water gargle.

- The practice of removing the tonsils, particularly during childhood, is now fortunately far less common than it was 20 or 30 years ago and if natural treatments with essential oils and nutritional measures are followed, it should only very rarely be necessary.

Chapter 22

Musculoskeletal System

This chapter summarises an holistic approach to the treatment of many common ailments and conditions associated with the musculoskeletal system.
Not only have the aromatherapy procedures for each condition been outlined, but details have also been included on other forms of treatment such as diet, herbs, acupressure and exercise.

Conditions discussed in this chapter include:

Arthritis
Backaches
Bruises
Bunions
Bursitis
Cramps
Gout
Sciatica
Sports injuries

Introduction

Our skeleton, the connective tissue, our muscles and our joints hold us together, enable us to stand, to move and give us form. The musculoskeletal system is used and misused considerably, it often becomes the site of much physical wear and tear. Some of the diseases of the musculoskeletal system such as arthritis may be extremely disabling, having a major adverse impact on normal living and working.

If problems are due to muscular injury or structural misalignments, a great deal can be done to realign the body with the help of remedial massage techniques, osteopathy, chiropractic techniques, and psycho-physical adjustments like rolfing, alexander technique or feldenkrais.

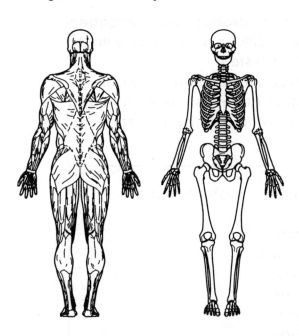

Muscular system and skeletal system

Aromatherapy considerations

Aromatherapy is very effective in treating musculoskeletal problems. Some essential oils bring warmth to the skin and can provide a considerable amount of pain relief through their analgesic effect.

In degenerative diseases like rheumatism or arthritis, the body has to be led back to a state of health and balance. To effectively treat problems that manifest in the bones and muscles, digestion and assimilation have to function correctly, as do the various aspects of elimination.

The particular therapeutic properties of essential oils which have a particular affinity for the musculoskeletal system are:

Analgesics

Many of the essential oils with anti-inflammatory or rubefacient properties also have analgesic effects. Some of these essential oils include *German chamomile, eucalyptus, cajeput, lavender, sweet* or *Spanish marjoram, peppermint, rosemary* and *thyme*.

Anti-inflammatory or antiphlogistic

Many essential oils such as *German chamomile, lavender, and yarrow* are used to reduce inflammation. These essential oils are known to have a non-irritant effect on the skin. The antiphlogistic effects of skin irritant essential oils such as thyme, clove and cinnamon is caused by different mechanisms than that of German chamomile. (1) Wagner suggests that the irritation caused by oils such as thyme and cinnamon triggers the release of (anti-inflammatory) corticoid substances.

Antirheumatics

Many essential oils prevent or relieve rheumatic problems. Antirheumatics are selected according to the specific action on the body such as detoxifying, anti-inflammatory, rubefacient, and diuretic. Oils with antirheumatic properties include: *black pepper, cajeput, German* or *Roman chamomile, eucalyptus, ginger, juniper berry, lemon, sweet* and *Spanish marjoram, nutmeg, pine, rosemary, Spanish sage* and *thyme* .

Detoxifiers or depurative

Essential oils that detoxify, also referred to as depuratives gradually cleanse and correct the 'polluted' condition of the body. The main clinical use of depuratives is in the treatment of chronic inflammatory disease, especially of the joints and connective tissue. Essential oils of *grapefruit, juniper berry, carrot seed, lemon, sweet fennel* and *rosemary* are some examples.

Rubefacients

Essential oils with a rubefacient effect cause better local blood-circulation, which can easily be observed by a redness of the skin. The local skin irritation which occurs triggers the release of free mediators which in turn causes vasodilation. Thus the result promotes not only circulation to the muscle tissue and skin but also brings an agreeable feeling of warmth and relief from pain and an anti-inflammatory effect.

For rheumatism of the joints, muscular stiffness, sciatica and lumbago use essential oils such as *black pepper, cajeput, eucalyptus, spike lavender, rosemary* and *sweet* or *Spanish marjoram.*

Associated conditions

Arthritis

Useful Oils

Black pepper, cajeput, cinnamon, clove bud, German chamomile, eucalyptus, ginger, juniper berry, lavender, lemon, sweet and Spanish marjoram, nutmeg, rosemary, thyme.

The term 'arthritis' means inflammation of a joint. There are many different types of arthritis. Some are due to infection and others are due to wear and tear; for many the cause is obscure. The two most common forms of arthritis are rheumatoid arthritis and osteoarthritis. Conventional treatment often reduces pain, but there is little improvement in the arthritic process itself.

The accepted medical view is that arthritis is incurable and treatment is confined to relief of pain with analgesic and anti-inflammatory drugs, often with undesirable side effects. Joint replacement surgery is often offered where there is very serious degeneration of the joint, but this can only be used for the largest joints such as the hips and knees, and involves major surgery.

John Harrison (2) states that two features of arthritic sufferers are fear and ensuing martyrdom. He has noticed that a high proportion of women afraid to become involved with new partners suffer arthritis as a way of alleviating the fear of socialising and perhaps finding a partner. Other women have developed arthritis in an effort to moderate bullying by their aggressive partner. Still others have developed arthritis to get some attention and care from their otherwise insensitive partners.

Psychogenic rheumatism is the name given when a client has arthritic symptoms but X-ray and pathology tests reveal no joint damage. People likely to suffer from psychogenic rheumatism tend to be chronic worriers and emotionally unstable. Regular massage can be beneficial for the nervous system, circulation and joints, however do not massage while the joints are in an acute, swollen, or inflamed state.

Rheumatoid Arthritis

Clinical features

Rheumatoid arthritis is often more severe and more generalised than osteoarthritis. It occurs more commonly in women but it is much more common in younger people. It characteristically affects the hands and the large knuckle joints as well as the wrists, elbows, knees and feet. It affects the hip joints less often than does osteoarthritis. In severe cases, there is considerable destruction of the joints, and other tissues including skin, lymph nodes, lungs, the heart, and even the liver and kidneys can be affected by the rheumatoid process.

Aetiology

There is evidence to prove that rheumatoid arthritis is an auto-immune reaction where antibodies develop against joint tissue. This causes an inflammatory response as the body's adaptation to protect itself from a hostile environment. What triggers this auto-immune reaction remains largely unknown.

The onset of rheumatoid arthritis is often associated with physical or emotional stress, however poor nutrition or bacterial infection may also be the cause. The synovial tissue experiences metabolic alterations primarily resulting in an acidic environment and a lack of fuel.

All these changes can be modified by holistic intervention, to decrease or normalise the inflammation reactions. Rheumatoid arthritis affects not only the joints but also many other bodily functions. These should also be treated to improve the patient's outcome.

According to Henry Osiecki (3) the following physiological variables have been observed:

- Many rheumatoid arthritic patients are anaemic. This may be due to a lack of iron absorption, or simply due to the chronic inflammation occuring throughout the body. Many patients are taking aspirin or NSAID (non-steroidal anti-inflammatory drugs) and this may produce bleeding in the bowel, and in turn anaemia.

- Many rheumatoid arthritic patients have an inefficient liver metabolism. Weakness and tiredness are common symptoms.

- 50% of rheumatoid arthritic patients have cold and wet hands, suggestive of a disturbed vegetative vaso-regulation.

- Females have an aggravation of symptoms during menses.

- The rheumatoid patient appears to have a reduced defence against the formation of toxic free radicals produced by inflammation.

General considerations

Rheumatoid arthritis requires a comprehensive therapeutic approach which focuses on reducing those factors known to be involved in the disease process.

The primary objectives in the management of rheumatoid arthritis are:

- reduction of inflammation and pain
- preservation of function
- prevention of deformity.

In addition to the above, natural therapies also aim at altering the body chemistry. Toxins must be eliminated and then new accumulation of toxins must be prevented. The body's own healing processes need to be stimulated to repair damaged tissue as much as possible. Circulation to the joints must be improved, both to drain off wastes and to improve nutrition to the affected tissue.

An holistic approach must also involve:

- dietary advice
- stress reduction
- weight control
- management of old injuries.

Exercise is an important physical therapy in the management of rheumatoid arthritis. Therapeutic exercises are designed to preserve joint motion, muscular strength and endurance. The most effective exercises are of the active-assistance type. As the tolerance for the exercise increases and the activity of the disease subsides, progressive resistance exercises may be introduced. (Specific instructions for exercises are contained in *Rheumatoid Arthritis: A handbook for patients*, a booklet published by the Arthritis Foundation of Australia.)

Remember that exercise should be done when the client is:

- least stiff
- has the least pain
- and is least tired.

Alternating hot and cold compresses are used for their muscle relaxant and analgesic effects. If the arthritis is long standing it may not be possible to undo major damage to the joint surface, but the pain and inflammation can be minimised, improving mobility and preventing further damage.

Aromatherapy treatment

Detoxifying essential oils such as juniper, cypress, fennel and lemon are essential in helping the body eliminate toxins. They should be used in massage oils and baths.

Analgesic and anti-inflammatory oils such as German chamomile, clove bud, eucalyptus, ginger, spike lavender, nutmeg, Spanish or sweet marjoram and rosemary can be used in baths, local massage and compress on the affected joints, while local circulation can be stimulated by the use of rubefacient oils such as black pepper, ginger, nutmeg and marjoram.

A typical massage blend can be made up as follows:

nutmeg	10 drops
spike lavender	15 drops
cajeput	20 drops
juniper berry	15 drops
carrier oil	100 ml.

Whenever heat is applied to a painful stiff joint, it is very important to move the joint as much as possible immediately afterwards, otherwise the heat can cause congestion which will make the condition worse rather than better.

Other treatments

In the management of rheumatoid arthritis, a number of different therapies can be used with varying effects. It is important to remember that different people will respond to different treatments. In young people with warm, swollen joints, the most effective treatment is an elimination diet.

For those who are underweight, have a poor appetite, or have a poorly balanced diet, supplements should be used before going on an elimination diet. Elimination of allergic foods has been shown to offer significant benefits to some individuals with rheumatoid arthritis. (4)

Older people often do not respond as well to an elimination diet. For these people it is best to make use of supplements such as zinc, evening primrose oil, fish oils and other nutrients such as vitamin C and B which are involved in the metabolism of essential fatty acids. Such supplements may have a general anti-inflammatory effect, but this may take several weeks or even months for its full effect to be felt.

- An elimination diet should be followed initially to determine the presence of any food sensitivities. Common sensitivities are to wheat, milk, dairy products, potato and beef.

- Avoid nutritional patterns that decrease immunity such as processed foods, alcohol, tea and coffee, smoking.

- Avoid all foods from nightshade plants such as potato, eggplant, tomato, chilli, and capsicum.

- Improve bowel flora by supplementing with acidophilus.

- Increase consumption of cold water fish (cod, tuna, mackerel), linseed oil and evening primrose oil.

- Ginger has anti-inflammatory effects by inhibiting prostaglandin synthesis. According to Leung (5) one patient took 50g/day of lightly cooked ginger while 6 others took either 5g of fresh or 0.1 to 1g of powdered ginger daily. All patients reported substantial improvement, including pain relief, increased joint mobility, and decreased swelling and morning stiffness.

- Physical therapy has a major role in the management of patients with rheumatoid arthritis. While not curative, proper physical management can improve patient comfort and preserve joint and muscle function. Heat is generally used to help relieve stiffness and pain, relax muscles, and increase range of motion. Moist heat such as moist packs and hot baths are more effective than dry heat. Cold packs are of value during acute flare-ups.

Osteoarthritis

Osteoarthritis or degenerative joint disease is characterised by joint degeneration, loss of cartilage and alterations of the subchondral bone. It is the most common form of arthritis. Although primarily seen in the elderly, degenerative changes in joints occur from as early as age 30. By the age of 65, 80% of people have radiographic evidence of osteoarthritis although only 25% may have symptoms. (6)

Osteoarthritis is divided into two categories: primary and secondary. In primary osteoarthritis, the degenerative 'wear and tear' process occurs after the 5th and 6th decade, with no apparent predisposing abnormalities.

Secondary osteoarthritis is associated with some predisposing factor which is responsible for degenerative changes. Predisposing factors in secondary osteoarthritis include:

- trauma (obesity, fractures and injuries along joint surfaces, surgery)

- crystal deposits

- presence of abnormal cartilage

- previous inflammatory diseases of the joints.

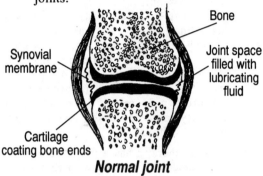

Normal joint

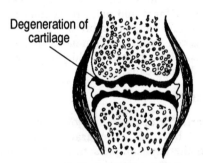

Early stages of disease

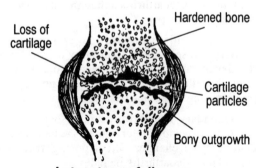

Later stage of disease

How osteoarthritis develops

The cartilage lining of the joint tends to soften, fragment and ulcerate as the damage progresses. In an effort to overcome this, the body manufactures new bone around the joint margins. This tends to have the effect of altering the mechanics of the joint, increasing the rate of damage and producing greater inefficiency of the joint.

The onset of osteoarthritis can be subtle. Morning stiffness is often the first symptom. As the disease progresses, there is pain on motion of the involved joint that is made worse by prolonged activity and relieved by rest. There is usually no sign of inflammation. (7)

According to Henry Osiecki (8), the primary chemical change observed is the loss of proteoglycan (a protein sugar or mucopolysaccharide). These 'proteoglycans' are responsible for cartilage resilience or bounce and their loss from cartilage results in a stiffer material that is more easily damaged by wear and tear. Proteoglycans account for 75-80% of normal cartilage. In osteoarthritis the percentage of proteoglycans is reduced to 35-40%.

Aromatherapy treatment

Oestoarthritis is less likely to be inflammatory in nature, but is characterised by degeneration of the smooth gliding surfaces of the joints, and occurs more often in middle-aged and elderly people, as a result of 'wear and tear'. The treatment principles using aromatherapy are similar to those that apply to rheumatoid arthritis, perhaps with more emphasis on essential oils with analgesic and rubefacient properties such as black pepper, ginger, nutmeg, lavender, sweet or Spanish marjoram, rosemary and thyme.

Other treatments

- Wear jogging shoes as this allows for better cushioning of knee and hip joints.

- Avoid foods from nightshade plants (ie. potato, tomato, egg plant, chilli, capsicum)which are known to aggravate the arthritic condition in some patients.

- Avoid the group of foods known as salicylates as they also have been shown to increase inflammation in arthritis.

- Many people with arthritis seem to improve if digestion is improved. This can be done by taking digestive enzymes or apple cider vinegar with meals. Improving digestion and the acidity of the stomach ensures complete breakdown of any antigenic food protein that may exacerbate the condition.

- Eat cold water fish (cod, tuna, salmon, mackerel) at least three times per week. These fish are rich in linoleic acid and EPA. Cod liver oil and cold pressed linseed oil (one dessertspoon per day) should also be taken.

- Increase consumption of whole grain cereals, hard nuts, and apple pectin. These foods are rich in silicon which has been found to be important in bone homeostasis.

- Reduce the intake of red meats and avoid tea, coffee, alcohol and processed or refined foods.

- According to Louise Hay, arthritis is a disease that comes from a constant pattern of criticism of self and criticism of other people.

Backaches

Useful Oils

Arnica infused oil, black pepper, cajeput, German and Roman chamomile, eucalyptus, ginger, juniper berry, spike lavender, lemon, peppermint, sweet and Spanish marjoram, nutmeg, rosemary, thyme.

Aetiology

Bachaches may originate from a multiplicity of causes. The cause of any backache must be established before any treatment can be undertaken. Apart from the obvious causes such as sport injuries, domestic or industrially related accidents involving heavy lifting, bad posture, faulty or poor seating, back pain can also result from mental, emotional or physical problems.

Backaches may also be a symptom of kidney infection or disease, or degenerative condition of the spine and these possibilities must be investigated by properly qualified specialists. A great deal of back pain arises from stress. Many people, without realising it, respond to stress by tensing muscles. The upper back, neck and shoulders are very often the sites of such tensions, and tension in the neck can also affect the lower sacral area of the back.

Massage can be a valuable way of re-educating tense muscles. Many people are not aware of just how much tension they are holding in some areas of the body, and relaxation can be achieved through massage.

Aromatherapy Treatment

Aromatherapy massage is a very effective treatment where the pain is due to muscular fatigue, spasm or tension. There are many essential oils that will help reduce pain in the short term and treat the muscular problem or injury in the longer term.

Spike lavender, Spanish or sweet marjoram, rosemary, eucalyptus and cajeput are commonly used in combination with warming oils such as black pepper, nutmeg, ginger and thyme where there is acute pain.

It is important to have a good knowledge of anatomy and decide whether to refer a patient to an osteopath or chiropractor for manipulation. When manipulation for any spinal displacement is required, aromatherapy massages before and after the manipulation can reduce pain and increase the effectiveness of the treatment.

Many back injuries arise because of poor muscle tone. The muscles are no longer capable of supporting the vertebrae, or the various joints associated with them. The best way of improving the condition of the back is to increase muscle tone, usually through exercise. However the exercise has to be carefully chosen to improve the condition of the back without placing further strain on it. If there is injury it is usually best to avoid exercise until the injury or displacement has been treated.

Baths using relaxing essential oils such as lavender and ylang-ylang are a very useful form of self-help when backache is caused by tension. The best form of treatment for backache is prevention, and regular massage with essential oils and baths will prevent pain by reducing stress, improving muscle tone, relaxing tight muscles and improving the general level of wellbeing.

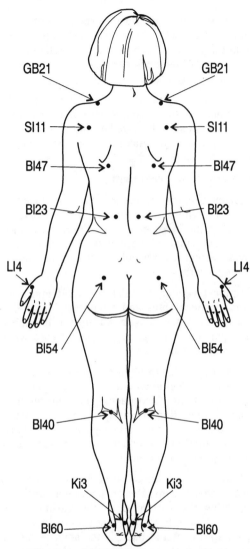

GB21 — GB21
SI11 — SI11
BI47 — BI47
BI23 — BI23
LI4 — LI4
BI54 — BI54
BI40 — BI40
Ki3 — Ki3
BI60 — BI60

Acupressure points to relieve backache

CAUTION

Never bend from your hips; bend your knees and hips.

Lift heavy objects to waist height only.

Face a heavy object you wish to carry.

Balance heavy loads on each side of you.

Keep heavy objects close to your body.

Seek help and use leverage when lifting heavy loads.

Move slowly when lifting.

Don't sit for long periods.

Other treatments

- Wear flat shoes.
- Use your abdominal muscles all the time.
- Stretch your muscles daily.
- Exercise regularly.
- The following acupressure points will tonify the lower back. Bl 40, located in the centre of the back of the popliteal crease, is a special trigger point for alleviating lower back pain. Bl 23, located on the lower back between the second and third lumbars, two finger widths away from the spine at waist level, is also recommended to tonify weak back. If this point is tender, stationary light touch, instead of deep pressure, can be quite healing. Bl 54, located 1 to 2 finger widths outside the sacrum and the base of the buttocks lateral to the midline of the lower third of the sacrum, is used to relieve lower back aches, sciatica, pelvic tension, hip pain and tension.

Bruises

Useful Oils

Infused arnica oil, black pepper, German chamomile, hyssop, fennel, spike lavender, lemon, rosemary.

Clinical Features

The skin is not broken when bruised, but the underlying tissue is injured, resulting in pain, swelling and black and blue marks due to blood that has collected under the skin.

Aetiology

Although body parts become bruised after contact with hard objects, there are several factors that predispose one to bruising. Anaemia, overweight, malnutrition, leukemia and excessive use of anticlotting drugs can lead to vessel rupture, resulting in bruising.

Aromatherapy treatment

Essential oils such as fennel, hyssop, rosemary or spike lavender are effective if applied to the area as soon as possible after the bruising has occurred, preferably in an ice cold compress. Arnica infused oil is a classic remedy for bruising and it can be applied neat to unbroken skin. In the case of severe bruising such as that resulting from an accident, oils which stimulate the spleen, such as black pepper, chamomile and lavender will be helpful.

Other treatments

- 3 000 to 10 000 mg of Vitamin C with bioflavonoids taken in divided doses during the day.
- Avoid aspirin.
- If bruising is frequent seek medical advice.
- The diet should include an abundance of dark green leafy vegetables and fresh fruit which are rich in vitamin C.
- Apply a comfrey ointment on a daily basis.

Bunions

Useful Oils

German chamomile, lavender, sweet or Spanish marjoram, peppermint.

Clinical features

Bunions are a very painful inflammation of the joint between the big toe and foot which can lead to a deformity of the joint of the big toe. Bunions are most common in middle-aged women and, in a majority of cases are the result of shoes that do not fit properly - too narrow, too tight or too high. Children and young people should always wear shoes that are the correct size and width, as their bones are more easily deformed than those of adults.

CAUTION
Bunions need to be distinguished from arthritis, gout and injuries.

Aromatherapy treatment

Essential oils can be used to relieve the pain, and sometimes reduce the amount of tender swelling around the joint, but they will be useless unless other physical measures are also included. If the joint is inflamed, very gentle massage with anti-inflammatory oils such as German chamomile may help. Lavender, sweet or Spanish

marjoram or peppermint may also be chosen for their analgesic properties. This combination may eventually cure a not-too-prominent bunion, but a severe deformity may need surgery to straighten the toe.

Other treatments

- Comfortable shoes which support the feet well are the answer, whether you have bunions or not.
- In hot weather, do not forget that your feet swell, therefore shoes that are not too tight are best. Go barefoot whenever possible, avoiding stockings and tights in summer.
- Severe cases should be treated by a podiatrist.

Bursitis

Useful Oils

Cajeput, eucalyptus, juniper berry, rosemary.

Clinical features

Bursitis is one of the most common rheumatic conditions. A bursa is a small sac containing lubricating fluid which is situated between moving joints. It often affects shoulders, but is well known for its appearance in elbows and knees (tennis elbow and housemaid's knee).

The symptoms can include sharp pain, hot and tender skin, and swelling. Some types of bursitis may require surgery.

Aetiology

It can become inflamed through injury, infection, repeated use or unusual pressure when the liquid content increases, causing pain and limiting movement.

Aromatherapy treatment

Essential oils such as rosemary, cajeput, juniper or eucalyptus blended in a massage oil and gently rubbed into the inflamed area will assist in reducing the inflammation and relieve pain.

Other treatments

- Avoid using the joint until the inflammation has diminished.

Cramps

Useful Oils
Black pepper, Roman chamomile, clary sage, cypress, geranium, lavender, sweet marjoram, thyme.

Clinical features

Cramp is the sudden involuntary contraction of a muscle or group of muscles, and can cause acute pain. Many people suffer from cramps in the legs or feet during sleep, said to be particularly common in young anaemic women, when the legs are not receiving sufficient blood; pregnant women suffer from this too.

While the smooth muscles of the body may also be prone to cramps, this section relates specifically to the skeletal muscles.

Aetiology

Muscle cramping in different parts of the body is commonly caused by dietary vitamin and mineral deficiencies, particularly calcium, potassium and magnesium.

Heat cramps are primarily due to salt depletion. The use of diuretic drugs for high blood pressure or heart disorders may also be the cause of muscle cramping. If someone is taking these drugs be sure to include potassium in the diet. Poor circulation contributes to leg cramps. If you have cramps during the day while you are active this may be a sign of impaired circulation.

Aromatherapy treatment

Rubbing the legs vigorously using black pepper, sweet marjoram, geranium, lavender, cypress and thyme in a massage oil will relieve cramps.

Other treatments

- Cramps in the leg can be relieved by bending the knee as far as it will go, or contracting the opposite muscle to that in contraction. If cramps are experienced while reclining, the flow of blood to the legs will be increased if you stand up.

- Yoga breathing is beneficial.

- Sodium chloride, 1 gm every 30-60 minutes with large amounts of water or a saline solution usually relieves heat cramps promptly.

- The patient should be placed in a cool place and sore muscles massaged.

- Hot foot baths are beneficial.

- Daily walking and regular exercise helps to increase circulation, reducing the incidence of cramps.

Gout

Useful Oils
Carrot seed, juniper berry, pine, rosemary.

Clinical features

Gout occurs when there is too much uric acid in the blood, tissues and urine. The uric acid crystallises in the joints, acting as an abrasive causing swelling and pain. Uric acid kidney stones may be an associated problem.

Approximately 90% of gout patients are male. The metatarsophalangeal joint of the great toe is the most susceptible joint, although others, especially those of the feet, ankles and knees, are commonly affected. Gout is characterised by sudden acute attack - the pain is usually intense. The involved joints are swollen and extremely tender and the overlying skin is tense, warm and dusky red. Fever, headache, malaise and tachycardia are common.

Subsequent attacks are common, with the majority having another attack within one year. This may lead to gouty arthritis in the long term, with progressive functional loss and disability. Hypertension, renal stones and renal failure may also be associated with gouty arthritis.

Aetiology

90% of sufferers are men, usually over 30 years of age. Gout is traditionally considered to be the result of excess rich food and alcohol.

Sometimes it is due to a particular enzyme defect or increased purine levels. Certain diseases can cause a decrease in the secretion of uric acid,. Some pharmaceutical drugs such as dyazide (an anti-hypertensive), cause high blood levels of uric acid leading to gouty conditions.

Uric acid is a by-product of certain foods, so this condition is closely associated with diet. It can be brought on by stress. Obesity and an improper diet increase the tendency for gout.

General considerations

A low purine diet is important. Purines are constituents of nucleoproteins from which uric acid is derived. (9)

Aromatherapy aims at detoxifying the body thus reducing the high levels of uric acid which cause gout.

Aromatherapy treatment

Massage will often not be appropriate for the treatment of gout due to the inflammatory nature of this condition. Foot baths and compresses are the better treatment methods.

Put several drops of carrot seed oil, pine oil, rosemary oil or juniperberry oil in a hot foot bath, keeping the feet in the bath for 10 minutes.

Other treatments

The dietary treatment of gout involves the following guidelines:

- Lose weight if overweight.
- Avoid alcohol completely.
- Avoid rich foods including red meat, game and fish roes. These foods are all high in uric acid.
- Eat only raw fruits and vegetables for two weeks. Juices are excellent. Also include grains, seeds and nuts. Cherries and strawberries are excellent as they help neutralise uric acid. Also drink celery juice diluted with purified water.
- Avoid purine rich foods such as anchovies, asparagus, herring, mushrooms, mussels, all organ meats, sardines and sweetbreads.
- Take vitamin C to increase the loss of uric acid via the kidneys.
- Anti-rheumatic herbs and herbs that aid the body's elimination, such as celery seed, burdock, and juniper berry, will be useful.

Sciatica

Useful Oils
Ginger, lavender, nutmeg, peppermint, rosemary.

Clinical features

This is an intense pain in the lower back sometimes accompanied by pain in the buttocks and on the outside of the leg. This denotes pressure on the sciatic nerve, which runs from the lower back to the foot. Sciatica is often accompanied by or precedes lumbago, and may be the first warning of a prolapsed or slipped vertebral disc. It is also caused by lifting heavy objects incorrectly or bending awkwardly.

General treatment

It is important to realise that the pain of sciatica is a symptom, and that treating the pain alone is no treatment. The cause must be found and treated.

Aromatherapy treatment

During the time when pain is intense, massage is not advisable, but cold compresses over the painful area with peppermint, ginger, nutmeg or lavender will reduce the pain. Gentle massage with either of these oils at times when there is less or no pain can be very beneficial, and baths can be helpful too - they should not be too hot.

Other treatments

- Exercises which gently stretch and strengthen the sciatic nerve are useful. Lie on the back with one knee placed over the other and pull the knees gently towards you using your hands. You will feel your lower back stretching. Change over knees to stretch the other side.
- The following acupressure points stimulate the lower back and relieve sciatica. Bl 40, the point behind the knee, is a special point for alleviating lower-back pain and sciatica. Bl 23 and Bl 47 relieve lower back aches and sciatica and strengthen the back. Bl 54 in the buttocks is an effective lower back point and sciatica pain point. These points can be used separately or together in a

sequence for relieving sciatica. See the diagram on page 320.

Sports injuries

Natural remedies go hand in hand with the standard methods of treating sporting injuries and maintaining the wellbeing of the body which is pushed by sport to the limits of endurance, stamina and skill.

Methods of treating injury

Heat

When heat is applied to an area of the body it dilates the capillaries and increases blood flow. Blood nourishes the tissues and can hasten healing, reduce muscular spasm and reduce pain, but applying heat does carry the risk of seepage of blood and plasma to the injured area. If this were to happen healing would be prolonged and swelling and fluid retention would be increased. It is important therefore that heat is not applied to an injured area until at least twelve hours have passed since injury.

Cold

Cold causes contraction of the small capillaries and this decreases the amount of blood collecting around the wound. Excessive bleeding could prolong the healing time. The application of cold to an area of injury reduces bruising, swelling, inflammation and pain.

RICE

'Rest, ice, compression and elevation' are words so often repeated by physiotherapists and sport therapists that they have been shortened to form the acronym 'RICE' which is drummed into anyone with an injury that needs care.

Rest

Resting an injury is extremely important to ensure that no further damage takes place.

Ice

Applying ice to all sorts of injuries, as long as it is done correctly, can stop internal bleeding, bruising, and inflammation and in doing so it reduces the healing time. Ice can be placed in a bowl or bucket into which you immerse the toes, feet, fingers, hands or elbows or any other parts of the body which are affected. Ice is often placed in a plastic bag, crushed and then placed between two towels and wrapped around the injured area.

Compression

Compressions can be made with a bandage or piece of material which is folded to form a pad. This should be wrapped firmly over the area to prevent swelling. A compress can be hot or cold and is needed to reduce the level of blood flowing to the area but should never be so tight that it impedes circulation and causes the injured person to experience pain, numbness or the skin turning blue.

Elevation

By raising the injured limb higher than the heart, swelling and pain can often be prevented or reduced. Elevation is important when injury occurs to the limbs.

Achilles tendonitis

Inflammation of the Achilles tendon. This restricts movement and the area may be hot and painful. Use cold compresses containing German chamomile and lavender to assist in the reduction of the inflammation. Massage using a massage oil blend of lavender, ginger and German chamomile with hypericum infused oil.

Ankle and heel bruising

Bruising of the tissues and skin as a result of a direct blow to the area. There is pain and swelling. Use the ice method at least three times a day for three days, and, in between, massage all over the foot and ankle, three times a day, with a blend of:

hyssop	10 drops
black pepper	20 drops
spike lavender	30 drops
arnica infused oil	30 ml
vegetable oil	70 ml.

It is also important to move the foot and ankle as soon as possible. This will prevent the swelling from becoming gelatinous and hard and prevents adhesive scars.

Ankle sprain

A slight tearing or stretching of the ligaments in the ankle. As soon as possible after the injury use an ice pack to control the swelling. Massage the whole foot and ankle and the leg to the calf muscle, using ginger, nutmeg, rosemary and hypericum infused oil. Keep the ankle bandaged to prevent further damage. Use ice packs followed by massage for three days several times a day.

If the pain continues use alternating hot and cold compresses containing peppermint or eucalyptus essential oil. While rest is imperative it is important that someone with an ankle strain should start trying to walk normally on the second day. This will not cause any damage and the heel-toe gait of ordinary walking will help to prevent adhesive scars.

Back: slipped or ruptured disc

This is a common cause of acute back pain. There may be no obvious reason for the pain, but many people can trace the start of the pain to an injury, a jolt or lifting a heavy object. Accurate diagnosis and correct early treatment is important. Discs are made from cartilage and are situated between the vertebrae, acting as shock absorbers. Each disc is made up of a hard outer ring with a soft jelly-like interior. If the pain has come on quickly, possibly with a click, the outer ring has cracked and 'slipped' out of place. This sometimes touches the nerves emerging from the spinal cord, and sends pain down the leg.

Slipped discs should be treated by a doctor, but additional care may be given. During the first three days ice packs may be used over the painful area to reduce inflammation.

A massage oil containing rosemary, peppermint and ginger can then be gently applied to the area as often as required.

Bruising

Bruising due to a fall or direct blow should be treated using the ice method three times a day and after three days using a hot compress. After each session use the following essential oils, gently massaging the area with a massage blend made of black pepper, cypress, hyssop and rosemary essential oils and arnica infused oil.

Carpal Tunnel Syndrome

A nerve disorder in both the hands and arms. The carpal tunnel is a space in the front of the wrist through which a nerve and various tendons pass from your forearm into your hand. There is no really effective treatment for this complaint though massaging both hands, arms and shoulders twice a day with a massage blend of Spanish marjoram, spike lavender and rosemary may relieve it temporarily.

Elbow sprain

Elbow sprain is caused by over stretching the ligaments in the elbow joint. Ice packs applied at least three times a day will help to reduce inflammation. Massage with a massage oil containing essential oils of ginger, nutmeg, rosemary and arnica infused oil.

Elbow tendonitis

Inflammation of the muscles, tendons, bursa or tissues of the elbow area which often causes pain in the arm as well. Use a hot compress of peppermint, cajeput or eucalyptus. Apply this to the elbow three times a day and massage the whole arm from the wrist to the shoulder with a massage oil containing peppermint, rosemary and German chamomile.

Finger sprain

Over stretching of the ligaments between the finger joints. Place the fingers in ice for at least ten minutes then massage over the whole hand using a massage oil containing essential oils of black pepper, nutmeg and ginger with arnica infused oil. After 24 hours use alternating hot and cold compress treatment using rosemary, spike lavender and black pepper several times a day. After applying the compresses, apply the massage oil.

Hip strain

Injury to the muscles and tendons that join the hip joint to the thigh bone. Rest and apply ice to the injured area and massage over the hips and thighs using ginger, black pepper, nutmeg and arnica infused oil. After 48 hours start to take alternate cold and hot baths, in which are placed three drops of rosemary and three drops of lavender essential oils blended in 10ml of essential oil dispersant.

Knee cartilage injury

A torn cartilage in the knee-joint is a very common injury among sports players, particularly footballers, and is caused by a twisting strain on a bent knee. If the knee is locked bent after the injury it will have to be manipulated straight. The knee should be bandaged to prevent further injury and kept elevated when the patient is sitting. Use the ice method three times a day, alternating with warm compresses. Massage the area with a massage oil blend made from essential oils such as ginger, nutmeg, and Spanish marjoram.

Knee synovitis (water on the knee)

Massage at least three times a day with a preparation made with juniper, fennel and Spanish marjoram. Massage from the ankle to the knee and from the knee to the top of the thigh.

Leg sprain

When over-stretching of the ligaments occurs, use an ice pack at least three times a day for ten minutes at a time. Prepare a massage oil containing rosemary, peppermint and cajeput. After 48 hours change to hot compresses, in which you place two drops of rosemary and spike lavender. Between treatments keep the leg supported by wrapping with an elastic bandage.

Shoulder strain

Injury to muscles or tendons. Use the ice method for ten minutes at a time and after 48 hours use the heat compress or flannel method. Massage all the arm and shoulder area three times a day with a massage blend made of German chamomile, black pepper, nutmeg and ginger.

Wrist sprain

Over-stretching of ligaments in the wrist. Apply an ice pack three or four times a day. Massage with a blend of ginger, nutmeg and black pepper. Movements that stretch the ligament will be painful, but use the wrist as normally as possible to avoid adhesive scars developing.

Chapter 23

Reproductive System

This chapter summarises an holistic approach to the treatment of many common ailments and conditions associated with the reproductive system.
Not only have the aromatherapy procedures for each condition been outlined, but details have also been included on other forms of treatment such as diet, herbs, acupressure and exercise.

Conditions discussed in this chapter include:

Pregnancy
Pre-menstrual syndrome
Dysmenorrhoea
Amenorrhoea
Menopause
Endometriosis
Thrush
Cystitis

Introduction

The focus of this chapter is primarily the reproductive system of women. By the nature of human anatomy, there is not the same degree of complexity of structure or function in the male reproductive system.

The cause of many problems associated with the reproductive system is partly psychological and partly physical. In many circumstances the dominance of male attitudes over female processes has led to certain natural functions being treated as illnesses or dispositions as in pregnancy, menstruation or menopause. It has been difficult to have a positive attitude to certain natural experiences because of the negative associations around them. For example, menstruation was and is often seen as a 'curse' or 'proof' of a woman's unreliability and changeability.

While attitudes are changing in the still largely male-dominated society, negative attitudes towards women's sexuality and role abound. Anyone who is in conflict with oneself as a creative and sexual being will develop negative patterns which will manifest in diseases. Breaking these negative patterns may require a natural therapy treatment such as aromatherapy.

As Valerie Ann Worwood (1) subtly explains, whether a woman has children or not, her body is a complex machine for making babies which guarantees her spending more than six years of her life having periods. That's five days, thirteen times a year for approximately 35 years. To this inconvenience, if not pain, some must add their days of pre-menstrual syndrome. The whole business continues until after menopause. The only break in this routine is pregnancy and, despite the myth that all women look and feel marvellous during pregnancy, this is when the body is going through dramatic hormonal changes and incurring great strains.

Dr Sandra Cabot (2) indicates that problems such as premenstrual syndrome, menopause and other sexual disorders have been treated as a 'Pandora's Box'. However, it is now realised that these conditions have huge psychological and economic implications for all societies and are worthy of public scrutiny.

Aromatherapy considerations

Aromatherapy is considered one of the most effective methods of dealing with menstrual, pregnancy and menopausal problems. Many essential oils can help to regulate hormone production, can relax or uplift, or are useful for reducing stress-related tension that often exacerbates symptoms.

Essential oils such as jasmine and rose have a general strengthening effect on the reproductive system and may be used to relieve specific complaints such as menstrual problems, genital infections and sexual difficulties.

The two most important female hormones are oestradiol, which is an oestrogen, and progesterone, which is a progestogen. Oestradiol controls the development and maintenance of the female sexual organs and gives a woman her essentially feminine shape and physiology. Progesterone prepares the uterine lining for pregnancy each month.

Some essential oil constituents have hormone-like behaviour because their structure is similar to the hormones, so they interact with the same receptors that identify hormones.

Oestrogenic activity has been found in essential oils of aniseed and sweet fennel. Anethole which is a methyl ether of oestradiol is responsible for the oestrogenic activity of these oils. There are no essential oils which have progesterone-like activity, nor are there any oils used in aromatherapy which have androgen-like activity.

The essential oils with oestrogenic activities influence the menstrual cycle, lactation and secondary sexual characteristics.

In treating conditions associated with the reproductive system the following properties are considered useful:

Antimicrobial

Essential oils with antiseptic and bactericidal properties may be used to treat leucorrhoea, vaginal pruritus and thrush. Examples include *bergamot, chamomile, myrrh, rose* and *tea tree.*

Antispasmodics

For menstrual cramp (dysmenorrhoea) and labour pain, essential oils such as *sweet marjoram, German* and *Roman chamomile, clary sage,* and *lavender* may be used.

Emmenagogues

Essential oils with emmenagogue properties have the ability to promote menstrual discharge, and may be used to treat amenorrhoea (lack of periods) and scanty periods. Examples include *German* and *Roman chamomile, sweet fennel, clary sage, juniper, lavender, sweet marjoram, rose* and *peppermint.*

Galactagogues

Essential oils with galactagogue properties may be used to increase milk flow. Examples include *sweet fennel, jasmine, aniseed* and *lemongrass.*

Parturients

Essential oils with parturient properties help to induce labour by stimulating uterine contraction, help to give a swift and relatively painless birth. Examples include *jasmine, rose* and *nutmeg.*

Uterine tonics

The uterine tonics have a specifically toning and strengthening effect on the whole system, both on the tissue of the organs and on their functioning. Whilst each may have its unique associated actions, which will be investigated in this chapter - they all aid the whole reproductive system, for example: *clary sage, jasmine, rose, myrrh* and *frankincense.*

Associated conditions

The conditions of the reproductive system are considered in four groups:

- those associated with pregnancy and child birth
- those associated with the menstrual cycle
- those associated with menopause
- those associated with infections.

Pregnancy

The experience of pregnancy and childbirth is one of the most exciting and challenging times in any woman's life. Pregnancy is the time between conception and childbirth in which the foetus grows and matures for nine months inside the mother's womb until it is ready to be born.

Many common problems occur during pregnancy and may be as life-threatening as a miscarriage or as simple as stretch marks. Most of these problems occur because of hormonal changes in the body, nutritional deficiencies in the mother, or a shift in weight distribution due to the sudden weight gain.

As long as certain oils are avoided, aromatherapy techniques and oils can be used safely and will be immensely beneficial to maintain the general health of the expectant mother and to help minimise the various discomforts of pregnancy.

CAUTION

During pregnancy do not use the following oils because they are toxic and will possibly harm the mother and foetus, or because they may involve some risk of miscarriage. aniseed, basil, clary sage, atlas and virginian cedarwood, cypress, sweet and bitter fennel, jasmine, juniper, sweet marjoram, myrrh, nutmeg, peppermint, rose, rosemary.

The following is a description of some problems encountered during pregnancy and the aromatherapy remedies and holistic advice that the pregnant woman can follow to overcome the problems.

Morning sickness

Approximately 50% of all pregnant women experience some degree of nausea and vomiting during the first three months of pregnancy and this usually ceases after the fourth to fifth month of gestation (3). This is commonly called morning sickness but it can occur at any time of the day. Eating and drinking should continue despite the nauseous feeling.

- Mothers suffering from morning sickness should eat small, frequent meals and snack on wholegrain crackers.

- The herb ginger taken in capsule form or freshly grated and drunk as a tea helps to relieve nausea.

- Red raspberry leaf and peppermint taken in tea form help relieve nausea.

- Avoid all fats, sugars, alcohols, caffeine, cigarette smoke, and processed orange juice.

- Taking a vitamin B complex with additional vitamin B6 and magnesium during pregnancy helps control morning sickness (4). Foods rich in vitamin B6 and magnesium include brewer's yeast or torula yeast, sunflower seeds, soya seeds, brown rice, walnuts, bananas, salmon, tuna, chicken and wheatgerm.

- Four to five drops of spearmint and/or ginger essential oils may be used as an inhalation and this will help keep the stomach calm.

A recent study of 86 pregnant women showed a significant increase in both nausea and vomiting in the first trimester in women who reported unplanned, undesired pregnancies and negative relationships with their own mothers (6).

Backache

Many women experience some lower back pain as their pregnancy advances, due not only to the increased weight of the baby, but also to the changing shape of their own body, and the way this increases the lumbar curvature of the spine. To minimise back pain during pregnancy, the mother should not stay in one position for too long, should not wear high-heeled shoes as they increase the likelihood of backache, and should not do any forward bending or strong upward stretching exercises.

Gentle exercise such as yoga and specific natal exercises are important. It is also a great help to rest for at least 20 minutes each day lying flat on the back, with the legs bent at the knees and supported on a chair. The thighs should be at right angles to the body, and the calves at right angles to the thighs. This position straightens out the lumbar curve and relaxes the overworked muscles of the lower back.

Massage with a massage oil blend containing:

spike lavender	15 drops
cajeput	5 drops
lemon	5 drops
carrier oil	50ml.

will give tremendous relief from pain, and help to tone the muscles which are carrying the increased weight. When massaging oils into a pregnant woman it is very important to ensure she is comfortable and relaxed. Finding comfortable positions in later pregnancy is often difficult. To facilitate back massage on a pregnant mother, she should sit forward over a straight-backed chair leaning onto a cushion. For head, neck or foot massage use a bean bag or cushions with the arms and legs supported.

Constipation

Bowel sluggishness is common in pregnancy. It is due to suppression of smooth muscle motility by increased steroid sex hormones and pressure upon and displacement of the intestines by the enlarging uterus. Constipation should not be allowed to continue untreated as it frequently leads to haemorrhoids and aggravates diverticulitis.

- Add more fresh and dried fruit such as prunes, raisins, and figs to the diet. Eat fresh vegetables and salads containing a variety of raw greens and vegetables daily.

- It is important to drink at least eight glasses of water a day.

- Wholegrain breads, cereals and whole bran flakes are helpful. Begin the day with two teaspoons of bran in a glass of apple juice.

- Do not take over-the-counter laxatives without a health care practitioner's approval.

- Walking at least a kilometre a day is very helpful in addition to setting a regular time each day for bowel movement.

- If the constipation persists take 500 mg of slippery elm after meals. The mucilaginous properties of this herb will line the mucous membrane of the intestines and assist the passing of the stool by removing dryness from the faeces and lubricating the intestinal wall.

Remember that the increased progesterone in the body makes the bowels less efficient.

The most effective aromatherapy treatment for constipation is massage of the abdomen, always in a clockwise direction. Essential oils to use for this massage are neroli, orange, tangerine and black pepper.

Flatulence

Keep a record of all the food eaten in order to determine what foods or food combinations are causing gas. Eat four to five small meals a day instead of three big meals. Walking a kilometre a day should assist the digestion and elimination.

Essential oils which are helpful in preventing flatulence and which can be used during pregnancy are dill, ginger and spearmint. Prepare a 2% dilution of one of these oils and massage over the abdomen several times a day.

Haemorrhoids

The worst thing about constipation is that it causes straining which in turn may cause haemorrhoids, especially in women who suffer from varicosities.

- Increase the intake of roughage in the diet with foods such as raw vegetables, fruit, whole bran, and whole grain bread. This often helps to soften stools and make elimination easier. Hard stools may be very painful and cause bleeding.

- Drink eight glasses of water a day.

- Cold witch hazel compresses will help shrink the haemorrhoids.

- Valerie Ann Worwood (6) suggests blending 15 drops of geranium and 5 drops of cypress essential oils to the contents of a small tube of KY jelly. This is done by squeezing the jelly into a small jar, to which you add the essential oils, mixing well and rubbing around the anal area when required. This treatment not only alleviates the symptoms but prevents haemorrhoids occurring in the first place.

Varicose veins

Varicose veins are enlarged veins close to the surface of the skin. They usually disappear after the birth of the baby and are due to:

- weakness of the vascular walls

- increased venous stasis in the legs due to the haemodynamics of pregnancy

- inactivity and poor muscle tone

- obesity, since the excessive tissue mass requires increased circulation and fatty infiltration of connective tissue impairs vascular support.

The following suggestions will help alleviate the condition:

- Do not wear restrictive knee socks, garters, belts or high heeled shoes.

- Do not stand for long periods of time or sit cross-legged.

- As often as possible, sit with the feet higher than the heart.

- Walking one kilometre a day is very helpful.

To make an oil that will prevent and alleviate varicose veins use the following:

calendula oil	20ml
wheatgerm oil	10ml
sweet almond oil	30ml
geranium	15 drops
cypress	5 drops
lemon	10 drops.

Stroke the legs very gently, working upwards from the ankle to the thigh. The geranium will help encourage the circulation of blood and the cypress and lemon have an astringent effect upon the whole venous system.

Swelling of the hands and feet (oedema)

A rise in oestrogen in the body causes swelling of the hands and feet. Some swelling is to be expected and is acceptable. Avoid all highly processed foods, while maintaining a well balanced diet. Wear loose, comfortable clothing. Be sure to wear properly fitting shoes, which may be larger than your normal size.

Using hand and foot baths containing a few drops of lime, orange, tangerine, grapefruit or geranium should relieve any fluid retention.

Stretch marks

Stretch marks are wavy reddish stripes , that gradually turn white, appearing on the abdomen, buttocks, breasts and thighs. They are caused by excessive and rapid weight gain typically associated with pregnancy, and appear when the skin becomes over stretched and the fibres in the deep layers tear. Unfortunately once they appear they are permanent, but they do become much less noticeable with time.

Stretch marks can be prevented by applying the following massage oil externally to the places in which they would commonly appear.

wheatgerm oil	10 ml
apricot kernel oil	40 ml
avocado oil	50 ml
neroli	5 drops
tangerine	20 drops
lavender	5 drops.

Other essential oils that can be used are rosewood and frankincense.

Heartburn

Heartburn occurs more often in pregnancy due to the re-entry of stomach fluids into the oesophagus, because of the expanded size of the uterus. Do not consume spicy or greasy foods, alcohol or coffee. Drink one tablespoon of milk before eating to coat and soothe the stomach. Eat four to six small meals a day. Heartburn can be relieved by gentle massage over the abdomen using a soothing and comforting oil such as chamomile, lavender or tangerine.

Leg cramps

Leg cramps in pregnancy are usually worse in the last months of pregnancy and can be caused by the position of the baby or due to reduction in the level of diffusible serum calcium or increase in the serum phosphorus level (or both).

To relieve the cramps try a foot bath made from:

geranium	5 drops
lavender	10 drops
cypress oil	2 drops.

in a bowl of hot water (not boiling) or rub and 'knead' the contracted, painful muscle using a massage oil with black pepper and ginger essential oils.

Other helpful hints are:

* Increase calcium and potassium intake by eating foods such as bananas, grapefruit, oranges, cottage cheese, yoghurt, salmon, sardines, soybeans, almonds, and sesame seeds.

* While sleeping or sitting, elevate the legs higher than the heart.

* Do not stand in one place for too long.

* Walk one kilometre a day to stimulate the flow of blood through the legs.

* When experiencing a cramp, apply a hot water bottle or heating pad to the cramping area and pressure (using your hands).

Skin problems

Common skin problems during pregnancy are pimples, acne, red marks, and mask of pregnancy (dark blotches on the skin and face). These skin changes will, however, disappear with the birth of the baby. Five milligrams of folic acid before each meal may help the pregnancy mask to disappear. Studies have shown an apparent correlation between pregnancy mask and adrenal gland depletion due to increased stress. Vitamin B complex and vitamin C are valuable supplements.

Avoid physical and emotional stresses. Some women experience skin problems when taking the contraceptive pill, which fools the body into believing it is pregnant, so there are obviously hormonal factors involved.

Exhaustion and faintness

Exhaustion can occur at any stage of the pregnancy. It is often associated with vasomotor instability, which results in transient cerebral hypoxia and pooling of the blood in the legs and in the splanchnic and pelvic areas, especially after prolonged sitting or standing in a warm room. Hypoglycemia before or between meals, more common during pregnancy, may result in 'lightheadedness' or even fainting. These attacks can be prevented by avoiding inactivity and utilising deep breathing, vigorous leg motions and slow change of position.

Bergamot, orange, tangerine, mandarin, lavender, lemon, grapefruit or geranium used in massage, baths or inhalations will help overcome exhaustion.

Miscarriage

Some women cannot carry a baby to full term and experience a miscarriage or spontaneous abortion. There may be many reasons for this, including emotional stress, malnutrition, general malaise, illness such as infection and glandular disorder.

A common contributing factor to miscarriage is an altered progesterone level. Progesterone is necessary for the maintenance of pregnancy. At about the third month of pregnancy the placenta takes over the major role of progesterone secretion from the corpus luteum. If the placenta fails to carry out this vital function, miscarriage will occur. The first symptom of a miscarriage is bleeding, sometimes accompanied by cramping. Slight bleeding, although alarming, does not necessarily mean that you will miscarry, and some women lose small amounts of blood regularly throughout their otherwise healthy pregnancy. You should seek urgent medical advice for persistent or heavy bleeding.

The emotional trauma experienced after miscarriage can be considerable, and the support of an experienced and caring practitioner can be a helpful addition to that of friends and family. Dr Bach's Rescue Remedy can have a very calming effect during this stressful time. Take a few drops as often as required.

The essential oils recommended for use after a miscarriage not only help the body back to its pre-pregnancy state, they also heal on the emotional and spiritual levels. Any of the following essential oils may be used in a massage blend: geranium, frankincense, jasmine, clary sage, neroli, rose or rosewood.

Preparing for birth

From about the seventh month you can prepare for childbirth by drinking raspberry leaf tea. Raspberry contains a substance called fragrine which relieves uterine pains by dilating the pelvic muscles. Use one teaspoon of raspberry leaf tea to one cup of boiling water.

Aromatherapy can be of great help during childbirth, since some essential oils strengthen and deepen contractions while at the same time having an analgesic effect. In the labour ward an anxiety-free atmosphere can be created with the help of vaporised essential oils. Oils such as bergamot, grapefruit, tangerine, neroli, jasmine, rose and lavender prove to be the most useful.

Labour

The birth process can be supported by the use of jasmine compresses or massages in the sacral area when suffering pain. Cooling refreshing compresses of rose water can be used for general relief.

Juliette Guenier (7) found lavender to be not only calming for the mother but also for the father and midwife. Aromatherapy is now being used by an increasing number of health professionals involved in childbirth.

A recent study conducted by Ethel Burns and Caroline Blamey (8) evaluated the benefits of essential oils in a labour ward. The essential oils chosen for the study were: lavender, clary sage, peppermint, eucalyptus, chamomile, frankincense, jasmine, rose, lemon and mandarin.

The results of the study were:

- Lavender was the most popular oil and was used to reduce maternal anxiety, for pain relief and to lighten the mood.

- Peppermint oil was the oil mostly used for nausea and vomiting during the later stages of labour.

- Clary sage was the oil used most to increase contractions. However once in labour, the tendency was for women to feel more anxious and lavender was once again the preferred oil to relax them.

This study indicated the high degree of overall satisfaction in using aromatherapy during labour/

delivery on the part of the women and midwives. Inge Stadelmann (9), recommends a perineum massage oil containing:

> rose essential oil
> clary sage essential oil
> hypericum infused oil
> wheatgerm cold pressed oil.

The expectant mother is instructed to massage the perineum with the massage oil during the last weeks of pregnancy. The aim of this treatment is to make it possible for women to give birth without the need of an episiotomy by making the perineum supple and elastic.

Labour is divided into three stages: the first is the dilation of the cervix, the second is the expulsion of the baby and the third is the delivery of the placenta. The average length of the first stage of labour with the first baby is about 12 hours, and with subsequent children about 7 hours. However, this stage may take anywhere from 2 to 24 hours, or more, depending on the size of the baby, the baby's position, the size of the mother's pelvic area and the behaviour of the uterus. During this stage massage oils with clary

---

Oils for the delivery room

Rose	• Uterine relaxant
	• Natural antiseptic
	• Slight analgesic effect
Neroli	• Facilitates easy breathing
	• Calming
	• Antiseptic
Lavender	• Circulatory stimulant
	• Slight analgesic effect
	• Calming
	• Antiseptic, anti-inflammatory
	• Promotes healing of wounds
	• Headaches and fainting
Clary sage	• Uterine tonic
	• Analgesic and antispasmodic
	• Euphoric
Jasmine	• Euphoric
	• Antidepressant
	• Uterine tonic

---

sage, jasmine, neroli or rose will help the mother relax between contractions. Use a few drops of bergamot or lavender added to a bowl of warm water to help refresh and disinfect the atmosphere.

Post-natal care

Breast and nipple care is very important, for the comfort of the mother and the wellbeing of the child. Cracked nipples are a common problem. They are not only painful but there is the possibility of infection. A good massage oil to prepare is:

Almond oil	40 ml
Infused calendula oil	5 ml
Wheatgerm oil	5 ml.

Post-natal depression

The uplifting properties of the essential oils are excellent to use after birth. Some of the essential oils recommended are bergamot, rose, neroli, clary sage, geranium, grapefruit, frankincense, mandarin, patchouli, rosewood, tangerine, vetiver and ylang-ylang.

Giving birth is not only the most profound chemical change that the human body undergoes in the space of several hours, but also the most profound social change for the mother. As well as the unrelenting demands of the baby, and the worry that the baby is healthy, there are the unremitting rounds of washing and cleaning, and relatives and friends all offering conflicting advice. It is far better to be prepared for these changes and difficulties. Profound changes have taken place hormonally, psychologically and socially. The essential oils will balance the hormonal and emotional levels.

Menstrual problems

Menstruation should not be considered as an illness although it is unusual to meet someone who does not suffer from at least a small amount of pre-menstrual syndrome, period cramping, some irregularities in the cycle or menopausal symptoms.

To ensure a normal and easy menstrual cycle, any of the uterine tonics may be used regularly or perhaps just for the time leading up to the expected onset of the period. 'Normal' is used here

Type	Description	Causes
PMS-A (Anxiety)	Symptoms of nervous tension, anxiety mood swings and irritability characterise this group. Biochemically this group shows a high oestrogen to progesterone ratio in the luteal phase.	Could be related to excess milk and animal fats. Also nervous excitability.
PMS-C (Craving)	This group shows increased appetite, sweet craving, headache, fatigue, dizziness, or fainting and heart pounding.	Low blood sugar, low prostaglandins.
PMS-D (Depression)	Depression, crying, forgetfulness, confusion and insomnia may characterise this group.	High progesterone, low oestrogen, high androgens. Also appears to be higher levels of lead in the body.
PMS-H (Hyper-hydration)	Fluid retention, weight gain, swelling of extremities, breast tenderness and abdominal bloating characterise this group.	These symptoms are attributed to increased retention of sodium in the body.

The main classifications of PMS

recognising that normality is relative and that each individual will have her own norm.

Pre-menstrual syndrome (PMS)

Useful Oils

Bergamot, German and Roman chamomile, clary sage, sweet fennel, geranium, juniper berry, lavender, neroli, rose, rosemary, ylang-ylang.

Clinical features

It is estimated that 50% of the premenopausal menstruating female population experiences premenstrual syndrome (10). The pre-menstrual syndrome is a recurrent (monthly) disorder characterised by physical and emotional upsets for some days before the onset of menstruation. PMS symptoms are: fluid retention, distended stomach, tender breasts, weight gain, constipation, insomnia, headaches and mood swings. In an attempt to bring some order to the clinically and metabolically confusing picture of PMS, Dr Guy Abraham has subdivided PMS into four distinct subgroups according to specific symptoms and hormonal patterns.

The four subgroups are detailed in the table above. Any woman may have a number of symptoms from each subgroup and not necessarily from one group only.

Aetiology

Imbalance in the hormones oestrogen and progesterone. This may only be to a subtle degree, but it is enough to produce PMS. It is this deficiency of female hormones that is the basic cause of all the physical and mental symptoms associated with PMS.

The secretion of oestrogen and progesterone is under the control of the pituitary gland. The pituitary is influenced by the hypothalamus which responds to stress and other psychological disturbances. This helps explain why PMS can vary from month to month.

According to Abraham (11), PMS sufferers consume 62% more refined carbohydrates, 275% more refined sugar, 79% more dairy products, 78% more sodium, 53% less iron, 77% less manganese and 52% less zinc. PMS patients given a multivitamin and mineral supplement containing high doses of magnesium and pyridoxine in an uncontrolled study showed a 70% reduction in premenstrual symptoms. (12)

Aromatherapy treatment

Various essential oils and aromatherapy techniques are very successful in reducing the severity of PMS and sometimes overcoming it, though for maximum benefit it is important to combine aromatherapy with a nutritional approach. The use of sweet fennel, juniper, rosemary and geranium in a massage oil in lymphatic drainage massage can minimise fluid retention.

Essential oils such as clary sage, sweet fennel, geranium and rose influence the production of hormones and are therefore beneficial for the treatment of PMS. Bergamot, Roman chamomile and rose may be used to reduce depression and irritability.

For aromatherapy to successfully treat PMS it is necessary to use daily a massage blend made up of any of the above essential oils in a massage base of evening primrose oil.

Other treatments

- Evidence suggests that that many of the symptoms of PMS are related to dietary imbalances and nutritional deficiencies. Over consumption of refined sugar, salt, animal fat, and dairy products may contribute to this variable symptom complex, whereas foods rich in linoleic acid such as cold pressed vegetable oils and seeds may be beneficial.

- Increase green leafy vegetable intake, except for the brassica family of foods (cabbage, brussels sprouts and cauliflower).

- Remove all refined starches, processed foods and additives from diet.

- Eat foods rich in vitamin B, particularly vitamin B6. Wholegrains and meat are rich sources of vitamin B6. Studies have shown that vitamin B6 (200-800 mg daily) helps reduce the amount of circulating oestrogen and elevates progesterone. (13)

- A high carbohydrate diet decreases hepatic clearance of estradiol while a high protein diet increases hepatic clearance of estradiol and may increase the half life of progesterone. The protein intake, however, should be derived largely from vegetable sources since vegetarian women are more able to clear oestrogen metabolites. (14)

- Evening primrose oil which contains GLA is a vital essential fatty acid for regulating menstrual problems. Evening primrose oil needs to be taken for two to three months, 2 x 500mg capsules three times a day which will decrease many PMS symptoms, particularly depression and irritability.

The results of scientific studies using evening primrose oil have been good, with more than 60% of women with PMS experiencing a reduction in depression, irritability, breast pain, bloating and headaches using evening primrose oil supplements. The study did not include any vitamins, minerals, dietary or lifestyle recommendations. The response rate is likely to have been higher if these had been included. (15)

- Sufferers should avoid tea, coffee, and alcohol and they should never resort to diuretics to banish excess fluid-related weight.

- Diet surveys have shown that people with PMS-A symptoms consume five times more dairy foods and three times more refined sugars than patients in other food groups. This consumption may contribute to calcium's interference with magnesium absorption and refined sugar's increase of the urinary excretion of magnesium. The combined effects of these may lead to a magnesium deficiency. Depletion in brain dopamine is associated with a deficiency of intracellular magnesium. (16)

- The Chinese herb dong quai has been found to relieve PMS symptoms.

- If progesterone is high then oestrogenic herbs such as alfalfa, red clover, sage, aniseed, sweet fennel and fenugreek are useful (17).

- If PMS is characterised by low levels of progesterone then herbs such as false unicorn and wild yam should be considered (18).

- Gentle exercise such as swimming, yoga, or just going for a walk when depression or irrational anger threaten, can also be a big help.

Dysmenorrhoea

Useful Oils
German and Roman chamomile, cypress, clary sage, geranium, jasmine, lavender, peppermint, Spanish sage.

Primary dysmenorrhoea

Pain that occurs with menstrual periods and with no organic cause accounts for 80% of cases of painful periods.

Aetiology

The pain is thought to result from uterine contractions, probably mediated by the effect of prostaglandins produced in secretory endometrium. Although primary dysmenorrhoea is particularly common during adolescence, it may continue well into adult life. Dysmenorrhoea and general menstrual discomfort are often described together as 'menorrhagia.'

Secondary dysmenorrhoea

Secondary dysmenorrhoea is menstrual pain for which an organic cause exists. It usually starts as late as the third or fourth decade of life.

Aetiology

In secondary dysmenorrhoea, a complete endometrial cast is sloughed, and pain is presumed to be the result of the local release of prostaglandins and of uterine expulsive contractions.

Aromatherapy treatment

Essential oils with antispasmodic, emmenagogue and analgesic properties such as Roman and blue chamomile, cypress, clary sage, geranium, jasmine, lavender, peppermint, and sage can be used to treat dysmenorrhoea.

The choice of essential oils also depends on the type of pain. For congestive pain, oils such as Roman chamomile and cypress are more useful, whereas spasmodic pain is relieved by peppermint, lavender and clary sage.

The method of application is massage, especially over the abdomen and lower back area. This should be done daily. Warm baths with a few drops of the essential oils such as cypress, lavender or clary sage are also recommended.

Other treatments

- Calcium and magnesium are most important for control of muscular contractions. A deficiency of either of these is indicated if the spasms are eased by heat. If only magnesium is lacking, then further relief can be gained by pressure or massage. If only calcium is missing no amount of pressure will make a difference.

- Increase the level of exercise. Many sufferers of dysmenorrhoea have found their symptoms improved after regular walking, exercise or swimming.

- Herbs such as ginger (for congestion); cramp bark (for spasmodic pain); pulsatilla (pain reliever for the female reproductive system); prickly ash (circulatory balancer) and dill and chamomile as teas for the pain.

- This pain usually responds to evening primrose oil, magnesium, B6, niacin, rutin and vitamin E. The effectiveness of niacin (200 mg/day) is enhanced by the addition of rutin and vitamin C. Supplements must begin 7 - 10 days prior to menses to be of any effect. (19)

Amenorrhoea

Useful Oils
German and Roman chamomile, sweet fennel, evening primrose, geranium, lavender, sweet marjoram, rose, Spanish sage, yarrow.

Clinical features

Amenorrhoea is the absence of menstrual periods at an age when regular menstruation is the norm. Many women will miss one or two periods during the fertile phase of their lives, perhaps during times of emotional stress, and if periods then return to normality there is nothing to worry about. It is obvious that amenorrhoea occurs during pregnancy.

Primary amenorrhoea refers to the failure to begin menstruating by the age of 18. A physical examination may be necessary just in case there is physical obstruction. If no physical blockage is evident then a constitutional treatment of essential oils and herbs should be considered to stimulate the sexual development and onset of menarche (the start of menstruation).

Secondary amenorrhoea refers to the disappearance of menstruation for more than three months after normal periods have been established, but before the onset of menopause. Missing periods during the several months following menarche is very common - it may take some young women several months or even years to establish a regular cycle. This should be taken into account when secondary amenorrhoea is being considered, as should the possibility of pregnancy and the early onset of menopause.

Aetiology

Other causes of amenorrhoea include: damage to the pituitary gland following postpartum haemorrhage or shock; ovarian cysts; drugs; extreme weight loss, very vigorous physical activity and severe stress.

One other common cause of amenorrhoea is an aftereffect of discontinuing the use of the contraceptive pill.

CAUTION
Always check for pregnancy.

Aromatherapy treatment

A blend of clary sage, geranium and rose in an evening primrose base is the most effective aromatherapy treatment when amenorrhoea is an after effect of discontinuing the use of the contraceptive pill, as it helps re-establish the hormonal balance.

Other useful essential oils for this treatment are German and Roman chamomile, sweet fennel, sweet marjoram, Spanish sage, rose, yarrow and geranium. Make a massage oil and massage over the abdomen and lower back every day for two weeks.

Other treatments

- Specific herbs to promote menstrual flow include false unicorn, blue cohosh and chaste tree.
- Oestrogenic herbs such as sage can also be taken as a tea daily.
- If there is no underlying medical problem, a good basic diet, and correction of any nutritional deficiencies with a broad spectrum nutritional program, should restore the periods to normal function within two to three months.

Menopause

Useful Oils
Bergamot, German and Roman chamomile, cypress, sweet fennel, geranium, jasmine, neroli, rose, ylang-ylang.

Clinical features

Menopause, also referred to as the change of life, is the point when women stop ovulating. Menopause affects each woman differently. The symptoms include hot flushes, dizziness, headache, difficult breathing, shortness of breathe, heart palpitations and depression.

While the average age of menopause is 50 years, some women go through a premature menopause in their 30s or early 40s, whilst others continue to menstruate up until their late 50s. Sweats and hot flushes are caused by the irregular function of the blood vessels when they constrict and dilate. This increases the blood flow, raises the temperature and slightly increases the heart rate.

Conventional treatment for menopause is HRT (hormone replacement therapy). This treatment introduces synthetic hormones into the blood stream to replace the oestrogen that is waning as a natural part of the menopausal process.

While HRT does relieve certain menopausal symptoms such as hot flushes, vaginal atrophy and slows down osteoporosis, it does not prevent cardiovascular disease, arthritis or depression. Moreover it only postpones menopausal symptoms which will reassert themselves whenever HRT is stopped.

Another argument against the use of HRT is that there are possible side effects associated with it. There is evidence that the use of oestrogen increases the risk of serious cardiovascular disease, especially potentially fatal blood clots. HRT is also linked to an increased risk of cancer of the breast and uterus (20).

Aromatherapy treatment

Every woman's experience is different, and the aromatherapist needs to take this into account when considering a treatment. The essential oils which help regulate menstruation earlier in life may minimise physical problems.

Oils such as geranium which is a hormonal balancer, rose which tones the uterus and regulates the menstrual cycle, and sweet fennel which is a natural plant oestrogen should all be considered. Chamomile, bergamot, jasmine, neroli, and ylang-ylang are calming and antidepressant so can be helpful when used in a massage, bath or in an oil burner.

The nurturing effects of rose and jasmine are immense especially when there is a loss of femininity. The following formulas may be helpful:

Problem	Aromatherapy formula	
Hot flushes:	clary sage	10 drops
	geranium	10 drops
	sage	5 drops
	lemon	5 drops
	evening primrose oil	50 ml
Day and night sweats:	cypress	10 drops
	sage	5 drops
	grapefruit	10 drops
	apricot kernel oil	50 ml
Water retention & bloating:	sweet fennel	5 drops
	juniper	5 drops
	lemon	10 drops
	geranium	10 drops
	apricot kernel oil	50 ml

Other treatments

- Fennel, liquorice, wild yam and sage may be helpful in stimulating oestrogen production.

- Exercise is very important. Avoid stress when possible.

- Diet is another important part of the lifestyle which needs to be addressed. Foods such as wholegrains, seeds, carrots, ripe bananas, apples, royal jelly and bee pollen are recommended. Foods to be avoided include coffee, tea, alcohol and refined foods, and foods with artificial additives.

- For hot flushes and sweating increase water intake to 2 to 3 litres a day.

- Take 500 iu of vitamin E once or twice a day, 1,000 mg of evening primrose oil 3 times a day, and herbs such as dong quai and sarsaparilla.

- For dry itching skin and dry vagina take a 1,000 mg capsule of evening primrose oil 3 times a day. Increase water intake to 2 to 3 litres a day.

- For fatigue, poor memory and reduced mental efficiency take siberian ginseng, ginkgo biloba and vitamin B complex tablets.

- For anxiety, irritability and insomnia take gentle sedative herbs such as passionflower, valerian, lime flowers, oats and skullcap, vitamin B complex tablets.

Endometriosis

Useful Oils
Clary sage, Roman chamomile, cypress, geranium, nutmeg, rose.

Endometriosis is a common gynaecological disorder affecting at least 8% of women (21). It is a unique disease in which the lining of the uterus which is called the endometrium develops in other sites of the body. In a healthy woman, this lining gradually thickens between periods under the influence of oestrogen, in preparation for the fertilised egg. If the egg doesn't arrive, the blood-rich lining is sloughed off and travels out of the body as a menstrual period. Endometriosis occurs when stray fragments of the endometrium somehow escape into the pelvic cavity and attack different pelvic organs.

Clinical features

The main symptom can be described in one word - PAIN. The pain may be a dull aching cramping or bearing down pressure felt in the lower abdomen or back. It tends to worsen with time and to begin progressively earlier in the cycle. Some sufferers may have as little as one pain-free week out of each month. There is pain during ovulation, pain during sexual intercourse, pain during urination or bowel movements. Other symptoms include infertility, abnormally heavy or irregular periods and inexplicable exhaustion and lethargy.

About 20% of sufferers have endometriosis close to the gastrointestinal tract, resulting in constipation, rectal bleeding and painful defecation during menstruation, with symptoms similar to irritable bowel syndrome (22). Symptoms can mimic conditions such as pelvic inflammatory diseases, diverticulitis, hernia, ovarian cysts and cancer.

Aetiology

The causes of endometriosis have not been identified. Dr Sampson's retrograde menstruation theory suggests that endometrial tissues from the uterus can flow upwards and outwards through the fallopian tubes into the abdominal cavity. Sampson recognised that a transference of endometrial tissue was taking place through fragments in the lymphatic glands (23).

Psychologically, endometriosis can have devastating effects on a women's sexuality and self-esteem. Dyspareunia (painful coitus) is a common symptom as lesions and implants behind the uterus can lock it in a retroverted position making sexual intercourse very painful. One third of endometriosis sufferers are infertile.

If endometriosis is suspected, the diagnosis is often confirmed through a hospital procedure called a laparoscopy. During a laparoscopy, a slender, telescope like instrument is passed into the abdominal cavity either through a small puncture wound beneath the navel, or through the upper vagina. This telescope allows the size and number of stray fragments of the endometrium tissue to be estimated.

Endometriosis has often been called the disease of the career woman, implying that delaying pregnancy may cause endometriosis, however, it has been diagnosed in females as young as 13. It is rare in post-menopausal women.

Conventional treatment

By creating a pseudomenopause, drug therapy can be effective, although lesions may recur when the therapy is discontinued. A commonly used drug is Danazol, a synthetic androgen thought to block the pituitary stimulation and production of leutenizing hormone (LH) and follicle stimulating hormone (FSH).

Synthetic androgens produce male characteristics and 85% of patients experience side effects such as deepening of the voice, alopecia, hirsutism, reduced breast size, clitoris enlargement and acne. Other side effects may include weight gain, high blood pressure and joint problems.

Pregnancy was long thought to halt the progress of the disease and is still suggested as an alternative to drug therapy. Pregnancy is not a panacea though; some women report no change, or even worsening of their problems.

Aromatherapy treatment

It is recommended that professional aromatherapy treatments be carried out over a three month period, with two visits a week initially. Lymphatic drainage must be avoided in the early stages due to the remote possibility of the endometrial cells being spread to other parts of the body. Gentle stress reducing aromatherapy techniques have no significant effect. However, neuromuscular and deep tissue massage can be very helpful. Many women with endometriosis have trigger points which contribute to the amount of pain they are experiencing.

Recommended essential oils are rose, geranium and cypress. Essential oils with analgesic and antispasmodic properties such as nutmeg, clary sage, and Roman chamomile should be used in a massage oil over the abdomen and the hips.

Use of essential oils in a bath should be encouraged and become part of a daily routine. Valerie Anne Worwood (24) recommends alternating hot and cold sitz or hip baths. Ideally you need to sit in waist-deep water. About 15 minutes should be spent in the hot sitz bath and 5 minutes in the cold sitz bath.

She recommends a blend of geranium, rose, cypress, nutmeg and clary sage to be added to the hot bath only. The entire treatment should ideally be repeated two to four times, depending on the severity.

CAUTION

It is advisable to avoid essential oils which are oestrogen imitators such as sweet and bitter fennel and aniseed.

Other treatments

- Diet is very important. Avoid caffeine, salt, sugar, animal fats, butter, dairy products, all hardened fats, fried foods, red meats and junk foods.

- The diet should include 50% raw vegetables and fruits. In addition eat plenty of wholegrain products, raw nuts, seeds and fish. Eliminate shellfish from the diet.

- There should be an emphasis on calcium-rich foods such as almonds, tahini, green leafy vegetables, sunflower seeds and hazelnuts. Calcium improves muscle tone and helps reduce menstrual cramps common in endometriosis sufferers.

- Evening primrose oil is rich in gamma linoleic acid, necessary to keep the cardiovascular and nervous systems healthy. Endometriosis patients find it helpful for dealing with depression and fatigue, especially when there are side effects from hormone therapy.

- Some herbal teas such as freshly grated ginger ease menstrual pain due to the anti-spasmodic effects. A strong brew of chamomile, lime blossom and passionflower is also effective for cramping; tension and irritability may also be reduced.

Thrush

Useful Oils

German chamomile, geranium, lavender, lemongrass, myrrh, petitgrain, tea tree, thyme.

Clinical features

Candida infections have been viewed for many years as minor infections that affect the mucous membranes such as the vaginal passages and the mouth. However, evidence presented recently suggests that it is more than an opportunistic infection. It has now been associated with a variety of conditions ranging from mental disorders, deranged immune system, food intolerance, gastric upsets and PMS (25).

Aetiology

The rise in this organism as a causative agent in many disease processes follows the increased use of broad spectrum antibiotics, oral contraceptives, steroid drugs and other immune suppressive drugs. *Candida albicans* suppresses both cellular and humeral defence systems.

All persons on long-term antibiotics are at greater risk of severe forms of candida. Oral contraceptives or corticosteroids should not be taken until the condition improves as they can upset the balance of the *Candida albicans* organism.

Aromatherapy treatment

The treatment consists of baths and local applications of essential oils. The oils chosen should have antiseptic, antifungal and immune-stimulant properties such as are found in German chamomile, geranium, lavender, lemongrass, petitgrain, thyme, myrrh or tea tree. A sitz bath is also very effective for vaginal irritation. 2-3 drops of the essential oil should be added to a bidet or large bowl of warm water twice a day whilst symptoms persist.

Valerie Ann Worwood (26) recommends a douche using whole milk, natural yoghurt containing live acidophilus culture.

German chamomile	5 drops
Lavender	5 drops
tea tree	5 drops

add to a 100gm carton of yoghurt and stir well.

The yoghurt combined with the above essential oils has the dual action of antibiotic and antifungal properties. This method is very effective if there is soreness and itching. Use either an applicator for inserting pessaries or a tampon applicator.

Another way of using yoghurt is by diluting it in warm spring water until a thin fluid has been obtained. Then add the essential oils and use this mixture in a douche, washing the vaginal tract twice a day.

Other treatments

- Avoid all yeast-containing foods such as breads, mushrooms, vegemite, marmite, cheese, soya products, miso, beer, wine, and all preserved and pickled meats.

- Avoid all refined carbohydrates - sugars, soft drinks, pastries, canned fruit, chocolate, honey and dried fruits. Candida thrives in a sugary environment.

- Eliminate citrus and acid fruits (eg oranges, grapefruit, lemons, tomatoes, pineapples) from the diet for one month; then add back only twice weekly. These fruit are alkalising and candida thrives in an alkaline environment.

- Garlic should be taken every day.

- Supplement the diet with vitamin B12, B6, biotin and folic acid as they maintain the candida in the non invasive form.

- Stimulate the immune system with the appropriate nutrients - see the section on colds and infections.

- Eat yoghurt which contains acidophilus and will help restore the natural balance of the bowel and vagina.

Cystitis

Useful Oils
Bergamot, German chamomile, lavender, sandalwood, tea tree.

Clinical features

Bladder infections are usually caused by bacteria, resulting in cystitis, an inflammation of the bladder. Kidney infections are more serious and often result from cystitis. Bladder inflammations are much more frequent in women than in men due to the closeness of the bladder and urethra to the vagina.

Aetiology

Sometimes the infection is caused by a bacterium *Escherichia coli*. Intense sexual activity can also trigger signs and symptoms - hence the term 'honeymoon cystitis'. Urinating before and after intercourse and washing afterwards with cool water can help to prevent this. It can also occur during pregnancy when the foetus is pressing down on the bladder, preventing it from emptying.

Often a yeast infection in the bowel is the culprit. Hyperacidity and stress can quickly bring on cystitis.

Aromatherapy treatment

The most valuable oils in the treatment of cystitis are bergamot and tea tree, used externally as a local wash and in the bath. As with all use of essential oils on delicate mucous membranes, a very low dilution should be made, between 0.5% and 1% of essential oil in warm water. Swab the opening of the urethra at frequent intervals.

A massage oil containing bergamot, lavender and German chamomile should be massaged over the lower abdomen. Sandalwood oil has been used as a urinary tract antiseptic in India for many centuries and may be a valuable alternative to bergamot or tea tree.

If there is pus or blood in the urine, or the temperature is high a medical doctor should be consulted, because cystitis can very quickly lead to more serious kidney infection. This is one situation in which antibiotics may be helpful.

Other treatments

- Beneficial herbs include burdock root, juniper berry, marshmallow root, and rosehips. Marshmallow root increases the acid content in the urine, inhibiting bacterial growth. Juniper berries will help restore kidney function. Goldenseal is an excellent herb to treat the bladder infection when there is bleeding.

- Diuretics can help cleanse the system. Dandelion tea acts as a liver cleanser and diuretic. Bearberry and uva ursi act as mild diuretics and antiseptics.

- Nutritionally, plenty of vitamin C and vitamin A are needed to repair the mucous linings of the bladder.

- Acidophilus will replace some of the 'friendly' bacteria especially if antibiotics have been prescribed.

- It is important to drink lots of water every day, but avoid tea and coffee.

- Avoid citrus fruit because these produce alkaline urine that encourages bacterial growth. Increase acid content in the urine to inhibit bacterial growth.

- Include celery, parsley, and watermelon in the diet. These foods act as natural diuretics.

- Do not delay emptying the bladder. Urination should occur every two to three hours. Research has shown that retaining the urine in the bladder for long periods increases the risk of urinary tract infection.

Chapter 24

Integumentary System

This chapter summarises an holistic approach to the treatment of many common ailments and conditions associated with the integumentary system.
Not only have the aromatherapy procedures for each condition been outlined, but details have also been included on other forms of treatment such as diet, herbs, acupressure and exercise.

Conditions discussed in this chapter include:

Boils and carbuncles
Acne
Dermatitis-eczema
Herpes simplex
Psoriasis
Sunburn

Introduction

Orthodox medicine classifies skin diseases according to histological changes occurring in the skin tissue. This approach often ignores the idea that skin problems can be manifestations of internal problems and should be treated as such and not as a local phenomenon. According to holistic principles, we can categorise the skin conditions into the following causes:

- internal causes, where the origins of a skin disease are the result of internal disharmony, as in psoriasis or eczema

- external causes, where the skin problem is a direct result of external influences, as with wounds, bruises or sunburns

- internal reactions due to external factors, where the skin problems are due to the body's inability to cope with external factors, such as allergic eczema or skin infections due to bacteria or fungi.

General considerations

In the treatment of skin diseases the following holistic approaches are essential:

- Attention to dietary and lifestyle factors is of paramount importance.

- Use holistic principles for restoring vitality and resistance, building health rather than killing a disease.

- Treat the obvious cause according to the properties of the essential oils and the pathology of the disease - for example use an antiseptic oil to treat an infection.

- Treat the underlying cause following philosophical or holistic principles applied to the observation of symptoms and what they reveal.

- Treat symptoms.

When treating skin problems, you need to have patience, as improvement is rarely dramatic and treatment needs to be continued for several months. Naturopath Nancy Beckham (1) recommends that an estimated time that it will take to treat certain skin conditions such as eczema and dermatitis is one month for every year suffered by the client.

Aromatherapy considerations

An extensive amount of research has been done on the use of essential oils for skin problems. Research conducted by Tubaro (2) has shown that German chamomile exerted anti-inflammatory activity after topical application. The effects of chamomile were tested on 14 patients after dermabrasion of tatoos. It was noted that the healing and drying process was significantly increased. (3)

A report in the medical journal of Australia in 1990 compared tea tree oil and benzoyl peroxide in the treatment of acne. It was found that tea tree reduced the number of inflamed and non-inflamed lesions more slowly, but fewer side effects were experienced by those treated with tea tree oil. (4)

From the above studies it can be seen that essential oils are particularly valuable because they are able to address skin complaints on a variety of levels. The therapeutic properties of essential oils which are beneficial for the integumentary system are:

Antimicrobial

For cuts, infections and insect bites use essential oils such as *eucalyptus, tea tree, lavender* and *lemon.*

Anti-inflammatory

For the treatment of eczema, infected wounds and bruises, essential oils such as *German chamomile, everlasting, lavender* and *yarrow* are highly beneficial.

Cicatrisant and cytophylactic

To encourage cell regeneration for the treatment of burns, cuts, scars and stretch marks, essential oils such as *everlasting, lavender, German chamomile, myrrh, rose, neroli, frankincense* and *geranium* are useful.

Fungicidal

For the treatment of fungal infections such as athlete's foot, candida and ringworm *lavender, tea tree, myrrh* and *patchouli* essential oils are highly effective.

Vulnerary

Vulnerary is a term used for a remedy which promotes healing of wounds, cuts and sores. Essential oils such as bergamot, cajeput, German and Roman chamomile, eucalyptus, frankincense, geranium, lavender, myrrh, niaouli, rosemary, tea tree, thyme and yarrow are recommended.

Associated conditions

Boils and carbuncles

Useful Oils
Bergamot, lavender, lemon, tea tree, thyme.

Clinical features

Inflamed, infected lumps - on or under the skin, as a result of *staphylococcus* infection. A carbuncle is a close collection of boils filled with pus. Carbuncles can be dangerous, can infect the blood stream (septicaemia) and so they should be treated and not ignored.

Symptoms of boil formation include itching, mild pain, and localised swelling. Boils appear suddenly. Within 24 hours they become red and filled with pus. Swelling of the nearest lymph glands often occurs and the glands become swollen and tender. General body aches and pains and lack of appetite are also common features. If the boils are very large, medical assistance may be required.

Aetiology

Boils may be caused by a bacterial infection, an airborne or food allergy, stress, poor hygiene, an illness, a lowered resistance, certain drugs, excessive consumption of junk foods, an infected wound, a toxic bowel and blood stream, or thyroid disorders. They may be caused when the deepest portion of the hair follicle becomes infected and the inflammation spreads, often with staphylococcus bacteria. Constipation is a common underlying cause.

Aromatherapy treatment

Hot compresses with essential oils can be used to 'draw out' a boil and speed healing, the most suitable being tea tree, bergamot and lavender because of their antiseptic properties. The area around the boil should be washed several times a day with a 1% to 3% dilution of lavender or bergamot.

If numerous or recurring boils are evident, there is a need to reduce the level of toxicity in the body. Regular massages and baths using detoxifying oils such as juniper berry, geranium, grapefruit, rosemary and carrot seed are valuable.

Other treatments

- Purifying the blood stream and enhancing immune function are the main goals in therapy. Lymphatic drainage is important.

- The diet should be especially high in fruit and vegetables. Restrict refined carbohydrates. It is possible that by restricting carbohydrates the glucose content of the sebaceous glands and sweat secretions can be reduced and the conditions for pathogenic growth made less favourable. It is likely that a diet low in fat and carbohydrates will reduce sebaceous gland activity and reduce the effect of follicular plugging.

- Garlic taken daily will help detoxify the body and stimulate the immune system.

- Prepare a detoxifying blend of herbs such as burdock root, red clover and yellow dock daily. Mix equal parts of each herb and place a teaspoon of the mixture into a cup of boiling water, allow to steep for 15 minutes, and drink. Repeat this routine three times per day.

- Poultices will bring the boil to a head much faster. Some poultices often used include (5):
  - Mix half a tablespoon of slippery elm with one tablespoon of linseed oil. Add a teaspoon of charcoal. Mix well, warm the mixture to a comfortable

- temperature, and apply to the boil as a poultice.
- Take a handful of comfrey roots, grind up into a pulp, and apply to the boil as a poultice.

Acne

Useful Oils

Bergamot, geranium, juniper berry, lavender, lemon, lime, mandarin, niaouli, palmarosa, petitgrain, rosemary, sandalwood, tea tree.

Clinical features

Acne vulgaris is commonly encountered in adolescence and pre-menstrually, but can proceed into adult life. It attacks regions containing large sebaceous glands, ie the face, back, and upper anterior chest. The lesion consists of closed (white) or open (black) comedones (black heads), papules, pustules, nodules and abscesses.

Aetiology

Acne may be related to both hormonal and dietary causes. The basic cause is an increase in androgen production in the male and oestrogen in the female in maturing teenagers which increases the secretion of the sebaceous glands.

The sebum produced may be broken down to fatty acids which may, in conjunction with bacteria present, provoke an inflammatory response in the sebaceous glands.

Aromatherapy treatment

Essential oils can be used to help clear the infection, reduce the amount of sebum produced and to minimise the extent of scarring and promote the growth of new skin tissue. Lavender, bergamot, lemon, niaouli and tea tree are highly antiseptic. Lavender is also soothing and healing, and promotes the growth of healthy new cells. Bergamot is astringent, as well as an anti-depressant (which is often useful for severe cases with young people who become depressed about their acne).

Geranium and palmarosa oil balance the production of sebum being secreted. All oils mentioned can be used in facial massages, using a light vegetable oil such as apricot kernel or rosehip oil as a base. The essential oils may also be mixed into creams or skin cleansing lotions so that they can be applied to the face.

A mild liquid castille soap may be used as a cleansing gel to which the following essential oils are added:

liquid castille soap	100 ml
lavender	7 drops
tea tree	5 drops
geranium	3 drops
neroli	5 drops.

Massage is useful as it stimulates the circulation and helps the body to eliminate toxins. Rosemary, mandarin and juniper can be used for body massage treatment to stimulate the lymphatic system. To minimise the possibility of scars use neroli, sandalwood and lavender in wheatgerm oil.

Other treatments

- Foods high in iodine should be eliminated, and milk consumption (due to high hormone content) should be limited. (6)

- Avoid all refined sugars, saturated fats and processed foods.

- Improve digestion by taking digestive enzymes or apple cider vinegar with meals.

- Increase the intake of foods rich in zinc and vitamin A. Retinols, including oral vitamin A, have been shown in many studies to reduce sebum production and the hyperkeratosis of sebaceous follicles. (7)

- Zinc is vitally important in the treatment of acne. It is involved in local hormone activation, retinol-binding protein formation, wound healing, immune system activity and tissue regeneration. (8)

- Menstrual related acne responds to vitamin B6. This reflects its role in the normal metabolism of steroid hormones. (9)

- Alfalfa, burdock root, dandelion root herbs will detoxify the body and echinacea will stimulate the immune system.

Dermatitis

Useful Oils

Bergamot, cedarwood, German chamomile, everlasting, juniper, lavender, myrrh, patchouli, sandalwood, yarrow, ylang ylang.

Clinical features

Superficial inflammation of the skin, characterised by vesicles (when acute), redness, oozing, crusting, scaling and usually itching. Scratching or rubbing may lead to lichenification.

The terms 'dermatitis' and 'eczema' are used synonymously. There is no general agreement among authorities as to the distinction between them. For diagnostic purposes the dermatitis - eczema group of skin diseases includes the following:

- contact dermatitis being either toxic or allergic in origin
- atopic dermatitis (eczema)
- seborrheic dermatitis
- photo-dermatitis.

Contact dermatitis

Most forms of dermatitis are associated with allergic tendencies - such as food allergies to dairy products or gluten. Other forms of dermatitis are the result of handling something with which the skin develops a reaction (eg washing-up liquid).

Dermatitis and eczema can appear for the first time or worsen during periods of emotional stress, or when overtired or run down. The patient may often develop hypersensitivity to many substances. Fortunately these hypersensitivities are mostly reversible. The treatment should include eliminating the causative agent and soothing the skin.

Atopic dermatitis or eczema

A chronic itching, superficial inflammation of the skin, usually occurring in individuals with a personal or family history of allergic disorders such as hay fever and asthma.

Seborrheic dermatitis

An inflammatory scaling disease of the scalp, face, and occasionally other areas of the body.

Despite the name, the composition and flow of sebum are normal. Onset in adults is gradual, and the dermatitis is apparent only as dry or greasy diffuse scaling of the scalp (dandruff) with variable itching. In severe cases yellow-red, scaling papules appear along the hairline, behind the ears, in the external auditory canals, on the eyebrows, on the bridge of the nose, in the naso-labial folds, and over the sternum. Seborrheic dermatitis does not cause hair loss.

Aetiology

As discussed, there are several forms, though little difference in the basic principles of treatment along holistic lines. Lifestyle and dietary factors are important. Check for allergies, both in diet and to contact. In particular be wary of dairy products, especially in childhood eczema.

Obesity, poor circulation and lack of exercise allow stagnation of the periphery to occur and will exacerbate eczematous condition. Constipation is often a common underlying problem.

Aromatherapy treatment

Since eczema is so varied there are many essential oils that are suitable for its treatment. The treatment should focus on removing the cause, and treating the skin according to its existing state. This often means:

- removing any known allergen (The anti-allergenic properties of German chamomile are well-documented.) (10)
- as eczema is an inflammatory skin condition, essential oils such as German chamomile, everlasting, yarrow and lavender may be used for their anti-inflammatory properties
- preventing infection from occurring by using antimicrobial essential oils such as lavender, myrtle, cajeput and tea tree
- eczema is often an attempt by the body to throw off accumulated toxins through the skin (In such cases detoxifying essential oils such as carrot seed, everlasting, geranium, juniper, rosemary, rock rose and yarrow are beneficial.)
- stress is usually involved in most cases of eczema, therefore essential oils such as lavender, bergamot, sandalwood,

patchouli, cedarwood and ylang ylang will play an important role in reducing the level of stress.

It is also important to treat the clinical type and stage of eczema appropriately. According to Weiss (11), the basic rule for treating acute weeping eczema is 'wet on wet'. This means using solutions, baths, wet dressing containing essential oils for 30 minutes 3 or 4 times a day. Moist compresses are needed until the weeping stage and acute inflammation have passed. The compresses or dressing should be loose, moist and allow plenty of evaporation. The most effective essential oils to use would be German chamomile, yarrow, everlasting, myrrh, lavender and juniper berry.

With chronic dry lesions the essential oils are best applied topically using ointments or creams. Essential oils such as German chamomile, yarrow, East Indian sandalwood, lavender, palmarosa and patchouli are helpful and should be used in a 1% dilution.

Other treatments

- The approaches to childhood and adult eczema are somewhat different. The severe exclusion diets used in adult eczema are not always suitable for children and care should be taken when using them. Children should not be put on rigid exclusion diets without expert guidance. However, the avoidance of common allergens such as cow's milk, eggs, cheese, food additives and sugar can safely be undertaken. Safe foods such as meat, vegetables, fruit, and rice can be eaten instead.

- Test or investigate for food or chemical hypersensitivity. Common contact sensitivities are as follows: cosmetics, hair dyes, shampoos, fragrances, insecticides, aerosol allergens such as polishes, nasal sprays, synthetic resins, earrings (nickel allergy), toothpastes, salicylate rich foods, deodorants, detergents, soaps, and lanolin derivatives.

- Reduce animal fat intake from dairy produce and remove the fat from meat. Also remember that all margarines may be chemically no better than animal fats.

- Include high quality cold pressed sunflower, safflower or linseed oil in the diet. The use of evening primrose oil normalises the essential fatty acid imbalances and reduces symptoms of eczema. (12)

- A diet rich in omega-3 fatty acids is recommended. This can be achieved by either fish oil supplements or by eating more cold water fish (eg mackerel, herring and salmon). This increases the eicosapentaenoic acid level which has been shown to reduce the incidence of eczema. (13)

- A diet high in fruit and vegetables is recommended.

- Detoxifying and blood purifying herbs such as burdock, nettle, yellow dock and red clover have been traditionally used for treating eczema.

Herpes simplex

Useful Oils

Bergamot, cajeput, geranium, lemon, melissa, niaouli, rose, tea tree.

Clinical features

There are two types of herpes virus.

- Type I (*Herpes simplex* or *Herpes labialis*) is recognised by cold sores and skin eruptions. It can also cause an inflammation of the cornea of the eye. If the eye becomes infected, see a doctor immediately.

- Type II (genital herpes) is sexually transmitted and is the most prevalent herpes infection. This viral infection can range in severity from a silent infection to a serious inflammation of the liver including fever, severe brain damage and stillbirths. Babies can pick up the virus in the birth canal, risking brain damage, blindness and death.

After entering the body, the virus never leaves. The virus enters the nerve cells where it hibernate and exists basically lifelong. From there the virus can resurface any time and cause an outbreak. Sickness, stress and unknown factors can cause the virus to break out in open sores again.

Aromatherapy treatment

Essential oils have been regularly used for the treatment of herpes. The antiviral properties of melissa extracts have now been recognised, and the immediate application of melissa and other essential oils, often prevents the viruses from replicating.

Professor Wabner (14) knows of some 500 cases of herpes simplex successfully treated with melissa oil. These include both acute and chronic cases. For adults he suggests three applications of undiluted melissa oil directly onto the blister, for one day only. The herpes then usually disappears within 24 hours.

Care must be taken to apply the oil only to the blister, as melissa may cause irritation on the surrounding skin. For children he suggests blending melissa with rose, to further reduce the risk of irritation. (15)

Other essential oils cited in various publications include bergamot, eucalyptus, cajeput, niaouli, geranium, lemon and tea tree. These oils are usually effective in treating the herpes blisters, particularly if applied very quickly at the first sign of an eruption. These oils are best applied in the form of an ointment or they can be diluted in an alcohol base and dabbed directly onto the cold sore with a cotton wool bud.

The aromatherapy treatment for genital herpes does not seem to be as spectacular and effective, unless it is combined with nutritional and attitudinal improvement. Bergamot plays an important role, as it is has antimicrobial and antidepressant properites.

Other treatments

- At least 1000 mg of vitamin C daily, together with bioflavinoids and zinc is beneficial as the role of these nutrients is to enhance cell-mediated immunity. (16)

- 300-1200 mg daily of the amino acid lysine, together with a diet low in its contrasting amino acid arginine (avoid peanuts, chocolate, seeds and cereals) is beneficial because lysine inhibits the

growth of *Herpes simplex* virus and arginine stimulates its growth. (17)

- Herbal treatment for herpes should include echinacea, golden seal, myrrh and red clover.

Psoriasis

Useful Oils

Bergamot, carrot seed, German chamomile, evening primrose, everlasting, lavender, sandalwood, yarrow.

Clinical features

This condition results from a greatly increased turnover of epidermal cells. A normal period from new cell to desquamation is 28 days, but for psoriasis sufferers this is reduced to 4 days. Psoriasis first appears on the body as small dull red patches covered with dry silvery scales. The definitive symptom is a tiny bleeding point under a scale when the lesion is scratched and a scale is removed.

Areas usually affected are the elbows, knees, lower back, ears and scalp. There may be itching and the finger nails can be affected. Remission is common. A stubborn and difficult problem to treat, psoriasis requires patience, diligence and long-term treatment with detoxifiers to observe lasting benefits.

Emphasis should be on convincing the patient that it is worthwhile to continue the treatment for a long period of time to see good results. Results are apparent in months, not days.

Aetiology

Causes are difficult to determine but they are generally regarded as metabolic disturbances as psoriasis affects the entire body, not just the skin. Indications according to Pizzorno (18) are:

- Some lesions are closely associated with linoleic acid deficiency.

- Incomplete protein digestion or poor intestinal absorption of protein breakdown products.

- A number of gut-derived toxins are implicated in the development of psoriasis. A diet low in dietary fibre is associated with increased levels of gut derived toxins.

- Attacks can be triggered by nervous tension and stress, illness, cuts, several viral and bacterial infections, sunburn, or drugs such as lithium, chloroquine, and beta blockers.

- Louise Hay states that psoriasis is associated with the fear of being hurt or refusing to accept responsibility for one's own feelings.

Aromatherapy treatment

Essential oils are very effective in dealing with the multi-dimensioned skin problem, psoriasis. A large number of patients (39%) report a specific stressful event occurring within one month prior to their intitial episode. (19)

Aromatherapy plays an important role in reducing stress. Any of the essential oils which help to alleviate stress and anxiety, such as bergamot, sandalwood, and lavender, are most suitable. These oils may be used as an inhalation, in a bath or prepared in a 1% massage blend.

When preparing a massage oil use evening primrose oil as a base. Wheatgerm oil also can be applied to patches of psoriasis on the face. Mix two to three drops of tea tree to every 10 ml of wheatgerm oil and apply to the skin morning and evening.

Any of the essential oils which have anti-inflammatory properties should also be considered, such as German chamomile, yarrow or everlasting.

Essential oils such as carrot seed and everlasting may be used to correct abnormal liver function which is often beneficial in the treatment of psoriasis. The connection between the liver and psoriasis relates to one of the liver's basic tasks of filtering and detoxifying the blood. If the liver is overwhelmed by an excessive level of toxins in the blood, or if there is a decrease in the liver's detoxification ability, the toxicity level in the blood will increase and the psoriasis will worsen.

Other treatments

- Attention should focus on diet and particularly:
  - All pork meat and pork fat (commonly used in the manufacture of pastry, biscuits, chocolate and ice cream) should be eliminated from the diet.
  - Benefit has been derived from eating a low-acid diet.
  - Fruit and vegetables are clearly beneficial to the condition.
  - Avoid saturated fats (milk, cream, butter, eggs), sugar, processed foods, white flour and citrus fruits. Avoid red meat and dairy products.
  - Increase the intake of fish oils, particularly those rich in EPA (eg cod, sardines, tuna or mackerel).

    Several double blind clinical trials have demonstrated that supplementing the diet with 10 to 12 grams of EPA results in significant improvement. The improvement is largely due to the inhibition of the production of inflammatory compounds known as leukotrienes. (20)
  - Take 1-2 tablespoons of linseed oil per day.

- Herbs such as St Mary's Thistle, sarsaparilla, red clover and burdock have all been reported to be of value in the treatment of psoriasis.

- Avoid stressful situations, fatigue, environmental changes (such as exposure to cold) and trauma to the skin as these can initiate new skin lesions.

- For symptomatic relief use chickweed as a lotion or a cream.

- Attention to nervous/emotional problems is also important.

- Sunlight is very beneficial in most cases. A standard medical treatment of psoriasis typically involves the use of a drug psoralen and exposure to UV light. (21)

Sunburn

Useful Oils
German chamomile, lavender, peppermint, tea tree.

Clinical features

This is an inflammation of the skin following exposure to the ultra-violet rays of the sun. Fair skinned people have little protective pigmentation in their skins, therefore their skin burns more easily than darker skinned people. Minor sunburn causes reddening of the skin and some discomfort, followed by increased pigmentation of the skin (ie. a tan). More serious sunburn can cause the skin and tissue to swell painfully and to blister and peel.

Aromatherapy treatment

Add lavender oil to water and dab on the burnt skin if no blistering is present and the skin is not broken. If blistering has occurred, you can gently apply lavender neat to the skin. German chamomile and tea tree oil can also be applied to soothe and cool burning skin.

A sunburn should be treated like any other burn, whether from prolonged exposure to the sun or from a hot iron. With all burns it is important to get the heat out of the skin. In order to do this simply fill a sink, bowl or bath with cold water (add ice if possible) and immerse the burn immediately. Add a few drops of peppermint and lavender to the water to help soothe and cool the burn.

Fresh aloe vera gel extracted from a leaf that has been kept in the refrigerator can be applied to the sunburn to help soothe, heal and cool the burn. If there has been a loss of body fluids these should be replaced by drinking water.

However, the best advice I can give on sunburn is:

Don't go out into the sun in the first place !!!!

If it is necessary to be outdoors, wear protective clothing and apply the maximum sun screen lotion regularly.

Chapter 25

Nervous System

This chapter summarises an holistic approach to the treatment of many common ailments and conditions associated with the nervous system.
Not only have the aromatherapy procedures for each condition been outlined, but details have also been included on other forms of treatment such as diet, herbs, acupressure and exercise.

Conditions discussed in this chapter include:
Stress
Anxiety
Depression
Insomnia
Mental Fatigue
Headaches
Migraines
Epilepsy
Shingles

Introduction

The nervous system is the body's control centre and communication network and it controls the actions and reactions of the body and its adjustment to the environment. The nervous system has three main functions:

- It senses changes within the body and in the outside environment.

- It interprets the changes.

- It responds to the interpretation by initiating action in the form of muscular contractions or glandular secretions.

Traditional allopathic medicine tends to reduce psychological problems to the mere biochemical level and assumes that 'appropriate' drugs will sort out or at least hide the problem sufficiently to allow 'normal' life to continue.

The over use of pharmaceutical sedatives and antidepressants has been well publicised. Dr Peter Breggin, author of Toxic Psychiatry, states that psychiatric drugs such as Prozac and other short-term 'solutions' are being prescribed by doctors as a quick antidote to depression, panic disorder and obsessive-compulsive disorders. He asserts that psychiatric drugs are spreading an epidemic of long-term brain damage and mental illness. (1)

While some help may be needed in extreme cases and for traumatic situations, the commonly prescribed tranquillisers do not cure the problems but often tend to dampen one's ability to think clearly. The result is that over a long period the person often loses the will to improve the general level of health and does not have the mental or physical energy to reduce the aggravating factors which probably caused the problem in the first place.

The nervous system is divided into two principal divisions, the central nervous system and the peripheral nervous system. The complete organisation of the nervous system is shown in the diagram on this page.

For example, in climbing stairs the muscles under conscious control receive orders from the brain via the somatic nervous system. However, the individual is not conscious of what the liver, pancreas or spleen are doing while climbing the

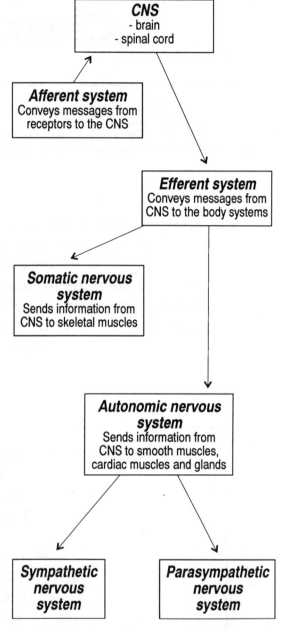

Organisation of the nervous system

stairs. The autonomic nervous system, part of the nervous system, normally operates without voluntary control. It controls the secretion of digestive enzymes, gastro-intestinal motility, constriction of blood vessels, urinary output, body temperature and heart rate. Its main function is the regulation, integration and control of the human body through homoeostasis.

The autonomic nervous system has two major divisions:

- sympathetic nervous system
- parasympathetic nervous system.

The sympathetic nervous system is associated with the secretion and effects of adrenaline and noradrenaline. Its primary role is to stimulate those functions that will be most useful for the fight-or-flight response. In general it produces the following effects:

- The heart rate increases.
- The blood vessels of the skin and viscera constrict.
- The remaining blood vessels dilate causing an increase in blood pressure and a faster flow of blood into the dilated blood vessels of the skeletal muscles, cardiac muscles, lungs and brain.
- Blood sugar levels rise as liver glycogen is converted to glucose to supply the body's additional energy needs.
- Processes that are not necessary for meeting the stress situation are inhibited. For example, muscular movements of the gastrointestinal tract and digestive secretions are slowed down or even stopped.

The parasympathetic system is primarily concerned with activities that restore and conserve body energy. Under normal body conditions the parasympathetic impulses reduce the heart rate and bronchial capacity and increase blood supply to the internal organs, digestive activity and glandular secretions.

It must be remembered that the autonomic nervous system is not a separate nervous system. Axons from the central nervous system are connected to the sympathetic and parasympathetic nervous systems. The hypothalamus is the major control and integration centre of the autonomic nervous system. The posterior and lateral portions of the hypothalamus appear to control the sympathetic division, while the anterior and medial portions of the hypothalamus seem to control the parasympathetic division.

While stress itself is not the problem, it is one's inability to handle stress and the way a person reacts to it which becomes injurious to one's health. To cope with stress, it is necessary to recognise one's limitations and become aware of the levels of anxiety or physical exhaustion. While nervous tension can give rise to many symptoms such as breathlessness, headaches, palpitations, skin irritations, respiratory problems, digestive and bowel problems, it can be the cause of more serious problems such as cancer and heart attacks.

Poor handling of stress should be dealt with immediately, before it leads to other problems. It is obviously not only a matter of using essential oils, but also the necessity to evaluate lifestyle habits, work and home situation and then take steps to eliminate, reduce or adapt to the aggravating factors. This might include an exercise program, meditation, yoga, a stress management course or developing a spiritual or philosophic belief.

This chapter does not discuss treatment strategies for severe mental problems or psychiatric disturbances although aromatherapy would be of assistance. These conditions need professional guidance.

General considerations

A relaxed body and mind are better able to deal with life situations than when stressed. Learning to control and balance stress with relaxation is an essential part of holistic health. While the care of oneself should involve a well balanced nutritional diet, regular exercise and plenty of sleep and rest, it should also be a process of life enrichment by doing what brings one satisfaction and a sense of wellbeing.

A holistic approach to the treatment of problems associated with the nervous system may involve the use of:

- a well balanced diet and nutritional supplements
- rest and sleep
- managing stress

- relaxation techniques

- aromatherapy and massage

- flower essences such as Bach Flowers or Australian Bush Flowers

- herbs

- and many other holistic therapies which address the body, mind and spirit.

It has also been shown that attitude and behaviour can influence one's resistance to disease. For many years positive imagery and thinking have been used in the treatment of cancer. Anslie Meares poetically describes the benefits of meditation (2):

'In meditation
There comes a calm,
A clarity,
Which enlightens
The inner depths of our being,
Brought to us
By the more harmonious function
Of nerve and endocrine cells
Which mastermind
The healing powers of the body.'

Aromatherapy considerations

Most aromatherapy sessions will involve a consultation followed by a massage with appropriately selected essential oils. This multi-dimensional approach involves:

- pharmacologically active essential oils

- massage

- a caring professional relationship between the therapist and the client

- the olfactory system which links memory, emotion, the autonomic nervous system and limbic brain.

It is now well known that essential oils have both a psychological and pharmacological effect on the nervous system and mind. (3) (4)

Torii (5), using an EEG to measure brain wave activity, confirmed many of the traditional uses of essential oils. He found that chamomile, bergamot, sandalwood, lavender and sweet marjoram have a sedative effect on the central

nervous system while jasmine, peppermint, basil and clove have a stimulating effect.

In this research, some essential oils such as geranium and rosewood were found to be either stimulating or sedating according to the individual's need. Thus these oils could be referred to as adaptogens.

Conversely, oils such as jasmine, ylang-ylang and neroli can be nerve stimulants yet, on a more subtle emotional level, they are soothing and relaxing.

Buchbauer (6) has shown that lavender used as an inhalation facilitates sleep and minimises stressful situations.

The benefits of massage have also been confirmed. Farrow (7) investigated the physical and psychological benefits of massage using 30 patients at St Mary's Hospital, London. The observed effects of the massage treatment included:

- reduction of pain levels

- reduction of anxiety

- reduction of muscle spasm and tension

- improved wellbeing and self worth.

In treating conditions associated with the nervous system the following properties of the essential oils are considered useful:

Antidepressants

Essential oils such as *basil, bergamot, clary sage, lavender, lemon, geranium, jasmine, neroli, rose, sandalwood* and *ylang-ylang* can be used to alleviate depression.

Antispasmodics

Essential oils such as *Roman chamomile, clary sage, lavender, sweet marjoram, peppermint* and *yarrow* help prevent or alleviate spasms or convulsions and may be beneficial for treating headaches, migraines and muscular spasms caused by nervous tension.

Nervine tonics (nervines)

Nervine tonics strengthen the nervous system. They are useful in cases of shock, stress or nervous debility. Some excellent nervine tonics include *angelica, basil, Roman chamomile, clary sage, juniper, lemongrass, vetiver, rosemary* and *peppermint.*

Nervine relaxants

Nervine relaxants can help alleviate stress and tension. Some excellent nervine relaxants include *Roman* or *German chamomile, bergamot, lavender, lemon, sweet marjoram, melissa, neroli, sandalwood,* and *valerian.*

Soporifics

Essential oils such as *hops, lavender,* and *valerian* help to induce sleep.

Associated conditions

Generally, conditions associated with the nervous system are categorised as:

* psychological disorders
* neurological disorders.

Psychological disorders

The connection between physical and psychological factors in illness is recognised by orthodox medicine as a psychosomatic illness. Psychological factors can predispose or aggravate physical problems, or physical factors can affect the psychological state. It would be more appropriate to view all illness as a relationship between body, mind and soul.

Society is plagued by self doubt, by fear and alienation, by de-humanisation and violence. It is not surprising that at least 25% of all hospitalisation is stress-related.

Stress

Useful Oils
Basil, bergamot, Roman and German chamomile, clary sage, frankincense, geranium, jasmine, lavender, lemon, sweet marjoram, melissa, palmarosa, peppermint, petitgrain, pine, rose, rosemary, sandalwood, vetiver, ylang-ylang.

Stress can be defined as a negative differential between a series of demands and ability to cope with them. We each have a personal comfort level, which may also vary from day to day. Everyone thrives and feels comfortable within this personal sphere, but placed outside of one's comfort zone, stress will quickly manifest.

The body's response to stress will depend on the individual's experience and coping ability, level of health, comfort, hormone balance and social support. Stress keeps the body's survival mechanisms in trim, increasing alertness, muscular strength and other abilities. At the end of a stressful situation, the body should return to its normal balanced state.

However long-term stress caused by worries about money, competition, difficult people, etc., leads to health complications.

The chemistry of stress

Once a stress or a danger has been identified, the hypothalamus secretes into the bloodstream a chemical known as corticotropin-releasing factor (CRF), which then triggers the pituitary gland to release a second chemical known as adrenocorticotropic hormone (ACTH).

As soon as the blood carrying ACTH reaches the adrenal glands, they in turn release adrenal hormones (principally adrenaline and cortisol) into the blood stream. These hormones circulate freely throughout the body to trigger different physiological responses in anticipation of an emergency.

CRF, ACTH, adrenaline and cortisol precipitate a large number of specific changes in neural activities, tissues and behaviour, all designed to prepare the body for the 'flight-fight' response.

This response is designed to get the body moving, usually out of trouble. However an increase in muscle tone, facilitation of sensory reflexes, increase in heart rate, blood pressure and blood sugar level are all of little use in an age when most stresses arrive in the mail, in a traffic jam or at the workplace in which most of us are sitting down. Therefore none of the body's stress responses can be safely diffused by accompanying physical exertion. The effects of sympathetic activity, adrenaline and noradredaline when there is no actual exercise exacerbates all the problems commonly referred to as 'stress diseases'.

Clinical features

Distress can cause psycho-biological reactions which, initially, produce warning signs such as palpitations, insomnia, fatigue and mild depression. This first stage of distress may lead one to resort to quick fix remedies such as coffee, alcohol or tranquillisers, but the long term effect of these 'remedies' has no beneficial properties and may even damage health.

If stress involves chronic nervous arousal, and tranquillisers reduce this arousal, why is it that they are not effective in the long term? Perhaps sedation alone is not sufficient, as it allows no emotional release.

Hans Selye (8) a leading researcher into the effects of stress has developed the notion of the 'General Adaption Syndrome':

- Stage 1 is the initial encounter with stress in which the body rises to meet the challenge of the stress.

- Stage 2 is when the body has adapted to the stress and there is a considerable expenditure of the body's adaptive energy, notably the function of the adrenal cortex.

- Stage 3 is finally one of exhaustion, in which many body functions become impaired.

Life changes can be stress-producing, whether they are negative or positive. To attempt to assess stress levels, two researchers Holmes and Rahe (9), have developed a list of arbitrarily-graded life events scoring from 1-100. The list on this page shows how to rate an individual's stress levels using their system.

Stress is a multi-dimensional syndrome because it involves mind, body and emotions. The symptoms of stress shown on the opposite page involve both behavioural and physiological problems, and the reason for the success of aromatherapy in dealing with stress is that it uses a multi-dimensional holistic approach.

death of a spouse	100	mortgage or loan over $10,000	31
divorce	73	change in work responsibilities	29
relationship or marital separation	65	son or daughter leaving home	29
jail term	63	trouble with parents or in-laws	29
personal injury or illness	53	outstanding personal achievement	28
loss of work	47	starting or finishing school	26
marriage	50	change in living conditions	25
relationship reconciliation	45	trouble with employer	23
retirement	45	change in residence	20
change of family member's health	44	change in school	20
pregnancy	40	change in social activities	18
sexual problems	39	mortgage or loan under $10,000	17
addition to family	39	change in sleeping habits	16
business readjustment	39	Christmas season	12
change in financial status	38	vacation	11
change in occupation	36		

This list indicates the relative numerical value of common stressors. To assess stress levels, an individual should add up the total 'score' of events experienced over the previous 12 months. If the total score is over 150, the individual has experienced a higher degree of stress than usual. If this is the case, stress reduction techniques will need to be employed to offset the negative effects of the stress.

Behavioural	Depression, irritability, aggression, loss of sense of humour
Mental	Depressing thoughts, difficulty concentrating
Physical	Headaches, indigestion, odd aches and pain, palpitations, lethargy, insomnia.

Aromatherapy treatment

Aromatherapy can help both physically and mentally. Aromatherapy's success is due to the benefits from:

- the essential oils
- the massage
- therapist/ client interaction.

The synergy of essential oils and massage is an extremely beneficial combination for dealing with stress. Other therapeutic modalities are often required and lifestyle advice given. Most stressed individuals initially do not feel comfortable visiting a counsellor and find an aromatherapy treatment more appealing and less confrontational. Aromatherapy is considered one of the most pampering of therapies.

According to Tisserand (10) the sensory aspects of aromatherapy are also significant in the treatment of stress. This involves the senses of touch and smell. It is interesting that these are perhaps the most intimate and sensual of our senses, and they are not the ones being stimulated in our work or environment. The fact that aromatherapy is a sensory experience is inherent in its de-stressing action. A lack of sensory input is in itself as stressful as a sensory overload from the senses of vision and hearing.

Many essential oils are available to cope with stress. Initially essential oils that are sedatives and antidepressant oils such as bergamot, Roman or German chamomile, clary sage, frankincense, lavender, petitgrain, palmarosa, orange, sandalwood, vetiver, ylang-ylang and sweet marjoram can be used to induce relaxation to soothe irritability and headaches and overcome insomnia.

After the initial reaction to stress, the body may adapt to the situation for some time and continue to function reasonably well. This adaptation stage places strain on the body, especially the adrenal glands, and if the level of stress increases further, the ability to adapt may break down. Some essential oils strengthen the action of the adrenals and may help in the short term. The most useful of these oils are basil, geranium, lemon, pine, rosemary and peppermint. These oils may also be used when stress has led to muscular aches, chronic aches and persistent infections.

When the stressed individual suffers from psychological problems such as chronic depression and persecution complexes, agoraphobia, guilt, apathy, melancholy and helplessness, essential oils such as rose, jasmine and neroli are recommended.

Other treatments

There are many different ways to relieve stress. The one which is best for the individual should be chosen. The following is a list of suggestions:

- Have a positive image of oneself. Find work or a hobby which gives a feeling of satisfaction or accomplishment.
- The best way to deal with stress is to remove the stressor(s). That is easier said than done, but a realistic perspective of the situation should be obtained, perhaps in consultation with an adviser - financial, psychological, or even just a good listening friend.
- Be positive: Recall successes; let them help through defeats.
- Physical activity can clear the mind and keep stress under control. Some people find running or walking beneficial; others prefer to play team sports. Any type of exercise will be ideal, as long as it is done regularly.
- Meditation is ideal for some people.
- Rest and get enough sleep. This may be difficult, because stress often interrupts sleep patterns. The less sleep obtained, the more stress generated, and the higher the chance of becoming ill, because the immune system will be weakened.

- Herbs such as catnip, chamomile, hops, lemon balm, passionflower, rosemary, Siberian ginseng, skullcap, and valerian which are known as nervine tonics or relaxants may be used.

- Avoid foods that place stress on the system such as cola drinks, fried foods, junk foods, sugar and white flour products. A quality diet, exercise and proper rest are very important.

Anxiety

Useful Oils

Bergamot, cypress, jasmine, lavender, lime, sweet marjoram, neroli, patchouli, rose, ylang-ylang.

Most people have experienced anxiety at some time. Normally the feeling lasts only a short time and is caused by some relevant external problem. Sometimes though, it becomes an habitual pattern, influencing thoughts and behaviour. The world is then perceived as filtered through the attitude of anxiety and people act accordingly. They enter a vicious circle where anxiety produces more anxiety.

Anxiety may reflect the result of a maladaptive attempt to resolve internal conflicts. These conflicts may include unresolved childhood problems such as dependency, insecurity, hostility, excessive need for affection, concerns for intimacy, and overly strong drives for power and control.

The principal components of anxiety are:

- psychological (tension, fears, difficulty concentrating, apprehension)
- somatic (tachycardia, palpitations, tremors, sweating and gastrointestinal upset).

Aromatherapy treatment

Aromatherapy offers a valuable alternative to psychotropic drugs and muscle relaxants that are commonly used in treating anxiety allopathically. Any of the essential oils that act as sedatives may be used. According to Rovesti (11) the following essential oils are used to relieve anxiety: bergamot, cypress, lavender, lime, marjoram, neroli, patchouli and rose.

With such a wide range of essential oils to choose from the aromatherapist should be guided by the client's personality, lifestyle and background and the source of anxiety and the client's individual preference for the smell of the different oils. The individual preference is often revealing. The client will often instinctively select the oil that corresponds to the present state.

Shirley Price suggests the following guidelines in selecting the most appropriate essential oils: (12)

- Top notes are indicated when the mind needs a lift, as in poor concentration and despondency.

- Middle notes are balancing, so are often indicated for mood swings and confusion.

- Base notes are more relaxing and are usually more suited to relieving intense feelings which are difficult to let go, such as grief, panic or fear and are often 'grounding'.

The caring approach of the therapist will be important in dealing with anxiety. Massage and essential oils should be the basis of the treatment because it will allow reassurance and concern to be expressed in the most direct, non-verbal way. Baths using essential oils are very valuable between treatments, as well as having clients wear their favourite essential oils as perfumes or using them in oil burners.

Other treatments

- Avoid all tea, coffee, alcohol or stimulants.

- Avoid all sweets, refined foods, and processed foods.

- Supplement the diet with ginger or use in cooking.

- Avoid monosodium glutamate (MSG).

- Relax by using techniques such as yoga, tai-chi and meditation.

Depression

Useful Oils
Bergamot, Roman chamomile, clary sage, geranium, jasmine, lavender, lemon, mandarin, melissa, orange, palmarosa, petitgrain, rose, sandalwood, tangerine, ylang-ylang.

Depression is a condition which affects most people at some time or another. Often depression is a normal response and part of a process of adapting to loss, grief or crisis.

Aetiology

There are many reasons for depression; among them failure at work, loss of a lover, or death of a relative or friend. Unrelieved anxieties about work, loss of a job, money, health and living conditions can ultimately contribute to a more acute depression. Sadness, general despondency and tearfulness are common symptoms. If there are no signs of these conditions diminishing after a week, proper treatment is required.

Depression may be caused by tension, upset stomach, stress, headache, nutritional deficiencies, poor diet, sugar, thyroid disorders, endometriosis (linked to depression in women), any serious physical disorder, or allergies. It has been discovered that foods greatly influence the brain's behaviour. Diet is often the cause of stress, related to poor eating habits and constant snacking on junk foods. The brain's neurotransmitters which regulate behaviour, are controlled by what is eaten.

The neurotransmitters are dopamine, serotonin and norepinephrine. When the brain produces serotonin, tension is eased. When it produces dopamine or norepinephrine, people tend to think and act more quickly and are generally alert.

Clinical features

The symptoms of depression include:

- present in most depressions
  - lowered mood, varying from mild sadness to intense feelings of guilt and hopelessness

  - difficulty in thinking, including inability to concentrate and lack of decisiveness
  - loss of interest, with diminished involvement in work and recreation
  - headaches, lessened or excessive sleep, decreased sexual drive
  - anxiety.
- present in severe depression:
  - withdrawal from activities
  - physical symptoms worsen, eg, anorexia, insomnia, reduced sexual drive, weight loss
  - suicidal thoughts.

In many cases the client comes to the practitioner to find out if the depression is abnormal, and in a significant number of cases all that is needed is reassurance that the client's depression is not significantly abnormal.

The psychology of depression

I have noticed how depressed people seem to be surrounded by complex, no win, dead end situations. A car may be needed to earn money, but the car is broken down and there's no money to fix the car. There is a desire to exercise but perpetual ill health and fatigue may make it impossible.

There are two important factors to overcoming this initial obstacle. Firstly, the need for change must be accepted and efforts begun in the areas which are found to be least difficult. It may be helpful to list the changes to be achieved and order them from the least to the most difficult.

Secondly there is a need to be prepared to examine and re-evaluate oneself and belief systems and relationships. This process needs to be shared with an impartial and trusted individual, who may or may not be a professional.

The longer depression continues, the more crystallised it becomes. The most serious complication is suicide, which usually includes aggression. The immediate intervention is to seek psychiatric evaluation and counselling to assess the suicidal risk.

When there is a lack of self confidence or an identity problem, individual psychotherapy is oriented towards helping the person change some life situations. In many cases, repressed anger or guilt underlies the depression. Verbalisation and facing these feelings will tend to lessen depression. When depression is secondary to interpersonal problems, family or couple therapy is warranted.

When there is a material loss, welfare services may be recommended and utilised, and when depression is associated with loss of work, vocational rehabilitation is valuable.

Medical treatment

Behavioural disorders such as depression are often associated with fluctuating amounts of particular neurotransmitters present within the brain synapses. It is well known that many drugs and many food constituents may modify normal and abnormal behaviour by changing the amounts of particular neurotransmitters. There are at least forty known types of neurotransmitters available for the brain to use as chemical communicators. These include monoamines such as dopamine, serotonin, noradrenaline and the amino acids glutamate, aspartate, tryptophan, tyrosine, glycine and histidine.

Breggin (13) a leading critic of psychiatric drugs has this to say about the treatment of depression using drugs.

> *'Although it is often possible to help depressed people through caring, enthusiastic psychotherapy, biopsychiatrists typically reject psychological approaches and instead make extraordinary claims for the efficacy of drugs.'*

Many of the traditionally used medications such as the tricyclics and MAO (monoamine oxidase inhibitors) have been recently overshadowed by a new generation of 'selective serotonin re-uptake inhibitors'. Since the introduction of the first of these drugs, Prozac in 1988, there have been at least seven separate serotonin receptors discovered.

However Breggin (13) comments on the pharmacology of Prozac:

> *'Some drugs are used to treat depression on the theory that they enhance serotonergic neurotransmission, this is especially true of the widely used antidepressant, Prozac, but in reality they cause extreme imbalance in the system, including a relative compensatory shutdown of serotonergic neurotransmission.'*

Prozac selectively affects the neurotransmitter serotonin possibly making it more limited in its impact on the brain and mind and less likely to produce complex or dangerous side effects. Breggin suggests that this is a false conclusion, because serotonin nerves spread throughout most of the brain - including the limbic system which governs emotions - thus he says that when a biochemical imbalance is created, many other related neurotransmitter systems, such as dopamine, are forced to undergo changes as well, creating more widespread disruptions.

According to Osiecki (14) nutritional factors may influence neurotransmitters. Dietary alterations in precursor availability may modify neural activity, eg tryptophan influences brain serotonin levels, tyrosine influences brain dopamine and noradrenaline.

A deficiency in vitamin B6 which is involved in converting dihydroxy-phenylalanine to dopamine and 5-hydroxytryptophan to serotonin may result in a decrease of a particular neurotransmitter.

Aromatherapy treatment

An honest look at the factors involved and a courageous re-appraisal of one's life is called for, as essential oils by themselves will not solve the underlying problem. Aromatherapy treatments do have a wonderful energising, uplifting effect on the nervous system and help lift the spirits. The essential oils can help balance, relax and restore the nervous system.

When prescribing an essential oil, care needs to be taken not to use a sedative oil when a depressed person is feeling abnormally fatigued or lethargic. On the other hand, if the depression is taking the form of restlessness, irritability and inability to sleep, such an oil would be ideal. Roman and German chamomile, clary sage, lavender, sandalwood and ylang-ylang are essential oils that are both sedative and antidepressant, while bergamot, geranium, jasmine, neroli, tangerine, orange, and rose are antidepressant but at the same time uplifting.

When anxiety is associated with depression, neroli is considered one of the most valuable essential oils to use. Jasmine should always be used to help boost one's self-confidence.

Massage is an important part of the treatment, because of the contact with the therapist. Baths are ideal home treatment and can be taken every day.

Other treatments

- Depressed people need to talk about themselves, so a sympathetic ear is always useful, as is reassurance of worth, effectiveness and that the bad times will pass. Cheerful companions can help bring a depressed person out of their low state.

- Keep the mind active and get plenty of rest. Avoid stressful situations as much as possible.

- Exercise is a great booster for the spirit, even if it is only a brisk walk with the dog.

- The body will react more quickly to the presence of sugar than it does to the presence of complex carbohydrates. The increase in energy supplied by sugar is quickly accompanied by fatigue and depression. Therefore increase complex carbohydrate intake and reduce sugar intake.

- Vitamin B3 (niacin) deficiency is often associated with anxiety and depression. Vitamin B3 is metabolised into the amino acid trypotophan which has mild sedative qualities. Trypotophan is a precursor of a neurotransmitter, serotonin, which regulates the transmission of electrical impulses within the central nervous system. Irregular serotonin levels are associated with depression, mania and schizophrenia.

- Mineral deficiencies of calcium and magnesium are also likely to lead to nervousness and depression.

- High fat intake can also contribute to depression through slowing the metabolism.

- For women there is the additional complication of premenstrual syndrome. This may be the prime cause of depression and needs to be treated.

Insomnia

Useful Oils

Bergamot, Roman chamomile, lavender, sweet marjoram, petitgrain, neroli, orange, valerian.

Clinical features

Insomnia is a very common complaint and at one time or another everyone has a sleepless night; stress during the day or anxiety about the next day can keep one awake and restless during the night, preventing a peaceful sleep. When this occurs only once in a while, there is nothing to worry about. However, when it becomes a repeated situation in which the whole body suffers then it is classified as insomnia. Very often the inability to sleep is caused by easily remediable factors such as lack of exercise, too many stimulants like alcohol and cigarettes, or eating too late at night.

Since insomnia is largely due to psychological factors, these should be considered and dealt with before inducing sleep pharmacologically.

Aromatherapy treatment

Lavender, Roman chamomile, sweet marjoram and neroli are some of the more effective essential oils. Any of the oils classified as a sedative can be helpful, and it is important to vary the essential oils that are used from week to week.

Bergamot and orange are good oils to be used when insomnia is linked with depression. Any of these oils may be used in a warm bath before bedtime. The water should not be too hot, as this can be stimulating rather than relaxing.

Massage is also very effective in breaking the stress cycle. Most people feel relaxed and possibly drowsy, after a massage, and an evening massage given at home is obviously the very best therapy. A single massage session will often break the vicious circle of sleeplessness though a course of treatment is obviously better if the insomnia has persisted for a long time.

Clinical trials have found lavender to be effective as a nocturnal sedative for elderly patients with sleeping disorders (15). According to observations made by the nursing staff at The

Old Manor Hospital, lavender was found to be very effective (16):

> 'After the aromatherapy started, residents exhibited less restlessness during the night, their sleep was deeper and so they would not be woken while the staff made their rounds, there were fewer periods of simple insomnia and the mood of residents on waking was more pleasant.'

Other treatments

- Reduce stress.

- Foods high in tryptophan, such as bananas, figs, dates, yoghurt and wholegrain crackers, promote sleep. The amino acid tryptophan is a precursor for the neurotransmitter serotonin and has been found to increase total sleep time.

- Avoid consumption in the evening of - caffeine, alcohol, sugar, cheese, chocolate, wine, ham, sausage, potatoes, spinach and tomatoes. These foods contain tyramine, which increases the release of norepinephrine, a brain chemical stimulant.

- Herbs with relaxant properties such as catnip, hops, chamomile, passionflower, skullcap and valerian root are all excellent herbs which can be drunk at bedtime.

- Exercise is important. Try to have an hour's brisk walk during the day, and take a walk after the evening meal. Do some gentle stretching exercises - yoga is particularly beneficial - to help relieve some of the tension of the day.

- Try not to sleep in a room which is too warm, cold or airless as this can lead to sleeplessness.

- Infants with sleeplessness will often respond positively to the removal of cow's milk from the diet.

Mental fatigue

Useful Oils
Basil, bergamot, ginger, grapefruit, lemon, peppermint, rosemary, thyme.

There are many factors including aromatherapy that play a vital role in maintaining memory and reducing mental fatigue. These factors are discussed below.

Blood sugar fluctuations

Of all the factors influencing brain function, blood sugar fluctuation is the most important. The brain cannot store its nutrients and relies almost entirely upon blood glucose for energy. This is why we should never skip a meal. Everyone has experienced brain fatigue and mood swings associated with low blood sugar. Hence to improve brain energy, it is best to eat whole foods, carbohydrates and proteins in balance.

Avoid refined sugars and fats and favour 'low glycaemic response' carbohydrates. These are sugar stabilising whole grains (such as brown rice, wholemeal bread, millet, oats, corn and barley), whole legumes (lentils, chickpeas, kidney beans, peas, peanuts) and whole fruit rather than juice. Combine these with good quality protein (seafood, eggs, chicken, beef) and this will facilitate stable blood sugar. Remember; coffee, teas, cola drinks, chocolate and alcohol will give a quick burst of blood sugar but will ultimately result in fatigue.

Blood flow to the brain

With age the blood flow to the brain is reduced from 106 ml/100 gm of brain tissue per minute for a six year old to 58 ml/100 gm in the elderly. Surprisingly, cerebral blood flow and oxygen consumption by the brain are not affected by mental effort, such as solving a mathematical problem. They are, however, affected by emotional stress which causes muscle tension, changes in breathing, heart rate and other physiological parameters which are under hormonal control.

The greatest effect on blood flow to the brain is caused by atherosclerosis (hardening of the arteries). One of the major causes of atherosclerosis is free radical-induced damage to the vessel walls. Two major sources of these free radicals are chemicals from cigarette smoke and alcohol which trigger oxidation of cholesterol and other dietary fats. These oxidised fats are the danger which initiate a chain of events which cause the arteries to harden. By preventing or minimising atherosclerosis not only will we drastically reduce the possibility of coronary failure but also reduce presenile dementia, short-term memory loss and the incidence of tinnitus just to mention a few.

A diet rich in anti-oxidant nutrients which include vitamins C, E, A and beta-carotene is recommended. The best natural sources of vitamin C are parsley, blackcurrants, green capsicum, broccoli and all fresh fruit and vegetables. Beta-carotene is especially high in dandelion greens, carrots, dried apricots, sweet potato, spinach and mango and plenty of vitamin A is found in liver, eggs and butter. The best sources of vitamin E are sunflower seeds, hazelnuts, vegetable oils and almonds.

Brain micro-nutrients

Nutrients such as vitamin B12, folic acid, magnesium, calcium, selenium and zinc play an important role in facilitating brain function. Low folic acid levels are associated with apathy, disorientation, poor concentration and short term memory loss. This situation is most likely to occur in people who do not eat enough fruit, salads and vegetables, all of which are high in folic acid. As well as poor dietary intake, malabsorption or digestive problems can cause low levels of folic acid and B12.

Herbs

Ginkgo biloba leaf extract is used to treat disorders associated with insufficient blood flow to the brain. There have been many studies demonstrating a statistically significant regression of the major symptoms of cerebral vascular insufficiency and impaired mental performance, including short-term memory loss, vertigo, dizziness, headache, ringing in the ears, hearing loss, lack of concentration, depression and delayed reaction time.

Gotu kola is a natural nerve tonic. It slowly builds stamina, is an excellent treatment for

nervous breakdown and is used to improve memory (17).

Another herb traditionally used in Ayurvedic medicine is *Bacopa monniera* which is used to improve memory and learning and to promote longevity. It is also used for nervous breakdowns and exhaustion. (18)

Panax ginseng and Siberian ginseng, *Eleutherococcus senticosis* contain adaptogenic (stress-overcoming) substances called ginsenosides. Both herbs aid mental function and restore mental abilities. (19)

Skullcap is one of the best nervines in the plant kingdom and is traditionally used to treat insomnia, nervous tension and pain. It is also used to remove nervous tension which probably interferes with learning, recall, logical thinking and memory formation. (20)

Exercise

Deep relaxed breathing is fundamental to mental health. This is why a brisk daily 30 minute walk or equivalent (ie, swimming, jogging, bike riding) is one of the best ways to increase oxygenation of the blood. Unfortunately most daily physical movements are anaerobic (ie, they do not require much oxygen). Minor oxygen starvation can cause a build-up of carbon dioxide and lactic acid in the muscles and blood. People suffering from anxiety and panic attacks have been found to have elevated lactic acid in their blood and would benefit from increased oxygenation.

Meditation

Most people experience an incessant flow of thoughts from one day to another. The more complex life becomes, and the faster the pace, the greater the mental and emotional pressures. Personal relationships become strained, the pressures to succeed and to secure personal power, money and status tend to dominate one's thoughts while at the same time the fear of failure is just around the corner.

Through meditation one can facilitate a state of mind which allows this incessant mental activity to subside. There are many ways to meditate, but the objective remains the same. That is, to give the mind and body deep rest, thus facilitating a richer, more conscious, stress-free life.

Meditators tend to become mentally very alert; have a wider perspective and are free from mental chaos; have an improved mental activity; have a better ability to concentrate; and have fewer memory lapses. When the brain is not bogged down with mental clutter it operates more smoothly and, above all, with greater reliability.

Aromatherapy treatment

Essential oils classified as cephalics or stimulants can help reduce mental fatigue, though it would be very unwise to over-use any of them. Basil, peppermint and rosemary are considered the best essential oils to use as an inhalation if preparing for examinations.

If your client wakes up feeling tired a bath with five drops of rosemary provides a wonderful lift. Other essential oils which have an uplifting and restorative effect include lemon, grapefruit, ginger and thyme. Please avoid using peppermint or basil in a bath because they are skin irritants.

Neurological disorders

So far we have discussed problems manifesting mainly through psychological causes. We now turn to aromatherapy treatment of problems that manifest themselves within the nerve tissue itself.

Headaches

Useful Oils
Cajeput, Roman chamomile, clary sage, eucalyptus, lavender, sweet marjoram, peppermint, rosemary, rosewood, thyme.

Clinical features

Headaches are a common symptom that may be due to a wide variety of causes, including emotional disorders, head injuries, migraine, fever, intracranial vascular disorders, dental disease, diseases of the eyes, ears, or nose, or intracranial masses.

Certain types of headaches are frequently observed to be associated with specific clinical entities. Throbbing, pulsating headaches are more likely to be encountered in vascular diseases such as migraine, arterial hypertension, and intracranial vascular malformations.

Pressure headaches, a sensation of tightness with a constricting band-like feeling about the head, are often due to emotional stress. A steady dull headache is often encountered in patients with intracranial masses or head injuries. Muscular contraction or spasm associated with excessive fatigue or emotional tension is most frequently involved in 'occipital' headaches. There may be a feeling of pressure or tightness or band-like constriction around the head associated with emotional tension. Tension headaches are by far the most commonly encountered headaches.

Aromatherapy treatment

There are many essential oils that can be used to relieve headaches. The most effective essential oils are lavender, rosemary and peppermint. A drop of lavender rubbed on the temples or a cold compress of peppermint or lavender is useful. Lavender is a sedative and would be more useful for headaches in which there is much muscular and emotional tension, while cajeput, rosemary, eucalyptus or peppermint which are stimulants, is better used for headaches due to mental fatigue or caused by catarrh or sinus infection.

Other treatments

- A good night's sleep, a nap, exercise, fresh air, a change of scenery, general relaxation, deep breathing, a wet compress on the face and neck, cold water on the forehead and back of the neck may all help to dispel a simple headache.

- Those who frequently suffer from headaches may have a food allergy to wheat, chocolate, monosodium glutamate, sulphites, sugar, luncheon meats, citric acid, fermented foods, alcohol, vinegar or marinated foods.

- Herbs such as lemon balm, chamomile, peppermint, rosemary, skullcap, thyme, valerian and sage may relieve headache pain.

- Acupressure will not bring about permanent relief for headaches, but it will relieve the symptoms and take away the sharp edge of the pain. However in the case of nervous and influenza headaches, acupressure can work miracles, often clearing up the headache in a matter of minutes.

  - Frontal headaches can be relieved by pressing LI 4 which is located in the webbing between the thumb and the index finger.

  - The following points are also recommended for the treatment of headaches: GB20, Bl 2, Tai Yang and Lv 3.

  - Yin tang, located directly between the eyebrows, in the indentation where the bridge of the nose meets the forehead relieves hay fever, headaches and eye strain.

Migraines

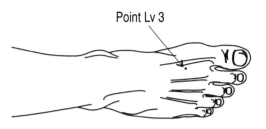

Useful Oils

Roman chamomile, clary sage, lavender, sweet marjoram, peppermint, valerian.

Clinical features

Migraine is a particular type of headache which occurs paroxysmally. Constriction of certain cerebral arteries takes place at the onset of the attack, but later these vessels dilate and cause characteristic headache.

There are three characteristic groups of symptoms:

- Visual disturbances may occur at the beginning of the attack. Usually they take the form of flashes of light, spots or patterns before the eyes, but sometimes partial loss of vision.

- A severe throbbing headache which usually commences on one side of the head and may last for several hours.

- Nausea and vomiting are frequently associated with the headache.

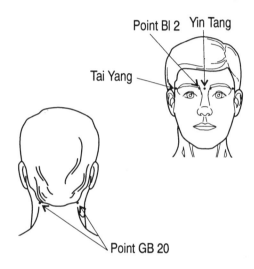

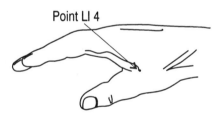

Acupressure points used to relieve headaches

Aetiology

The cause is unknown. However a number of triggers have been identified:

- injury to the head associated with contact sports such as football or boxing

- sudden changes in weather, particularly thunderstorms or hot dry winds

- hypoglycaemia and missing meals

- emotional stress may precipitate an attack

- fluctuations in hormonal levels - drops in oestrogen levels, particularly premenstrually
- food allergies have been identified as a precipitating factor in 80 to 90% of cases.

Aromatherapy treatment

Aromatherapy is better used as a preventative measure than as an attempted treatment for migraine. Once a migraine attack has begun, many sufferers find the smell of most essential oils overbearing or can't bear being touched.

A cold compress made with equal parts of peppermint and lavender should be placed across the forehead and temples and frequently changed as soon as it starts to warm up. Extremely light massage of the temples with lavender oil might be useful if touching the head does not make the pain worse. Many migraines seem to be due to restricted blood supply to the brain, and hot or warm compresses with sweet marjoram on the back of the neck will increase the flow of blood to the head. Sweet marjoram is a vasodilator, and warmth itself also helps.

Other treatments

- Feverfew, ginkgo biloba extract, peppermint and rosemary are very effective herbs in the treatment of migraines. A recent survey found that 70% of 270 migraine sufferers who had eaten feverfew daily for prolonged periods claimed that the herb decreased the frequency of their attacks (note that fresh feverfew leaves may cause mouth ulcers). (21)
- Foods such as chocolate, cheese and alcohol have been reported to trigger migraine attacks. They contain the amino acids phenylalanine and tyramine which are considered vasoactive amines. (22)
- Avoid stimulants such as coffee, tea, coke, nicotine and alcohol.
- Avoid nitrates (preservative found in hot dogs and salami), aspirin, and monosodium glutamate (MSG), a common seasoning.
- Increase consumption of cold water fish or fish oils.

- The use of acupuncture in the treatment of migraine headache has received considerable research attention. Acupuncture appears to have some success in reducing the frequency of migraine attacks. One study found that 40% of the subjects experienced a 50-100% reduction in the severity and frequency. (23)

Epilepsy

Useful Oils
Roman chamomile, cedarwood, clary sage, lavender, neroli.

Clinical features

Epilepsy is characterised by seizures, which are caused by electrical disturbances in the nerve cells in one section of the brain. These seizures vary in their severity. Petit mal seizures are mild - the person will stare into space and may twitch slightly. Grand mal seizures are more extreme - the person will have convulsions, falling to the ground, often becoming unconscious.

Aetiology

Epilepsy can be caused by infections, meningitis, rickets, rabies, tetanus, malnutrition, hypoglycaemia, sports injuries, head injuries, fever or allergies. It may result from scar tissue from an eye injury or a stroke, lack of oxygen, spasm to the blood vessels and arteriosclerosis. It is thought that it may be hereditary.

There are several types of seizures classified as follows (24):

- *Absence (petit mal)*. Most common in children and characterised by a blank stare. During these seizures children are unaware of their surroundings.
- *Atonic (drop attack)*. A childhood seizure in which the child loses consciousness for about ten seconds after the legs have collapsed.
- *Complex partial (temporal lobe)*. Blank stares, random activity, and chewing motion are characteristic of this type of seizure. The person may be dazed and

unaware of the surroundings, and may act oddly. There is no memory of this seizure.

- *Generalised tonic-clonic (grand mal).* Characterised by sudden cries, a fall, rigidity and muscle jerks, shallow breathing and bluish skin. Loss of bladder control is possible. The seizure usually lasts two to five minutes, and is followed by confusion, fatigue, or memory loss.

- *Myoclonic.* Brief, massive muscle jerks occur.

- *Simple partial (Jacksonian).* Jerking begins in the fingers and toes and progresses through the body while the person is conscious.

- *Simple partial (sensory).* The person may see, hear, or sense things that do not exist. May occur as a preliminary symptom of a generalised seizure.

Aromatherapy treatment

There are a number of essential oils that can provoke epileptic fits in people who are susceptible, so before any aromatherapy treatment be certain that the person does not suffer from epilepsy.

+---+
| **CAUTION** |
| Any person prone to epileptic seizures should avoid use of the |
| following oils: |
| Hyssop, sage, fennel, wormwood and rosemary. |
+---+

Tim Betts (25) a consultant neuropsychiatrist suggests that the conventional medical approach which uses medications, surgery and occasional dietary measures does not take into account the psychosomatic condition associated with epilepsy. Betts used essential oils as an effective counter measure in a trial conducted at the Seizure Clinic of the University of Birmingham. Patients who were anxious and didn't know how to relax selected a relaxing essential oil and used it in conjunction with self hypnosis techniques to effectively prevent seizures from occurring.

Essential oils such as lavender are anti-convulsive, however do not attempt to treat epilepsy unless you have formal medical qualifications.

Robert Tisserand (26) presents case studies in the use of essential oils for people with epilepsy. He suggested that some essential oils have particular characteristics that have specific actions on the psychological state. All the oils used (Roman chamomile, cedarwood, clary sage, neroli, melissa) were calming.

According to Tisserand the conclusion was that essential oils significantly reduce seizure rates, although maintenance of orthodox treatment was still necessary. It was not possible to identify the anti-convulsive properties of the oils used, or the relaxed state induced by the treatment. There was an excellent relaxation response to aromatherapy, and it helped the individuals to learn to relax.

High anxiety levels and traumatic or stressful life events can precipitate seizures for individuals with epilepsy. It is at this level that aromatherapy can help. Aromatherapy can be used for balancing and harmonising so that the individual's ability to deal with intrinsic and extrinsic dis-ease improves. As a result there appears to be a decrease in the seizure rate.

Other treatments

First Aid for seizures is as follows:

- Move sharp or dangerous objects away from the person.

- Place the person on a bed or the floor.

- Loosen tight clothes.

- Turn the person on the side, if possible.

- Do not put anything in the person's mouth. Swallowing objects is more dangerous than biting the tongue.

- Stay calm and remember that the person feels nothing during the seizure.

Other general recommendations to reduce the frequency of seizures are:

- Avoid alcoholic beverages, animal protein, caffeine, artificial sweeteners such as nutrasweet, and nicotine. Avoid refined sugars and foods.

- Eat small meals, don't drink a lot of fluid at once.

- Stay away from pesticides.

Shingles

Useful Oils
Bergamot, lavender, melissa, rose, tea tree.

Clinical features

Herpes zoster, or shingles, is an acute infection of the sensory nerve roots. The disease is caused by a virus which is closely related or identical to the chicken pox virus. It most commonly affects middle-aged or elderly people. The virus affects the sensory nerves before they enter the spinal cord and causes clusters of blisters on the area of skin served by the affected nerves. The pain is usually felt before the blisters appear and will persist sometimes for weeks or months after the blisters have disappeared.

Aetiology

- Burning pain and hypersensitivity of the skin in the affected segments are the first symptoms. There may be associated fever or malaise.

- After three or four days there is a skin eruption consisting of papules which later become vesicular and crusted.

- The skin of the affected area may become insensitive, although pain may persist for several months.

- The trunk and the face are the regions most commonly affected. When the trigeminal nerve is affected, eruptions may appear on the cornea of the eye. Unless treated promptly, blindness may ensue.

Aromatherapy treatment

The analgesic and anti-viral properties of bergamot, tea tree, melissa, rose and lavender are very helpful in easing the pain, soothing the irritation, combating the virus and drying the blisters.

It is interesting to note that bergamot which is one of the most active oils in inhibiting the herpes virus also has the benefit of being one of the finest anti-depressants.

The best way of applying the essential oils is to make a 3% dilution in apricot kernel oil and gently apply it to the areas of blisters and pain. If large areas are affected use the essential oils in a bath. When the pain persists long after the blisters have disappeared, lavender and chamomile can be used.

Chapter 26

Lymphatic System

This chapter summarises an holistic approach to the treatment of many common ailments and conditions associated with the lymphatic system.
Not only have the aromatherapy procedures for each condition been outlined, but details have also been included on other forms of treatment such as diet, herbs, acupressure and exercise.

Conditions discussed in this chapter include:

The effects of poor lymphatic circulation
Cellulite
Lymphoedema

Introduction

The role of the lymphatic system has always been of paramount importance in holistic therapies. The tissues of the body and organs excrete waste products as a result of their daily work. The waste products must be quickly removed or the tissues will suffer damage. The cleansing process of the body is performed by a mechanism called lymphatic circulation. This chapter will investigate the structure and the function of the lymphatic system and how the use of essential oils and specific massage techniques can increase its efficiency.

Structure of the lymphatic system

The lymphatic system comprises a network of both superficial and deep vessels which are found in all parts of the body except the brain, spinal column and areas such as bone marrow and cartilage that receive nutrition through diffusion rather than from blood vessels.

The two main structures of the lymphatic system are the lymph capillaries, vessels and larger ducts, which make up the network for the transport of lymph, and the lymph nodes, which are the filtering devices. Unlike the circulatory system, the lymphatic system has no pump and relies on muscular compression and general body activity for moving the lymphatic fluid around the body.

The lymph nodes are the filtering sites for the lymphatic fluid, which resembles blood plasma but contains less protein and more lymphocytes. The lymph nodes are composed of lymphoid tissue, and are found near veins. There are about 600 to 700 lymph nodes found singly or in groups throughout the body. Those most easily felt on the body surface are the cervica (in the groin), the popliteal fossa (behind the knee), the occipital area (base of the skull), and the cupital area (at the elbow).

The spleen, thymus and tonsils are considered lymphatic organs, and the breast is largely made up of lymphatic glands and vessels.

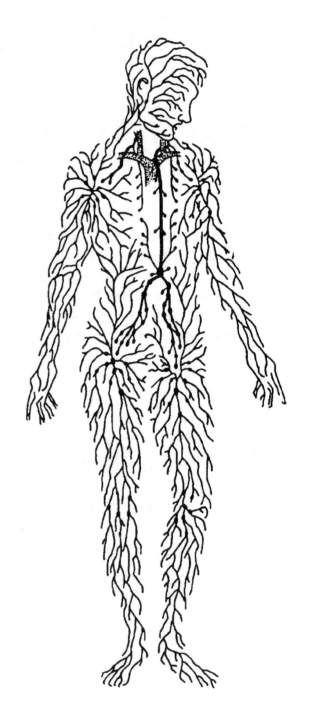

The lymphatic system

The functions of the lymphatic system

The lymphatic system serves three major functions in the body:

- draining excess fluid from the body cells and tissues
- helping provide immunological defences
- absorbing and distributing fat soluble nutrients.

Draining excess fluid from the body cells and tissues

One of the main functions of the lymphatic system is to control the volume of fluid circulating in the body. Interstitial fluid consists of blood plasma, which filters through the thin walls of the capillaries into the surrounding connective tissues. Most of the proteins in the plasma remain in the blood, and this helps to draw some of the fluid back into the capillaries by osmosis.

The interstitial fluid is vital to the cells. It brings moisture and nutrients, picks up waste products of cell metabolism, excess proteins, bacteria, viruses and inorganic materials such as chemicals, to be transported to the organs of elimination. At rest the lymph system will drain away about 1.2-2.0 ml of 'dead fluid' per minute. Not all the fluid is drawn back into the capillaries, and this becomes lymph, which is absorbed into the lymphatic vessels and transported to the lymph nodes for filtering. During activity the lymph system can drain away about 20 ml of 'dead fluid' per minute. (1)

Poor lymphatic drainage results in excessive fluid in the tissues, which causes oedema and a strain on all the organs responsible for excretion of fluids. Pronounced oedema may in fact be a sign of heart or kidney disease and should not be neglected. If this is suspected, a medical practitioner should be consulted.

Because the lymph system does not have a pump like the heart it can become sluggish and inefficient, particularly if we get little exercise and have a poor diet, which strains the cells with waste products that are difficult to eliminate.

Helping provide immunological defences

The lymphatic system helps fight infections in two ways:

- Lymph nodes manufacture lymphocytes, which make up 23% of the white blood cells. Lymphocytes in turn manufacture antibodies, which are complex proteins with the capacity to neutralise invading organisms. The enlargement of lymph nodes indicates the production of large numbers of lymphocytes when an infection is present, or when the body is on the defensive. Granulocytes, which are white blood cells made in the bone marrow, also help in this process, and ingest foreign bacteria in a process known as phagocytosis. They migrate out of the capillaries and accumulate around areas of infection to engulf the invading microbes.

Fever is a natural rise in the metabolic rate which allows the body to produce increased white blood cells and antibodies. Lymphocytes and antibodies are also produced in the spleen and thymus gland. The spleen also filters lymph like a large lymph node, and contains considerable lymphoid tissue.

- Lymph nodes also filter the lymphatic system. They comprise a network of fibres in which are found white blood cells called macrophages which ingest foreign bodies as the lymph passes through the nodes.

Absorbing and distributing fat soluble nutrients

In the small intestine, small lymphatic vessels are in contact with the intestinal wall. The villi, which are minute projections on the wall, enclose lacteal ducts which are also in contact with small lymphatic vessels. Blood capillaries are also found in the villi. Sugars, minerals, amino acids, water soluble vitamins and a few fatty substances are absorbed into the blood stream via these capillaries. Fatty nutrients and the fat-soluble vitamins are absorbed into the lymphatic system via the lacteals, directly via the hepatic portal system of the circulatory system, or indirectly via the lymphatic system. These nutrients are carried to the liver, where fat soluble vitamins are stored. They are also carried to the cells for nourishment. There are also small lymph nodes in the small intestine which provide antibodies against micro-organisms that may find their way there.

The effects of poor lymphatic performance

When the lymphatic system does not work well, the resulting condition is known as congestion. Congestion is a form of lymphatic stagnation. The lymph is filled with waste products that pass through the lymph nodes. The lymph nodes fulfil the function of filter beds. These nodes form secretions and possess cells which have the ability to neutralise, dissolve, destroy or take up debris or waste products which may be in the body.

The liver, one of the biggest detoxification plants in the body, is responsible for neutralising and eliminating a large number of toxins. However, when the lymph nodes and the liver are unable to cope with the toxins, the toxins are diverted towards and can ooze through the mucous membranes and other emergency elimination sites. This 'oozing' is a common condition known as catarrh or inflammation of the mucous membranes. This is the cause of every form of 'itis'.

This serves as the basis for understanding how the essential oils and naturopathic principles can be applied in eliminating toxins from the body, treating many conditions associated with toxic overload and restoring the body to good health.

Even though the lymph system acts as a modern sewage treatment plant, it is literally vital for the maintenance of life because when this system fails to function properly, excessive fluid and toxins build up in the body causing pain, loss of energy, infection and various diseases.

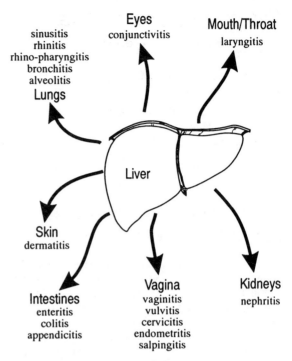

When the liver is overloaded with toxins the above emergency elimination pathways are utilised.

How aromatherapy can assist lymphatic problems

Aromatherapy can help overcome some of the problems associated with the lymphatic system. Essential oils with the following properties are recommended.

Diuretics

Any essential oil which increases the flow of urine has diuretic properties which stimulate the kidney and accelerate the detoxification process. Typical oils include fennel, grapefruit, cypress, lemon, juniper, mandarin, orange and tangerine and they are often employed in conditions where water is retained in the body.

CAUTION
Excessive use of juniper oil has been known to cause kidney irritation.

Circulatory stimulants

Stimulating the circulation will also stimulate the flow of lymph. Oils such as black pepper, ginger or rosemary may be used in a lymphatic massage blend.

Increasing leucocytosis

Gattefosse (2) first commented on the cytophylactic (increased activity of leucocytes against infection) powers of the essential oils. He comments on observations made by Dr P. Sassard who used lavender oil:

Wounds to the scalp: healed in 10 days;
Infected herpes vesicle: healed in 5 days;
Firearm wound: healed in 15days;
Sacral bedsore due to a thigh fracture in a 68 year old woman: healed in 11 days.

In all cases, the following was noted: rapid disappearance of pus; decrease in the number of bacteria; powerful stimulation of healing; recovery in a very short time.

Apart from lavender, essential oils such as bergamot, lemon, rosemary, tea tree and thyme will increase the body's ability to manufacture white blood cells.

Alteratives, blood cleansers, depuratives or detoxifiers

Most essential oils will to some degree stimulate phagocytosis, that is, the ability of the white blood cells to 'gobble up' and clean up microbes and toxins.

According to Mills (3), tissues may be cleansed by improving the function of the major eliminatory channels in the body. These remedies are classed as 'blood purifiers', 'depuratives' or 'alteratives'. They may of course have conventional anti-inflammatory action or may otherwise change metabolic functions. All of these help in the elimination of excess waste products and make the job of the lymphatic system easier.

Oils such as angelica, carrot seed, German and Roman chamomile, everlasting, sweet fennel, juniper, geranium, lavender, lemon and rosemary may be used.

Bactericidal, antiviral and antifungal

Dr Jean Valnet (4) speaks at great length of the antiseptic powers of essential oils. He lists essential oils of eucalyptus, clove, niaouli, thyme, garlic, sandalwood, lemon, cinnamon, lavender, German chamomile and peppermint as being particularly beneficial.

> *'The essential oil of lemon for example according to the works of Morel and Rochaix can neutralise the meningococcus in 15 minutes, the typhus bacillus in less than an hour, pneumococcus in 1-3 hours and staphylococcus aureus in 2 hours.'*

Dr Kurt Schaubelt (5) discusses the fact that aromatherapy is proving to be an unrivalled modality for the management of chronic viral infections. He cites studies in the treatment of *Herpes simplex* virus.

> *'Immediate application of melissa or other essential oils prevents the viruses from replicating. If this is accomplished, the process is shortened considerably or a new outbreak is completely inhibited.'*

Stimulating lymph and tissue fluid circulation

Many essential oils such as orange, grapefruit, juniper berry, cold pressed lime, tangerine, peppermint and rosemary will stimulate lymph and tissue fluid circulation.

According to Dr Gumbel (6) peppermint is a key oil for the lymphatic system. He mentions that it stimulates lymph and tissue fluid circulation, and:

> *'has a special connection to everything aqueous, to blood, to tissue fluid, lymph, spinal and cerebral fluid. The refreshing effect on all tissues lies in the liberating influence on the lymphatic stream......The oil has a cleansing, purifying and antiseptic effect on mucous membranes. It accelerates and increases their resorption ability.'*

Other considerations

Lymphatic problems can also be helped by using specific lymphatic drainage massage techniques. Aromatherapy massage techniques developed by Maury and Arcier incorporate lymphatic massage.

The Micheline Arcier aromatherapy massage technique described in this book uses the neuro-lymphatic reflexes. These reflexes are also called 'Chapman's reflexes' (7). The positions of the reflex points do not necessarily correspond to the positions of the lymph glands. The reflex points act like circuit breakers in that they 'turn off' when the system is overloaded. By gently massaging these points the lymphatic function will be stimulated.

The best known system of lymphatic massage was developed by Dr Emil Vodder. Dr Vodder developed a system of movements which drained the lymph nodes and relieved the symptoms. He spent 40 years developing a system of lymphatic drainage massage which is now taught all over the world.

It is important that the contraindications of lymphatic massage must be observed rigidly. Lymphatic massage should not be performed on anyone who has active cancer, heart problems, thrombosis, phlebitis, high blood pressure, varicose veins, pregnancy, any acute inflammation or infection, or any other severe medical problem. Do not use these techniques on anyone who has recently undergone chemotherapy, since the toxins stored in the blood and liver will be released into the bloodstream and make the person feel very ill.

In all work on the lymphatic system, diet is of utmost importance, because a highly refined diet full of chemicals and potentially toxic by-products makes the job of waste removal much more difficult. Anyone serious about improving the lymphatic system must stop smoking, eliminate junk food, red meat, coffee, tea, alcohol, refined white sugar, flour and milk products from their diet.

An exercise program is also important. Baths with the appropriate essential oils and adding epsom salts can be useful and brisk friction over the body using a loofah or body brush should also be incorporated.

In conclusion, Simon Mills (6) suggests in his 'Toxic Thesis of Disease' that:

'The process of removing waste materials from the body is essential to health;

several eliminatory functions share the task: failure in supression of one will lead to extra burdens and possible signs of distress in others, and will have potentially widespread implications for general health.'

Cellulite

Useful Oils
Carrot seed, cypress, fennel, ginger, juniper berry, grapefruit, geranium, lemon, cold pressed lime, mandarin, orange, rosemary, sage, thyme.

Cellulite is an accumulation of water and toxic wastes in the connective tissue surrounding the fat cells, which in turn forms nodules. It starts with a build up of toxins which cause the body to react via water retention in an effort to dilute the toxins and prevent self poisoning. The tissue around the fat cells tends to harden, imprisoning the water and causing the unsightly bulges.

Cellulite is seen almost exclusively in women. The reason for this is the basic structure of the subcutaneous tissue which is disturbed in cellulite. The basic construction of the subcutaneous tissue of the thighs in men and women is shown below:

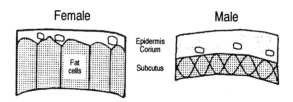

The anatomical basis of cellulite

In women, the uppermost subcutaneous layer consists of what are referred to as 'large standing fat-cell chambers', which are separated by radial and arching dividing walls of connective tissue anchored to the overlying connective tissue of the skin (epidermis). In contrast, in men the uppermost part of the subcutaneous tissue is thinner and has a network of crisscrossing connective tissue walls. The epidermis is also thicker in men.

A simple test to demonstrate these differences is the 'pinch test'. Pinching the skin will result in the 'mattress phenomenon,' pitting, bulging and deformation of the skin as shown below.

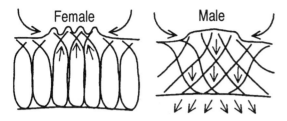

The 'Pinch' test

As women age, the epidermis becomes progressively thinner and looser (8). This allows fat cells to migrate to this layer. In addition, the connective tissue walls between the fat cell chambers also become thinner, allowing the fat cell chambers to enlarge excessively. The breakdown or the thinning of connective tissue structures is a major contributor to the development of cellulite. Histological examination reveals distension of the lymphatic vessels of the upper epidermis and a decrease in the number of subepidermal fibres (9).

Other contributing factors to cellulite include:

- hormonal imbalance
- poor blood circulation
- accumulation of wastes
- unbalanced diet
- abuse of stimulants (coffee, tea, cigarettes, alcohol)
- lack of correct exercise
- stress and emotional upheaval
- poor breathing
- constipation
- incorrect posture.

Medical statistics show that when there is greatest hormone fluctuation, cellulite may occur in women (10). Typically this is:

- at the onset of puberty (12%)
- when first going on the pill (19%)
- during pregnancy (17%)
- during menopause (27%).

Oestrogen is responsible for female sexual development. Another important role of oestrogen is that it helps to eliminate waste materials from the vital organs and deposit them into areas where they will be relatively harmless. Therefore it may be assumed that cellulite forms when there is a general circulatory problem in the body because the lymphatic system is unable to dispose of the body's wastes in the normal way. Cellulite was first thought to have a hormonal component when French doctors realised that cellulite does not normally occur in men.

Since the mid-1960s, with the introduction of the contraceptive pill and hormone replacement therapy for post-menopausal women, the amount of oestrogen present in women's bodies has increased enormously. The more oestrogen present, it seems the more likely it is that cellulite will develop.

Therapeutic considerations

It must be kept in mind that cellulite is not a 'disease' per se. While there is little that can be done to decrease the amount of oestrogen circulating in the body, it is possible to reduce the level of toxins that the body has to deal with. Therefore the holistic approach to the treatment of cellulite is to reduce the level of toxins by incorporating the following techniques into the treatment regime:

- exercise
- massage
- diet
- aromatherapy.

Exercise

Exercise can be very effective once most of the cellulite has been eliminated. Although cellulite is partly caused by a sedentary lifestyle, vigorous exercise will not make the slightest difference to cellulite deposits that are already there. In fact, many forms of exercise, particularly impact sports such as jogging or aerobics may place extra pressure on the joints and encourage the cellulite to harden and become even more compacted.

Massage

Massage, particularly lymphatic, is very beneficial, as is self-administered massage with hand or brush. The physical effects of massage improve circulation of the blood and lymph. The direction of the massage should always be from the periphery to the heart.

Diet

Dietary considerations are basic:

- A diet high in complex carbohydrates and low in refined carbohydrates and fats is very important.

- Cut out junk food, anything greasy, fatty, refined, sugary or salty.

- Natural diuretic herbs such as fennel and dandelion tea work as blood cleansers by stimulating the liver and kidneys.

- Celery juice and lemon juice are also worthwhile taken daily.

The anti-cellulite diet should contain lots of green leafy vegetables and basic whole foods and should follow these general rules:

- To make digestion easier, eat a limited number of foods at each meal.

- Reduce salt intake as salt tends to promote the retention of fluids in the tissue; cellulite is partly a result of excess water storage in the connective tissue.

- Avoid taking fluids with meals or for half an hour afterwards, as liquids cause food to pass into the blood stream before it has been sufficiently digested. Drink liquids 20 minutes before or between meals.

- Drink purified water or mineral water with a low salt content, and fresh vegetable and fruit juices rich in minerals that cleanse the body.

- The following foods are recommended as they are easily digested and provide varied nutrition needed for maintenance, regrowth, repair and detoxification:

  - proteins of animal origin: lamb, poultry, fish, eggs; meat should be lean and prepared by roasting or grilling

  - proteins of vegetable origin: wholegrains, cereals, legumes, lentils, soya beans

  - dairy products: skim milk, natural cottage and fetta cheese, natural yoghurt.

Aromatherapy

Essential oils which are detoxifying, stimulating to the lymphatic system, hormone balancing and which have diuretic properties need to be used. The essential oils must be used in a massage and bath. While daily self massage will be necessary, regular professional aromatherapy massage which uses lymphatic drainage techniques is also recommended.

The following aromatherapy detoxifying bath formula is suggested:

epsom salts	100gm
grapefruit	10 drops
geranium	20 drops
rosemary	10 drops
juniper berry	20 drops.

Add 50 gm of this preparation to a bath. Another suggestion is to add the above essential oils to 100ml of dispersing bath oil and add 10ml of this preparation to a bath.

The following massage oil blends should be alternated weekly, making sure the massage oil is used at least once a day and a professional aromatherapy massage is obtained once a week. Blend into 100 ml of apricot kernel or other suitable carrier oil:

Formula 1

juniper berry	15 drops
rosemary	10 drops
lemon	20 drops
geranium	15 drops.

Formula 2

fennel	10 drops
cypress	10 drops
grapefruit	20 drops
juniper berry	20 drops.

Formula 3

cypress	10 drops
juniper berry	15 drops
cold pressed lime	10 drops
rosemary	20 drops.

A complete anti-cellulite programme should consist of:

Pre-programme

Cut out:

- smoking
- alcohol
- coffee.

Programme

Take up:

- detoxifying diet for 3 weeks
- dry skin brushing daily before bath
- massage daily after bath.

Post-programme

Keep up:

- exercise
- healthy diet
- skin brushing daily
- regular massage.

Lymphoedema

Useful Oils

Carrot seed, cypress, fennel, juniper berry.

Lymphoedema, a swelling of subcutaneous tissues due to obstruction, destruction, or increase in the lymph fluid in the lymph vessels. Lymphoedema may be primary or secondary. The primary type can be present from birth, or may occur during puberty or, less frequently, later in life. It is due to an abnormal increase in the number of normal cells in the lymph vessels. The sufferer complains of swelling of the foot, leg, or entire extremity. It is usually unilateral and it is worse during warm weather and prior to menstruation.

Secondary lymphoedema is often a result of infection. The onset is explosive, with chills, high fever, toxicity, and a red, hot, swollen leg. The treatment for secondary lymphoedema is to immediately treat the infection.

Therapeutic considerations

The aromatherapy treatment strategy is reduction of the swelling by stimulating the lymph flow by using lymphatic drainage massage techniques, and using cool compresses of essential oils such as juniper berry, fennel seed and cypress. The legs should be elevated and the use of firm elastic support to be worn during the day is also recommended.

Chapter 27

Immune System

This chapter summarises an holistic approach to the treatment of many common ailments and conditions associated with the immune system.
Not only have the aromatherapy procedures for each condition been outlined, but details have also been included on other forms of treatment such as diet, herbs, acupressure and exercise.

Conditions discussed in this chapter include:

Infection
Tissue inflammation
Fever
Allergies
Candida albicans
Myalgic encephalomyelitis

Introduction

Twenty-four hours a day our body is at war. Millions of micro-organisms are continually attempting to invade and occupy our organs and tissues. If it was not for the highly sophisticated immune system, we would succumb.

However our immunity often succumbs when exposed to deadly viruses such as the one in the book *The Hot Zone* (1) by Richard Preston in which he describes the anguish that the character Monet suffers from the ebola virus:

'The headache begins, typically on the seventh day after exposure to the agent.....His eyeballs ached, and then his temples began to ache, the pain seemed to circle around inside his head. It would not go away with aspirin, and then he got a severe backache.........Then on the third day after the headaches started, he became nauseated, spiked a fever and began to vomit. His vomit grew intense and turned into dry heaves. At the same time, he became strangely passive. His face lost all expression of life and set itself into an expressionless mask, with eyeballs fixed, paralytic, and staring. The eyelids were slightly droopy......The eyeballs themselves seemed almost frozen in their sockets, and they turned bright red. The skin of his face is yellowish, with brilliant starlike red speckles. He began to look like a zombie.'

The story continues as Monet finds himself on a small plane on the way to hospital:

'He is holding an airsickness bag over his mouth. His eyes are the colour of rubies, and his face is an expressionless mass of bruises.......The connective tissue in his face is dissolving, and his face appears to hang from the underlying bone, as if the face is detaching itself from the skull. He opens his mouth and gasps into the bag, and the vomit goes on endlessly. The bag fills to the brim with a black vomit. The black vomit is not really black; it is a speckled liquid of two colours, black and red, a stew of tarry granules mixed with fresh red arterial blood. It is haemorrhage, and it smells like a slaughter house.'

This is the true account of one of the world's most deadly viruses - the Ebola virus. As the author explains, the virus is multiplying in its host. It can saturate the body with virus particles, from the brain to the skin. When this amplification peaks, an eyedropper of the victim's blood may contain a hundred million particles of virus. During this process the body is being transformed into virus particles. In other words, the host is possessed by a life form that is attempting to convert the host into itself. The transformation in Monet's case was not entirely successful and the end result was a great deal of liquefying flesh mixed with virus. This occurred in Monet, and the sign of it is the black vomit. To find out the fate of Monet I suggest you read *The Hot Zone*, by Preston as he describes the virus which kills nine out of ten of its victims.

Why was Monet's immune system not able to deal with the ebola virus? Why are we encountering many problems that the immune system cannot cope with, such as AIDS, cancers, allergies and viral infections?

With this in mind let us begin our discussion on the immune system. What we often refer to as pathogens or micro-organisms may actually be:

- viruses
- bacteria
- fungi
- parasites.

The common misconception is that these pathogens that produce many diseases are malevolent little beasts out to destroy higher forms of life. In fact, all they are trying to do is survive and reproduce, just as we are. Human suffering and death are merely unfortunate by-products. The table opposite lists the number of people killed by infectious diseases in 1990, according to the World Health Organisation. (2)

In order to understand how our immune system deals with these pathogens, it is necessary to discuss each of the above micro-organisms individually.

Viruses

Viruses are very adaptable and successful life forms (or near-life forms; they cannot survive on their own). For a virus to grow and multiply it must enter an environment of specific cells that will become unwilling hosts. Viruses are therefore parasites, living off other organisms.

A virus is composed of genetic material in the form of DNA. Once it has invaded a cell, it can

Infectious disease	Cause	Annual deaths
Acute respiratory infections	Bacterial or viral	4,300,000
Diarrhoeal diseases	Bacterial or viral	3,200,000
Tuberculosis	Bacterial	3,000,000
Hepatitis	Viral	approx 2,000,000
Malaria	Parasite	1,000,000
Measles	Viral	880,000
Neonatal Tetanus	Bacterial	600,000
AIDS	Viral	550,000
Pertussis (Whooping cough)	Bacterial	360,000

The number of people killed by infectious diseases in 1990

then reprogram the cell's DNA inside the nucleus to manufacture copies of the virus. The infected cell will then fill up with new viral particles, the cell membrane bursts, releasing the viruses which happily go on invading other cells causing extensive damage. When a virus is reproduced by a cell it has just invaded, it is often wrapped in an envelope made of a combination of protein and fatty material. This often allows the virus to live undamaged for extended periods of time outside the body.

Unfortunately there are very few effective antiviral agents that have been developed. Therefore viral infections are essentially private battles fought between the virus and the immune system. To date, most success in handling viruses has come from developing vaccines that stop the infection in the first place.

The most common way that a virus enters the human body is through direct contact with the infected secretions of another infected organism. We can easily inhale viral particles as a good sneeze will often expel millions of viral particles.

While vaccines have been relatively successful in taming viral organisms such as smallpox, measles and polio, viruses which have gone undetected for centuries keep being discovered. Many of these viruses such as the ebola virus described in the introduction have made the jump from monkeys to humans, simply because people

are slowly destroying the natural habitat of the animals and the viruses. Dr Robert Shope (2), a Yale epidemiologist says,

'We know of at least 50 different viruses that have the capacity of making people sick that inhabit the Brazilian rainforest. There are probably hundreds more that we have not found'.

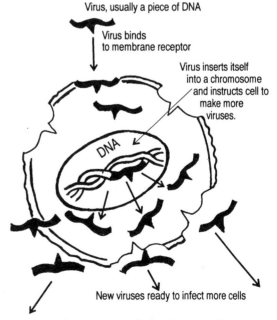

A virus invading a host cell

Bacteria

Bacteria are very different from the viruses discussed previously, mainly because bacteria are complete life forms. Unlike viruses, they are not parasites and do not need a host to reproduce. The bacteria that cause tetanus by secreting a toxin that can paralyse nerves live just as happily in the soil as they do inside the human body. Bacteria consist of one or more cells, and are much bigger than viruses. Bacteria just eat and divide constantly, and they thrive when the conditions are right. Bacteria can harm us in at least three ways:

- As they multiply in the body, they may secrete poisonous chemicals (toxins) and disturb one or more bodily functions. Some may block the ability of the cells in our intestinal tract to absorb water into our body which would lead to diarrhoea, or others may paralyse our nerves.

- Bacteria may invade body tissue such as the lungs and multiply so quickly that staggering numbers of them can accumulate, interfering with the function of the lungs, causing pneumonia.

- When our immune system comes to the rescue and mounts a vicious attack on the invading bacteria, our own tissue is often caught up in the battle and may be damaged. Such tissue destruction results in an abscess, and the chemically digested remains of the bacteria and those parts of our cells that were accidentally destroyed are known as pus.

There are thousands of species of bacteria. Bacteriologists can identify bacteria and then doctors can apply a treatment (usually antibiotics) known to be effective against the specific organism. However, bacteria are especially wise in the ways of evolution (3):

'Bacteria develop resistance to antibiotics for the same Darwinian reason that gazelles evolved speed in response to lions. When a colony of bacteria is dosed with, say, penicillin, most die. But a few lucky microbes, by chance,

Microbe	Disease caused	Antiobiotics that no longer work
Enterococcus	blood poisoning, surgical infections	aminoglycosides, cephalosporins, tetracycline,
Haemophilus influenzae	meningitis, ear infections, pneumonia, sinusitis	chloramphenicol, penicillins, tetracycline, trimethoprim/ sulfamethoxazole
Mycobacterium tuberculosis	tuberculosis	aminoglycosides, ethambutol, isoniazid, pyrazinamide, rifampin
Neisseria gonorrhoeae	gonorrhoea	penicillins, spectinomycin, tetracycline.
Plasmodium faciparum	malaria	chloroquine
Shigella dysenteriae	severe diarrhoea	ampicillin, chloramphenicol, tetracycline, trimethoprim/ sulfamethoxazole
Staphylococcus aureus	blood poisoning, pneumonia, surgical infections	all but vancomycin
Streptococcus pneumoniae	meningitis, pneumonia	aminoglycosides, cephalosporins, chloramphenicol, erythromycin, penicillins, tetracycline, trimethoprim/ sulfamethoxazole

Some of the microbes that have now become resistant to antibiotics

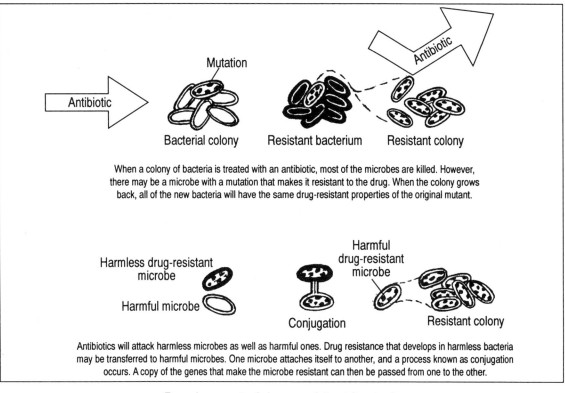

Development of drug-resistant bacteria

harbour mutant genes that make them immune to the drug. They survive, just as speedy gazelles live to romp another day, while the slower-footed herd mates become dinner. The mutants pass on their resistant genes to their progeny - one bacterium can leave 16,777,220 offspring within 24 hours.'

In the past, pharmaceutical companies typically found new antibiotics by chance. Nowadays rather than building antibiotics molecule by molecule, researchers are turning to nature. Most pharmaceutical companies are searching everywhere from the bottom of the sea to the jungles of Borneo for the next bacteria-killing compound.

While tea tree oil has been used since the 1920s recent research conducted at the Australian National University has proven that tea tree oil effectively treated 60 different varieties of *Staphylococcus aureus*, 29 of which had become immune to treatment with antibiotics. It was also

surprising to find that the tea tree oil concentration used was only 0.25%. (4)

Fungi

Everyone has come in contact with some fungi. Moulds are fungi and they can grow on a piece of bread or crawl up a shower curtain. There are thousands of fungi, the great majority of which are harmless to humans. Fungi possess a simple membrane-bound nucleus which contains their genetic information and the walls of the fungi are made up of polysaccharides.

As is true of bacteria, not all fungi cause disease, in fact some can be beneficial,such as the fungi that are used to make cheeses, yoghurt and fermented drinks. More than 200 species of fungi are known to cause disease in humans. In people with depressed immune systems fungal infections of the skin, intestinal tract, lungs and brain are frequent.

One particular fungus, known as candida has come under the spotlight. This fungus happily inhabits your intestinal tract. Defence mechanisms have been developed to ensure that bacteria found in the intestines will not harm us but work in our favour. The bacteria make vitamins for us and break down proteins to help us digest and reassimilate the essential nutrients that we eat.

However, the bacteria can get out of hand very easily and may grow so rapidly in our intestinal tract that they swamp our defence mechanisms. To prevent this from happening the candida organism, which is naturally found in human intestines, competes with bacteria for essential nutrients. An ecological balance is maintained that prevents excessive growth of either bacteria or fungi.

It is common for anyone who has been treated by antibiotics, that the bacteria in the gastrointestinal tract may have been killed. As a result the candida fungus can spread up and down the intestinal tract. Candida may emerge in the mouth as a white coating on the tongue (commonly referred to as thrush).

Parasites

A parasite is anything that depends on others in one way or another for its ability to survive without contributing to the wellbeing or the survival of the organism on which it depends. In biological terms, a virus could be a parasite. However, the term parasite often refers to those usually large and complicated organisms that produce long-standing infections in humans and other animals, particularly in the developing countries.

According to Professor John Dwyer, one of the world's most experienced immunologists, diseases such as malaria, trypanosomiasis, leishmaniasis and filariasis are usually responsible for most human sickness and death (5).

Parasites can be divided into two major groups, the protozoans and the helminths. The protozoan family is made up of many different types of organism. One of these is responsible for malaria which is one of the world's most serious infectious diseases, although the hepatitis B and AIDS viruses are closing in on the title.

'Helminth' is the technical term for worms. There are three major types of worms that are found in humans. Some are round worms, while others are flat, commonly known as flatworms or tapeworms. The latter can cause dogs and humans much trouble. The third type of worm is the fluke. This type of worm produces the disease schistosomiasis in 200 million people around the world.

The parasite that causes malaria matures in the salivary glands of a particular family of mosquito which is the host for the parasite. When a mosquito bites it secretes and injects saliva which contains a substance which stops the blood from clotting before it begins to feast on the blood. Of course the malaria parasites in the mosquito's saliva now find themselves in the victim's bloodstream.

Many deaths from malaria occur because the parasitic organism produces severe anaemia, destroying too many red blood cells. Most victims develop an uneasy truce with the parasite. It does not kill them, nor are they able to kill it and a chronic state of ill health is established.

The organisation of defence

The body's protection against intrusion from outside may be compared to a high security system for a very important industrial complex. This system is designed to keep intruders out and detect immediately any that do make it into the complex. The security problem is made more difficult by the fact that, during the day, the complex employs thousands of people. These employees need to be readily identifiable, and of course provoke no response from the security forces.

The human body continually attempts to maintain balance by counteracting harmful stimuli in the environment. These harmful stimuli are often disease-producing organisms, referred to as pathogens. Defence against pathogens is grouped into two broad areas:

- non-specific resistance
- specific resistance.

Non-specific resistance

The first line of defence is the physical barrier such as the skin which makes it physically difficult for an intruder to get in. Unfortunately if the skin has been damaged the intruders are able to easily enter. Moreover, when the skin is moist, as in hot humid climates, dermal infections, especially fungal infections such as athlete's foot, are quite common. The mucous membranes and mucus also inhibit the entrance of many intruders, and trap microbes in the respiratory and digestive tracts.

Chemical barriers such as the high acidity of gastric juice, which is a collection of hydrochloric acid, enzymes, and mucus produced by the glands of the stomach, are sufficient to preserve the usual sterility of the stomach and destroy almost all bacterial toxins.

The acid pH of the skin, the unsaturated fatty acids and lysosomes (antimicrobial substance in perspiration, tears, saliva, nasal secretions and tissue fluids) also discourage the growth of many microbes that come in contact with the skin. In addition to the mechanical and chemical barriers of the skin and mucous membranes, the body produces certain antimicrobial substances. These include interferon, complement and properdin.

Host cells infected with viruses produce a protein called interferon. Once released from virus-infected cells, it diffuses to uninfected cells and binds to surface receptors, allowing the uninfected cell to synthesise another antiviral protein that inhibits intracellular viral replication. Interferon appears to be effective in reducing the virulence of viruses associated with chickenpox, genital herpes, rabies, rubella, chronic hepatitis, shingles, eye infection and at least one type of common cold.

Complement is a group of eleven proteins found in normal blood serum. This group is called complement because it 'complements' certain immune and allergic reactions involving antibodies. Properdin, like complement, is also a protein found in serum. Working together with complement, properdin is able to destroy several species of bacteria, increase phagocytosis and trigger inflammatory responses.

Phagocytosis

When microbes penetrate the skin and mucous membranes or bypass the antimicrobial substances in the blood, there is another non-specific resistance of the body called phagocytosis. Phagocytes are able to ingest and destroy any microbes or any foreign particles.

When an infection occurs phagocytes appear on the scene. Phagocytes include neutrophils and monocytes (which later develop into macrophages). Both are types of white blood cells. Neutrophils have the most prominent phagocytic activity. Monocytes follow the neutrophils into the infected area. Once in the tissue they become transformed into wandering macrophages. They are named as such because they leave the blood and migrate to the infected area. Other macrophages, called fixed macrophages are found in the liver, lungs, brain, spleen, lymph nodes, subcutaneous tissue and bone marrow.

Since fixed macrophages can be either reticular (forming a supporting network) or endothelial (lining a mucous membrane) they are referred to as cells of the reticuloendothelial system (RES). Wandering macrophages augment the phagocytic activity of fixed macrophages. In addition, fixed macrophages mobilise under the stimulus of inflammation and wandering macrophages also migrate to the infected area. The neutrophils predominate in the early stages of infection, but tend to die off rapidly. Macrophages enter the scene during the infection. They are several times more phagocytic than neutrophils, and are large enough to engulf tissue, and invading microbes.

Specific resistance: immunity

The mechanisms involved in non-specific resistance are designed to protect the body from any kind of pathogen. The specific resistance to disease, called immunity, involves the production of a specific antibody to destroy a particular antigen. The ability of the body to defend itself against invading agents such as bacteria, toxins, viruses and foreign tissues consists of two closely allied components, known as cellular (cell-mediated) immunity and humoral immunity.

- Cellular (cell-mediated) immunity consists of the formation of specially sensitized lymphocytes that have the ability to attach to the foreign agent and destroy it.
- Humoral immunity consists of circulating antibodies which are able to attack an invading agent.

Cellular immunity and humoral immunity are the product of the body's lymphoid tissue. The lymphoid tissue consists primarily of T cells which are responsible for cellular immunity and B cells that provide humoral immunity. Both types of lymphocytes are originally derived in the embryo from lymphocytic stem cells in the bone marrow.

About half of these cells migrate to the thymus gland, which is often referred to as the university where the cells will undergo rigorous training after which they will be able to react to a specific antigen. Cellular immunity is activated when the T- lymphocytes recognise the foreign antigen or another cell membrane, releasing lymphokines and activating macrophages to ingest the offending cell vigorously.

The thymus gland actually graduates four functionally and physically distinct types of T cells. They are the:

- **Killer T cell.** These are equipped with arsenol which is able to damage/or kill cells which are harbouring an organism such as a virus. The killer cells also secrete a substance which attracts macrophages to the site of the invasion where they can destroy the antigens by phagocytosis.
- **Helper T cell.** These are the scouts which will sound the alarm as soon as they recognise a foreign invader.
- **Suppressor T cell.** These are also known as the immunoregulatory cells. They can be seen as the Generals in charge of the intensity and duration of the battle waged by the attacking cells. They are responsible for determining appropriate

vigour of the immunological attack and for restraining the uncontrollable natural killing urge of the Killer T cells.

- **Delayed Hypersensitivity Producing T cell.** These T cells, once activated, call the macrophages in for help by secreting chemicals which attract the macrophages to assist in battle. This process, in humans, can require 48 hours of preparation.

While the function of T cells is impressive they do have some limitations. The body not only contains thousands of different T cells, it also contains thousands of B cells, each capable of responding to a specific antigen. Whereas Killer T cells leave their reservoirs of lymphoid tissue to attack a foreign antigen, B cells are less likely to patrol the body looking for trouble. They are based

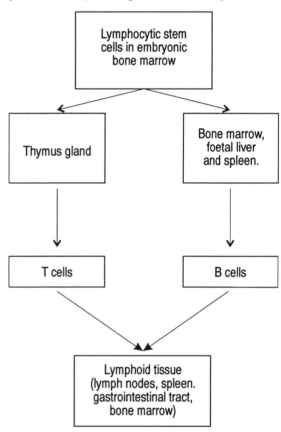

Origin and differentiation of T cells and B cells

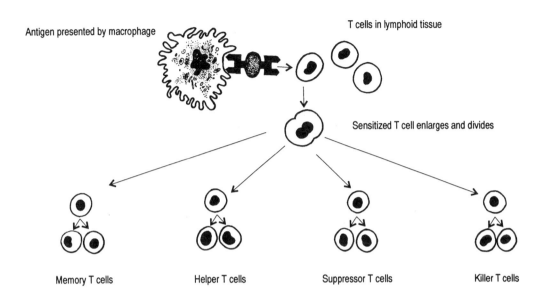

Antigen presented by macrophage

T cells in lymphoid tissue

Sensitized T cell enlarges and divides

Memory T cells

Helper T cells

Suppressor T cells

Killer T cells

The role of T cells in cellular immunity

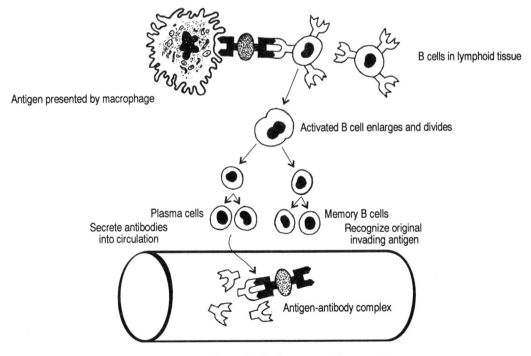

B cells in lymphoid tissue

Antigen presented by macrophage

Activated B cell enlarges and divides

Plasma cells
Secrete antibodies
into circulation

Memory B cells
Recognize original
invading antigen

Antigen-antibody complex

The role of B cells in humoral immunity

in the lymph nodes, where they wait for foreign antigens to be presented by the macrophages. When this occurs, B cells specific for the antigen presented are activated. The activated B cells then enlarge and divide into plasma cells which secrete the antibodies.

Plasma cells are factories that produce and secrete about 2,000 antibody molecules per second for each cell, and this occurs for several days until the plasma cell dies. The idea is to flood the body with these antigens which can attack any antibody that has been lucky enough not to be trapped in a lymph node. These cells, unlike the majority of T cells, have a relatively short lifespan and thus our bone marrow must replenish the supply constantly throughout life. The activated B cells that do not differentiate into plasma cells remain as memory cells, ready to respond more rapidly and forcefully should the same antigen appear at a future time.

For thousands of years, doctors have pondered the mechanisms of immunity. The ancients knew that a patient who had recovered from a specific infectious disease would usually not succumb to it again. Towards the end of the 19th century scientists discovered that serum (serum is the blood without the cells that circulate in it) contained a protective element. They noticed the ability of serum to damage micro-organisms, leading to the discovery of antibodies. The term humoral was derived from the fact that early scientists referred to the chemicals in the serum as the 'humors'. The 'humors' were in fact composed of antibodies and chemicals belonging to the complement system. Today we know that antibodies are specifically made up of globulins such as gammaglobulins or immunoglobulins.

When a baby is given a first shot of vaccine against diphtheria, pertussis and tetanus, the vaccine stimulates the baby's B cells that can recognise these organisms.

Immunity and the mind

There is now considerable anecdotal evidence that immunity and resistance to disease are linked to attitudes and behaviour. For many years positive imagery and positive thinking have been used in the treatment of cancer. However it has been only recently that sufficient scientific evidence has been collected to confirm this association. David Felton, a Professor of Neurobiology and Anatomy, discusses the physical link between the nervous system and the immune system (6):

'Why would a lymphocyte have a receptor for a neurotransmitter? So we started studying immunologic changes that occur when you use drugs to affect the neurotransmitters. Much to our surprise, we found that if you took the nerves away from the spleen or the lymph nodes, you virtually stopped immune responses in their tracks....The practical implication was that the many stressors we face in life, which affect the autonomic nervous system, might have an impact on the immune system.'

He continues his discussion by saying that at this stage we still do not understand some of the brain chemistry of emotion. However, it is quite clear that the higher centres of the brain can generate signals that very clearly influence hormonal production. There is a huge production of adrenaline and noradrenaline from the sympathetic nervous system and the adrenal gland under certain conditions. One study at UCLA used actors and actresses who were told to think of a scenario, and generate in their own minds a feeling that comes with it. While they did this, their hormones in the blood were tested, and changes in hormone levels and subtle changes in the immune system were noted.

Recent studies have shown that depression as a psychological state is not sufficient on its own to predict a diminished immune system. However, depression does play a role in that the more severe the depression, the more likely it is that a decreased measure of immune response will be found.

One study, using medical students during examinations, was surprised to find chronically diminished immune responses not in those at risk of failing their exams but in those students who were lonely and had poor social support. (7) The same reference discusses the benefits of college students visiting someone in a nursing home on a weekly basis. Most family members and social workers probably don't realise the effect their interaction is having on the chemistry and pharmacology of the nervous and immune systems of a person they are visiting in hospital or in a nursing home.

Dr Kidman, a Sydney psychologist (8), is hoping that therapy designed to boost self-esteem and improve state of mind can be used to help people with diseases such as cancer to live longer. People diagnosed with cancer frequently suffer

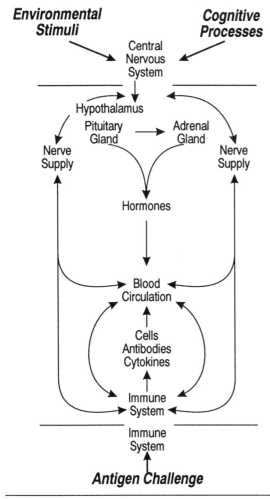

Environmental Stimuli

Cognitive Processes

Central Nervous System

Hypothalamus

Pituitary Gland → Adrenal Gland

Nerve Supply

Nerve Supply

Hormones

Blood Circulation

Cells Antibodies Cytokines

Immune System

Immune System

Antigen Challenge

The brain and central nervous system interact with the immune system via a number of pathways. It is now well documented that the activities of one system can profoundly influence the outcome of responses in the other.

stress-related symptoms such as depression, anxiety and anger.

> *'The stress that accompanies cancer may actually impede the recovery process. For this reason, many psychologists feel it is important that patients learn to develop effective coping skills that will help maintain a positive state of mind.'*

Dr David Spiegel, a Professor of Psychiatry and Behavioural Science at Stanford University, made a major breakthrough in this area by conducting weekly therapy sessions for women with advanced breast cancer with the aim of helping the women deal with emotional distress and manage pain. He taught the women relaxation techniques and how to better express their emotions. Ten years later Dr Spiegel found that those who had received the therapy had survived twice as long as those who hadn't. (9)

It has been proven that touching during early development, before weaning, greatly increases the number of small neurons in certain parts of the brain. (10)

Therefore holistic aromatherapy treatment may be considered effective for people with a weakened immune system since it offers:

- pharmacologically active essential oils
- aromatherapy massage which stimulates the mind/body connection
- psychotherapeutically active essential oils.

When immunity fails

Infection

Useful Oils
Bay, bergamot, cajeput, clove, cinnamon, eucalyptus, lavender, spike lavender, lemon, lemongrass, niaouli, oregano, pine, rosemary, tea tree, thyme.

The role of infection by micro-organisms is often over emphasised. The details of this have already been discussed in Chapter 8.

As Simon Mills indicates (11):

'any attitude that says that bacteria, fungi, viruses, every form of mosquito, fly and other pest, is always evil, always to be attacked, is unimaginative and counter-productive as any jingoistic nationalism.'

Mills sees the role of these pathogens as the fungus on the forest floor, whose role it is to help decompose all the flora that die and fall to the forest floor. This vital role played by these 'saprophytic' organisms ensures that fallen dead trees decompose, releasing nutrients into the ground and thus maintaining the delicate ecocycle.

Most pathogens are also classified as saprophytes. They do not come out of the blue to strike down an unwary victim. Rather, they colonise only where there is unhealthy tissue. The common cold is considered the cause of much misery, however searching for its cure is like searching for the Holy Grail. Antibiotics, of course, have no effect on viral infections. However the misuse of antibiotics has created many problems and a recent survey found that seven out of ten Americans receive antibiotics when they seek treatment for the common cold. (12)

A recent article revealed that Golden Staph *(Staphylococcus aureus)* is one of several staph bugs which have become immune to antibiotics and which thrive in state-run hospitals, killing otherwise healthy patients indiscriminately. The article reported that one-third of all staph bacteria was now antibiotic resistant.

However new research conducted at the Australian National University has reported on the excellent wide spectrum antimicrobial activity of tea tree oil. The research team tested 60 different varieties of the staph bugs, 29 of which had become immune to treatment with antibiotics. All 60 varieties were successfully treated with a tea tree oil concentration of 0.25 percent. (13)

Essential oils can be effectively used in treating conditions of the immune system:

- Through their anti-microbial action they work directly against micro-organisms.

- Through their immune-stimulant action they boost the body's own defences.

- Through their depurative properties they eliminate accumulations of waste material and toxins that become a prime environment for microbes to breed.

According to Dr Daniel Penoel (14) who has extensively used essential oils in the medical treatment of infectious diseases, the following conclusions can be drawn:

- There are close relationships between the bacteria that live inside the organism and the general state of health, not only physically but also psychologically.

- Each organism has its specific bacterium, even if the bacteria of different organisms are identified by the same name.

- Essential oils respect the protective commensal flora of the organism, which is of the utmost importance for genuine and long-lasting results. Antibiotics, which are still being used or misused by most doctors, on the contrary, generate bacterial organisms with immunity to the antibiotic, having far-reaching consequences.

While antibiotics have played an important role in modern medicine in the battle against bacterial infections, the development of antiviral drugs has not lived up to the same expectations. This is largely because a virus does not show all the qualities of a living organism until it invades the host cell. This means that:

- Viruses are difficult to inactivate chemically and usually require highly toxic agents to do so.

- Once a cell is infected it is difficult to selectively inhibit the virus without harming the cell.

Viruses also exhibit rapid rates of mutation which can make immunity difficult to sustain. The world is currently facing the prospects of major chronic viral epidemics in the form of AIDS, hepatitis B and Epstein-Barr. The holistic approach to viral infections is to support the immune system.

Much interest has focussed on plants as strong allies in restoring immune strength and inhibiting the spread of virus-mediated diseases. The immune enhancing properties of echinacea have been well documented. (15) (16) (17)

While most of the studies have examined water or alcohol extracts, more recently studies have commenced on the antiviral properties of essential oils. Dr Pierre Franchomme in France has used essential oil of *Thymus vulgaris,* thuyanol 4 chemotype, for the treatment of chlamydia infections (18). According to Franchomme's studies, enveloped viruses are sensitive to essential oils with a predominance of terpene-alcohols and phenols. Naked viruses are sensitive to essential oils with a large proportion of terpenoid-ketones. (19)

Dr Penoel suggests using essential oils with high proportions of terpene alcohols, such as α−terpineol, and oxides, such as 1,8-cineole commonly found in the oils of *Laurus nobilis, Eucalyptus radiata,* and *Melaleuca quinquenervia viridiflora,* for the treatment of influenza caused by the myxovirus. (20) Other oils suggested by him include *Melaleuca alternifolia, Eucalyptus globulus* and *Lavendula spica.* The recommended methods of application are external applications in the form of aerosols and internal applications in the form of suppositories. Dr Penoel claims that if such an aromatic treatment starts at the onset, the disease can be defeated in the first day. (21)

As discussed previously, the essential oils have a two fold effect. One is the direct action of the oil on the pathogen and the other is the powerful action on the host. The effect of the essential oil on the host's immune system is known as the immune-stimulant effect. Comparative tests show that clients who received essential oils of *Melaleuca alternifolia, Origanum vulgaris, Melaleuca quinquenervia viridiflora* or *Thymus vulgaris* (thuyanol 4 chemotype) had higher levels of immunoglobulins after the test period than before.

Dr Penoel stresses the importance of using sufficient amounts of essential oil. The oils are used internally and externally. However, as the bulk of essential oil is applied externally, the actual quantity in the course of the day may reach 12 ml without any problem. This type of intensive treatment should produce significant improvements within two to three days. (22)

If inflammatory conditions also exist, essential oils with high aldehydes will be required, and excess mucus treated with essential oils with a high proportion of ketones. As can be seen essential oils not only control the pathogen but also strengthen the client's immune system.

Tissue inflammation

Useful Oils
German chamomile, clove, cinnamon, everlasting, ginger, lavender, nutmeg, thyme, yarrow.

Many disease states have inflammation as a component of distress. In order to successfully deal with inflammation it is necessary to understand the actual process that leads to it. The initial stages of inflammation are:

- dilation of blood vessels in the area with consequently greatly increased blood flow

- increased permeability of the capillaries in the area allowing fluid to leak into the tissues

- migration of leucocytes (and later macrophages) through the leaky capillary wall into the tissues.

The total effect leads to the breakdown of damaged tissue and foreign material with sufficient pain and immobility, so that the area is protected from further damage. If this is completely successful, healing occurs.

If on the other hand, healing cannot keep pace with the rate of damage, the inflammation becomes chronic, and inflammatory and repair processes occur simultaneously. The inflammation becomes increasingly counter-productive. This can often result from:

- persistence of some foreign material at the inflamed site, such as chemicals, metabolites (eg uric acid), insoluble particles such as silica and asbestos, etc.

- infection by certain pathogens, such as tuberculosis or syphilis, where phagocytic activity is compromised and hypersensitivity develops to persistent allergens

- autoimmune diseases, also marked by hypersensitivity to persistent antigens.

In all cases of chronic inflammation there is a shift in the population of phagocytes. The neutrophil leucocytes that are responsible for resolving acute inflammation are replaced by macrophages, and also by eosinophil leucocytes. Most cases of inflammation are conditions whose names end in 'itis'. Chronic conditions such as arthritis, bronchitis, sinusitis, rhinitis, colitis, gastritis, hepatitis and dermatitis, to name a few, are the most common problems in clinical medicine.

Modern medicine is primarily concerned with treating these 'itis' as if inflammation is the core of the problem. In traditional natural therapies, inflammation is an indication that the body has recognised a problem and is engaging it. It is a call for support of the active participants in inflammation, those mediators responsible for increasing blood flow, and the phagocytes responsible for resolving the damage. It may be seen as the body's resolving what could possibly be a long-standing malady.

Unfortunately chronic inflammations are usually resistant to conventional drug treatment. Anti-inflammatory drugs such as steroids and aspirin-derived drugs often alleviate the symptoms while they are being administered but have possible negative long-term effects. The prospects for a sufferer of chronic arthritis, ulcerative colitis or sinusitis are not improved by conventional medicine, although the symptoms may be eased, and patch-up surgery often used to repair damaged tissue.

Traditional remedies used in inflammatory diseases have been found to possess circulatory stimulating, diuretic, laxative, choleretic, digestive stimulating or any other eliminating effects. (23)

The topical application of German chamomile has been well documented for its anti-inflammatory properties. The presence of both the lipophilic (principally the sesquiterpenes) and the hydrophilic (principally the flavonoids) groups greatly contribute to the anti-inflammatory action. (24) The flavenoids in particular are involved in the suppression of histamine release. (-)-α–bisabolol promotes granulation and tissue regeneration. Originally much attention was paid to the presence of chamazulene as the primary anti-inflammatory constituent, but in recent years both the flavonoids and (-)-α–bisabolol have been acknowledged as the primary constituents. (25)

Other essential oils such as nutmeg, thyme, clove and cinnamon oil also have been reported as having pronounced anti-inflammatory effects (26). However these oils are also well known as skin irritants and the anti-inflammatory effect has not been fully explained. It seems that through skin irritation the skin reflexes release binding endogenous substances, whereby the local inflammation process is influenced.

Osiecki (27) recommends the following for their anti-inflammatory effects:

- avoiding all processed and refined foods
- not smoking and avoiding all tea, coffee and alcohol
- taking supplements of vitamins C and E
- taking supplements of evening primrose oil and fish oils
- taking supplements of fresh or dried ginger.

Fever

Useful Oils
Cinnamon, eucalyptus, ginger, peppermint.

Fever can promote much fear in a patient and can be equally troubling to the practitioner. Fevers have in the past been the most common cause of death, and some, such as the plague, smallpox, typhoid and cholera, have been notoriously destructive.

The traditional naturopathic approach is that fever plays a major role in the body's defence against infection. Its effect up to a point is beneficial. The higher temperature is believed to inhibit the growth of some bacteria and viruses. Morever, the heat speeds up the rate of chemical reactions and the activity of some white blood cells.

According to Mills the following points will assist in interpreting the results (28):

- Feeling cold, having a pale cyanosed skin and shivering means that the body temperature is lower than the thermostat setting in the hypothalamus, and is most likely to be still rising.

- Feeling hot, having a flushed skin and sweating means that the body temperature is higher than the thermostat setting, and is most likely coming down.

- Having no dominant feeling of being hot or cold suggests relative equilibrium between thermostat and body temperature.

Apart from the usual techniques for bringing temperature down, such as cold wet face flannels or tepid baths, there is aspirin. This simply switches the thermostat controls down without attending to any of the other aspects of the fever. Essential oils and herbal remedies by contrast appear to be beneficial.

If fever is in the safe and optimal range (38.9° to 39.4°C), or if a high fever (above 39.4°C) is accompanied by sweating, which is a sign that the temperature is dissipating, and there are no contraindications, the fever is best left to run its course naturally. When treatment is indicated, the following approaches are recommended:

- The classic treatment for fever is bed rest.

- The digestive system rests when temperature exceeds 38.1°C. Gastric acid secretion decreases as fever intensifies, reaching zero in most persons when the temperature reaches 39.4°C, and resuming when temperature falls to normal. (29)

Fasting, which febrile people tend to do automatically, is the treatment of choice in moderate to high fevers (30). Clinical evidence shows that fasting prevents the temperature from rising too high. In adults, fever rarely exceeds 39.8°C if they are not fed. In children, a properly managed fever may occasionally reach 40°C for a short time. (31)

- Increase water intake to prevent dehydration.

- Light, nourishing, easily digestible foods are recommended to promote recovery after the fever.

According to Holmes, remedies that induce sweating to release 'external' conditions are used to treat fever. External conditions are acute conditions with rapid onset, which are triggered by bacterial or viral infection and are said to belong to the initial or alarm stage of general adaption. These symptoms are typically found at the onset of colds, influenza, laryngitis and other acute upper respiratory infections. (32)

The nature of the fever is dependent upon the virulence of the pathogen and the vigour of the individual's own immune system response. If the defences are weak, then no matter what the virulence of the offensive pathogen, the result will be a slight fever. If on the other hand active defence response is good, then the fever will accurately reflect the virulence of the pathogen itself. The pathogen merely triggers the immune system.

It is known that a high temperature actually assists in the struggle against micro-organisms, while the act of sweating itself not only keeps the temperature under control, but also speeds up the removal and elimination of toxic debris resulting from the conflict. The treatment strategy for resolving external conditions is to support the body's own active defences. Since the initial stage involves a fever, it follows that diaphoretics or sudorifics are required. Sweat inducing remedies are divided into warming and cooling types.

Holmes (33) states that rubifacients such as peppermint, ginger, and cinnamon are known as warm circulatory stimulant diaphoretics because they generate warmth. He also states that essential oils such as eucalyptus, spearmint and chamomile are known as warm peripheral vasodilatory diaphoretics, and are used to carefully control and resolve the warmth response.

Apart from monitoring body temperature there are other symptoms of fever that need to be observed. Nausea, vomiting, diarrhoea, headaches, coughing, pains and spasms can be addressed using the appropriate essential oils. However, accepting the potential value of the febrile reaction does not mean the client should undergo any unnecessary discomfort.

CAUTION

A practitioner must not attempt to take responsibility for treatment of any fever condition which might actually be a more serious infection. For example a pulse rate that does not rise with temperature, as expected, might indicate meningitis.

Allergies

Useful Oils
German and Roman chamomile, everlasting, lavender, yarrow.

A person who is overly reactive to an antigen is said to be hypersensitive or allergic. Whenever an allergic reaction occurs, there is tissue injury. The antigens that induce an allergic reaction are called allergens.

Common allergens include certain foods, antibiotics such as penicillin, cosmetic ingredients, chemicals in certain plants such as poison ivy, pollens, dusts, moulds and even microbes. (34) These allergens can be divided into three common groups:

- food
- chemicals
- inhaled allergens.

What is an allergy?

Allergic reactions are caused by an antibody called IgE circulating within the body. To understand the mechanism behind an allergic reaction, let us assume you have just received a scratch on your hand. Cells and antibodies are rushed to the infected scratch site by increasing the blood flow to the area.

Certain chemicals known as histamines which allow the blood flow to be controlled are released by the body. Nature has designed a series of little chemical mines, i.e. cells full of different chemicals, that can be exploded in the tissues when needed. Such cells are called mast cells and they are liberally scattered throughout our tissues.

To release these chemicals, IgE is needed. The mast cells, which contain histamine, have an outer membrane that can bind IgE. Once an antigen has been bound to two IgE molecules, the mast cell is activated, releasing histamine and other chemical mediators. These chemical mediators act on the shock organs (eg skin, bronchioles) and are responsible for the clinical manifestations of the immediate hypersensitivity reaction as shown in the diagram.

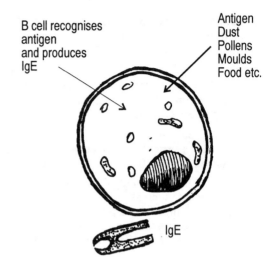

B cell recognises antigen and produces IgE

Antigen
Dust
Pollens
Moulds
Food etc.

IgE

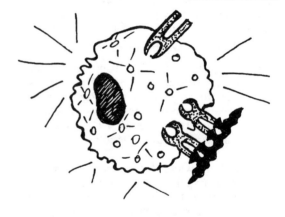

IgE plus antigen produces immediate reaction

Histamine-like Chemicals

Blood vessels swell	Airways constrict
Fluid leaks out	Difficult breathing
HIVES	ASTHMA

Immediate hypersensitivity

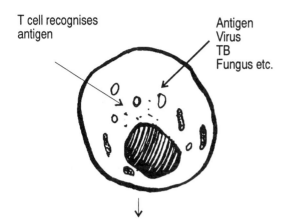

T cell recognises antigen

Antigen
Virus
TB
Fungus etc.

↓

Activating Chemicals

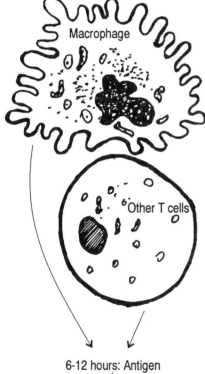

Macrophage

Other T cells

↓ ↓

6-12 hours: Antigen

↓

12-24 hours: Attack starts

↓

24-48 hours: Maximum intensity

Delayed hypersensitivity

Delayed hypersensitivy reactions are based upon a longer interval for the reaction to occur following a challenging antigen. These are mainly due to cell-mediated immunity and include most immunologic responses not dependent upon circulating IgE. Tuberculin response and various forms of contact dermatitis are examples of delayed reactions, which usually take hours or even days to occur.

According to Chris Green the mind plays a major part in allergy-related conditions. His approach, which uses simple healing procedures which combine the practical use of reflexology, bioenergetics, meditation, neuro-linguistic programming, dreamwork, relaxation and time line therapy, has resulted in many spectacular successes. One of his clients successfully treated was Kristy McFadden who was allergic to almost every conceivable product made in the 20th century. (35)

The recommended treatment is to avoid contact with the allergenic substance. However, Chris Green suggests that the buried emotional issue is the real cause of the allergic reaction.

Holistic approach

- The suspected allergens should be totally withdrawn at least initially.

- If food allergies exist, a food diary should be kept.

- Treat the liver using cholagogues.

- Promote immunostimulation.

- Promote elimination using depuratives.

- Promote relaxation and removal of stressors which are known to trigger allergic reactions.

- For specific aromatherapy treatment refer to the appropriate sections eg hayfever, sinusitis, psoriasis, of this book.

Candida

Useful Oils
Bergamot, German chamomile, lemon-scented eucalyptus, lavender, lemongrass, melissa, myrtle, rosemary, tea tree.

Candida albicans infection is a yeast-like fungus that inhabits the intestine, genital tract, mouth and throat. Normally this fungus lives in healthy balance with the bacteria and other fungal yeasts in the body, however certain conditions can cause this fungus to multiply, weakening the immune system and causing the infection candidiasis.

Because this fungus travels through the blood stream to many parts of the body, various symptoms may develop. When it infects the oral cavity, it is called thrush. White sores may form on the tongue, gums, and inside the cheeks. When it infects the vagina, it results in vaginitis, also commonly known as thrush. The most common symptoms include a large amount of white discharge and intense itching.

If thrush persists, other symptoms which may develop include depression, poor memory, pre-menstrual syndrome, recurrent cystitis and fungal infections such as athlete's foot. It can also cause food intolerances which result in abdominal distention, bloating, diarrhoea or constipation.

Aetiology

- Broad-spectrum antibiotics, given for bacterial infections, will destroy the friendly bacteria in the bowel. This will allow the candida organism to pass through the bowel wall by a process of presorption and be transported to other organs by the blood and lymphatic systems.

- Steroid therapy for asthma and rheumatoid arthritis has a depressant effect on the immune system.

- Excessive consumption of sugar and foods with sugar helps the candida organism to multiply.

- The contraceptive pill changes the hormonal balance of the body.

- Immune-suppressant drugs used for cancer lower the immune system capability.

Therapeutic strategy

There are several important steps in successfully controlling *Candida albicans*:

- Eliminate the use of antibiotics, steroids, immune-suppressing drugs, and birth control pills (unless a medical necessity).

- Follow the candida control diet given below.

- Enhance digestion.

- Enhance immune function.

- Enhance liver function.

- Use herbs and aromatherapy which help control yeast overgrowth and promote a healthy bacterial flora.

- Eliminate candida toxins by using a water-soluble fibre such as psyllium seeds or pectin which can bind to the toxins in the gut and promote their excretion.

The candida control diet

- Avoid all yeast-containing foods such as: vegemite, melons, yeast breads, fermented beverages, beer, wine, brandy, scotch, mouldy cheeses, fermented vinegars, salad dressing, nuts, biscuits, old cereals, apple cores, canned citrus fruit juices, cake mixes, hamburgers, ice cream, all dried fruit, oranges, pickles, tomato sauce, sugars, fungi, yeast powder, buttermilk, sour milks, processed and smoked meats, malt products, barbecue sauce, olives, mayonnaise, chillies.

- Avoid all refined carbohydrates such as refined sugars, soft drinks, pastries, fruit juices, honey and canned fruits.

- Avoid all known or suspected allergic foods.

- Avoid milk and milk products with a high content of lactose.

- One clove of garlic and one teaspoon of olive oil should be taken daily. Garlic is especially active against *C. albicans*, having been found more potent than nystatin, gentian violet, and many other antifungal agents in both *in vivo* and *in vitro* studies. (36)

- *Lactobacillus acidophilus* has been shown to retard the growth of candida in culture media (37). Since many individuals react unfavourably to the traditional milk-based sources of *L. acidophilus* (due to lactose intolerance or milk protein allergy), many practitioners recommend milk free *L. acidophilus* supplements.

- Foods which can be eaten freely include all vegetables, protein sources (legumes, fish, poultry and meat) and whole grains.

- Gentian is a good herb which aids gastric secretions and is a good digestive stimulant.

- Other herbs that are recommended include barberry and golden seal. These herbs contain berberine and have been used in herbal medicine as antidiarrhoeal and anti-infective agents. Berberine is an effective antimicrobial agent against a wide range of organisms, including *Candida albicans*. Its action on candida prevents the overgrowth of yeast that commonly follows antibiotic use. (38)

Aromatherapy treatment

Many essential oils have been investigated for their action upon *Candida albicans*. *Melaleuca alternifolia* has demonstrated remarkable activity in both in vitro (39) and in vivo (40). In Australia this has lead to the development of the phyto-pharmaceutical products, 'Vaginol' range of creams, douches and pessaries for vaginal infections (41).

Other essential oils which have been found to be effective include *Matricaria recutita*, *Melissa officinalis* (42), *Eucalyptus citriodora* (43), *Rosmarinus officinalis* (44), *Cymbopogon citratus* (45) and *Myrtus communis* (46).

Valerie Ann Worwood (47) suggests using :

German chamomile	5 drops
lavender	5 drops
tea tree	5 drops.

These essential oils are added to 100 gm of acidophilus yoghurt and mixed well. Then use an applicator for inserting pessaries or a tampon applicator to get the mixture into the vagina. This method is very effective if there is a lot of soreness and itching.

Another way of using yoghurt is to dilute it in warm spring water until a thin fluid has been obtained. Then add the essential oils. This mixture is added to a douche and the vagina is washed once a day.

If a douche is not available, a sitz bath may be used, however this method is not as effective.

For oral thrush, gargle and mouthwash - 2 drops of tea tree oil in warm water after meals.

Immune stimulating oils such as lavender, lemon and rosemary may also be used in massage. If the candida patient suffers from depression as is often the case, uplifting oils such as grapefruit, clary sage or bergamot can be used in massage, baths or oil burners.

Chronic fatigue syndrome (CFS)

Useful Oils
Basil, geranium, lavender, lemon, orange, rosemary.

CFS has also been called myalgic encephalomyelitis (ME), immune dysfunction syndrome and post-viral fatigue syndrome. It remains uncertain whether there is a specific disease, or syndrome called CFS, what its causes or cause may be, what treatment is most effective, and whether or not it is the same as post-viral fatigue syndrome.

Many believe that it is not a condition as such, but a set of symptoms which can be produced by more than one causative factor. When CFS affects a person, the immune system 'goes on red alert', and the suppressor T-cells often become overactivated. This event often exacerbates allergies, which further weakens the immune system. A recent study by Chaney and Bell (48), found that CFS sufferers have a very high level of interleukin 2 in their blood. Interleukins are protein messenger molecules which stimulate the defences of the T cells, B cells and macrophages against toxins and pathogens. This high level of interleukins indicates the presence of disease-causing pathogens.

CFS seems to be largely restricted to the 'civilised' First World and, in the main does not appear to be mortal (49).

The principal symptoms of CFS often include:

- forgetfulness, inability to concentrate

- mild fever or chills

- headaches

- sleep disturbances - insomnia, or too much sleep

- extreme and protracted muscle fatigue following exertion

- mood disturbance and depression

- digestive disturbances

- general aches and pains.

Few patients have all the symptoms, and similar patterns may be due to other conditions such as MS and glandular fever. Some people believe that CFS sufferers have a candida problem. This may be caused by the immune system disturbance in CFS, and it may be a contributing factor to the condition.

Until recently, the most common treatment offered to CFS patients was antidepressant medication. Although some sufferers claim that low doses of antidepressants are helpful, it is possible that the antidepressants further challenge their already fragile immune systems, giving the liver one more chemical to detoxify. (50)

The best advice is to rest. The viral factor in CFS has to be balanced with the emotional factor. The majority of CFS sufferers experience moderate to severe depression. Many sufferers have found help from meditation, positive thinking and other spiritually uplifting modes of treatment. Therefore it is not surprising to find aromatherapy as one of the ideal forms of treatment.

As in AIDS and cancer, CFS can be greatly relieved by a concerted effort to enhance immunity, and by natural therapies, such as aromatherapy, nutrition, visualisation and massage.

Hoffman, a medical practitioner (51) who specialises in the treatment of CFS, suggests using intravenous vitamin C. Vitamin C is very important for the functioning of the immune system, and when it is offered intravenously it bypasses the digestive system, which may be faulty in CFS sufferers, going directly to the cells where it is needed. He also suggests that 'Ester C', an oral form of vitamin C, produced significantly higher concentrations of the vitamin in the blood as long as 24 hours after ingestion. Some CFS patients have shown only 20% of normal levels of vitamin C.

Other herbs and nutrients that boost the immune system, such as garlic and echinacea, should also be included. Ginkgo biloba may be used to stimulate circulation, thus improving memory and concentration.

Steve Wilkens (52) believes that aromatherapy is one of the most consistently successful therapies. Lemon and orange oil are recommended for their uplifting and refreshing effects on the mind. Rosemary and basil oil are suggested to relieve lethargy. Geranium oil is recommended for its harmonising influence on the body and mind. Lavender oil is ideal as it has a soothing and relaxing influence suitable for physical and mental fatigue. The essential oils used for the treatment of CFS address the problem at all levels.

Chapter 28

Digestive System

This chapter summarises an holistic approach to the treatment of many common ailments and conditions associated with the digestive system.

Not only have the aromatherapy procedures for each condition been outlined, but details have also been included on other forms of treatment such as diet, herbs, acupressure and exercise.

Conditions discussed in this chapter include:

Irritable bowel syndrome
Constipation
Diarrhoea
Dyspepsia
Flatulence
Nausea and vomiting

Introduction

Food is vital to life. It is required for all the chemical reactions that occur in every cell. However, most of the food that we eat is simply too large to pass through the plasma membranes of the cells. Therefore the food needs to be broken down into molecules small enough for the body cells to use. This process is called digestion and the organs that collectively perform this function comprise the digestive system.

The digestive system prepares food for consumption by the cells through five basic activities.

1. **Ingestion.** Taking food into the body (eating).
2. **Peristalsis.** The movement of food along the digestive tract.
3. **Digestion.** The breakdown of food by both mechanical and chemical processes.
4. **Absorption.** The passage of digested food from the digestive tract into the cardiovascular and lymphatic systems for distribution to the cells.
5. **Elimination.** The elimination of indigestible substances from the body.

The digestive functions are considered, in both traditional herbal medicine and Chinese medicine, as the *'throne of the vital powers'* which means that digestion and metabolism, are literally central to any medical treatment.

Therefore health and vitality depend on the digestive system's ability to provide nutrients for the body. It is not just a matter of what substances are being eaten, but essentially one of what is properly processed so that it can be assimilated and used by the body. If there is a functional problem in the digestion, then no matter what is eaten it will not be properly absorbed, and a deficiency will occur.

An example of a functional problem, as opposed to an organic problem, is eating rapidly and at irregular intervals. This leads to indigestion; when food enters an unprepared gut too fast it causes malabsorption and discomfort. The fault lies usually in poor eating habits, insufficient digestive enzymes or in a dysfunction of the intestinal walls, causing the food not to be properly absorbed through the lining of the gut.

Besides the function of assimilation, an equally important activity of the digestive system is elimination. Not all food that is eaten is absorbed. Some food is not digestible and needs to be excreted. The body produces metabolic waste products that have to be eliminated, partly through the digestive system. The condition of the bowel and the state of its contents will fundamentally affect the rest of the body.

In addition to the physiological influences affecting the functioning and the health of the digestive system, there is a profound influence exerted by the emotions and state of the mind. There is an immediate response to anger, anxiety, fear and all forms of stress and worry. To treat digestive problems holistically, these psychological influences must be considered. Most digestive problems that commonly occur are easily avoidable by changes of lifestyle and habits.

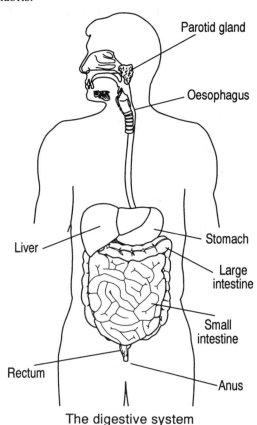

The digestive system

General considerations

The holistic treatment includes soothing and healing; supporting nervous balance; restoring digestive and absorptive mechanisms; correcting liver and gall bladder functions; cleansing and correcting eliminative functions. Some general guidelines include:

- Avoid over eating, particularly rich fatty and fried foods.

- Do not eat too fast, as this taxes the system.

- A number of commonly ingested substances and drugs may cause or aggravate digestive problems; for example coffee, smoking, alcohol, excess orange juice and certain pharmaceutical drugs.

- Avoid drinking with meals. It does not seem sensible to dilute the gastric enzymes more than necessary, especially if there is a digestive problem.

- Regular exercise is essential to the health of the digestive system.

- Meals should be eaten in a relaxed environment and all food should be chewed thoroughly.

- The diet should be as natural and as high in roughage as possible.

- Artificial chemical additives should be avoided.

- Beware of fad diets and restrictive dietary recommendations.

CAUTION

Changes in bowel patterns and rectal bleeding must always be checked by a medical practitioner.

Aromatherapy considerations

The antispasmodic, carminative, and digestive stimulating properties of essential oils are well known, and many essential oils are still currently used in pharmacopoeias. Peppermint oil is used in 'Mintec' and 'Colpermin', both of which are licenced as medicines to treat irritable bowel syndrome. These products contain peppermint oil in an enterically coated capsule designed not to dissolve until it reaches the large intestine.

Research has proven that peppermint essential oil can be effectively used to treat irritable bowel syndrome. (1)(2) These tests concluded that peppermint oil was a carminative with potent antispasmodic properties, and is particularly valuable for the symptomatic treatment of irritable bowel syndrome.

Lavender, peppermint, spearmint, sweet fennel, coriander, thyme and German chamomile are cholagogic (stimulating bile). (3)

Mills (4) suggests that many herbal preparations used for treating the digestive system are either 'cooling and drying' bitters or 'warming and drying' aromatic digestives. The emphasis on 'drying' is not surprising as the main organ responsible for digestion in Chinese medicine is the spleen and it is particularly vulnerable to 'damp'. Essential oils which have a 'warming and drying' effect and which have traditionally been used to tonify the digestive system include: black pepper, sweet fennel, coriander, sweet marjoram, myrrh and peppermint.

The therapeutic properties of essential oils which have a particular affinity for the digestive system include:

Antispasmodics

Antispasmodics are remedies that quickly relax any nervous tension that may be causing digestive spasms or colic.

Antispasmodic oils to use are *angelica, aniseed, bay, black pepper, cajeput, cardamom, German* and *Roman chamomile, cinnamon, clary sage, dill, sweet fennel, ginger, nutmeg, orange, peppermint, rosemary* and *rose.*

Carminatives

Essential oils such as *angelica, aniseed, basil, black pepper, carrot seed, cinnamon, clove, cardamom, Roman* and *German chamomile, coriander, dill, sweet fennel, ginger, sweet marjoram, peppermint, rosemary* and *thyme* affect the digestive system by relaxing the stomach muscles, increasing the peristalsis of the intestine and reducing the production of gas in the system.

Cholagogues

Cholagogues increase the flow of bile and stimulate the gall bladder. Essential oils such as *Roman* and *German chamomile, everlasting, lavender, peppermint, rosemary, rose* and *yarrow* can be used.

Hepatics

Hepatics strengthen, tone and stimulate the secretions of the liver. This causes an increase in the flow of bile. Essential oils such as *bay, carrot seed, German and Roman chamomile, cypress, grapefruit, everlasting, lemon, peppermint, rose, sage* and *rosemary* stimulate the liver.

Aromatherapy treatment for digestive disorders may be given by aromatherapy massage, inhalation and by local compresses. I do not recommend the internal ingestion of the essential oils as is often recommended in some books, unless it is being supervised by a medical practitioner or professionally trained herbalist with a clinical aromatherapy background.

Associated conditions

Irritable bowel syndrome

Useful Oils

Black pepper, Roman chamomile, sweet fennel, lavender, lemongrass, mandarin, sweet marjoram, neroli, peppermint.

Clinical features

Irritable bowel syndrome is a term used to identify a clinical condition that is characterised by a combination of:

- abdominal pain
- altered bowel function, constipation or diarrhoea
- hypersecretion of colonic mucus
- dyspeptic symptoms (flatulence, nausea, anorexia)
- varying degrees of anxiety or depression.

These common disorders have several names eg nervous indigestion, functional dyspepsia, irritable colon, or colitis. Colitis is an inflammatory condition of the colon. The mucous membranes of the colon become inflamed, and small, pouch like areas are formed. Colitis may be acute or chronic. It often strikes young and early-middle-aged adults. Its symptoms include cramps in the abdominal area, diarrhoea, and an almost continual need to eliminate. Often there is blood in the stool. There are several types of colitis, and they range from mild to serious. Enteritis and ileitis are types of inflammation of the small intestine often associated with colitis. Severe colitis is called ulcerative colitis. With this condition, the colon is both inflamed and lined with ulcers.

Aetiology

Three main factors appear significant in the pathogenesis of irritable bowel syndrome:

- **Colonic motor activity** - Colonic motor activity is abnormally high in patients with colonic pain, eg after meals or after emotional stress.
- **Psychological stress** - Many patients with irritable bowel syndrome exhibit colonic symptoms at times of stress. It is very often associated with a nervous disorder and anxiety.
- **Diet** - Irritable bowel syndrome has been linked to allergies to certain foods. A food sensitivity test is advised. The foods which commonly provoke symptoms include:
  - wheat
  - corn
  - dairy products
  - coffee and tea
  - citrus fruits.

General treatment

There is a choice of different therapeutic strategies to be adopted, depending on the origin of the symptoms:

Diet: No single diet is applicable to all clients with irritable bowel syndrome. Some clients respond to an increase in dietary fibre. Others who suffer from lactose intolerance will benefit from exclusion of dairy products. Lactose intolerance is caused by a deficiency of the naturally occurring enzyme lactase, which breaks down the sugar lactose in the gut.

Personal habits: Regular hours and meals and adequate sleep, exercise and recreation are important. Restriction of alcohol and tobacco are also necessary.

Stress: The gut is very sensitive to stress and individuals prone to IBS might develop an irritable bowel when stressed. Relaxation techniques and essential oils which assist the client in dealing with the stress usually settle an irritable bowel.

Symptomatic treatment: Sedative - antispasmodic essential oils may be of value.

Vegetable mucilages: Mucilages such as slippery elm or psyllium seeds may be useful. Slippery elm is a soothing demulcent which is ideal for sensitive or inflamed mucous membrane linings in the digestive system. Place a teaspoon of powdered slippery elm into a half litre of boiling water and allow to steep for ten minutes. Drink a cup before breakfast and dinner.

Aromatherapy treatment

Essential oils which have antispasmodic properties such as: black pepper, sweet fennel, peppermint, Roman chamomile and sweet marjoram may relieve the symptoms of irritable bowel syndrome if used in an abdominal massage.

Essential oils such as neroli, lavender, frankincense and mandarin should be used because they allow the client to relax.

Other treatments

- Rest and treat the diarrhoea if present (see Diarrhoea).

- A simple bland diet should be followed. Avoid raw fruits and vegetables (especially their skins and seeds), whole cereals, fresh bread, sugar, fried or fatty foods and game meat. Do not eat dairy products as these can often be painful to digest. Do not drink alcohol and sparkling or soda drinks.

- Increase intake of fibre. However the addition of wheat bran fibre to the Western diet, often without reduction in the amount of refined carbohydrate being consumed

will exacerbate the problem. Some individuals who have wheat sensitivities will experience a worsening or a precipitation of their IBS symptoms. In these situations it is worth trying soya bran or rice bran.

- Increase fluid intake and correct any mineral imbalance that may have occurred with persistent diarrhoea.

- Chamomile, dandelion root, red clover and yarrow are beneficial herbal teas for colitis.

- Stretching exercises are important for improved digestion. Partially digested starches may allow food to pass through the colon too rapidly.

Constipation

Useful Oils
Black pepper, sweet fennel, sweet marjoram, rosemary.

Clinical features

Constipation results when defecation is difficult and infrequent. Many ailments arise from constipation including haemorrhoids, flatulence, insomnia, headaches, bad breath, varicose veins, obesity, indigestion, diverticulitis, appendicitis, hernia and bowel cancer.

Aetiology

The cause of constipation could be something simple such as stress, insufficient dietary fibre, excess protein, refined foods or poor bile flow. It could also be related to liver or thyroid under-activity. Other causes include inadequate fluids, pregnancy, antacids, metabolic disorders, tumours, strokes, old age and constant use of enemas and laxatives. The causes are generally classified as follows:

Atonic constipation   weakness of colon due to neglect, chronic disease, advanced age or immobility

Spastic constipation   due to colonic spasm which inhibits forward peristalsis

Compaction of faecal mass   due to insufficient dietary fibre or fluid

Dyschezia   habitual failure to heed the call to defecate.

General treatment

Check for the possible cause of constipation. Including fibre in the diet is now a widely accepted practice and will often help eliminate constipation. It is better to increase consumption of fibre rich foods, such as wholegrains, vegetables, fruit, nuts and seeds rather than take high fibre supplements. It is also important that intake of refined carbohydrate foods is reduced at the same time.

Aromatherapy treatment

The most effective aromatherapy treatment for constipation is massaging the abdomen, always in a clockwise direction. This is something that the patient can be easily taught to carry out daily at home. The most effective oils to use for massage are sweet fennel, sweet marjoram and rosemary, together or on their own. Black pepper also stimulates peristalsis.

Other treatments

- Exercise is important. Physical activity speeds the movement of waste through the intestines and reduces the time that potential cancer-causing waste is in contact with tissues.

- Avoid foods that stimulate secretions of mucous membranes. Eat fresh fruits, raw leafy vegetables and brown rice daily. Avoid dairy products, white flour and sugar. It is important to drink extra amounts of water since you are adding fibre to the diet.

- Increase water intake to at least 2 litres per day.

- Include foods in the diet which have a natural laxative effect, such as figs, prunes and apricots.

- Some people find that a glass of hot water with the juice of half a lemon is helpful when taken first thing in the morning.

- The following herbs will help relieve constipation: flaxseed, aloe vera juice, golden seal, barley juice, pepsin, psyllium seed and yellow dock.

- A heavy laxative user will have cleaned out the intestinal bacteria causing chronic constipation. Acidophilus yoghurt will replace the friendly gut bacteria.

- According to Harrison (5):
  'In general, relief of physical constipation will rapidly follow relief of mental constipation.

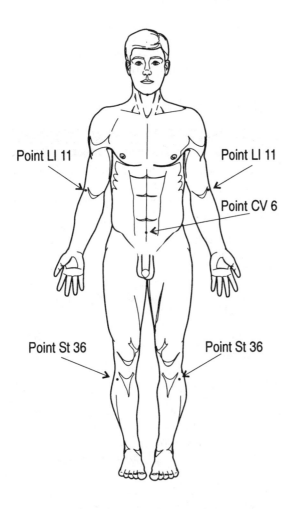

Point LI 11   Point LI 11

Point CV 6

Point St 36   Point St 36

Location of acupressure points to relieve constipation

Flexible minds make flexible bodies, capable of adjusting to environmental change.'

- Louise Hay (6) suggests that people with constipation refuse to release old ideas and are stuck in the past.

- Acupressure points CV 6, St 36, LI 11 and LI 4 are used to relieve abdominal pain, constipation and stomach disorders.

Diarrhoea

Useful Oils
Black pepper, German and Roman chamomile, cinnamon leaf, cypress, eucalyptus, sweet fennel, ginger, mandarin, neroli, peppermint.

Clinical features

Diarrhoea is characterised by frequent and loose watery stools, and is sometimes accompanied by severe vomiting. Symptoms include runny stools, cramping, frequent bowel movements, thirst and abdominal pain.

Aetiology

Most cases of diarrhoea are self-limiting and pose no special problem. They are often due to dietary indiscretions or mild gastrointestinal infections. Other causes of diarrhoea are (7):

- psychogenic disorders: 'nervous' diarrhoea

- intestinal infections: viral enteritis, salmonellosis, cholera, giardiasis, amoebiasis, staphylococcal infections etc.

- other intestinal factors: heavy metal poisoning, antibiotic therapy, faecal impaction, inflammatory bowel disease, carcinoma

- malabsorption: coeliac sprue, short bowel syndrome

- pancreatic disease: pancreatic insufficiency, pancreatic endocrine tumours

- reflex from other viscera: pelvic disease (extrinsic to gastrointestinal tract)

- neurological disease: diabetic neuropathy

- metabolic disease: hyperthyroidism

- immunodeficiency

- malnutrition: marasmus

- food allergy

- dietary factors: excessive fresh fruit intake.

General treatment

- Determine the cause and treat appropriately (eg laxative abuse, drugs, alcohol etc.).

- Improve digestion.

- Check for food sensitivities.

- Increase intake of fluids and electrolytes.

- Re-establish gut flora by supplementing with acidophilus.

Aromatherapy treatment

Essential oils may be useful in treating diarrhoea because of their antispasmodic action on the intestinal muscles, because of their astringent properties and because of their ability to calm the nervous system.

German and Roman chamomile, cypress, mandarin, neroli and peppermint are among the most effective antispasmodics that can be used to treat diarrhoea. Eucalyptus is recommended if a viral infection is the cause of the diarrhoea, as it has anti-viral properties.

German and Roman chamomile are anti-allergenic, and should be used if a food allergy is involved. Warming and carminative essential oils, such as ginger, sweet fennel or black pepper are used to relieve the pain in diarrhoea. Massaged gently over the abdomen, they can be helpful in easing the griping pains caused by spasmodic contractions of the intestinal walls.

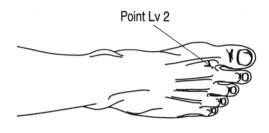

Point Lv 2

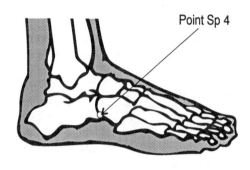

Point Sp 4

Location of acupressure points to relieve diarrhoea

Other treatments

- A high fibre diet is important. Eat oat bran, rice bran, raw foods, yoghurt daily.

- Do not consume milk products - they are highly allergenic. Also limit fats, wheat, and foods containing gluten.

- Diarrhoea is especially serious in babies and old people, as it causes dehydration. Make them drink plenty of water.

- Occasional bouts of diarrhoea may be treated by drinking teas made from chamomile or raspberry leaves. Ginger tea is good for cramps and abdominal pain. Slippery elm bark powder is also beneficial.

- The abdominal acupressure points St 16 and CV 6 tone the abdominal area, while St 36, Sp 4 and Lv 2 on the legs and feet harmonise the digestive system. These points should be pressed three to four times a day to alleviate diarrhoea.

Dyspepsia

Useful Oils
Aniseed, black pepper, cardamom, German and Roman chamomile, cinnamon leaf, sweet fennel, ginger, mandarin, sweet marjoram, neroli, nutmeg, orange, peppermint, rosemary, spearmint.

Clinical features

Indigestion may be a symptom of a disorder in the stomach or small or large intestine or it may be a disorder in itself. Symptoms can include gas, abdominal pain, heartburn, a bloated feeling, belching, nausea, vomiting, and a burning sensation after eating. Heartburn is a burning sensation in the stomach. It often occurs when hydrochloric acid, which is used by the stomach for digestion, backs up into the oesophagus.

Aetiology

Chewing with the mouth open, talking while chewing, swallowing too much air by gulping down food, and drinking liquids with meals can flush away enzymes needed for digestion thus causing indigestion. Food allergies can also be a cause. Food allergies cause fermentation of food in the colon that produces hydrogen and carbon dioxide.

Carbohydrates are the main food source responsible for gas because of the bacteria they contain. It is important to find out which foods the body cannot digest. Indigestion can be caused by excessive consumption of spicy or fatty and fried foods, alcohol, coffee, citrus fruit, chocolate, and tomato based food, gall bladder problems, stress, allergies and enzyme deficiency.

Stress has been known to affect the digestive process, and this should be considered when treating persistent indigestion. Although gastritis is commonly thought to be caused by too much gastric acid, many people with dyspepsia do not get better when they take antacids such as magnesium or aluminium hydroxide.

In fact, gastritis can be associated with too little as well as too much gastric acid. In such circumstances hydrochloric and pepsin supplements are useful.

The chronic presence of candida yeast organism can cause gastric burning following eating. Reflux oesophagitis and hiatus hernia can also cause dyspepsia. Gall bladder disease, be it stones in the gall bladder or chronic infection or inflammation of the gall bladder, can cause abdominal pain and discomfort just under the ribs on the right side, and even into the upper central part of the abdomen.

Other situations that can cause indigestion include cancer of the stomach, coronary heart disease (angina) and acute pancreatitis. These should be investigated fully and thoroughly by a doctor.

> ### CAUTION
> Anyone with severe or persistent pain, weight loss, vomiting or who develops resistant diarrhoea or constipation should consult a doctor immediately.

General advice

There are many ways of treating indigestion. More importantly there are many ways of preventing indigestion.

- **Eating slowly**
  Most cases of indigestion are caused by eating quickly which sets up several imbalances leading directly to indigestion. Eating quickly results in a tendency to swallow quantities of air which in turn causes gas and abdominal bloating.

  The other problem is that eating quickly overloads the stomach, causing much of the surplus to pass through the intestine without receiving adequate enzyme breakdown. This results in further trouble when the food reaches the lower bowel.

- **Chewing food well**
  The process of digestion begins in the mouth. By carefully masticating food the enzymes in the saliva are able to do their job thoroughly so that by the time the food reaches the stomach it is in an easily assimilated form.

- **Not drinking liquids with meals**
  Enzymes secreted in the saliva have a specific digestive function to perform. This process can be impaired by a surplus of liquids. The liquids will dilute the digestive enzymes, impairing the efficiency of the saliva.

- **Avoiding unhealthy or gas-producing food**
  Indigestion also results from eating unhealthy foods such as fried foods, carbonated beverages, fats, sugar, processed foods, or spicy or highly seasoned foods.

  Certain gas producing foods such as onions, beans and peas which are normally considered healthy may also cause indigestion. Avoid fatty meats as they are a primary cause of bloating.

- **Eating good foods**
  All soured milk products such as yoghurt are helpful for stomach and intestinal bacteria. Food combining is important. Protein and starch are a poor combination, as are vegetables and fruits. Milk should not be consumed with meals. Sugars must not be consumed with proteins or starches.

- **Avoiding iced drinks with meals**
  Whether one takes liquid with a meal or not, it is not wise to drink iced liquids with meals.

- **Not over-eating**
  Over indulgence accounts for many cases of indigestion. The best practice is to leave the table feeling slightly hungry.

- **Not eating when emotionally upset**
  Eating when nervous, angry, overtired or depressed can cause indigestion. It may not be easy to make these emotional states disappear just in time for dinner, thus when eating food in a stressed state the best procedure is to eat the food as slowly as possible and to eat little.

- **Not smoking**
  Smokers should not smoke immediately before a meal. Smoking slows down the peristaltic action of the stomach and intestines, and hence makes food stagnate throughout the alimentary system. The final result can be constipation, diarrhoea, or both.

Aromatherapy treatment

Indigestion can be helped by gentle massage over the stomach with carminative and antispasmodic essential oils such as peppermint, aniseed, cardamom, sweet fennel, ginger and sweet marjoram. A hot compress placed over the stomach can also help.

Other essential oils useful in the treatment of indigestion include mandarin, sweet orange, rosemary, spearmint, neroli, Roman and German chamomile and cinnamon.

Other treatments

- At the first sign of heartburn, drink a large glass of water. This often works.

- Do not lie down immediately after eating.

- Avoid stress.

- Relief from heartburn can be obtained by sipping one tablespoon of apple cider vinegar, mixed with water, while eating a meal.

- Do not drink liquids with meals.

- Drink the juice of a lemon first thing in the morning. It is a good healer and blood purifier.

- Herbal infusions of catnip, chamomile, golden seal, fennel, fenugreek and peppermint are beneficial.

- Garlic has antiseptic qualities, it stimulates gastric juices, relieves flatulence, helps detoxify the intestines and serves as a general aid to the entire digestive system.

- Acupressure is very effective for treating indigestion that results from emotional or psychological problems. The acupressure points commonly used for relieving abdominal pain and preventing indigestion are CV 12. St 36, Pe 6 and Sp 4. Precaution: Use CV12 only before eating.

Flatulence

Useful Oils

Aniseed, black pepper, cardamom, dill, sweet fennel, lavender, peppermint.

Clinical features

Flatulence is the medical term for excessive production of wind, which is then passed anally or orally.

Aetiology

Flatulence is usually the result of fermentation by bacteria in the gastrointestinal tract, which produces gas. It can cause abdominal distension, pain and disturbed bowel function. Increased fermentation can occur as a result of bacterial overgrowth of the gastrointestinal tract, constipation, irritable bowel syndrome, inflammatory bowel disease, food intolerance, chronic gastrointestinal candidiasis, and chronic gut infections with parasites.

Certain foods, especially beans, can cause flatulence. All these conditions are made worse by inadequate digestive juice secretion by the stomach, pancreas and gall bladder. So flatulence can be either 'normal' or a manifestation of almost any gastrointestinal disease.

Aromatherapy treatment

Essential oils described as carminatives will help reduce flatulence, and ease the pain that accompanies it. Aniseed, black pepper, cardamom, dill, sweet fennel, ginger or peppermint can be used in a 3% dilution of carrier oil and massaged into the abdomen area in a clockwise direction.

If the flatulence is a temporary problem, usually following a meal containing gas-producing foods, simply avoid those foods known to cause flatulence.

Other treatments

- Eliminate specific causes if known. For example people who experience flatulence after eating beans may experience relief if the beans are soaked in water for 24 hours before removal of the husks and thorough cooking.

- Reduce anxiety as this is often associated with deep breathing and sighing and consequent swallowing of considerable quantities of air.

- Eating slowly and avoiding over-eating will have a beneficial effect on flatulence.

Nausea and vomiting

Useful Oils
Black pepper, cardamom, Roman and German chamomile, fennel, ginger, peppermint.

Clinical features

Nausea and vomiting may be due to a wide variety of causes. Psychological causes may include disgusting smells and sights and physiological causes may include early pregnancy. Bad digestion, flu, a hangover, migraine, food allergies, travel motion or food poisoning can also cause nausea.

Aromatherapy treatment

Vomiting and nausea can often be relieved by gently massaging over the stomach area, or applying a warm compress to the area. Any of the essential oils listed above may be used to relieve nausea. Sweet fennel, peppermint, and ginger are the most commonly used oils.

Other treatments

- Chamomile, fennel, ginger and peppermint herbal teas will relieve nausea.

- The acupressure point Pe 6 is often used to relieve nausea.

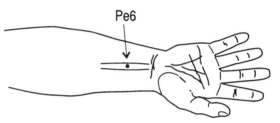

Location of acupressure point used for treating nausea

Chapter 29

Aromatherapy Skin Care

Skincare is a large and important branch of aromatherapy.

Aromatherapy which makes use of essential oils and cold pressed vegetable oils can contribute enormously to the health and appearance of the skin.

Topics discussed in this chapter include:

Skin structure
The skin's functions
Skin types
The effect of essential oils
Aromatherapy skin care
Skincare preparation recipes

415

Introduction

The use of essential oils in skin care is one of the most widely and commercially exploited branches of aromatherapy. Marguerite Maury helped establish the reputation of aromatherapy in skincare and the foundations of holistic aromatherapy. Many of her works, such as *Le Capital Jeunesse,* focussed on the healing and rejuvenating properties of the essential oils. Totally dedicated to her work, she gained a formidable reputation, as well as two international prizes in 1962 and 1967 for her research into essential oils and cosmeticology. (1)

Combined with a healthy diet and lifestyle, essential oils and other natural ingredients such as vegetable oils and waxes have the same results as the more costly cosmetics available on retail shelves.

Skin structure

The skin is the largest organ of the body in terms of surface area. For the average adult, the skin occupies a surface area of approximately 19 355 cm^2. It varies in thickness from 0.5 to 3 mm.

Structurally the skin is divided into 3 main layers.

- epidermis   first/outer layer
- dermis   second/inner layer
- hypodermis   third/supportive layer.

Epidermis

The epidermis is the outermost protective layer of the skin and consists of four distinct sub-layers.

- stratum germinativum ┬ spinosum
                       └ basale
- stratum granulosum
- stratum lucidum
- stratum corneum.

The stratum spinosum and stratum basale are collectively referred to as the stratum germinativum. The **stratum germinativum** or germinative layer is where all the new cells are produced. These cells gradually begin to die in the **stratum granulosum** or granular layer and by the time they reach the cornified layer or **stratum corneum** they are dead skin cells and desquamation takes place. The word *desquamation* means the natural removal of dead skin cells.

It usually takes between six to eight weeks for the cells to move from the stratum basale to the surface of the skin (2). This process slows down as we age. In an older person, it may take 50 days. In a psoriasis sufferer, it may take 3 days.

Keratinocytes are specialised cells that produce keratin, which toughens and waterproofs the skin. As keratinocytes are pushed away from the vascular nutrients and oxygen supply of the dermis, their nuclei degenerate, their cellular content is dominated by keratin, and the process of keratinization is complete.

The **stratum lucidum** is quite pronounced in the thick skin of the palms and soles. It consists of several rows of clear, flat, dead cells.

Melanocytes or melanin pigment cells are located in the germinative layer. These are dark coloured granules which, when triggered by UV rays, migrate to the surface giving the skin a tanned colour or freckled appearance.

Water is the key ingredient which keeps the skin soft and flexible. The skin's natural moisturiser is a combination of:

- extra-cellular fats (epidermal lipids)
- secreted sebum (sebaceous lipids) which form an oily protective film over the surface of the skin and prevent water from escaping
- the 'natural moisturising factor complex' within the skin's corneal layer which chemically combines with water.

Dermis

This is the major layer which lies beneath the epidermis and here are found the:

- sebaceous glands
- sweat glands
- hair follicles

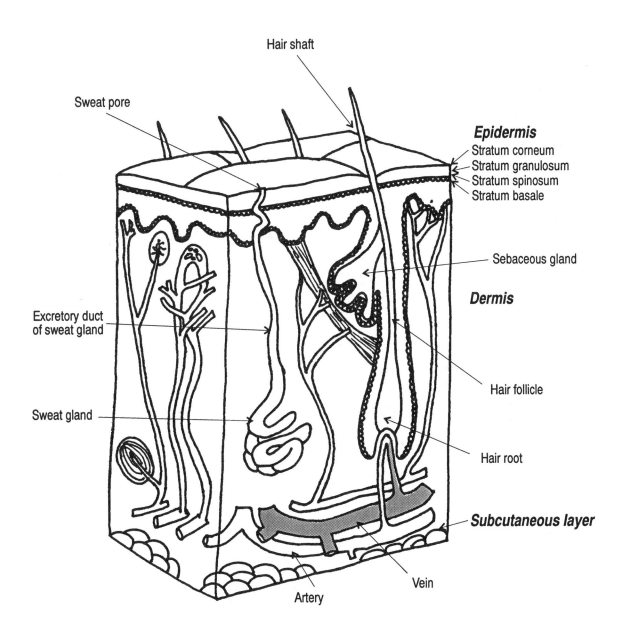

Schematic of cross section of the skin

- muscles
- blood and lymph capillaries
- nerves and nerve endings
- collagen and elastin fibres.

The dermis is the thicker underlying layer of the skin. It is a connective tissue layer composed of relatively few cells dispersed among great quantities of collagen and elastin fibres surrounded by an aqueous gel-like matrix. The dermis is held together with collagen fibres, which act like a support structure, and elastin fibres which provide elasticity. The aqueous gel-like matrix is a mixture of amino acids - mainly hyaluronic acid and other mucopolysaccharides and it acts as a lubricating fluid between the fibres and binds water to the dermal tissue.

The sebaceous glands

Running through the dermis and epidermis are hair follicles or pores. A pore is an empty hair follicle. Each hair follicle has a sebaceous gland, which produces an oil called sebum. The main constituents of sebum are free fatty acids (mostly palmitic and oleic acids), triglycerides, waxes, cholesterol and squalene. Traces of vitamin E and other fat-soluble vitamins are also present. Sebum lubricates the surface of skin and keeps it supple and moist.

The activity of the sebaceous gland determines skin type. Very active sebaceous glands produce a lot of oil resulting in greasy skin. If skin is well-balanced it produces just the right amount of sebum to prevent pimples from forming or drying out of the skin. The majority of people produce too much or too little sebum. Sebum production slows down in later years, so older people generally have drier skin.

The sweat glands

Each sweat gland is a tightly coiled tube buried deep inside the dermis and is connected to the skin surface by a tube about 5 mm long. This tube is called a sweat duct. The sweat duct reaches the surface to form a pore. The sweat glands excrete moisture to cool the body and also to throw out waste products in the form of perspiration. When sweat and sebum mix on the surface of the skin, they produce an acid mantle. This is the skin's first line of defence against bacteria and infection. It has a natural pH level of between 4.5 and 6 which should not be disturbed.

Hypodermis

This is the bottom skin layer, also known as the subcutaneous tissue, which separates the dermis from the muscles, allowing the skin to move freely over the underlying structures. It is the fatty layer of the skin containing fat cells, nerve fibres and blood vessels. The hypodermis protects the organs underneath from mechanical shock and also serves as a fat reservoir.

The skin's functions

The skin is a highly dynamic organ that not only protects the body from pathogens and external injuries but is also extremely important in maintaining body homeostasis. The main functions of the skin include:

- maintaining body temperature
- protecting the organs within our body from the environment, germs, damage
- eliminating waste
- producing vitamin D
- giving shape to the body structure and holding it together
- preventing excessive loss of inorganic and organic materials
- receiving stimuli from the environment.

Skin types

There is a generally accepted method of classifying the skin according to the balance of water and sebum in the tissues. It needs to be emphasised that skin may change its type often. Essential oils can be used to help correct the particular imbalances represented by the skin types.

Dry skin

Useful Oils
German chamomile, jasmine, neroli, rose, geranium, palmarosa, lavender, sandalwood, ylang-ylang.

Dry skin lacks the surface oils which give normal skin its smooth, velvety feel. This skin often looks attractive and delicately textured during youth, however it will often develop wrinkles and lines at an early age if the skin is not kept supple. Paula Begoun (3) suggests that dry skin and wrinkles have nothing to do with each other.

'Dry skin is caused by the inability of the surface layers of the skin to retain water and that dehydration does not affect or impact how a wrinkle is made. Wrinkling is solely the result of changes occurring in the underlying layers of the skin and the structure of the skin cell caused by sun damage, facial expressions, genetic predisposition and growing up.'

Dry skin tends to be:

* dull

* often flaky and chapped

* finely textured

* dry and coarse to touch

* 'tight' after washing

* prone to broken capillaries

* dehydrated.

Dry skin is often very delicate and sensitive, so essential oils such as German chamomile, jasmine, neroli and rose are recommended. Other oils such as geranium, palmarosa, lavender and sandalwood have a balancing effect on sebum production. These essential oils may also be used for treating oily skin because of their normalising effect and will reduce or increase the amount of sebum produced by the sebaceous glands.

The recommended base oils to use are avocado, wheatgerm, sweet almond, apricot kernel, jojoba, evening primrose oil and infused carrot oil.

Oily skin

Useful Oils
Bergamot, cedarwood, cypress, lavender, lemon, geranium, juniper, myrtle, palmarosa, tea tree, sandalwood.

Oily skin, a common skin condition in teenagers, is caused by over-active sebaceous glands which secrete too much sebum. The sebaceous glands are under hormonal control, being triggered by androgens. This skin type is subject to infections, as excess sebum clogs pores which develop into blackheads and acne.

Oily skin tends to have:

* a shiny look and be greasy to touch

* a coarse-grained texture

* dilated pores

* blackheads, acne and skin blemishes.

Essential oils can be used to reduce the amount of sebum being produced, and control the bacteria which thrive on the surface of the skin. The most effective essential oils are bergamot, cedarwood, cypress, lavender, lemon, juniper, tea tree and sandalwood. Cypress and juniper are astringents and help regulate the fluid levels. A blend of bergamot and lavender is very effective as bergamot directly reduces sebum production and lavender has a balancing effect and both essential oils are antiseptic, controlling bacteria on the surface of the skin.

If a carrier oil is used, a light polyunsaturated carrier oil such as apricot kernel or jojoba should be used. All traces of the carrier oil should be carefully removed using a cleanser and toner after the treatment. Geranium oil has a balancing effect on the sebaceous glands and makes a useful addition to bergamot and lavender. Because of its balancing effect, it is useful for combination type skins.

To treat oily skin, essential oils may be added to a liquid soap base, such as castille liquid soap, or compresses may be administered.

Normal skin

Useful Oils
German chamomile, geranium, lavender, rose, neroli, palmarosa, rosewood, ylang-ylang.

Normal skin tends to have:

- a soft, supple and smooth velvety feel
- no areas of excess oiliness or dryness and be balanced throughout with perhaps a slight oiliness in the T-zone
- a clear appearance, with a fine-grained texture
- an appearance similar to the skin of a young child.

Almost any essential oil that will not irritate the skin can be used on normal skin. Use sweet almond, apricot kernel oil and jojoba cold pressed oils as base oils and make a 2% dilution using any of the following oils: German chamomile, geranium, lavender, rose, neroli, palmarosa, rosewood and ylang-ylang.

Combination skin

Useful Oils
Geranium, palmarosa, sandalwood, lavender, neroli.

This type of skin is a mixture of dry skin with oily patches on the T-zone, where the sebaceous glands are most prevalent. Generally, it is best to treat each area separately, using the appropriate oils.

Combination skin tends to be:

- partly dry and partly oily
- subject to blackheads and dilated pores in the T-zone area, other areas being fine grained.

The most useful essential oils are geranium and palmarosa because of their balancing effect on the sebaceous glands. Other essential oils that can be used include sandalwood, lavender and neroli.

The recommended base oils are apricot kernel, jojoba or evening primrose oil.

Sensitive skin

Useful Oils
Lavender, neroli, everlasting, yarrow, German chamomile.

Many people seem to have skin sensitivities and allergies, particularly to the chemicals and fragrances found in many skin care products. While essential oils do not usually produce similar reactions to these chemicals and fragrances, it is always recommended that a patch test on a small part of the client's skin be conducted before using the essential oils on a large area, and that, in general, dilutions of 1% or less be used.

Sensitive skin tends to:

- be pale (Scottish/Irish complexion)
- be sensitive to many cosmetics (burning sensation)
- be sensitive to sunlight, developing red, scaly patches
- develop red blotches and broken veins in extreme temperatures
- be dry and fine textured
- be poorly protected due to insufficient epidermic oils.

Potentially, we all have sensitive skin. Our skin may become sensitive to certain substances, or sensitive in certain circumstances, such as when we are under stress. The ageing process can bring about increased sensitivity. Avoid hard water, harsh alkaline soaps or cleansers, alcohol in skin toners, skin abrasives and highly perfumed products. Patch tests should be used for several days before full use of new cosmetics, irrespective of how 'non-allergenic' the product is claimed to be.

Great care must be taken in selecting essential oils. The oils with anti-inflammatory qualities such as lavender, neroli, everlasting, yarrow and German chamomile should be used. It is advisable to use a 1% dilution of any of the above essential oils in a base of evening primrose, jojoba, apricot kernel and infused calendula oils.

Mature skin

Useful Oils
Carrot seed, everlasting, frankincense, jasmine, lavender, neroli, rose, sandalwood, rosewood, myrrh, patchouli.

This skin is usually very dry, lacking both oil and moisture and is developing wrinkles and lines. This could be due to exposure to the sun, wind and harsh climatic conditions.

Mature skin tends to have:

- expression lines around the eyes, nose and mouth

- slackness around the eyes

- a dull complexion with loss of skin elasticity and natural moisture

- a fine network of veins.

Most skins become less oily as they grow older. Massage oils made with oils such as geranium, jasmine, neroli, and rose will help restore this natural balance.

The cytophylactic properties of everlasting, frankincense, lavender, sandalwood, rosewood, myrrh and patchouli make these oils ideal for the treatment of older skin. Thread veins are sometimes a problem and daily application of German chamomile and rose essential oils over several months will see a great improvement.

Many essential oils are cytophylactic meaning that they stimulate the generation of new cells, and in doing so help preserve the health and beauty of the skin. The cytophylactic property is particularly evident in lavender oil which is also used for the treatment of burns.

Recommended carrier oils are avocado, carrot infused oil, evening primrose, jojoba, rosehip and wheatgerm.

The effect of essential oils

Essential oils are ideally suited to skin care because they are readily absorbed through the skin and are often used because they:

- are highly antiseptic

- help speed up the removal of old skin cells and stimulate the growth of new cells

- improve muscle tone and blood circulation

- help eliminate waste

- reduce inflammation

- regulate sebum production

- reduce the impact of emotional stress.

Essential oils can be easily incorporated into any base cream, lotions, ointments, gels, toilet waters, or perfumes, and of course most of the essential oils have an appealing scent. When giving a facial treatment the effect of the scent is important in itself, as it is possible to achieve a considerable degree of relaxation.

The skin is designed to prevent the absorption of many substances by the body. The determining factor is molecular size. The small molecular size of the essential oils allows them to penetrate the skin. Many substances such as lanolin and mineral oils, often found in skincare products, have a large molecular size and will not be absorbed.

Antiseptic properties

The skin is continually exposed to micro-organisms such as bacteria and fungi. If the skin's natural defences fail, infections, boils and other skin disorders can result. One way that the skin protects itself is its acid mantle. The acid nature of the sebum helps to neutralise bacteria.

Essential oils, such as cajeput, eucalyptus, lemon, myrtle, niaouli, tea tree, lavender and myrrh, that are either antiseptic, bactericidal or anti-fungal, may be used to help the skin's protective functions and are excellent for treating acne and a wide variety of common skin infections.

Stimulating growth of new cells

This refers to the cytophylactic property of essential oils, which helps to increase the speed at which skin cells in the germinative layer of the skin reproduce, hence promoting the rapid healing of wounds and burns and thus eliminating scarring. The ability of an essential oil to eliminate scarring is known as its cicatrisant action.

Essential oils such as carrot seed, lavender, everlasting, myrrh, frankincense, neroli, patchouli and yarrow can be used to maintain a healthy and youthful complexion, minimise stretch marks and scarring.

Circulatory stimulants

The skin has the ability to control temperature through expansion or contraction of the superficial capillaries. It also controls the production of sweat which regulates body temperature by the evaporation of perspiration. Rubefacient essential oils such as ginger, black pepper and rosemary help increase circulation and can be used to assist the skin's body temperature regulation being useful for general 'detoxification' of congested skin thus improving dull complexions.

By increasing the micro-circulation in the skin, and by strengthening the capillaries, essential oils such as cypress, German chamomile, rose and geranium are useful for the treatment of spider veins and varicose veins.

Helping eliminate waste

Up to 25% of the body's waste products are eliminated via the skin. Problems with the elimination of wastes will place a burden on the three main organs of elimination: kidneys, lungs and bowels. Alternatively if these organs are not functioning efficiently, the skin takes over some of their work, and this can give rise to congested skin, boils, rashes and other skin problems.

Any of the essential oils known as lymphatic stimulants or hepatics, such as grapefruit, sweet orange, peppermint, rosemary, carrot seed, can assist the skin, as can essential oils which stimulate the kidneys such as juniper and fennel, or essential oils such as ginger which will increase perspiration.

Reducing inflammation

The anti-inflammatory properties of essential oils such as German chamomile have been thoroughly investigated and documented. Other essential oils which reduce inflammation are lavender, neroli, yarrow, and everlasting. German chamomile and everlasting have anti-inflammatory and anti-allergenic properties, and have been shown to be effective in the treatment of eczema and dermatitis.

Regulating sebum production

Sebum is produced by the oil glands to keep the skin supple. Essential oils such as geranium, palmarosa and rosewood may be used to help balance the secretions of the glands. For example dry skin is caused by too little sebum, while oily skin is caused by excessive sebum production.

Reducing the impact of emotional stress

The skin provides an interface with the world. The sensory nerves in the skin respond to the environment. The sense of touch is considered one of the most powerful and important senses, physically, emotionally and psychologically.

The skin reflects the emotional state. Poor skin may not necessarily represent poor living habits, but may indicate the level of stress, anxiety, lost love, spiritual crisis or any other problem. In these cases, the oils can be used to reduce and soothe the underlying disharmony on the emotional, psychological or spiritual level.

In traditional Chinese medicine the facial features and skin tissue are used as a diagnostic aid. Over the years, grief, depression, anxiety, fear, apathy as well as joy, laughter and contentment all leave their mark. Excessive grief and depression may affect the heart, which in turn causes redness and inflammation to appear. This

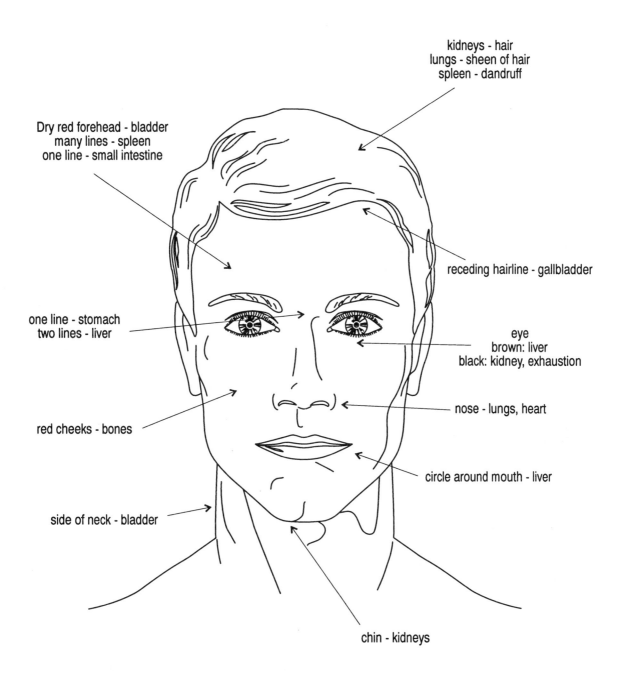

kidneys - hair
lungs - sheen of hair
spleen - dandruff

Dry red forehead - bladder
many lines - spleen
one line - small intestine

receding hairline - gallbladder

one line - stomach
two lines - liver

eye
brown: liver
black: kidney, exhaustion

nose - lungs, heart

red cheeks - bones

circle around mouth - liver

side of neck - bladder

chin - kidneys

Facial diagnosis according to traditional Chinese medicine

does not mean that broken capillaries are always a result of grief, but it is obvious that the condition of the heart and blood vessels affects the redness and blueness of the skin.

Essential oils such as neroli and lavender are used to soothe and calm not only the skin, but also the mind. Anger and frustration affect the liver. This may result in poorly assimilated food, often leading to dry skin. Rose, ylang-ylang and rosemary will help to correct the imbalance of the mind-body relationship, while rose, sandalwood and chamomile will also help the skin directly.

Dehydrated skin is usually associated with fear and the kidneys. The kidneys regulate the amount of water in the body, which in turn affects the water content of the skin. A dehydrated skin may indicate a dehydrated body, which may be due to insufficient fluid intake or kidney dysfunction. Essential oils that may be used to assist dehydrated skin are sandalwood and geranium.

Oily skin is physically related to the large intestine and worry. Worry tends to affect the diet. Worried people will often eat too much, especially the wrong foods. Constipation often results from the tension of continual thinking and worrying. Essential oils such as lemon, geranium and lavender may be of assistance.

Aromatherapy skin care

Finding the appropriate skin care routine is a combination of using the correct products for a particular skin type and finding products which are enjoyable to use. Despite all the advertising hype, there are no instant solutions for a problem skin. The only way to improve the skin is to treat it well. Aromatherapy skin care is simple and based on the age-old routine of

- cleansing
- toning
- moisturising.

Remember that it takes between 21 to 28 days for skin to renew itself, so the skin-care routine must be followed for at least three weeks before results can be seen.

Cleansing

The basis of cleansing is simple - to remove excess sebum, make-up, dirt etc. from the skin in a gentle manner. According to Paula Begoun (4) the most important part of cleaning the face is using water. This makes a lot of sense, especially since water:

- is one of the most abundant natural resources in our environment, making it inexpensive to use!

- reduces friction (Hands will glide over a wet face preventing pulling at the skin. Constant wiping and pulling on the skin eventually weakens the skin's elasticity.)

- is gentle, as long as it is used tepid (Hot water will burn and cold water will shock the skin.).

However, water alone is not suitable if mascara, lipstick or heavy foundation are worn. Water and soap may be suggested, however this is not totally effective. The alkalinity of most soaps disrupts the acid mantle of the skin and some soaps have synthetic fragrances that can cause irritation and sensitisation. The individual is the best judge of the soap or cleanser which best suits the skin. Indications of use of the wrong soap include a sensation of excessive tightening of the skin, drying and scaling, redness, irritation and itching.

Many commercial products use surfactants such as sodium lauryl sulphate, which is quite 'aggressive' as it removes all traces of sebum from the skin, creating a dry and sensitive skin. An all-time favourite is liquid castille soap which is made using potassium hydroxide and olive oil to create a liquid soap. To make a cleansing wash using castille soap add 1ml of essential oil to each 100ml of castille soap.

Depending on the skin type a cleansing soap, a liquid lathering cleanser, cleansing milk or cleansing cream may be appropriate.

Make-up should be removed with a cream or lotion cleanser. The first cleansing cream was developed by the Greek physician, Galen, in AD 150. It was a mixture of melted beeswax, olive oil, water and rosewater. He found that it had a cooling sensation to the skin (hence the name 'cold cream'). Galen's formula has been refined over the years but the combination of water and oil remains the basis of cleansing creams.

For cleansing, use a simple lotion that does not contain lanolin or mineral oil and as few emulsifiers and preservatives as possible. Cold pressed jojoba oil often makes a good cleanser.

A basic cleansing cream recipe is as follows:

> 15 ml of beeswax
> 90 ml almond oil
> 75 ml purified water or herbal infusion
> 20 gm of vegetable emulsifying wax
> 5 drops of an appropriate essential oil according to skin type
> 2 drops of benzoin tincture.

Melt the waxes in a bain marie and add the oil to it at a low heat until they have combined. Heat the purified water to the same temperature in a separate container.

Slowly add the water to the oil/wax mixture and beat the mixture continuously. Lastly add the essential oil and the benzoin tincture, and pour into a container.

Toning

Toners are used to:

- remove all traces of the cleanser

- act as gentle astringents

- brighten the skin and restore its acidity level which is inevitably altered by cleansing and washing

- heal the skin.

For toning, use simple floral waters such as rosewater or orange flower water or herbal infusions. Floral waters can be used as facial sprays on hot days to freshen and hydrate the skin. The finest floral waters are by-products of essential oil production.

Keep a spray bottle of floral water in the clinic. It is an excellent way to finish a facial treatment when the client appears a little too dreamy after the massage. As with essential oils floral waters vary considerably in quality. Some are alcohol and water mixes, some are distilled water with a little oil or perfume added, some are glycerine and water with essential oils. Check with your supplier

that you are buying the genuine residual distillate or distilled floral water.

The following table lists the commonly-available floral waters and their uses:

Floral water	Function
Rose	ideal for all skin types as a freshener or toner
Orange flower	ideal for combination and sensitive skin types
Lavender	ideal for normal and sensitive skin types
Chamomile	ideal for dry, sensitive and inflammed skin
Witch hazel	astringent, ideally suited for oily skin

Another alternative is to dissolve the essential oil in water using a dispersant. The dispersant, often a fractionated glyceride of a vegetable oil, is used to dissolve the essential oil in water. The solution is made by mixing 5 drops of essential oil to 5ml of dispersant and then adding this to 100ml of water.

Moisturising

A moisturiser will:

- prevent moisture loss by adding a protective film to the skin

- protect the skin against dirt, damage, pollution and harsh climatic and living conditions

- give the skin a plump, smooth, supple appearance.

Moisturing creams are emulsions of water, oil and wax. The oil softens, smoothes, prevents moisture loss and protects the skin while the water adds moisture to the skin and the wax acts as an emulsifier. As water and oil do not blend, emulsifiers are used which allow for very small droplets of oil to be suspended in water.

A basic moisturising cream, suitable for all skin types is as follows:

> 20 ml (4 tsps) emulsifying wax
> 60 ml of cold pressed vegetable oil or oils to suit your skin type
> 90 ml of purified water.

To prepare, melt the wax in a bowl in a bain marie and add in the oils. Bring the water to the same temperature in a separate bowl. Remove both bowls from the heat and beat the water into the oil/wax mixture. Add five drops of an essential oil suitable for skin type and add two drops of benzoin tincture to help preserve the cream. This recipe is designed to be adapted to an individual's requirements.

Moisturisers are particularly beneficial for people with dry skin who suffer from low sebum production. If the body is not able to produce an effective acid mantle which is a combination of sebum and perspiration, the skin will be unprotected causing moisture loss. Adding a topical moisturiser creates an artificial barrier that combines with the sebum on the skin to retain the moisture.

Facial oils are often used as rich formulations of a regular moisturiser. They are based on pure cold-pressed vegetable oils and essential oils. As the skin becomes older and drier, vegetable oils such as wheatgerm oil, avocado oil and infused carrot oil should be used.

Appendix 1 Glossary

Absolute: Products obtained from a concrete, a pomade or a resinoid by extraction with ethanol at room temperature. The resulting ethanol solution is generally cooled and filtered to eliminate the waxes. The ethanol is then eliminated by distillation.

Anosmic: Complete loss of sense of smell. May be temporary or permanent.

Anaerobic: A type of organic respiration which does not require oxygen. Many bacteria are anaerobic.

Aromatic water: Aqueous distillates, remaining from water or steam distillation after essential oils have been separated.

Arrhythmia: Irregular or loss of rhythm of the heartbeat.

Arteriosclerosis: A loss of elasticity of the arteries.

Atherosclerosis: An accumulation of fatty deposits on the inner walls of the arteries.

Balsam: An oily or resinous substance exuded by a plant in response to injury to its tissue.

Chemotype: Variation in the chemical composition of an essential oil produced from two or more plants of the same species.

Chi or Qi: A term used in traditional Chinese medicine and holistic therapies, referring to the lifeforce.

Colonoscopy: Examination of the upper portion of the rectum with an elongated speculum.

Concrete: Extracts obtained with non-aqueous solvents from fresh, natural raw materials. A concrete consists mainly of waxy components of plant materials. Mainly prepared for the production of absolutes.

Defensive Qi: The Qi that permeates the surface of the body and wards off external pathogens.

Endocrine: A gland without a duct.

Essential oil: A product obtained from natural raw materials by distillation or expression.

Exocrine: A gland, with a duct, which secretes directly onto the outside surface of an organism.

Functional group: The smallest part of an organic molecule consisting of a single atom or group of atoms that substitutes for a hydrogen atom and has a profound effect upon the properties of the molecule as a whole.

Hepatotoxicity: Having a harmful or toxic effect on the liver.

Hypoxia: Deficiency of oxygen.

Isomers: Compounds that have the same molecular formula but different structures and hence different properties.

Lichenification: Cutaneous thickening and hardening from continued irritation.

LD_{50}:   This stands for 'lethal dose 50%'. It is a traditionally accepted method of determining toxicity. The value is the dosage required to kill 50% of the group of animals used in the test (usually rats or mice). LD_{50} values are usually expressed in grams of the toxic substance per kilogram of body weight.

Menarche: Onset of menses.

Myelin: A fatty material enveloping the majority of nerve cells.

Neurotoxic: Having a harmful or toxic effect on the nervous system.

Occlusions: The covering of the skin with an impermeable material which prevents evaporation of a volatile substance from the skin.

Oxidation: The addition of oxygen to, or the removal of electrons or hydrogen from, an organic molecule.

Pomade: Perfumed fat obtained as a result of enfleurage.

Pheromone: A chemical messenger used as a signal between individuals.

Polar: A term used to describe a molecule which has a partial positive and negative charge. Polar molecules are generally water-soluble.

Rectification: The process in which an essential oil is distilled a second time to remove unwanted constituents (also known as redistillation).

Resinoid: An extract obtained from dried, natural, raw materials by use of non-aqueous solvents.

Terpeneless oil: Essential oils from which the monoterpene hydrocarbons have been removed.

Terpenoid: Essential oil constituents based on the isoprene skeleton, but containing a functional group.

Tincture: Solutions obtained by maceration of natural raw materials in ethanol. Such products are commonly used in herbal medicine.

Appendix 2

List of Properties

Abortifacient	An agent capable of inducing abortion.
Alterative	An agent which cleanses the blood and corrects impure blood conditions.
Analgesic	Loss of sensation - pain relieving.
Anaphrodisiac	Diminishing sexual desire.
Anthelmintic	A vermifuge, destroying or expelling intestinal worms.
Anti sudorific	Reduces sweating.
Anti-allergenic	Reduces symptoms of allergy.
Anti-arthritic	An agent which combats arthritis.
Anti-emetic	Reduces the incidence and severity of vomiting.
Anti-inflammatory	Alleviates inflammation.
Anticonvulsive	Helps arrest or control convulsions.
Antidepressant	Uplifting, counteracting melancholy.
Antimicrobial	An agent which resists or destroys pathogenic organisms.
Antiphlogistic	Reduces inflammation.
Antipruritic	relieves sensations of itching or prevents its occurrence.
Antirheumatic	Helps to relieve rheumatism.
Antiseptic	Helps control infection.
Antispasmodic	Prevents and eases spasms and relieves cramps.
Aphrodisiac	Exciting sexual desire.
Astringent	Contracts, tightens and binds tissues.
Bactericide	An agent that destroys bacteria.
Balsamic	A soothing substance having the qualities of a balsam.
Cardiac	Stimulating effect on the heart.
Carminative	Settles the digestive system, expulsion of gas from the intestines.
Cephalic	Stimulating and clearing the mind.
Cholagogue	Increases the secretion and flow of bile production into the duodenum.
Choleretic	Aids excretion of bile by the liver, so that there is a greater flow of bile.
Cicatrisant	Helps formation of scar tissue.
Cordial	A stimulant and tonic for the heart.
Cytophylactic	Encouraging growth of skin cells.
Decongestant	An agent which relieves or reduces congestion, eg nasal mucus.
Demulcent	Soothes, softens and allays irritation of mucous membranes.
Deodorant	Destroying odour.
Depurative	Helps to purify the blood, detoxifying.
Diaphoretic	Promotes perspiration.
Digestive	A substance that aids the digestion of food.

Disinfectant	Prevents and combats the spread of germs.
Diuretic	Increases urine flow.
Emetic	Induces vomiting.
Emmenagogue	Promotes and regulates menstrual flow.
Emollient	Soothes and softens skin.
Expectorant	Helps to expel mucus from the respiratory system.
Febrifuge	Cooling and reducing high body temperature.
Fungicide	Destroying fungal infections.
Galactagogue	Increasing secretion of milk.
Germicidal	Destroys germs or micro-organisms.
Haemostatic	Arrests bleeding haemorrhage.
Hepatic	Stimulates and aids function of liver and gall bladder.
Hypertensive	Increases blood pressure.
Hypoglycaemiant	Lowers blood sugar levels.
Hypotensive	Lowers blood pressure.
Insecticide	Kills insects.
Laxative	Aiding bowel evacuation.
Mucolytic	Dissolves or breaking down mucus.
Nervine	Strengthening or toning to the nerves and nervous system.
Parturient	Helping delivery in childbirth.
Prophylactic	Helping prevent disease.
Relaxant	Soothing, causing relaxation, relieving strain or tension.
Rubefacient	Warming and increasing blood flow.
Sedative	An agent that reduces functional activity; calming.
Soporific	A substance which induces sleep.
Spasmolytic	See antispasmodic.
Splenetic	A tonic to the spleen.
Stimulant	An agent which increases the physiological functions of the body.
Stomachic	Digestive aid and tonic, improving appetite.
Styptic	Arrests external bleeding.
Sudorific	Increases perspiration.
Tonic	Strengthens and improves bodily performance.
Uterine	Tonic to the uterus.
Vasoconstrictor	Contraction of blood vessel walls.
Vasodilator	Dilation of blood vessels.
Vermifuge	Expulsion of worms.
Vulnerary	Prevents tissue degeneration and arrests bleeding in wounds.

Appendix 3   Therapeutic Cross Reference

Skin care

Acne   Bergamot, cajeput, German and Roman chamomile, *geranium*, juniperberry, *French alpine lavender*, lemon, lemongrass, lime, palmarosa, rosemary, rosewood, sandalwood, *tea tree*

Allergies   *German and Roman chamomile, everlasting, French alpine lavender*

Athlete's foot   Eucalyptus, lavender, lemon, *myrrh*, patchouli, tagetes, tea tree

Burns   German and Roman chamomile, *lavender, tea tree*, yarrow

Cold sores   Bergamot, eucalyptus, *tea tree*

Congested and dull skin   *Geranium*, grapefruit, *lavender*, palmarosa, rosemary

Cuts/sores   German and Roman chamomile, cistus, eucalyptus, geranium, lavender, lemon, *tea tree*, yarrow

Dermatitis   Carrot seed, *German chamomile,* Roman chamomile, *everlasting*, infused calendula oil, juniperberry, *lavender*, palmarosa, patchouli

Dry and sensitive skin   German and Roman chamomile, infused calendula oil, jasmine, *lavender, neroli, patchouli, rose otto, rosewood, sandalwood*

Greasy and oily skin   Bay, *bergamot*, cajeput, cedarwood, clary sage, cypress, *geranium, juniperberry, lavender*, lemon, mandarin, myrtle, niaouli, palmarosa, patchouli, rosemary, rosewood, sandalwood, tea tree, ylang-ylang

Insect repellent   Cedarwood, *citronella*, clove bud, eucalyptus, spike lavender, lemongrass, *peppermint*, tea tree, thyme

Psoriasis   Bergamot, carrot seed, *German chamomile, lavender,* juniperberry, tea tree

Scars and Stretch marks   Frankincense, *lavender, neroli*, palmarosa, rosewood, sandalwood

Mature and aging skin   Carrot seed, infused carrot oil, frankincense, geranium, jasmine, lavender, *myrrh*, neroli, palmarosa, *patchouli*, rose, rosewood, sandalwood, sweet fennel, ylang-ylang

Musculoskeletal system

Aches and pains   Cajeput, German and Roman chamomile, clove bud, eucalyptus, fir, ginger, lavender, *spike lavender*, lemongrass, peppermint, Spanish marjoram, sweet marjoram, nutmeg, *black pepper, rosemary*, Spanish sage, pine, red thyme

Arthritis   *Cajeput*, carrot seed, clove bud, *German chamomile*, eucalyptus, ginger, *juniperberry, spike lavender*, lemon, Spanish marjoram, sweet marjoram, nutmeg, black pepper, pine, *rosemary*, Spanish sage, thyme, vetiver, yarrow

Poor muscle tone   Ginger, grapefruit, *lemongrass*, sweet marjoram, *black pepper*, pine, rosemary

Gout   Carrot seed, juniperberry, *lemon*, rosemary, thyme

Circulatory system

Oedema and water retention   Carrot seed, cypress, *sweet fennel*, grapefruit, *juniperberry*, lemon, cold pressed lime, mandarin, orange, tangerine

Palpitations   melissa, *neroli*, rose, ylang-ylang

Poor circulation and low blood pressure Bay, cinnamon leaf, cypress, eucalyptus, geranium, *ginger*, lemon, lemongrass, niaouli, nutmeg, *black pepper*, pine, rose, *rosemary*, Spanish sage, *thyme*

Cellulitis   *Cypress, sweet fennel, geranium, grapefruit, juniperberry, lemon*, rosemary, thyme

High blood pressure   Melissa, garlic, *lavender, sweet marjoram*, yarrow, *ylang-ylang*

Respiratory system

Asthma   Cajeput, clary sage, cypress, eucalyptus, *frankincense*, hyssop, *lavender*, lemon, mandarin, sweet marjoram, peppermint, spearmint, myrrh, niaouli, pine, tea tree

Bronchitis   Aniseed, cajeput, cedarwood, cypress, *eucalyptus*, fir, frankincense, hyssop, lavender, spike lavender, sweet and Spanish marjoram, peppermint, *myrrh, myrtle*, niaouli, *sandalwood*, tea tree, thyme

Catarrh   Cajeput, cedarwood, everlasting, *eucalyptus*, frankincense, ginger, hyssop, *lavender, spike lavender, peppermint, pine*, myrtle, niaouli, black pepper, pine, sandalwood, *tea tree, thyme*

Chronic coughs   Atlas cedarwood, cypress, eucalyptus, *frankincense, hyssop*, peppermint, myrrh, myrtle, sandalwood, *sweet marjoram, pine*, rosemary, tea tree

Sinusitis   Basil, cajeput, eucalyptus, everlasting, fir, ginger, peppermint, niaouli, pine, tea tree

Digestive system

Colic   Aniseed, black pepper, cardamom, carrot seed, *German and Roman chamomile*, sweet fennel, ginger, *sweet marjoram, peppermint*, neroli, rosemary

Constipation and sluggish digestion
Cinnamon leaf, sweet fennel, sweet marjoram, nutmeg, sweet or bitter orange, *black pepper*

Heartburn   Cardamom, black pepper

Indigestion/ flatulence   Aniseed, black pepper, *cardamom, sweet fennel*, sweet marjoram, *peppermint*, spearmint, orange

Nausea/vomiting   *Sweet fennel*, ginger, *peppermint*, spearmint, black pepper

Genito-urinary and endocrine system

Amenorrhoea   Basil, carrot seed, *clary sage*, Roman chamomile, sweet fennel, hyssop, sweet marjoram, myrrh, rose, *Spanish sage* , yarrow

Dysmenorrhoea   *Clary sage, German and Roman chamomile*, cypress, geranium, lavender, jasmine, juniperberry, *sweet marjoram*, rose, rosemary, yarrow

Cystitis   *Bergamot*, Atlas, Texas and Virginian cedarwood, German and Roman chamomile, juniperberry, lavender, *sandalwood, tea tree*

Menopausal problems   Clary sage, cypress, *sweet fennel, geranium*, jasmine, juniperberry, rose

Premenstrual syndrome   Bergamot, *German and Roman chamomile*, clary sage, *geranium*, juniperberry, *lavender*, sweet marjoram, neroli, rose, ylang-ylang

Thrush/candida   Bergamot, lavender, lemongrass, melissa, myrrh, rose, rosemary, tea tree

Nervous system

Anxiety   Basil, bergamot, frankincense, jasmine, lavender, neroli, ylang-ylang

Depression   Basil, bergamot, grapefruit, jasmine, lavender, orange, neroli, rose, pine, vetiver, ylang-ylang

Headache   German and Roman chamomile, *lavender*, sweet marjoram, peppermint, *rosemary*, rosewood, thyme

Insomnia   *Lavender*, sweet marjoram, neroli, sandalwood, orange

Nervous exhaustion   *Basil, cinnamon leaf*, citronella, eucalyptus, ginger, jasmine, lemongrass, peppermint, petitgrain, *rosemary*, vetiver, thyme

Appendix 4 — List of Essential Oils

Essential Oil	Botanical Name	Origin	Part of Plant	Method of Extraction
Ajowan	*Trachyspermum copticum*	India	Seeds	Steam distillation
Ambrete seed	*Abelmoschus moschatus*	India	Seeds	Steam distillation
Amyris	*Amyris balsamifera*	Haiti	Wood and branches	Steam distillation
Amyris	*Amyris balsamifera*	West Indies	Wood	Steam distillation
Angelica	*Angelica archangelica*	Europe	Roots or seeds	Steam distillation
Anise, Star	*Illicium verum*	China	Seeds and dried flowering tops	Steam distillation
Aniseed	*Pimpinella anisum*	Spain	Seeds and dried flowering tops	Steam distillation
Asafoetida	*Ferula asafoetida*	Afghanistan	Oleoresin from roots	Steam distillation
Balsam, Fir	*Abies balsamea*	Canada	Oleoresin	Steam distillation
Basil (linalool)	*Ocimum basilicum*	France	Leaves and flowering tops	Steam distillation
Basil (Methyl chavicol)	*Ocimum basilicum*	Comoro Islands	Leaves and flowering tops	Steam distillation
Bay Laurel	*Laurus nobilis*	Mediterranean region	Leaves	Steam distillation
Bay, West Indian	*Pimenta racemosa*	West Indies	Leaves	Steam or water distillation
Benzoin	*Styrax benzoin*	South East Asia	Resin	Solvent extraction
Bergamot	*Citrus aurantium* ssp. *bergamia*	Italy	Fruit rind	Steam distillation
Birch	*Betula lenta*	USA	Bark	Steam distillation
Black Pepper	*Piper nigrum*	Indonesia	Dried black peppercorns	Steam distillation
Boldo Leaf	*Peumus boldus*	Chile	Leaves	Steam distillation
Buchu	*Agothosma betulina*	South Africa	Dried leaves	Steam distillation
Cade	*Juniperus oxycedrus*	Europe	Branches and heartwood	Destructive distillation
Cajeput	*Melaleuca cajeputi*	Australia	Fresh leaves and twigs	Steam distillation
Calamus	*Acorus calamus* var. *angustatus*	India	Roots	Steam distillation
Camphor	*Cinnamomum camphora*	China	Wood, root stumps and branches	Steam distillation
Cananga	*Cananga odorata*	Indonesia and Philippines	Flowers	Water distillation
Caraway	*Carum carvi*	Europe	Ripe seeds	Steam distillation
Cardamom	*Elettaria cardamomum*	India and Sri Lanka	Dried ripe seeds	Steam distillation
Carrot Seed	*Daucus carota*	Europe	Seeds	Steam distillation
Cassia	*Cinnamomum cassia*	China	Leaves, twigs, or bark	Steam or water distillation
Cassie	*Acacia farnesiana*	East Indies	Flowers	Solvent extraction
Cedarwood Atlas	*Cedrus atlantica*	Morocco	Wood	Steam distillation
Cedarwood, Himalayan	*Cedrus deodorata*	Nepal	Wood	Steam distillation
Cedarwood, Texas	*Juniperus ashei*	USA	Heartwood	Steam distillation
Cedarwood, Virginian	*Juniperus virginiana*	North America	Wood	Steam distillation
Celery Seed	*Apium graveolens*	Southern Europe	Whole or crushed seeds	Steam distillation
Chamomile, Blue	*Matricaria recutita*	Europe	Flower heads	Steam distillation

Essential Oil	Botanical Name	Origin	Part of Plant	Method of Extraction
Chamomile, Maroc	*Ormenis multicaulis*	Morocco	Flower heads	Steam distillation
Chamomile, Roman	*Chamaemelum nobile*	Western Europe	Flower heads	Steam distillation
Cinnamon	*Cinnamomum zeylanicum*	Sri Lanka	Leaves and twigs or bark	Steam or water distillation
Cistus	*Cistus ladaniferus*	Mediterranean region	Resin or the leaves and twigs	Steam distillation
Citronella	*Cymbogon winterianus*	Java	Fresh or partly dried grass	Steam distillation
Citronella	*Cymbogon nardus*	Sri Lanka	Fresh or partly dried grass	Steam distillation
Clary Sage	*Salvia sclarea*	Europe	Leaves and flowering tops	Steam distillation
Clove	*Eugenia caryophyllata*	Indonesia, Molucca Is. Madagascar	Buds, leaves, stalks or stems	Water distillation
Coriander	*Coriandrum sativum*	Europe	Seeds	Steam distillation
Costus	*Saussurea costus*	India	Dried mascerated roots	Maceration, steam distiilation
Cubeba	*Piper cubeba*	Indonesia	Unripe berries	Steam distillation
Cypress	*Cupressus sempervirens*	Europe	Needles, cones and twigs	Steam distillation
Dill	*Anethum graveolens*	Mediterranean region	Seeds or herb	Steam distillation
Elecampane	*Inula helenium*	Europe	Dried roots	Steam distillation
Elemi	*Canarium luzonicum*	Indonesia, Phillipines	Resin or gum	Steam distillation
Eucalyptus, Australiana	*Eucalyptus radiata*	Australia	Leaves and twigs	Steam distillation
Eucalyptus, Blue Gum	*Eucalyptus globulus*	Australia	Leaves and twigs	Steam distillation
Eucalyptus, Lemon-scented	*Eucalyptus citriodora*	Australia	Leaves and twigs	Steam distillation
Eucalyptus, Peppermint	*Eucalyptus dives*	Australia	Leaves and twigs	Steam distillation
Everlasting	*Helichrysum angustifolium*	Mediterranean region	Flowering tops	Steam distillation
Fennel, Bitter	*Foeniculum vulgare var. amara*	Europe, Tasmania	Seeds	Steam distillation
Fennel, Sweet	*Foeniculum vulgare var. dulce*	Europe	Seeds	Steam distillation
Fir Canadian	*Abies alba*	Canada	Needles and young twigs	Steam distillation
Fir, Siberian	*Abies siberica*	Siberia	Needles and young twigs	Steam distillation
Fir, Silver	*Abies alba*	Europe	Needles and young twigs	Steam distillation
Frankincense	*Boswellia carteri*	Somalia	Resin or gum	Steam distillation
Galbanum	*Ferula galbaniflua*	Middle East	Resin or gum	Steam distillation
Geranium	*Pelargonium graveolens*	Reunion, Egypt, China	Leaves, stalks and flowers	Steam distillation
Ginger	*Zingiber officinale*	China, India	Dried, ground roots	Steam distillation
Grapefruit	*Citrus paradisi*	USA	Fruit peel	Cold pressed
Hops	*Humulus lupulus*	Europe	Dried cones	Steam distillation
Horseradish	*Armoracia rusticana*	Russia, Europe	Ground roots	Steam or water distillation
Hyssop	*Hyssopus officinalis*	Europe	Leaves and flowering tops	Steam distillation
Jasmine	*Jasminum officinale*	France, Morocco, Egypt, India	Flowers	Solvent extraction, enfleurage
Juniper	*Juniperus communis*	Europe	Berries, or needles and wood	Steam distillation
Labdanum	*Cistus ladaniferus*	Spain	Resin or gum	Steam distillation
Lavandin	*Lavendula burnatii*	France	Fresh flowering tops	Steam distillation
Lavender, Spike	*Lavendula latifolia*	Spain	Fresh flowering tops	Steam distillation
Lavender	*Lavendula angustifolia*	Tasmania, France	Fresh flowering tops	Steam distillation

Essential Oil	Botanical Name	Origin	Part of Plant	Method of Extraction
Lemon verbena	*Lippia citriodora*	France	Leaves	Steam distillation
Lemon	*Citrus limon*	USA, Mediterranean region	Citrus peel	Cold pressed
Lemongrass	*Cymbopogon citratus*	Sri Lanka	Grass	Steam distillation
Lime, Cold Pressed	*Citrus medica*	USA	Citrus peel	Cold pressed
Lime, Distilled	*Citrus medica*	USA	Fruits	Steam distillation
Mandarin	*Citrus reticulata*	USA	Citrus peel	Cold pressed
Marjoram, Spanish	*Thymus mastichina*	Spain	Dried flowering herb	Steam distillation
Marjoram, Sweet	*Origanum majorana*	Europe	Dried flowering herb	Steam distillation
May Chang	*Litsea cubeba*	China	Fruits	Steam distillation
Melissa	*Melissa officinalis*	Europe	Leaves	Steam distillation
Mugwort	*Artemisia vulgaris*	Europe	Leaves and flowering tops	Steam distillation
Mustard	*Brassica nigra*	Europe	Black mustard seeds	Steam distillation
Myrrh	*Commiphora myrrha*	Somalia	Resin or gum	Steam distillation
Myrtle	*Myrtus communis*	North Africa	Leaves and twigs	Steam distillation
Neroli	*Citrus aurantium var. amara*	France, Morocco	Flowers	Steam distillation
Niaouli	*Melaleuca viridiflora*	Australia	Leaves and twigs	Steam distillation
Nutmeg	*Myristica fragrans*	Indonesia	Dried nutmeg seeds	Steam distillation
Oakmoss	*Evernia prunastri*	Europe	Lichen	Solvent extraction
Opopanax	*Commiphora erythraea*	East Africa	Oleogum resin	Steam or water distillation
Orange Sweet	*Citrus sinensis*	Brazil, Australia, USA	Citrus peel	Cold pressed
Orange, Bitter	*Citrus aurantium var. amara*	France	Citrus peel	Cold pressed
Oregano, Common	*Origanum vulgare*	Europe	Dried flowering herb	Steam distillation
Oregano, Spanish	*Thymus capitatus*	Spain	Dried flowering herb	Steam distillation
Palmarosa	*Cymbopogon martinii*	India, Indonesia, Comoro Is.	Grass	Steam or water distillation
Parsley	*Petroselinum sativum*	Europe	Seeds or herb	Steam distillation
Patchouli	*Pogostemom cablin*	Indonesia	Dried leaves	Steam distillation
Pennyroyal	*Mentha pulegium*	Europe or USA	Herb	Steam distillation
Peppermint, Japanese	*Mentha arvensis*	China	Herb	Steam distillation
Peppermint	*Mentha piperata*	USA	Flowering herb	Steam distillation
Petitgrain	*Citrus aurantium var. amara*	France	Leaves and twigs	Steam distillation
Pine, Dwarf	*Pinus mugo var. pumilo*	Austria	Needles and twigs	Steam distillation
Pine, Longleaf	*Pinus palustris*	USA	Wood chips	Steam distillation
Pine, Scotch	*Pinus sylvestris*	Baltic States	Needles and twigs	Steam distillation
Rose, Cabbage	*Rosa centifolia*	France, Morocco	Flowers	Water distillation or solvent extraction
Rose, Damask	*Rosa damascena*	Bulgaria, France, Turkey	Flowers	Water distillation or solvent extraction
Rosemary (Camphor)	*Rosmarinus officinalis*	Spain	Leaves and flowering tops	Steam distillation
Rosemary (Cineole)	*Rosmarinus officinalis*	Tunisia	Leaves and flowering tops	Steam distillation
Rosemary (Verbenone)	*Rosmarinus officinalis*	France	Leaves and flowering tops	Steam distillation

Essential Oil	Botanical Name	Origin	Part of Plant	Method of Extraction
Rosewood	*Aniba rosaeodora*	Brazil	Wood	Steam distillation
Rue	*Ruta graveolens*	Europe	Fresh herb	Steam distillation
Sage, Common	*Salvia officinalis*	Europe	Dried leaves	Steam distillation
Sage, Spanish	*Salvia lavendulaefolia*	Spain	Leaves	Steam distillation
Sandalwood, Australian	*Santalum spicatum*	Australia	Wood	Steam distillation
Sandalwood, East Indian	*Santalum album*	India	Wood	Steam distillation
Sandalwood, West Indian	*Amyris balsamifera*	Haiti	Wood and branches	Steam distillation
Sassafras	*Sassafras albidum*	USA	Dried roots bark chips	Steam distillation
Savine	*Juniperus sabina*	North America	Twigs and leaves	Steam distillation
Savory, Summer	*Satureja hortensis*	Europe	Whole herb	Steam distillation
Savory, Winter	*Satureja montana*	Spain	Whole herb	Steam distillation
Spearmint	*Mentha spicata*	USA	Leaves and flowering tops	Steam distillation
Spikenard	*Nardostachys jatamansi*	India	Dried and crushed roots	Steam distillation
Spruce	*Tsuga canadensis*	USA	Needles and twigs	Steam distillation
Styrax	*Liquidamber orientalis*	Asia	Oleogum resin	Steam distillation
Tagetes	*Tagetes minuta*	South America	Fresh flowering herb	Steam distillation
Tangerine	*Citrus reticulata blanco*	USA	Fruit rind	Cold pressed
Tansy	*Tanacetum vulgare*	Europe	Leaves and flowering tops	Steam distillation
Tarragon	*Artemisia dracunculus*	Europe	Leaves	Steam distillation
Tea Tree	*Melaleuca alternifolia*	Australia	Fresh leaves and twigs	Steam or water distillation
Thuja	*Thuja occidentalis*	North America	Fresh leaves and twigs	Steam distillation
Thyme, Lemon	*Thymus citriodorus*	Mediterranean Region	Leaves and flowering tops	Steam or water distillation
Thyme, Red	*Thymus vulgaris*	Mediterranean Region	Leaves and flowering tops	Steam or water distillation
Thyme, Spanish	*Thymus zygis*	Spain	Leaves and flowering tops	Steam or water distillation
Thyme, Wild	*Thymus serpyllum*	Mediterranean Region	Leaves and flowering tops	Steam or water distillation
Tuberose	*Polianthes tuberosa*	France	Flowers	Solvent extraction
Turmeric	*Curcuma longa*	Indonesia	Roots	Steam distillation
Turpentine	*Pinus palustris* and other pinus species	USA	Oleoresin	Steam distillation
Valerian	*Valeriana officinalis*	Europe	Roots	Steam distillation
Vanilla	*Vanilla planifolia*	Madagascar	Beans	Steam distillation
Vetiver	*Vetiveria zizanoides*	Indonesia and Sri Lanka	Roots	Steam distillation
Violet Leaf	*Viola odorata*	Europe	Fresh leaves	Solvent extraction
Wintergreen	*Gaultheria procumbens*	North America	Leaves	Steam or water distillation
Wormseed	*Chenopodium ambrosioides*	South America	Whole herb	Steam distillation
Wormwood	*Artemisia absinthium*	Europe	Leaves and flowering tops	Steam distillation
Yarrow	*Achillea millefolium*	Europe	Dried herb	Steam distillation
Ylang Ylang	*Cananga odorata* var. *genuina*	Madagascar	Flowers	Steam distillation

Introduction

Several different kinds of acupressure techniques are currently practiced, although the same pressure points are used for all of them. Varying rhythms, pressure, and techniques create different styles of acupressure. Shiatsu, for example, a form of acupressure originating from Japan, can be quite vigorous, with firm pressure applied to each point for only three to five seconds. Other styles of acupressure gently hold the points for a minute or more. Pressing with an intermittent, fast beat is stimulating, while light pressure creates a sedating effect on the body.

How acupressure works

The acupressure points are junctions along special pathways called meridians which carry human energy, known in traditional Chinese medicine as Qi. In traditional Chinese medicine tension and pain are caused when the Qi does not flow freely through the meridians. Acupressure will promote the free flow of Qi, thus relieving tension and pain.

Western scientists have found that, when these points are stimulated by pressure or needles, endorphins - neurotransmitters that relieve pain - are released.

How to apply pressure

A general guideline to follow is that the pressure should be firm enough so that it 'hurts good', in other words, something between pleasant, firm pressure and outright pain. The more developed the muscles are, the more pressure can be applied. If the client is sensitive to the pressure, gradually decrease the pressure until balance is found.

Apply firm pressure on the specified point at 90° to the surface of the skin. If the skin is being pulled then the angle of the pressure is not correct.

How to find a point

Acupressure points are located by referring to anatomical landmarks. To help in finding the points, all of the points mentioned in this book are highlighted in illustrations with descriptions of the anatomical landmarks contained in the accompanying text.

Acupressure techniques

The following techniques are commonly used:

- Firm pressure is the most fundamental technique, using thumbs, fingers, palms, the side of the hand, or knuckles to apply steady, stationary pressure. To relax the area or relieve pain, apply pressure gradually and hold without any movement for several minutes.

- Slow motion kneading uses the thumbs and fingers along with the heels of the hands to squeeze large muscle groups firmly. The motion is similar to that of kneading a large mass of dough. This relieves general stiffness, shoulder and neck tension, constipation and spasms in the calf muscles.

- Brisk rubbing back and forth with the thumb, finger or palm uses friction to stimulate the blood and lymph, as well as to benefit the nerves and tone of the skin.

- Quick tapping with the finger tips stimulates muscles on unprotected, tender areas of the body such as the face. For larger areas of the body such as the back or buttocks, use a loose fist. This can improve the stimulation of energy flow and improve muscle tone.

Do not be tempted to rub or massage the entire area, unless specifically mentioned to do so. It is best to hold the point steadily with direct pressure.

Aromatherapy Courses

For a list of schools and teachers in your area offering practitioner training contact:

> The International Federation of Aromatherapists
> *on*
> National Info Line 190 224 0125
> *or at*
> 1/390 Burwood Rd.,
> Hawthorn, Vic., 3122

For introductory courses and post graduate training on aromatherapy contact:

> The Perfect Potion Training Centre
> PO Box 273,
> Zillmere Qld 4034
> Tel: (07) 3216 2763; Fax: (07) 3865 1483

Practitioners

Aromatherapists

The IFA has published a directory of accredited schools and practitioners. For details of accredited aromatherapists in your area, contact:

> The International Federation of Aromatherapists
> *on*
> National Info Line 190 224 0125
> *or at*
> 1/390 Burwood Rd.,
> Hawthorn, Vic., 3122

Herbalists

For a list of accredited herbalists in your area, contact:

> The National Herbalists Association of Australia
> PO Box 61
> Broadway NSW 2007
> Tel: (02) 211 6452

Natural therapists

For a list of accredited Natural therapists in your area, contact:

> Australian Traditional Medicine Society Ltd
> PO Box 442,
> Ryde, NSW, 2112
> Tel: (02) 809 6800

Essential oil suppliers

To ensure that you are buying the best quality essential oils available choose a supplier that meets the criteria for quality control specified in this book (Chapter 5).

Aromatherapy Journals and Newsletters

Aromatherapy Today Journal, a journal for the professional aromatherapist co-edited by the author of this book, is published quarterly:

Aromatherapy Today
PO Box 273
Zillmere Qld 4034.
Tel: (07) 3216 2263; Fax: (07) 3865 1483

perfect potions, a periodical which contains much practical information for those interested in aromatherapy, is edited by the author of this book and is published quarterly:

The Perfect Potion
PO Box 273
Zillmere Qld 4034.
Tel: (07) 3216 2263; Fax: (07) 3865 1483

International Journal of Aromatherapy, a journal for the professional aromatherapist edited by Robert Tisserand, is published quarterly:

The International Journal of Aromatherapy
Aromatherapy Publications
PO Box 746
Hove, East Sussex, BN3 3XA, UK
Tel: 01273-772479 Fax: 01273-329811

References

Chapter 1 Introduction to Aromatherapy

1. Buchbauer, G., Cited from AROMA'95 conference. Guildford, UK, (1995).

2. Kusmirek, J., *Perspectives in Aromatherapy: Fragrance: The psychology and biology of perfume.* Edited by S. Van Toller and G.H. Dodd, Elsevier Applied Science, UK, (1992), pp.277-285.

3. Tisserand, R., *Aromatherapy Today.* The International Journal of Aromatherapy, AROMA '93 Harmony from Within Conference Proceedings, p.3.

4. *Anti-bacterial Constituents in the Essential oil of Cymbopogon Citratus* Journal of Ethnopharmacology 12 (1984), pp.279-286.

5. Montague, A., *Touching - The Human Significance of the Skin.* Harper and Row, New York, (1986), p.46.

6. Prescot, J., Cited in Montague, A. *Touching - The Human Significance of the Skin.* Harper and Row, New York, (1986), p.326.

7. Hooper, A., *Massage and Loving.* Unwin Hyman Ltd, London, (1988).

8. Field, T., et al, *Massage reduces anxiety in child and adolescent psychiatric patients.* Int. Journal Alternative and Complementary Medicine, Vol. 11, No. 7, (1993), pp.22-27.

9. Bell, G., *The New Healers.* The Independent, April 1994, pp.38-42.

10. Sapira, J., *The Art and Science of Bedside Diagnosis.* Williams & Wilkins, Baltimore, (1990).

11. Husband, A., *Stress, behaviour and the immune system.* Current Affairs Bulletin Aug/Sept 1994, pp.25-31.

12. Meares, A., *A Way of Doctoring.* Hill of Content Publishers, Australia, (1985).

13. O'Neill, J., *Some People will swallow anything.* The Independent, April 1994, pp.36-37.

14. Bach, E., *Heal Thyself.* C.W.Daniel Company, Great Britain, (1931).

15. Cited from *Aroma: The Cultural History of Smell.* By Classen, C., Routledge, London, (1994), p.40.

16. Lapraz, J., *In Profile.* IJA, Vol. 3. No 4, (1991), pp.12-14.

17. Tisserand, R., *Aromatherapy Today.* The International Journal of Aromatherapy, AROMA '93 Harmony from Within Conference Proceedings, (1993), p.8.

Chapter 2 History of Aromatherapy

1. Tisserand, R., *Essential oils as psychotherapeutic agents: Perfumery: The Psychology & Biology of Fragrance.* Chapman & Hall, UK, (1987).

2. Morris, E.T., *Fragrance: The Story of Perfume from Cleopatra to Chanel.* Products of Nature and of Art, USA, (1984).

3. Tisserand, R., *Aromatherapy for Everyone.* Penguin Publications, UK, (1988).

4. Holmyard E.J., *Alchemy.* Dover Publications, New York, 1990, First published in 1957. p. 93.

5. Griggs, B., *Green Pharmacy: A History of Herbal Medicine.* Robert Hale Limited, Great Britain, (1981).

6. Suskind, P., *Perfume*. Penguin Books, England, (1987).

7. Potterton, D., *Culpeper's Colour Herbal*. W.Foulsham & Company Limited, UK, (1983), p.159.

8. Squire, P., F.L.S., J. & A., *Squire's Companion to The British Pharmacopoeia*. Churchill, (1885), 13th Edition.

9. Valnet, J., *The Practice of Aromatherapy*. Destiny Books, USA, (1980).

10. Gattefosse, R., *Gattefosse's Aromatherapy*. From the original French text *'Aromatherapie; Les huiles essentielles hormones vegetales'*, First published in 1937, English version published by C.W Daniel, UK, (1993).

11. Valnet, J., *The Practice of Aromatherapy*. Destiny Books, USA, (1980).

12. Maury, M., *Marguerite Maury's Guide to Aromatherapy: The secret of life and youth*. First published in French as *'Le Capital Jeunesse'* in 1961. English version published by C.W.Daniel, UK, (1964), p.158.

Chapter 3 What Are Essential Oils?

1. Brud, W., *Blending and compounding: Where is the true essential oil?* AROMA '93 Conference Proceedings, IJA, UK, (1993), p.44.

2. Francomme, P., *Phytoguide No. 1: Aromatherapy, Advanced Therapy for Infectious Illnesses*. La Courtete, France: International Phytomedical Foundation, (1985).

3. Hall, R., et al., *The H&R Book: Guide to Fragrance Ingredients*. Johnson Publications Limited, London, 1985.

4. Guenther, E., *The Essential Oils Vol. 1*. D. Van Nostrand Comp. Inc., New York, (1953).

5. Singh, N., and Luthra, R., *Sucrose metabolism and essential oil accumulation during lemongrass leaf development*. Plant Science, Vol. 57, (1987), pp.127-133.

6. Maffei, M., *Photosynthesis, photorespiration and herbicide effect on terpene production in peppermint*. The Journal of Essential Oil Research, Vol. 2, No. 6 Nov/Dec 1990. pp.275-286.

7. Penfold, A.R., and Willis, J.L., *The formation of essential oils in plants*. Aust. J. Pharmacy, Sept, (1955).

8. Gumbel, D., *Principles of Holistic Skin Therapy with Herbal Essences*. Karl F. Haug Publishers, Germany, (1986), p. 131.

9. Erman, W.F., *Chemistry of monoterpenes. In: Studies in Organic Chemistry. Vol. II A and B*. Marcel Dekker, New York, (1985).

10. Morris, E.T., *Fragrance*. Products of Nature and Art, New York, (1984).

11. Dell, B., et al, *Plant resins - their formation, secretion and possible functions*. Adv. Bot. Res., Vol. 6, (1978), pp.277-316.

12. Simon, J., et al, *Water Stress-Induced Alterations in Essential Oil Content and Composition of Sweet Basil*. The Journal of Essential Oil Research Vol. 4, No 1., Jan/Feb 1992.

13. Bhaskaruni R. et al, *Variation in yields and quality of geranium under varied climatic and fertility conditions*. The Journal of Essential Oil Research Vol. 2, No. 2, Mar/Apr 1990.

14. Piccaglia, R., *Effect of mineral fertilisers on the composition of Salvia officinalis oil*. The Journal of Essential Oil Research, Vol. 1, No. 2, Mar/Apr 1995, p.73.

15. Gasic, O., *The influence of Sowing and Harvest Time on the Essential Oils of Chamomilla recutita*. The Journal of Essential Oil Research Vol. 3, No 5, Sep/Oct 1991, pp.295-302.

16. Bonnardeaux, J., *The Effect of Different Harvesting Methods on the Yield and Quality of Basil Oil in the Ord River Irrigation Area.* The Journal of Essential Oil Research Vol. 4, No 1., Jan/Feb 1992.

17. Perrin and Colson, *Timing of the Harvest Date for Mentha piperita Based on the Observations of the Floral Development.* The Journal of Essential Oil Research, Vol. 3. No 1., Jan/Feb 1991.

18. Stahl-Biskup, E., *The Chemical Composition of Thymus Oils.* The Journal of Essential Oil Research, Vol. 3, No. 2., Mar/Apr 1991.

19. Soulier, J., *The Thymus Genus.* Aromatherapy Records, No.1, September, (1995), pp.38-49.

20. Lawrence, B., *Rosemary Oil.* Essential Oils 1981-1987, Allured Publishing, USA, (1989), pp.60-62.

Chapter 4 Methods of Essential Oil Extraction

1. Holmyard, E.J., *Alchemy.* Dover Publications, USA, (1990).

2. Lawrence, B., *Clary Sage Oil.* Perfumer & Flavorist, Oct/Nov 1986, Vol. 11, No. 5, p.111.

3. Holmes, P., *Clary Sage.* IJA. Vol. 5, No. 1, (1993), pp.15-17.

4. Lawrence, B., *Clary Sage.* Perfumer & Flavorist, Vol. 11, No. 5, Oct/Nov 1986, p.111.

5. Lawless, J., *The Essential Oil Catalogue.* Aqua Oleum, Great Britain, (1983).

6. Suskind, P., *Perfume.* Penguin Books, Great Britain, (1986).

7. Wilde, P., *In Profile.* IJA. Vol. 6. No. 2 (1994), pp.3-7.

Chapter 5 Quality Control and Assurance

1. Fleischner, A.M., *Plant extracts: to accelerate healing and reduce inflammation.* Cosmetic Toilet, Vol. 100, (1985), pp.45-58.

2. Carle, R., et al., *The medicinal use of Matricaria Flos.* Br J. Phytother 2, Vol. 4, (1992), pp.147-153.

3. Gershbein, L., *Regeneration of rat liver in the presence of essential oils and their components.* Food Cosmet Toxicol, Vol. 15, No. 3, (1977), pp.173-182.

4. Deans, S.G., et al., *Antibacterial properties of plant essential oils.* International Journal Food Microbiology, Vol. 5, (1987), pp.165-180.

5. Lawrence, B., *Chamomile Oil, Wild.* Perfumer & Flavorist, April/May, Vol. 11, No. 2, (1986), p.75.

6. Lavabre, M., *Aromatherapy Workbook.* Healing Art Press, USA, (1990).

7. Buckle, J. *Aromatherapy. Does it matter which lavender essential oil is used?* Nursing Times 89(20), (1993) pp.32-35.

8. Soulier, J., *The Thymus Genus.* Aromatherapy Records, No.1, September, (1995), pp.38-49.

9. Lawrence, B., *Marjoram Oil.* Perfumer & Flavorist, October/November 1981 Vol. 6, No. 5, p.27.

10. Lavabre, M.,*Aromatherapy Work Book,* Healing Arts Press. Rochester, Vermont, (1990) p.128.

11. Lawrence, B., *Spanish Marjoram Oil.* Perfumer & Flavorist, June/July 1980 Vol. 5, No. 3, p. 63.

12. Lawless, J., *The Encyclopedia of Essential Oils.* Element Books Limited Great Britain, (1992) pp.164-165.

13. Lawrence, B., *Sage Oil.* Perfumer & Flavorist, February/March 1980 Vol. 5, No. 1, p. 55.

14. Lawrence, B., *Spanish Sage Oil.* Perfumer & Flavorist, October/November 1980 Vol. 5, No. 6, p. 27.

15. Lassak, E.V., *Australian Medicinal Plants.* Methuen Australia, (1983) p. 195.

16. Beylier, M.F., *Proceedings of the 10th I.F.S.C.C. Congress.* Sydney, (1978).

17. Stahl-Biskup, E., *The Chemical Composition of Thymus Oils.* The Journal of Essential Oil Research. Vol. 3, No. 2 March/April 1991, p.61.

18. Soulier, J., *Thyme Folder.* Aromatherapie Records, September 1995, No 1., pp.38-49.

19. Stahl-Biskup, E., *The Chemical Composition of Thymus Oils.* The Journal of Essential Oil Research. Vol. 3, No. 2 March/April 1991, p.65.

20. Soulier, J., *The Thymus Genus.* Aromatherapy Records, No.1, September, (1995), pp.38-49.

21. Lawrence, B., *Basil Oil.* Perfumer & Flavorist December/January 1980, Vol. 4, No. 6, p. 31.

22. Lawrence, B., *Rosemary Oil.* Perfumer & Flavorist December/January, 1982/1983, Vol. 7, No. 6, p. 20.

23. Lawrence, B., *Ylang Ylang.* Perfumer & Flavorist, Oct/Nov, 1986, Vol. 11, No. 5, p. 195.

24. Lawrence, B., *Adulteration of an Oil.* Perfumer & Flavorist, Oct/Nov, 1980, Vol. 5, No. 6, p.27.

25. Brud, W., *Blending and Compounding.* AROMA'93 Conference Proceedings. IJA. pp.44-54.

26. Fraisse, C.S., et al. *SPECMA Bank Applications of the Study of Geranium Oils of Various Origins.* IXth International Essential Oil Congress, Singapore (1983).

27. Tisserand, R. *The Art of Aromatherapy*, C.W. Daniel, London (1985).

28. Muller, J., et al. *The H&R Book of Perfume.* Johnson Publishers, London (1984).

29. Dodd, G.H., *Perfume Oils and Aromatherapy.:Perfumery: The psychology and biology of fragrance.* Chapman & Hall London (1988). pp. 27-30.

30. *Ibid.*

Chapter 6 Research

1. Benor, D., *Healing Research Vol. 1.* Helix Editions Ltd. London (1993).

2. Woolfson, A., and Hewitt, D., *Intensive Aromacare.* IJA, Vol. 4, No. 2, (1992), pp.12-13.

3. Rangelov, A., et al, *Experimental study of the cholagogic and choleretic action of some of the basic constituents of essential oils on laboratory animals.* Folia Med (Plovdiv) Vol. 30, No. 4, (1988), pp.30-38.

4. Jager, W., et al, *Evidence of the Sedative Effect of Neroli oil, Citronellal and Phenylethyl Acetate on Mice.* J. EE. Oil Res., Vol.4. No.4, July/August, 1992, pp.381-385.

5. Aldridge, D., *Clinical Research Methodology For Complementary Therapies.* Hodder & Stoughton, Great Britain, (1993).

6. Stevenson, C., *Orange Blossom Evaluation,* I.J.A Vol. 4. No. 3, (1992).

7. Mills, S., *Out of the Earth.* Penguin Group, England, (1991).

8. Jager, W., et al, *Evidence of the Sedative Effect of Neroli oil, Citronellal and Phenylethyl Acetate on Mice.,* J. EE. Oil Res., Vol. 4. No. 4, July/August, 1992, pp.381- 385.

Chapter 7 Essential Oil Chemistry

1. Price, S., *Shirley Price's Aromatherapy Workbook.* Thorsons, Great Britain, (1993).

2. Lassak, E., *Australian Medicinal Plants.* Methuen, Australia, (1983).

3. Tisserand, R., & Balacs, T., *Essential Oil Safety*. Churchill Livingstone, UK, (1995).

4. Cited from Mediherb Monitor, No. 7, December 1993.

5. Schnaubelt, K., *Friendly Molecules*. IJA, Vol. 2, No. 2, (1989), pp.20-23.

6. Knobloch, K., et al, *Antibacterial and Antifungal Properties of Essential Oil Components*, J. Ess. Oil Res. 1, (May/June 1989), pp.119-128.

7. Bowles, E.J., *The Basic Chemistry of Aromatherapeutic Essential Oils*. Australia, (1991).

8. Knobloch, K., et al, *Antibacterial and Antifungal Properties of Essential Oil Components*, J. Ess. Oil Res. 1, (May/June 1989), pp.119-128.

9. Jager, W., et al, *Evidence of the Sedative Effect of Neroli Oil, Citronellal and Phenylethyl Acetate on Mice.*, J. EE. Oil Res., Vol. 4., No. 4, (July/August 1992), pp.381-385.

10. Isaac, O., *Pharmacological investigations with compounds of chamomile.* , Planta Med 35 (1979), pp.188-194.

11. Lassak, E.V., *Australian Medicinal Plants*. Methuen Australia Pty Ltd., Australia, (1983), p.99.

12. Buchbauer, G., et al, *Evidence of the sedative effect of neroli, citronellal and phenylethyl acetate on mice*. J. Essent. Oil Res., Vol. 4, No. 4, (Jul/Aug 1992), pp.387-394.

13. Onawunmi, G.O., *Antifungal activity of lemongrass*. Int. J. Crude Drug Research, Vol. 27, No. 2, (1989), pp.121-126.

14. Lavabre, M., *Aromatherapy Workbook*. Healing Art Press, USA, (1990).

15. International School of Aromatherapy. *A safety guide on the use of essential oils*. Nature by Nature Oils Ltd, (1993), p.61.

16. Penoel, D., *Winter Shield*. I.J.A. Vol. 4, No. 4, UK, (1992), pp.10-12.

Chapter 8 Traditional Pharmacology

1. Gennis, F., *Alternative Roads to Hell?* Nursing Standard, Vol. 6, No. 44, July 22 (1992), pp.42-3.

2. Long, N., *Business is booming for alternative treatments*. The Weekend Independent, August 11 to 24, 1995, p.14.

3. Holmes, P., *The Energetics of Western Herbs*. Artemis Press, USA, (1986).

4. Mills, S., *Out of the Earth*. Viking Arkana, England (1991).

5. Buchbauer, G., Jirovetz, L., Jager, W., Dietrich, H., Plank, C., *Aromatherapy: evidence for sedative effects of the essential oil of lavender after inhalation*. Z Naturforsch C Nov - Dec; 46(11-12), (1991) pp.1067-1072.

6. Jager, W., et al, *Evidence of the Sedative Effect of Neroli Oil, Citronellal and Phenylethyl Acetate on Mice*. J. EE. Oil Res., Vol. 4. No. 4 (July/August, 1992), pp.381-385.

7. Tisserand, R., *POP'91 Conference Report*. IJA Vol. 3, No. 3, (1991), p.10.

8. Della Loggia, R., *Paper presented at the 24th International Symposium on Essential Oils,* Berlin, (1993).

9. Isaac, O., *Pharmacological investigations with compounds of chamomile*. Planta Med 35, (1979) pp.188-124.

10. Wagner, H., Wierer, M., Bauer, R., *In vitro inhibition of prostaglandin biosynthesis by essential oils and phenolic compounds*. Planta Med Jun:(3) (1986) pp.184-187.

11. Merk, H., *Dermatopharmacological Properties of Eugenol and Eugenol Containing Oils*. 24th International Symposium Essential Oils. Programme Abstracts. (1993).

12. Valnet, J., *The Practice of Aromatherapy*. Healing Art Press, (1980).

13. Penfold, A.R., and Grant, R., Journal and Proceedings of the Royal Society of New South Wales, (1923), pp.57-80.

14. Knobloch, K., et al, *Antibacterial and Antifungal Properties of Essential Oil Components.* J. Ess. Oil Res. 1, (May/June, 1989), pp.119-128.

15. Larrondo, J.V., Calvo, M.A., *Effect of essential oils on candida albicans: a scanning electron microscope study.* Biomed Letters 46:184 (1991), pp.269-272.

16. Department of Genito-urinary Medicine, Swansea, *Tea tree oil and anaerobic (bacterial) vaginosis.* Lancet 337(8736) (1991), p.300.

17. Pena, E.F., *Melaleuca alternifolia: Its use for trichomonal vaginitis and other vaginal infections.* Obstet Gynecol 19(6), (1962) p.7.

18. Bassett, I.B., Pannowitz, D.L., Barnetson, R.S., *A comparative study of tea tree oil versus benzoyl peroxide in the treatment of acne.* Medical J Aust Oct 15, 1990; 153(8) pp.455-458.

19. Hmamouch, M., *Illustration of antibacterial and antifungal properties of eucalpytus oils.* Plantes Med Phytotherapie, 24(4) (1990) pp.278-289.

20. Rangelov, A., Pisanetz, M., Toreva, D., Kosev, R., *Experimental study of the cholagogic and choleretic action of some of the basic constitiuents of essential oils on laboratory animals.* Folia Med (Plovdiv) 30(4), (1988) pp.30-38.

21. Rangelov, A., *An experimental characterisation of cholagogic and cholesteric activity of a group of essential oils.* Folia Med (Plovdiv) 31(I), (1989) pp.46-53.

22. Mills, S., *Dictionary of Modern Herbalism.* Lothian Publishing Company Pty Ltd, UK, (1985).

23. Cited from Mediherb Monitor No.7 December, 1993.

24. *Ibid.*

25. Schafer, D., Schafer, W., *Pharmacological studies with an oinment containing menthol, camphene and essential oils for broncholytic and secretolytic effects.* Arzeimittelforschung 31(I), (1981) pp.82-86.

26. Glowania, H.J., Raulin, C., Swoboda, M., *Effect of chamomile on wound healing - a clinical double blind study.* Z Hautkr Sept 1; 62(17), (1987) pp.1267-71.

27. Kloucek-Popova, E. et al, Acta *Physiologica et pharmacolgica.* Bugarica (8) (1982),p. 63.

28. Gattefosse, R., *Gattefosse's Aromatherapy.* C.W. Daniel. First published in French in 1937, reprinted in English in 1993.

29. Guillemain, J., Rousseau, A., Delaveau, P., *Neurodepressive effects of the essential oil of lavendula angustifolia mill.* Ann Pharm Fr 47(6), (1989) pp.337-343.

30. Buchbauer, G., Jirovetz, L., Jager, W., Dietrich, H., Plank, C., *Aromatherapy: evidence for sedative effects of the essential oil of lavender after inhalation.* Z Naturforsch C Nov - Dec; 46(11-12), (1991) pp.1067-1072.

31. Jager, W., et al, *Evidence of the Sedative Effect of Neroli Oil, Citronellal and Phenylethyl Acetate on Mice.* J. EE. Oil Res., Vol. 4. No. 4 (July/August, 1992), pp.381-385.

32. Henry, J., et al, *Lavender for night sedation of people with dementia.* International Journal of Aromatherapy, Vol. 6. No. 2, pp.28-30.

33. McKenzie, J., Gallacher, M., *A sweet smelling success: use of peppermint oil in helping patients accept their colostomies.* Nursing Times 85(27), (1989) pp.48-49.

34. Leicester, R.J., Hunt, R.H., *Peppermint oil to reduce colonic spasm during endoscopy.* Lancet Oct 30; 2(8305), (1982) p.989.

Chapter 9 The Biology and Psychology of Essential Oils

1. Kallan, C., *Probing the power of common scents.* Prevention No. 43, (1991), p.10.

2. Tisserand, R., *Lemon fragrance increases office efficiency.* IJA. Vol.1 No.2, p.2.

3. Steele, J., *Environmental Fragrancing.* IJA. Vol. 4. No.2, pp.8-11.

4. Hirsch, A., *Dollars and scents.* Glamour. (July 1991).

5. Tortora, G.J., *Principles of Anatomy and Physiology.* 4th Ed., Harper & Row, p.374.

6. Calvin, W., *Conversations with Neil's Brain.* Addison-Wesley Publishing Company. (1994), p.148.

7. Knasko, S.C., *Ambient odor's effect on creativity, mood and perceived health.* Chem Senses 17(I), (1992), pp.27-35.

8. Hines, D., *Olfaction and the right cerebral hemisphere.* Journal of Altered States of Consciousness, 3(1), (1977), pp.47-59.

9. Lawless, J., *Aromatherapy and the mind.* Harper Collins Publishers, U.K., (1994).

10. Gatti, G., and Cayola, R., *Azione terapeutica degli olii essenziali.* Rivista Italiana delle Essenze e profumi, 5(12), (1923), pp.133-5

11. Rovesti, P., *Aromatherapy and aerosols.* Soaps, Perfumery and Cosmetics, 46, (1973), pp.475-7.

12. Van Toller, S., et al, *Skin conductance and subjective assessments associated with the odour of androstan-3-one.* Biol. Psychol., 16, (1983), pp.85-107.

13. Lorig, T.S., et al, *Brain and Odor: Alteration of Human EEG by Odor Administration.* Psychophysiology No. 24, (1987), p.599

14. Watts, G.O., *Dynamic Neuroscience: Its Application to Brain Disorders.* Harpers and Row, New York, (1975).

15. Warren, C, & Warrenburg, S., *Mood Benefits of Fragrance.* IJA, Vol. 5, No. 2, (1993), pp.12-16.

16. Stoddart, DM., *The Scented Ape.* Cambridge University Press, New York, (1990).

17. Ehrlichman, H., and Bastone, L., *The use of odour in the study of emotion. Fragrance: The Psychology and Biology of Perfume.* (1992), pp.143-159.

18. Baron, R., *Environmentally induced positive effect: Its impact on self-efficacy, task performance, negotiation and conflict.* J of Appl. Soc. Psych. Vol. 16, (1990), pp.16-28.

19. Steele, J., *Brain research and essential oils.* Aromatherapy Quarterly, Spring 1984.

20. Torii, S., et al, *Contingent negative variation and the psychological effects of odour.* Perfumery: The psychology and biology of fragrance. Chapman & Hall, London, (1988), pp.107-120.

21. Klemm, W.R., Lutes, S.D., et al, *Topographical EEG maps of human responses to odours.* Chem Senses, 17(3), (1992). pp.347-361.

22. Van Toller, S., *Emotion and the Brain.* Perfumery: The psychology and biology of fragrance. Chapman & Hall, London, (1988), pp.140-3.

23. Buchbauer, G., et al, *Aromatherapy: evidence for sedative effects of the essential oil of lavender after inhalation.* Z Naturforsch C, Nov-Dec; 46 (11-12), (1991), pp.1067-72.

24. King, J.R., *Have the scents to relax?* World Medicine, 19, (1983), pp.29-31.

Chapter 10 Pharmacokinetics

1. Zatz, J., *Skin Permeation: Fundamentals and Application.* Allured Publishing Corporation. (1993).

2. Jager, W., et al., *Percutaneous absorption of lavender oil from a massage oil.* J. Soc. Cosmetic Chem, Vol. 43, No. 1, (1992), pp.49-54.

3. Buchbauer, G., *Molecular Interaction.* IJA Vol. 5 No. 1. (1993), p.11.

4. Balac, T., *Essential Oils in the Body.* AROMA '93 Conference Proceedings. IJA. (1993), p.13.

5. Zatz, J., *Skin Permeation: Fundamentals and Application.* Allured Publishing Corporation. (1993), p.15.

6. *Ibid*, p.116.

7. Klemp, P., et al., *Local variation in cutaneous and subcutaneous blood flow measured by CdTe(Cl) mini-detectors in normal and psoriatic skin.* J. Invest Dermatol, No. 86, (1986), p.109.

8. *Ibid.* p.116

9. Tisserand, R., and Balac, T., *Essential Oil Safety.* Churchill Livingstone, Uk, (1995).

10. Cronin, E., et al, *Percutaneous absorption, regional variations and the effect of hydration and epidermal stripping,* Br. J. Dermatology, Vol. 74, (1962), p.265.

11. Malkinson, FD., *Permeating the stratum corneum,* Ch XXI in Epidermis, W Montagna and WC Lobitz, Academic Press, New York, (1964).

12. Fritsch, WC., et al, *The effect of temperature and humidity on the penetration of C14 acetylsalicylic acid in excised human skin.* J. Invest. Dermatology, Vol. 41, (1963), p.307.

13. Bronaugh, R., et al, *Comparison of percutaneous absorptions of fragrances by humans and monkeys.* Food Chemical Toxicity, Vol. 23, No. 1, (1985),p. 111.

14. Loth, H. *Vehicular Influence on Transdermal Drug Penetration,* Int J Pharm. No. 68. (1991) pp. 1-10.

15. Breuer, M.M. *The Interaction between Surfactants and Keratinous Tissues.* J. Soc. Cosm. Chem. Vol. 30. (1979), pp. 41-64.

16. Yackovich, F., et al, *Validation of the agar patch test using soap bars which deposit different amounts of triclocarbon.* J. Society Cosmetic Chemists, No. 26, (1985), p.411-425.

17. Zatz, J., *Skin Permeation: Fundamentals and Application.* Allured Publishing Corporation. (1993), p.117.

18. Bickers, D.R., *The skin as a site of drug and chemical metabolism,* in Cutaneous Toxicity, V.A. Drill and P. Lazar, editors, Academic Press, New York, (1980).

19. Tisserand, R., and Balac, T., *Essential Oil Safety.* Churchill Livingstone, UK, (1995).

20. Zatz, J., *Skin Permeation: Fundamentals and Application.* Allured Publishing Corporation. (1993), p.117.

21. Danon, A., et al., *Effect of exercise and heat exposure on percutaneous absorption of methyl salicylate.* Eur J. Clin Pharmacol, Vol. 31, No. 49, (1986)

22. Buchbauer, G., et al, *Aromatherapy: Evidence for Sedative Effects of the Essential Oil of Lavender after Inhalation.* Z Naturforsch C Nov-Dec; 46 (11-12), (1991), pp.1067-72.

23. Falk-Filipsson, A., *d-limonene exposure to humans by inhalation: uptake, distribution, elimination, and effects on the pulmonary system.* J Toxicology & Environmental Health. No. 38, (1993), pp.77-88.

24. Kovar K.A.,et al, *Blood levels of 1,8-cineole and locomotor activity of mice after inhalation and oral administration of rosemary oil.* Planta Med Aug; 53(4): (1987), pp. 315-8.

25. Buchbauer, G., *Molecular Interaction.* IJA Vol. 5 No. 1. (1993), p.11.

26. Balac, T., *Essential Oils in the Body.* Aroma '93 Conference Proceedings, Aromatherapy Publications, UK, (1994), pp.11-20.

27. Zatz, J., *Skin Permeation: Fundamentals and Application.* Allured Publishing Corporation. (1993).

447

28. Jori, A., et al, *Effects of Essential Oils on Drug Metabolism.* Biochem Pharmacol Sept; 18(9), (1969), pp. 2081-5.

29. Tisserand, R., and Balac, T., *Essential Oil Safety.* Churchill Livingstone, UK, (1995).

30. Truitt, EB., et al, *Evidence of monoamine oxidase inhibition by myristicin and nutmeg.* Proceedings of the Society for Experimental Biology and Medicine. No. 112, (1963) p.117-120.

31. Reynolds, JEF., *Martindale: The extra pharmacopoeia.* The Pharmaceutical Press, London, (1993).

Chapter 11 Essential Oil Safety

1. Tisserand, R., Balacs, T., *Essential Oil Safety.* Churchill Livingstone, UK. (1995).

2. Wabner, D., *Purity and Pesticides.* IJA., Vol. 5, No. 2, pp.27-29.

3. Orafiduja L.A., *The effect of autoxidation of lemongrass oil on its antimicrobial activity.* Phytotherapist No. 7, (1993), pp.269-71.

4. Tisserand, R., Balacs, T., *Essential Oil Safety.* Churchill Livingstone, UK. (1995).

5. Australian Health Ministers' Advisory Council. *Standard for the Uniform Scheduling of Drugs and Poisons. No. 10.* Australian Government Publishing Service, Canberra, 1995.

6. Price, S., *Aromatherapy Workbook.* Thornsens, UK, (1993), p.123.

7. *Ibid,* p.74.

8. Tisserand, R., *The Essential Oil Safety Data Manual.* Tisserand Aromatherapy Institute, Brighton, England, (1988), p.22.

9. Schnaubelt, K., *Aromatherapy Course Notes.* Pacific Institute of Aromatherapy, USA, (1991).

10. Tisserand, R., *The Essential Oil Safety Data Manual.* Tisserand Aromatherapy Institute, Brighton, England, (1988), p.22.

11. *Ibid*

12. Tisserand, R., *New Perspectives on Essential Oil Safety.* Aroma '95 Conference presentation, July 1995.

13. Hotchkiss, S., *How Thin Is Your Skin.* New Scientist, 29th January 1994, pp. 24-27.

14. Tisserand, R., Balacs, T., *Essential Oil Safety.* Churchill Livingstone, UK. (1995), p.158.

15. Dragoco Report 7th May 1982.

16. *Study of Skin irritation caused by perfume materials.* Perfumer & Flavorist Vol. 4 No. 4 (1979).

17. Maury, M., *Marguerite Maury's Guide to Aromatherapy: The Secret of Life and Youth.* C.W. Daniel Company, First published in French in 1961, First published in English in 1964.

18. Tisserand, R., *The Essential Oil Safety Data Manual.* Tisserand Aromatherapy Institute, Brighton, England, (1988), p.52.

19. *Ibid*

20. *Perfumer & Flavorist.* Vol.1 No.2 (1976), pp.32-4.

21. *Hazardous Substances- Supplementary Definition of Strong Sensitisers.* (Aug.14th 1986) U.S. Federal Regulation.

22. Tisserand, R., Balacs, T., *Essential Oil Safety.* Churchill Livingstone, UK. (1995).

23. *The IFRA's guidelines and recommendations on citrus oils.* Perfumer & Flavorist Vol. 5 No. 1 (1980). pp.1-17.

24. Miller, J.A., *The metabolic activation and carcinogenicity of alkenylbenzenes that occur naturally in many spices.* Carcinogens and Mutagens in the environment.Vol. 1 (1982) pp.83-6.

25. Tisserand, R., Balacs, T., *Essential Oil Safety*. Churchill Livingstone, UK. (1995).
26. Tisserand, R., *The Essential Oil Safety Data Manual*. Tisserand Aromatherapy Institute, Brighton, England, (1988), p.50
27. Tisserand, R., Balacs, T., *Essential Oil Safety*. Churchill Livingstone, UK. (1995).
28. Mann, J., *Murder, Magic and Medicine*. Oxford University Press, USA, 1994.
29. Tisserand, R., Balacs, T., *Essential Oil Safety*. Churchill Livingstone, UK. (1995), p.72.
30. Del Castillo, J., et al, *Marijuana, Absinthe and the CNS*. Nature, No. 253, (1975), pp.365-366.
31. Truitt, EB., *The Pharmacology of Myristicin and Nutmeg*. Public Health Service Publications Washington No. 1645, p.215-222.
32. Weil, AT., *Nutmeg as a Narcotic*. Economic Botany, No. 19, (1965), pp.194-217.
33. Truitt, EB., et al., *The Pharmacology of Myristicin*. Journal of Neuropsychiatry. No. 2 (1961), pp.205-210.29.
34. Ryman, D., *Aromatherapy*. Piatkus, UK, (1991).
35. Balac, T., *Safety in Pregnancy*. IJA Vol. 4, No. 1, (1992), pp.12-15.
36. Tisserand, R., Balacs, T., *Essential Oil Safety*. Churchill Livingstone, UK. (1995).

Chapter 12 The Essential Oils

1. Lawrence, B., *Angelica Root Oil*. Perfumer & Flavorist, Dec/Jan 1977, Vol. 1, No. 6, p.31.
2. Grieve, M., *A Modern Herbal*. Penguin Books, Great Britain, (1984).
3. Fischer-Rizzi, S., *Complete Aromatherapy Handbook*. Sterling Publishing Co. USA, (1990)
4. Holmes, P., *The Energetics of Western Herbs. Vol. II*. Artemis Press, USA, (1989)
5. Lawrence, B., *Anise Oil*. Perfumer & Flavorist, June/July 1983, Vol. 8, No. 3, p. 65.
6. Jian-Qin Cu, et al, *GC/MS Analysis of Star Anise Oil*. J.Ess. Oil Res., (March/April 1990), p.91-92.
7. Lawless, J., *Aromatherapy and the Mind*. Harper Collins Publishers, (1994), p.118-9.
8. Holmes, P., *The Energetics of Western Herbs. Vol. II*. Artemis Press, USA, (1989), p.468.
9. Weiss, R.F., *Herbal Medicine*, Beaconsfield Publishers Ltd, England, (1988), p. 69.
10. Balacs, T., *Hormones and Health*. IJA.Spring 1993, Vol. 5, No. 1, pp.18-20.
11. Lawrence, B., *Basil*. Perfumer & Flavorist, December/January 1980, Vol. 4, No. 6, p. 31.
12. Lawless, J., *Aromatherapy and the Mind*. Harper Collins Publishers, 1994. p.120-1.
13. Holmes, P., *The Energetics of Western Herbs. Vol. II*. Artemis Press, USA, (1989), p.660.
14. *Ibid*. p.662.
15. Miller, J.A., et al, *The Metabolic activation and carcinogenicity of alkenylbenzenes that occur naturally in many spices*. Carcinogens and Mutagens in the Environment. Vol. 1. (1982) pp.83-6.
16. Tisserand, R., and Balac, T., *Basil & Methyl Chavicol New Data*. IJA. Vol. 3, No. 1 (1991).
17. Lawrence, B., *Bay Oil*. Perfumer & Flavorist, April/May 1980, Vol. 5. No. 2, p.33.
18. Lawrence, B., *Bay Oil*. Perfumer & Flavorist, November 1977, Vol. 2, No. 6, p.36.
19. Lawless, J., *Aromatherapy and the Mind*. Harper Collins Publishers, (1994), pp.122-1.
20. Lawrence, B., *Bergamot Oil*. Perfumer & Flavorist, October/November, 1982, Vol. 7, No.5, p.43.
21. Fischer-Rizzi, S., *Complete Aromatherapy Handbook*. Sterling Publishing Co. USA, (1990), pp.70-6.

22. Holmes, P., *The Energetics of Western Herbs. Vol. II.* Artemis Press, USA, (1989), p.466.

23. *A Safety Guide on the Use of Essential Oils.* Compiled by The International School of Aromatherapy. Nature by Nature Oils Ltd, UK. (1993), p.75.

24. Lawrence, B., *Major Tropical Spices - Pepper.* Essential Oils Journal 1979-1980. p. 141.

25. Lawless, J., *Aromatherapy and the Mind.* Harper Collins Publishers, (1994), pp.184-5.

26. Davis, P., *Subtle Aromatherapy.* C.W. Daniel Company, Great Britain, (1991), p.201.

27. Holmes, P., *The Energetics of Western Herbs. Vol. I.* ArtemisPress, USA, (1989), p.328.

28. Lassak, E.V., *Australian Medicinal Plants.* Methuen, Australia, (1983), p.38.

29. Williams, L., *The Composition and Bactericidal Activity of oil of Melaleuca alternifolia.* The International Journal of Aromatherapy, Vol. 1, No.3, p. 15.

30. Lawrence, B., *Major Tropical Spices - Cardamon: Essential Oils 1976-1978.* Allured Publishing, USA, pp. 105-155.

31. Lawrence, B., *Carrot Seed Oil.* Perfumer & Flavorist, August/September 1980, Vol. 5, No. 4, p.29.

32. Lawless, J., *The Encyclopedia of Essential Oils.* Element Books, Great Britain, (1992).

33. Fischer-Rizzi, S.. *Complete Aromatherapy Handbook.* Sterling Publishing Co, USA, (1990), pp.77-9.

34. Lawrence, B., *Virginian and Texan Cedarwood Oil.* Perfumer & Flavorist, June/July 1980, Vol. 5, No. 3, p. 63.

35. Lawrence, B., *Chamomile Oil.* Perfumer & Flavorist, February/March 1987, Vol. 12, No. 1, p. 35.

36. Harris, B., and Lewis, R., *Chamomile-Part 1.* IJACM, Vol. 12, No. 9, Sept 1994, p.12.

37. Holmes, P., *The Energetics of Western Herbs. Vol. II.* Artemis Press, USA, (1989), p.462.

38. Valnet, J., *The Practice of Aromatherapy.* Destiny Books, (1980), p. 105.

39. Isaac, O., *Pharmacological investigations with compounds of chamomile.* Planta Med, Vol. 35, (1979), pp.118-124.

40. Gershbein, L., *Regeneration of rat liver in the presence of essential oils and their components.* Food Cosmet Toxicol, Vol. 15, No. 3, (1977), pp.173-182.

41. Isaac, O., *Pharmacological investigations with compounds of chamomile. On the pharmacology of (-)-a-bisabolol and bisabolol oxides.* Planta Medica. Vol. 35. (1979), pp.118-124.

42. Grieve, M., *A Modern Herbal.* Penguin Books Ltd., England, (1931).

43. Lawrence, B., *Roman Chamomile Oil.* Perfumer & Flavorist, April/May 1981, Vol. 6, No. 2, p. 59.

44. Fischer-Rizzi, S., *Complete Aromatherapy Handbook.* Sterling Publishing Co., USA, (1990), pp.80-5.

45. Lawless, J., *Aromatherapy and the Mind.* Harper Collins Publishers, (1994), pp.133-5.

46. Fleichner, A. M., *Plant extracts: to accelerate healing and reduce inflammation.* Cosmet toilet, Vol. 100, (1985), pp.45-58.

47. Mc George, B.C., et al., *Allergic Contact Dermatitis of the Nipple from Roman Chamomile Ointment.* Contact Dermatitis, Vol. 24., No. 2, (1991), pp.139-140.

48. Lawrence, B., *Cinnamon Leaf and Bark Oil.* Perfumer & Flavorist, August/September 1978.Vol. 3, No. 4, p.54.

49. Valnet, J., *The Practice of Aromatherapy.* Destiny Books, (1980), p. 110.

50. Holmes, P., *The Energetics of Western Herbs. Vol. I.* Artemis Press, USA, (1989), p.335.

51. Lawrence, B., *Citronella Oil.* Perfumer & Flavorist, June/July 1985, Vol. 10 No. 3, p. 27.

52. Lawrence, B., *Clary Sage Oil.* Perfumer & Flavorist, October/November 1986, Vol. 11, No. 5, p. 111.

53. Holmes, P., *Clary Sage.* IJA., Vol. 5, No. 1, (1993), pp.15-17.

54. Davis, P., *Subtle Aromatherapy.* C.W. Daniel Company, Great Britain, (1991), p.202.

55. Fischer-Rizzi, S., *Complete Aromatherapy Handbook.* Sterling Publishing Co. USA, (1990), pp.86-90.

56. Burns, E., and Blamey, C., *Soothing scents in childbirth.* IJA, Vol. 6, No. 1, pp.24-28.

57. Lawrence, B., *Major Tropical Spices - Clove.* Essential Oils: 1976-19 77. Allured Publishing Corporation, (1979), pp.84-145.

58. Cited from Schnaubelt, K., *Aromatherapy Course. Part III,* Pacific Institute of Aromatherapy, San Rafael, CA, p.14.

59. Hartnoll, G., et al, *Near fatal ingestion of oil of clove.* Arch. Diseases in Childhood. Vol. 69, (1993), pp.392-393.

60. Tisserand, R., *Essential Oil Safety.* Churchill Livingstone, UK, 1995.

61. Lawrence, B., *Cypress Oil,* Perfumer & Flavorist, December/January 1977, Vol. 1, No. 6, p. 31.

62. Fischer-Rizzi, S., *Complete Aromatherapy Handbook.* Sterling Publishing Co. USA, (1990), pp.91-93.

63. Davis, P., *Subtle Aromatherapy.* C.W. Daniel Company, Great Britain, (1991), p.203.

64. Boland, D.J., *Eucalyptus Leaf Oils.* Inkata Press, Australia, (1991).

65. Lassak, E.V., McCarthy, T., *Australian Medicinal Plants.* Methuen, Australia, (1983).

66. *Ibid.*

67. Boland, D.J., *Eucalyptus Leaf Oils.* Inkata Press, Australia, (1991).

68. Holmes, P., *The Energetics of Western Herbs: Vol. I.* Artemis, Boulder, USA, (1989).

69. Valnet, J., *The Practice of Aromatherapy.* Destiny Books, (1980).

70. Lassak, E.V., McCarthy, T., *Australian Medicinal Plants.* Methuen, Australia, (1983).

71. Cited by Dr Lyall Williams, *Australian Eucalyptus Oils.* Simply Essential, No.12, April (1994), pp.21-5.

72. Lassak, E.V., McCarthy, T., *Australian Medicinal Plants.* Methuen, Australia, (1983).

73. Valnet, J., *The Practice of Aromatherapy.* Destiny Books. 1980. p. 122.

74. Penoel, D., *Winter Shield.* IJA. Vol.4, No.4, (1992), pp.10-12.

75. *Ibid.*

76. Lawless, J., *The Encyclopedia of Essential Oils.* Element, Great Britain, (1992), p.95.

77. Lassak, E.V., McCarthy, T., *Australian Medicinal Plants.* Methuen, Australia, (1983), p.47.

78. Lawrence, B., *Everlasting Oil.* Perfumer & Flavorist, Febuary/March 1978, Vol. 3, No. 1, p. 54.

79. Fischer-Rizzi, S., *Complete Aromatherapy Handbook.* Sterling Publishing Co., USA, (1990), pp.100-3.

80. Lawless, J., *Aromatherapy and the Mind.* Harper Collins Publishers, (1994), p.154.

81. Lawrence, B., *Fennel Oil.* Perfumer & Flavorist, April/May 1979, Vol. 4, No. 2, p. 53.

82. Holmes, P., *The Energetics of Western Herbs. Vol. I.* Artemis Press, USA, (1989).

83. Balacs, T., *Hormones and Health.* IJA.Spring 1993, Vol. 5, No. 1, pp.18-20.

84. *Ibid.*

85. Lawrence, B., *Fir Oil.* Perfumer & Flavorist December/January 1979 , Vol. 3, No. 6, p. 54.

86. Lawrence, B., *Frankincense Oil.* Perfumer & Flavorist, Febuary/March 1982, Vol. 7, No. 1, p.45.

87. Lawless, J., *Aromatherapy and the Mind.* Harper Collins Publishers, (1994).

88. Lawrence, B., *Geranium Oil.* Perfumer & Flavorist, October/November 1984, Vol. 9, No. 5, p.87.

89. Lawrence, B., *Ginger Oil.* Perfumer & Flavorist, February/March 1982, Vol. 7, No. 1, p. 30.

90. Holmes, P., *The Energetics of Western Herbs. Vol. I.* Artemis Press, USA, (1989), p.110.

91. Lawrence, B., *Grapefruit Oil.* Perfumer & Flavorist, December/January 1983, Vol. 8, No. 6, p.69.

92. Lawrence, B., *Hyssop Oil.* Perfumer & Flavorist, June/July 1984, Vol. 9, No. 3, p.35.

93. *Ibid.*

94. Lawrence, B., *Jasmine Oil.* Perfumer & Flavorist, November 1977, Vol. 2 No. 6, p. 36.

95. Fischer-Rizzi, S., *Complete Aromatherapy Handbook.* Sterling Publishing Co., USA, (1990), pp.104-9.

96. Lavabre, M., *Aromatherapy Workbook.* Healing Art Press, USA, (1990), p.69.

97. Lawrence, B., *Juniper Berry Oil.* Perfumer & Flavorist, December/January 1987/1988, Vol. 12, No. 6, p.59.

98. Davis, P., *Subtle Aromatherapy.* C.W. Daniel Company, Great Britain, (1991), p.209.

99. Cited from Mediherb Monitor. No. 7, December 1993.

100. Lawrence, B., *Lavender Oil.* Perfumer & Flavorist, December/January 1987/1988, Vol. 12, No. 6, p. 59.

101. Holmes, P., *Lavender Oil.* IJA. Vol.4, No.4, (1992), pp.20-2.

102. Tisserand, R., *The Art of Aromatherapy.* Destiny Book, USA, (1977), pp. 243-248.

103. Lawrence, B., *Spike Lavender Oil,* Perfumer & Flavorist, June/July, 1987, Vol. 12, No. 3, p 58.

104. Von Frohlich, E., *A review of clinical, pharmalogical and bacteriological research into Oleum spicae.* Wein Med Wochenschr Vol. 15, (1968), pp.345-350.

105. Lawrence, B., *Lemon Oil.* Perfumer & Flavorist, August/September 1984, Vol. 9, No. 4, p.37.

106. Tisserand, R., *Lemon Fragrance Increases Office Efficiency.* IJA. Vol. 1, No. 2, (1988), p.2.

107. Valnet, J., *The Practice of Aromatherapy.* Destiny Books, (1980), pp. 150-55.

108. Lawrence, B., *Lemongrass Oil.* Perfumer & Flavorist, June/July, 1984, Vol. 9, No. 3, p 35.

109. Buchbauer, G., et al., *Fragrance compounds and essential oils with sedative effects upon inhalation.* Journal of Pharmaceutical Science, Vol. 82, No. 6, (1993), pp.660-64.

110. Gumbel, D., *Principles of Holistic Skin Therapy with Herbal Essences.* Karl F. Haug Publishers, Germany, (1986), pp.200-4.

111. Orafidiya, LA., *The effect of autoxidation of lemongrass oil on its antibacterial activity.* Phytotherapy Res, No. 7, (1993), pp.121-26.

112. Steltenkamp, RJ., et al., *Citral: a survey of consumer patch-test sensitisation.* Food Cosmetic Toxicology, Vol. 18, No. 4, (1980), pp.413-17.

113. Lawrence, B., *Lime Oil.* Perfumer & Flavorist, August/September 1976, Vol. 1, No. 4, p 31

114. Lawrence, B., *Mandarin Oil.* Perfumer & Flavorist, August/September 1987, Vol. 12, No. 4, p 69.

115. Davis, P., *Subtle Aromatherapy.* C.W. Daniel Company, Great Britain, (1991), p. 211

116. Lawrence, B., *Sweet Marjoram Oil.* Perfumer & Flavorist, February/March 1984, Vol. 9, No. 1, p. 49.

117. Lawrence, B., *Spanish Marjoram.* Perfumer and Flavorist, June/July 1980, Vol. 5, No.5, No. 3, p.63.

118. Lawrence, B., *May Chang.* Perfumer & Flavorist, June/July 1981, Vol. 6, No. 3, p.46.

119. Tisserand, R., *May Chang.* IJA. Vol. 4, No. 3, (1992), pp.25-7.

120. Tisserand, R., *In Praise of Melissa.* IJA, Aromatherapy Publications, Vol. 1, No. 4, (1989), pp.10-11.

121. Lawrence, B., *Lemonbalm oil in Progress in Essential Oils.* Perfumer & Flavorist, Vol. 3 No. 4, (1978), p.58.

122. Fischer-Rizzi, S., *Complete Aromatherapy Handbook.* Stirling Publishing Co., New York, (1990).

123. Tisserand, R., *In Praise of Melissa.* IJA, Vol. 1, No. 4, (1989), pp.10-11.

124. Guenther, E., *The Essential Oils Vol. 4.* D Van Nostrand Company INC, New York, (1952), pp.344-348.

125. Ryman, D., *Aromatherapy.* Piatkus Publishers, Great Britain, (1991), p.151.

126. Lawrence, B., *Myrtle Oil.* Perfumer & Flavorist, June/July 1977, Vol. 2, No. 3, p.53.

127. Fischer-Rizzi, S., *Complete Aromatherapy Handbook.* Sterling Publishing Co. USA, (1990), pp.138-41.

128. Guenther, E., *The Essential Oils: Volume 3.* D Van Nostrand Company Inc, New York, USA, (1952), pp.228-245.

129. Fischer-Rizzi, S., *Complete Aromatherapy Handbook.* Sterling Publishing Co., USA, (1990), pp.142-5.

130. Stevenson, C., *Orange Blossom Evaluation.* IJA. Vol. 4, No. 3, (1992), pp.22-4.

131. Lassak, E.V., *Australian Medicinal Plants.* Methuen Australia, Australia, (1983), p.166.

132. Lawrence, B., *Nutmeg Oil.* Essential Oils: 1976-1978, Allured Publishing, USA, (1979), p. 51.

133. Bennett, A., et al, *The biological activity of eugenol, a major constituent of nutmeg.* Phytother Res, Sept, Vol. 2, No. 3, (1988), pp.124-30.

134. Truitt, EB., *The Pharmacology of Myristicin and Nutmeg.* Public Health Service Publications Washington No. 1645, p.215-222.

135. Weil, AT., *Nutmeg as a Narcotic.* Economic Botany, No. 19, (1965), pp.194-217.

136. Truitt, EB., et al., *The Pharmacology of Myristicin.* Journal of Neuropsychiatry. No. 2 (1961), pp.205-210.

137. Lawrence, B., *Orange Oil.* Perfumer and Flavorist, June/July 1987, Vol. 12, No. 3, p. 58.

138. Fischer-Rizzi, S., *Complete Aromatherapy Handbook.* Sterling Publishing Co., USA, (1990), p.146.

139. Lawrence, B., *Palmarosa Oil.* Perfumer and Flavorist, October/November 1987, Vol. 12, No. 5, p.54.

140. Lawrence, B., *Patchouli Oil.* Perfumer and Flavorist, August/September 1981, Vol. 6, No. 4, p.73.

141. Davis, P., *Subtle Aromatherapy.* C.W. Daniel Company, Great Britain, (1991), p.216.

142. Lawrence, B., *Peppermint Oil.* Perfumer and Flavorist, February/March 1986, Vol. 11, No. 1, p.29.

143. Gallacher, M., et al., *A Sweet Smell of Success.* Nursing Times July 5, Vol. 85, No. 27, 1989, p.48.

144. Leicester, R., et al., *Peppermint oil to reduce colonic spasm during endoscopy.* The Lancet, October 30, 1982, p. 989.

145. Gumbel, D., *Principles of Holistic Skin Therapy with Herbal Essences.* Karl F. Haug Publishers, Germany, (1986), pp.204-6.

146. Lawrence, B., *Petitgrain Oil.* Perfumer and Flavorist, December/January 1977, Vol. 1, No. 6, p.31.

147. Davis, P., *Subtle Aromatherapy.* C.W. Daniel Company, Great Britain, (1991), p.217.

148. Bauer, K., *Common Fragrance and Flavor Materials.* VCH., Germany, (1990), p.172.

149. Lawrence, B., *Cistus Leaf Oil.* Perfumer and Flavorist, August/September 1986, Vol. 11, No. 4, p.73.

150. Fischer-Rizzi, S., *Complete Aromatherapy Handbook.* Sterling Publishing Co., USA, (1990), pp.151-3.

151. Wabner, D., and Wurdack, I., *Rose Oil: Its use in Therapy and Cosmetics.* IJA Vol. 1, No. 4 and Vol. 2. No. 1 (1989), pp.28-31.

152. Fischer-Rizzi, S., *Complete Aromatherapy Handbook.* Sterling Publishing Co., USA, (1990), pp.154-9.

153. Holmes, P., *Rose: The Water Goddess.* IJA. Vol. 6, No. 2., (1994), pp.8-11.

154. Wabner, D., and Wurdack, I., *Rose Oil: Its Use in Therapy and Cosmetics.* IJA. Vol. 1, No. 4 and Vol. 2. No.1, (1989), pp.28-31.

155. Lawrence, B., *Rosemary Oil.* Perfumer and Flavorist, April/May 1986, Vol. 11, No. 2, p.75.

156. Davis, P., *A-Z of Aromatherapy.* C.W. Daniel Company, Great Britain, (1988), pp.291-4.

157. Lawrence, B., *Bois-de-Rose Oil.* Perfumer and Flavorist, Oct/Nov 1984, Vol. 9, No. 5, p.87.

158. Davis, P., *Subtle Aromatherapy.* C.W. Daniel Company, Great Britain, (1991), p.220.

159. Lawrence, B., *Sage Oil.* Perfumer & Flavorist, October/November 1984, Vol. 9, No. 5, p. 87.

160. Valnet, J., *The Practice of Aromatherapy.* Destiny Books, 1980, pp.181-3.

161. Lawrence, B., *Spanish Sage Oil.* Perfumer and Flavorist, December/January 1984/1985, Vol. 9, No. 6, p.61.

162. *Ibid.*

163. Chana, J., *Sandalwood Production.* IJA., Winter 1994 Vol. 6, No.4, pp.11-13.

164. Fischer-Rizzi, S., *Complete Aromatherapy Handbook.* Sterling Publishing Co., USA, (1990), pp.168-171.

165. Lawrence, B., *Spearmint Oil.* Perfumer and Flavorist, December/January 1977, Vol. 1, No. 6, p.31.

166. Lawrence, B., *Tangerine Oil.* Perfumer & Flavorist October/November 1980, Vol. 5, No. 6, p.27.

167. Morris, H., *A New Australian Germicide.* Medical Journal of Australia, 26 January 1930, p.417.

168. Williams, L., *The Composition and Bactericidal Activity of oil of Melaleuca alternifolia.* The International Journal of Aromatherapy, Vol. 1 No. 3, p.15.

169. Soulier, J., *The Thymus Genus.* Aromatherapy Records, No.1, September, (1995), pp.38-49.

170. Cunningham, S., *Magical Aromatherapy.* Llewellyn Publications Inc., USA, (1989).

171. Mailhebiau, P., *Approach to the Characterology of Thymes.* Aromatherapy Records, No.1, September, (1995), pp.57-60.

172. Valnet, J., *The Practice of Aromatherapy.* Destiny Books, (1980), pp.194-7.

173. Guenther, E., *The Essential Oils Vol. 4.* D Van Nostrand Company INC, New York, (1952).

174. Fischer-Rizzi, S., *Complete Aromatherapy Handbook.* Sterling Publishing Co., USA, (1990), pp.178-181.

175. Arcier, M., *Aromatherapy.* Hamlyn Publishing Group, UK, (1990), p.45.

176. Davis, P., *A-Z of Aromatherapy.* C.W. Daniel Company, Great Britain, (1988), p.223.

177. Holmes, P., *Vetiver.* IJA. Vol. 5, No. 3, (1993), pp.13-15.

178. Lawrence, B., *Yarrow Oil.* Perfumer and Flavorist, August/September 1984, Vol. 9, No. 4, p.37.

179. Fischer-Rizzi, S., *Complete Aromatherapy Handbook.* Sterling Publishing Co., USA, (1990), pp.182-185.

180. Lawrence, B., *Ylang Ylang Oil.* Perfumer & Flavorist, October/November 1986, Vol. 11, No. 5, p.195.

181. Fischer-Rizzi, S., *Complete Aromatherapy Handbook.* Sterling Publishing Co., USA, (1990), pp.186-191.

Chapter 13 Carrier Oils

1. Erasmus, U., *Fats and Oils: The complete guide to fats and oils in health and nutrition.* Alive Books, Canada (1986), p.104.

2. Krause, B.S., et al., *Food, Nutrition and Diet Therapy.* W.B. Saunders Company, USA, (1979).

3. Graham, J., *Evening Primrose Oil.* Thornsons Publishing Group, U.K, (1984).

4. Stanton, R, *Eating for Peak Performance.* Allen & Unwin, Australia, (1994), pp.19-20.

5. Erasmus, U., *Fats and Oils: The complete guide to fats and oils in health and nutrition.* Alive Books, Canada (1986), p.104.

6. *Ibid.* p.104.

7. Erasmus, U., *Fats that Heal, Fats that Kill.* Alive Books, Canada, (1993), p.113.

8. Erasmus, U., *Fats and Oils: The complete guide to fats and oils in health and nutrition.* Alive Books, Canada (1986), p.104.

9. *Ibid.* p. 95.

10. *Ibid.* p. 95.

11. Erasmus, U., *Fats that Heal, Fats that Kill.* Alive Books, Canada, (1993), p.113.

12. Earle, L., *Vital Oils.* Ebury Press, U.K, (1991).

13. Graham, J., *Evening Primrose Oil.* Thornsons Publishing Group, U.K, (1984).

14. Cited from *Research on Rosehip Oil.* Primal Nature Products, Australia.

15. Bone, K., *The real value of herbal preprations in cosmetic products.* 29th Annual Conference of the A.S.C.C., May 1994.

16. Kleinschmidt, H.E., et al., *Weeds of Queensland.* Queensland Department of Primary Industries, (1987), p.219.

17. Southwell, I.A., et al., *Hypericin content variation in hypericum perforatum in Australia.* Phytochemistry, No. 39, (1991), pp.475-478.

18. Cited from *Hypericum perforatum* in ATMS Newsletter, Issue 6, July 1993, p. 18.

19. Castleman, M., *The Healing Herbs.* Rondale Press, USA, (1991).

Chapter 14 Hazardous Essential Oils

1. Lawrence, B., *Ajowan Oil.* Perfumer & Flavorist April/May 1979, Vol. 4, No. 2, p.53.

2. *A Safety Guide on the Use of Essential Oils.* Compiled by The International School of Aromatherapy. Nature by Nature Oils Ltd, UK. (1993), p.96.

3. Lawrence, B., *Boldo Oil*. Perfumer & Flavorist February/March 1977, Vol. 2, No.1, p.3.

4. *A Safety Guide on the Use of Essential Oils*. Compiled by The International School of Aromatherapy. Nature by Nature Oils Ltd, UK. (1993), p.97.

5. *Ibid* p.130.

6. *Ibid*. p.95.

7. *Ibid*. p.95.

8. Lawrence, B., *Camphor Oil*. Perfumer & Flavorist August/September 1979, Vol. 4, No. 4, p.49.

9. *A Safety Guide on the Use of Essential Oils*. Compiled by The International School of Aromatherapy. Nature by Nature Oils Ltd, UK. (1993), p.61.

10. *Ibid*.

11. *Ibid*.

12. Lawrence, B., *Cassia Oil*. Perfumer & Flavorist August/September 1978, Vol. 3, No. 4, p.54.

13. Lawrence, B., *Cinnamon leaf and bark Oil*. Perfumer & Flavorist August/September 1978, Vol. 3, No. 4, p.54.

14. *A Safety Guide on the Use of Essential Oils*. Compiled by The International School of Aromatherapy. Nature by Nature Oils Ltd, UK. (1993), p.90.

15. Lawrence, B., *Major Tropical Spices - Clove*. Essential Oils: 1976-1978, Allured Publishing Co., USA, p.106.

16. *A Safety Guide on the Use of Essential Oils*. Compiled by The International School of Aromatherapy. Nature by Nature Oils Ltd, UK. (1993), p.79.

17. Balacs, T., *Research Reports*. IJA., Vol. 6, No. 2, (1994), p.33.

18. *A Safety Guide on the Use of Essential Oils*. Compiled by The International School of Aromatherapy. Nature by Nature Oils Ltd, UK. (1993), p.90.

19. *Ibid*.

20. Lawrence, B., *Horseradish Oil*. Perfumer & Flavorist, 1981, Vol. 6, No. 1, pp.45-6.

21. Grieve, M., *Modern Herbal*. Penguin Books, Great Britain, First published in 1931.

22. Lawrence, B., *Mugwort Oil*. Perfumer & Flavorist, 1989, Vol. 14, No. 3, pp.71-4.

23. Grieve, M., *Modern Herbal*. Penguin Books, Great Britain, First published in 1931.

24. Lawrence, B., *Oregano Oil*. Perfumer & Flavorist, 1989, Vol. 14, No. 1, pp.36-9.

25. Lawrence, B., *Parsley Seed Oil*. Essential Oils: 1981-1987, p.27.

26. Tisserand, R., and Balacs, T., *Essential Oil Safety*. Churchill Livingstone, UK. (1995), p.158

27. Lawrence, B., *European Pennyroyal Oil*. Perfumer & Flavorist, 1978, Vol. 3, No. 5, p.36.

28. Allen, W.T., Lancet No. 1, (1897) pp.1022-1023.

29. Vallance, W.B., Lancet No. 2, (1955) pp.850-851.

30. Buechel, D.W., et al, JAOA. 793, (1983) p.129.

31. Lewis, W., *Focus on American Pennyroyal*. IJA, Vol. 3, No. 2, (1991), pp.18-19.

32. Lawrence, B., *Rue Oil*. Perfumer & Flavorist April/May 1978, Vol. 3, No. 2, p.45.

33. *A Safety Guide on the Use of Essential Oils*. Compiled by The International School of Aromatherapy. Nature by Nature Oils Ltd, UK. (1993), p.88.

34. *Ibid*.

35. Lawrence, B., *Sassafras Oil*. Perfumer & Flavorist June/July 1978, Vol.3, No.3, p.46.

36. Tisserand, R., & Balacs, T., *Essential Oil Safety*. Churchill Livingstone UK, (1995), p. 168.

37. *A Safety Guide on the Use of Essential Oils.* Compiled by The International School of Aromatherapy. Nature by Nature Oils Ltd, UK. (1993), p.94.

38. *Ibid.*

39. Lawrence, B., *Savin Oil.* Perfumer & Flavorist August/September 198 2, Vol. 7, No. 4, p.41.

40. *A Safety Guide on the Use of Essential Oils.* Compiled by The International School of Aromatherapy. Nature by Nature Oils Ltd, UK. (1993), p.118.

41. Lawrence, B., *Savory Oil.* Perfumer & Flavorist August/September 1981, Vol. 6, No. 4, p.73.

42. Lawrence, B., *Tansy Oil.* Perfumer & Flavorist February/March 1976, Vol. 1, No.1, p.1.

43. *A Safety Guide on the Use of Essential Oils.* Compiled by The International School of Aromatherapy. Nature by Nature Oils Ltd, UK. (1993), p.83.

44. Lawrence, B., *Thuja Oil.* Perfumer & Flavorist February/March 1979, Vol. 4, No. 1, p.48.

45. Tisserand, R.. *The Essential Oil Safety Data Manual.* Tisserand Aromatherapy Institute, England, (1988), p.110.

46. *A Safety Guide on the Use of Essential Oils.* Compiled by The International School of Aromatherapy. Nature by Nature Oils Ltd, UK. (1993), p.117.

47. *Ibid.*

48. Tisserand, R., *The Essential Oil Safety Data Manual.* Tisserand Aromatherapy Institute, England, (1988), p.96.

49. *A Safety Guide on the Use of Essential Oils.* Compiled by The International School of Aromatherapy. Nature by Nature Oils Ltd, UK. (1993), p.97.

50. Tisserand, R., *The Essential Oil Safety Data Manual.* Tisserand Aromatherapy Institute, England, (1988), p.96.

51. *A Safety Guide on the Use of Essential Oils.* Compiled by The International School of Aromatherapy. Nature by Nature Oils Ltd, UK. (1993), p.97.

52. Lawrence, B., *Wormwood Oil.* Perfumer & Flavorist, (1992), Vol. 17, No. 2, p.32.

53. Turner, R., *Absinthe: The Green Fairy.* IJA (1992), Vol. 5, No. 2. p.6.

54. Del Castillo, S., et al., *Marijuana, Absinthe and the CNS.* Nature, Vol. 253, pp.365-366.

Chapter 16 The Consultation

1. Sapira, J., *The Art and Science of Bedside Diagnosis.* Williams and Wilkens, USA, (1990).

2. Harrison, J., *Love Your Disease: It's Keeping You Healthy.* Angus and Robertson Publishers, Australia, (1984).

Chapter 17 Guidelines to Prescribing

1. Bach, E., *Heal Thyself.* C.W. Daniel Company, First published in 1931, last published in 1994, UK.

2. Engen, T., et al, *Long term memory of odours with and without verbal descriptors.* Journal of experimental Psychology, Vol. 100, 1973, pp.221-7.

3. Classen, C., *Aroma: The Cultural History of Smell.* Routledge, London (1994).

4. Muller, J., et al. *The H & R Book of Perfume: Volume 1.* Johnson Publications Limited, England, (1984).

5. Stoddart, M., *The Scented Ape.* Cambridge University Press, Great Britain, (1990).

6. Mensing, J., and Beck,. C., *The Psychology of Fragrance Selection*. Perfumery: The Psychology and Biology of Fragrance. Edited by S. Van Toller and George H. Dodd, Chapman and Hall, UK, (1988), pp. 185-216.

7. Tisserand, R., *Essential Oils as Psychotherapeutic Agents*. Perfumery: The Psychology and Biology of Fragrance. Edited by S. Van Toller and George H. Dodd, Chapman and Hall, UK, (1988), pp.168-181.

8. Stoddart, M., *The Scented Ape*. Cambridge University Press, Great Britain, (1990).

9. Fischer-Rizzi, S., *Complete Aromatherapy Handbook*. Stirling Publishing Company, USA, (1990).

10. *Ibid*.

11. Mailhebiau, P., *The Characterology of Essences*. Aromatherapy Records, No.1, September, (1995), pp.54-56.

12. Schnaubelt, K., *Less is More*. IJA. Vol. 1, No. 3, p.4.

13. Tisserand, R., *The Art of Aromatherapy*. C.W. Daniel Company, U.K., (1977).

14. Holmes, P., *Lavender Oil*. IJA, Vol. 4, No. 2, (1992), pp.20-22.

15. Schnaubelt, K., *Less is More*. IJA. Vol. 1, No. 3, p.4.

16. Schnaubelt, K., *Aromatherapy Course Notes*. Pacific Institute of Aromatherapy, USA, (1991).

17. Jellinek, J.S., *Perfumery: Practice and Principles*. John Wiley & Sons, USA, 1994. p.88.

18. Appell, L., *Cosmetics, Fragrances and Flavors: Their Formulation and Preparation*. Novox Inc, USA, (1982).

Chapter 18 Methods of Application

1. Jager, W., et al, *Percutaneous absorption of lavender oil from a massage oil*. J. Soc Cosmetic Chemists, Jan-Feb 1992, Vol. 43, No. 1, pp.49-54.

2. Tisserand, R., *Essential Oils as Psychotherapeutic Agents*. Perfumery: The Psychology and Biology of Fragrance. Edited by S. Van Toller and George H. Dodd, Chapman and Hall, UK, (1988), pp.168-181.

3. Buchbauer, G., *Molecular Interaction*. IJA, Vol. 5, No. 1, (1993), pp.11-14.

4. Maury, M., *Marguerite Maury's guide to aromatherapy: The secret of life and youth*. First published in French as '*Le Capital Jeunesse*' in 1961. English version published by C.W.Daniel, UK. 1964.

5. Lassak, E.V., *Australian Medicinal Plants*. Methuen Australia Pty Ltd, Australia (1983), p.46.

6. Bardeau, F., *Use of essential aromatic oils to purify and deodorise the air*. Chir Dent France, (1976), Sept 29, Vol. 46, No. 319, p.53.

7. Maury, M., *Marguerite Maury's Guide to Aromatherapy: The Secret of Life and Youth*. First published in French as '*Le Capital Jeunesse*' in 1961. English version published by C.W.Daniel, UK. 1964.

Chapter 19 The Aromatherapy Massage

1. Chaitow, L., *Soft-Tissue Manipulation*. Thorsons Publishing Group. UK. (1988), p.32.

2. Ebner, M., Connective Tissue Manipulations. Robert E. Krieger Publishing Co. USA (1985), p.214.

Chapter 20 Circulatory and Cardiovascular System

1. Bennett, A., et al, *Sugar consumption and cigarette smoking.* Lancet, (1970), pp.1011-4.

2. Pelletier, O., *Smoking and vitamin C levels in humans.* Am J. Clinical Nutrition 21, (1968), pp.1254-8.

3. Stevenson, C., *Orange Blossom Evaluation.* IJA. Vol. 4. No. 3. (1992), pp.22-4.

4. Tisserand, R., *May Chang.* IJA. Vol. 4. No. 3. (1992), pp.25-7.

5. Janssens, J., et al, J. Enthnopharmacol. Vol. 29. (1990), pp.179-188.

6. Pizzorno, J., *A Textbook of Natural Medicine. Vol. II.* Bastyr College Publications, USA. (1993).

7. Petkov, V., *Plants with hypotensive, antiatheromatous and coronary dilating actions.* A.J. Chinese Med 7, (1979), pp.197-236.

8. Rao, R., et al, *Effect of polyunsaturated vegetable oils on blood pressure in essential hypertension.* Clin Exp Hypertension 3, (1981), pp.27-38.

9. Pizzorno, J., *A Textbook of Natural Medicine. Vol. II.* Bastyr College Publications, USA. (1993).

10. Holmes. P., *The Energetics of Western Herbs.* Artemis Press, USA. (1989).

11. Kuhnau, J., *The flavonoids. A class of semi-essential food components: Their role in human nutrition.* World Review Nutrition and Dietetics 24, (1976), pp.117-91.

12. Pizzorno, J., *A Textbook of Natural Medicine; Volume II.* Bastyr College, USA. (1993).

Chapter 21 Respiratory System

1. Gumbel, D., *Principles of holistic skin therapy with herbal essences.* Karl F. Haug Publishers, Germany, (1986), p.119.

2. Valnet, J., *The Practice of Aromatherapy.* Destiny Books, USA, (1982), pp.33-48.

3. Cited from Mediherb Monitor No. 7, December, 1993.

4. Haas, M., Schnaubelt, K., *Breathing Space.* IJA. Vol. 4, No. 4, (1992), pp.13-15.

5. Ogle, K.A., *Children with allergic rhinitis and/or bronchial asthma treated with elimination diet.* Ann Allergy, (1980), pp.377-81.

6. Garrison, R., Somer, E., *The Nutritional Desk Reference, Vitamin Research: Selected Topics.* Keats Publications, Canada, (1985), pp.93-4.

7. Tan, Y., Collins-Williams, C., *Aspirin-induced asthma in children.* Ann Allergy, Vol. 48, (1982), pp.1-5.

8. Vanderhoek, J., et al, *Inhibition of fatty acid lipoxygenases by onion and garlic oils.* Bioch. Pharmacol. Vol. 29, (1980), pp.3169-73.

9. Cyong, J., et al, *A pharmacological study of the anti-inflammatory activity of Chinese herbs.* Acupunc Electro-Ther Res Int, Vol. 7, (1982), pp.173-202.

10. Hay, L., *You can heal your life.* Specialist Publications, Australia, (1987).

11. Weiss, R.F., *Herbal Medicine.* Beaconsfield Publishers Ltd., England, (1988), pp.194-207.

12. Balch, J., *Prescription for Nutritional Healing.* Avery Publishing Group, USA, (1990), pp.113-114.

13. Hay, L., *You can heal your life.* Specialist Publications, Australia, (1987).

14. Balch, J., *Prescription for Nutritional Healing.* Avery Publishing Group, USA, (1990).

15. Harrison, J., *Love your disease: It's keeping you healthy.* Angus & Robertson Publishers, Australia, (1984), p. 136.

Chapter 22 Musculoskeletal System

1. Wagner, H., *Phytotherapy*. Vol. 9. (1988) pp.11-14.

2. Harrison, J., *Love Your Disease: It's Keeping You Healthy*. Angus and Robertson. Australia, (1984).

3. Osiecki, H., *The Physician's Handbook of Clinical Nutrition*. Bioconcepts Publishing. Brisbane, (1990), pp.17-19.

4. Darlington, L.G., et al, *Placebo-controlled, blind study of dietary manipulation therapy in rheumatoid arthritis*. Lancet, (1986), pp.236-8.

5. Leung, A.Y., *Encyclopedia of common natural ingredients used in food, drugs, and cosmetics*. John Wiley & Sons, New York, (1980).

6. Robbins, S.L., et al, *Pathologic Basis of Disease*. W.B Saunders, (1984), pp.1356-61.

7. Macleod, J., et al, *Davidson's Principles and Practice of Medicine*. Churchill Livingstone, United Kingdom, (1987), pp.582-6.

8. Osiecki, H., *The Physician's Handbook of Clinical Nutrition*. Bioconcepts Publishing. Brisbane, (1990), p.22.

9. *Ibid*. p.24.

Chapter 23 Reproductive System

1. Cabot, S., *Women's Health*. Pan Macmillan, Australia, (1987).

2. Worwood, V., *The Fragrant Pharmacy*. MacMillan, London, (1990).

3. Pizzorno, J., *Morning Sickness: A Textbook of Natural Medicine Vol. II*. Bastyr College Publications, USA, (1993).

4. Weinstein, B., *Oral administration of pyridoxine hydrochloride in the treatment of nausea and vomiting in pregnancy*. Am J. Ob Gyn, No. 47 (1944), pp.389-394.

5. FitzGerald, C.M., *Nausea and Vomiting in Pregnancy*. Br J. Med Psycho No. 57, (1984), pp.159-65.

6. Worwood, V., *The Fragrant Pharmacy*. MacMillan, London, (1990), p.271.

7. Guenier, J., *Essential Obstetrics*. IJA. Vol. 4, No. 1., (1992), pp.6-8.

8. Burns, E., and Blamey, C., *Soothing Scents in Childbirth*. IJA. Vol. 6, No. 1., (1994), pp.24-8.

9. Stadelmann, I., *Dedicated to Better Birth*. IJA. Vol. 4, No. 1., (1992), pp.9-11.

10. Abraham, G.E., *Nutritional Factors in the Etiology of the Premenstrual Tension Syndromes*. J. Repro Med. No. 28, (1983), pp.446-64.

11. *Ibid*.

12. Goei, G.S., et al, *Effect of Nutritional Supplement, Optivite, on Symptoms of Prementstrual Tension*. J. Repro Med. No. 28, (1983), pp.527-31.

13. Pizzorno, J., *Morning Sickness: A Textbook of Natural Medicine Vol. II*. Bastyr College Publications, USA, (1993).

14. *Ibid*.

15. Graham, J., *Evening Primrose Oil*. Thorsons Publishing Group, England, (1984).

16. Abraham, G.E., *Nutritional Factors in the Etiology of the Premenstrual Tension Syndromes*. J. Repro Med. No. 28, (1983), pp.446-64.

17. Mowrey, D., *The Scientific Validation of Herbal Medicine*. Keats Publishing, USA, (1986).

18. *Ibid.*

19. Osiecki, H., *The Physician's Handbook of Clinical Nutrition.* Bioconcepts Publishing, Qld, (1990).

20. Kearsley, E., *Female Menopause.* Tasmania, (1983).

21. Cabot, S., *Endometriosis.* What's News: The Newsletter of Women's Health Advisory Network, October 1993.

22. Worwood, V., *Silently Bleeding Tears.* IJA. Vol. 2, No. 4, UK, pp.16-17.

23. *Ibid.*

24. Worwood, V., *Fragrant Pharmacy.* MacMillan, London, (1990), p.301.

25. Kroker, G.F., *Chronic Candidiasis and Allergy.* Food Allergy and Intolerance, W.B. Saunders, Philadelphia, (1987), pp.850-72.

26. Worwood, V., *Fragrant Pharmacy.* MacMillan, London, (1990), p.309.

Chapter 24 Integumentary System

1. Beckham, N., *The Family Library Guide to Natural Therapies.* Greenhouse Publications, (1992) p.106.

2. Tubaro, A., et al, *Evaluation of anti-inflammatory activity of a chamomile extract topical application.* Planta Medica Aug; 50(4), (1984) p.359.

3. Glowania, H.J., *Effect of chamomile on wound healing- a clinical double-blind study.* Z Hautkr, Sept 1987; 62 (17). p.1262.

4. Bassett, I.B., *A comparative study of tea tree oil versus benzoyl peroxide in the treatment of acne.* Med J Aust. Oct 15; 153(8), pp.455-8.

5. Vogel, A., *Swiss Nature Doctor.* Druckerei und Verlagsanstalt, (1952) p.41.

6. Ayres, S., Mihan, R., *Acne Vulgaris: Therapy directed at pathophysiological defects.* Cutis 28, (1981) pp.41-2.

7. Kugma, A., et al, *Oral Vitamin A in Acne Vulgaris.* Int J. Dermatol 20, (1981) pp.278-85.

8. Michaelson, G., et al, *Effects of oral zinc and vitamin A on acne.* Arch. Dermatol., No. 113, (1977), pp.31-6.

9. Snider, B., Dieteman, D., *Pyridoxine Therapy for Premenstrual Acne Flare.* Arch Dermatol 110, (1974) pp.101-3.

10. Tubaro, A., et al, *Evaluation of anti-inflammatory activity of a chamomile extract topical application.* Planta Medica Aug; 50(4), (1984) p.359.

11. Weiss, R., *Herbal Medicine.* Beaconsfield Publishers Ltd, England, (1988) p.328.

12. Wright, S., et al. *Oral evening primrose improves eczema.* Lancet 2, (1982) p.1120.

13. Lee, T., et al, *Effect of dietary enrichment with EPA and DHA on in vitro neutrophil and leukotriene generation.* NEJM. 312 (1985) pp.1540-3.

14. Schnaubelt, K., *Aromatherapy and Chronic Viral Infections.* Aroma '93 Conference Proceedings, Aromatherapy Publications. England. (1994) pp.33-41.

15. Tisserand, R., *In Praise of Melissa.* IJA. Vol. 1, No. 4. (1988) pp. 10-11.

16. Brody, I., *Topical treatment of recurrent herpes simplex and post-herpetic erythema multiforme with low concentrations of zinc sulphate solution.* Br. J. Dermatol 104, (1981) pp.191-213.

17. Griffth, R., et al, *Relation of arginine-lysine antagonism to herpes simplex growth in tissue culture.* Chemotherapy 27, (1981) pp.209-13.

18. Pizzorno, J., *A Textbook of Natural Medicine. Vol. II.* Bastyr College Publications, USA, 1993.

19. Seville, R.H., *Psoriasis and Stress*. Br J. Dermatol, Vol. 97. (1977), p.297.

20. Bittiner, S.B., et al, *A double-blind, randomised, placebo-controlled trial of fish oil in psoriasis*. Lancet (1988) pp.378-80.

21. Parrish, J., *Phototherapy and photochemotherapy of skin disease*. J. In. Dermatol. (1988) pp.167-71.

Chapter 25 Nervous System

1. Breggin, P., *Toxic Psychiatry*. St Martins Press, USA, (1991).

2. Meares, A., *A Way of Doctoring*. Hill of Content, Australia, (1985).

3. Harris, R., and Lewis, R., *Psychophysiological Effects of Odour - Part 1*. JACM, Vol. 12, No. 1, (1994), p.16.

4. Harris, R., and Lewis, R., *Psychophysiological Effects of Odour- Part 2*. JACM, Vol. 12, No. 3, (1994), p.23.

5. Torii, S., et al., *Contingent negative variation and the psychological effects of odour. Perfumery: The psychology and biology of fragrance*. Chapman and Hall, UK, (1988), pp.107-118.

6. Buchbauer, G., *Aromatherapy: evidence for sedative effects of the essential oil of lavender after inhalation*. Z. Naturforsch c. Nov-Dec; 46, (1991), pp.1067-72.

7. Farrow, J., *Massage Therapy and Nursing Care*. Nursing Standard, Vol. 7, No. 17, (1990) pp.26-28.

8. Mills, S., *Out of the Earth*. Viking Arkana, England, (1991).

9. Mason, L., *Stress Reduction*. The Holistic Health Life Book, Penguin Books, USA, pp.127-130.

10. Tisserand, R., *Success with Stress*. IJA. Vol. 4, No. 2, (1992), pp.14-16.

11. Rovesti, P., *Aromatherapy and Aerosols*. Soaps, Perfumery and Cosmetics, 46, (1973), pp.475-7.

12. Price, S., *Aromatherapy Workbook*. Thorsons, (1993), p.179.

13. Breggin, P., *Toxic Psychiatry*. St Martins Press, USA, (1991).

14. Osieki, H., *The Physician's Handbook of Clinical Nutrition*. Bioconcepts Publishing, Brisbane, (1990).

15. Hardy, M., *Sweet Scented Dreams*. IJA. Vol. 3 No. 1. (1991), pp.12-13.

16. Henry, J., et al, *Lavender for night sedation of people with dementia*. IJA. Vol. 6 No. 2 (1994), pp.28-30.

17. Mowrey, D., *The Scientific Validation of Herbal Medicine*. Keats Publishing, USA, (1986), p.193.

18. Bone, K., *How to Prescribe Herbal Medicines*. Mediherb Pty Ltd., Australia, (1992), p.10.

19. Mowrey, D., *The Scientific Validation of Herbal Medicine*. Keats Publishing, USA, (1986), p.192.

20. *Ibid*. p.193.

21. Johnson, E.S., et al, *Efficacy of feverfew as prophylactic treatment of migraine*. Br Med J. Vol. 291, (1985), pp.569-73.

22. Egger, J., et al, *Is migraine food allergy?* Lancet (1982), pp.1-4.

23. Lenhard, L., *Acupuncture in the prophylactic treatment of migraine headache*. NZ Med J., (1983), pp.663-6.

24. Rubenstein, E., et al, *Scientific American Medicine*. Scientific American, NY, (1989), p.11.

25. Betts, T., Cited from presentation *Practical Experience of Using Aromatherapy in People with Epilepsy* at Aroma '95 Conference, July 1995, Guilford, UK.

26. Clouston, T., *Oils for Epilepsy*. IJA Vol. 3 No. 3. (1991), pp.22-23.

Chapter 26 Lymphatic System

1. West, C., *The Golden Seven Plus One.* Samuel Publishing Co, USA, (1981), p.40.

2. Gattefosse, R., *Gattefosse's Aromatherapy.* C.W. Daniel Company Limited, (1993), first published in France in 1937 by Girardot & Cie.

3. Mills, S., *Out of the Earth: The Essential Book of Herbal Medicine.* Viking Arkana, England, (1991).

4. Valnet, J., *The Practice of Aromatherapy.* Destiny Books, USA, (1980).

5. Schnaubelt, K., *Aromatherapy and Chronic Viral Infections.* Aroma '93 Conference proceedings, IJA, UK, (1994).

6. Gumbel, D., *Principles of Holistic Skin Therapy with Herbal Essences.* Karl F. Haug Publishers, Germany, (1986).

7. Chaitow, L., *Soft-Tissue Manipulation.* Thorson's Publishers Limited, England, (1988).

8. Nurhberger, F., and Muller, G., *So-called Cellulite: An Invented Disease.* J. Dermatol Surg Oncol, 1978, pp.221-9.

9. Scherwitz, C., and Braun-Falco, O., *So-called Cellulite.* J. Dermatol Surg Oncol, 1978, pp.230-4.

10. Hodgkinson, L., *How to Banish Cellulite Forever.* Grafton Books, UK, (1989).

Chapter 27 Immune System

1. Preston, R., *The Hot Zone.* Random House, New York, (1994).

2. Lemonick, M., *The Killers all Around.* Time magazine, Sept 12, 1994, No. 37, pp.58-65.

3. Begley, S., *The End of Antibiotics.* The Bulletin, April 19, (1994), pp.55-60.

4. Cited from The Courier Mail, *Tea tree oil answer to staph.* January 29, 1995, p.91.

5. Dwyer, J., *The Body at War.* Allen & Unwin, 2nd Edition, Australia, (1993).

6. Moyers, B., *Healing and the Mind.* Doubleday, USA, (1993).

7. *Ibid.*

8. Towers, M., *Mood Linked with Cancer.* The Courier Mail, 10 Feb 1995.

9. Moyers, B., *Healing and the Mind.* Doubleday, USA, (1993).

10. *Ibid.*

11. Mills, S., *Out of the Earth.* Viking Arkana, England, (1991).

12. Begley, S., *The End of Antibiotics.* The Bulletin, April 19, (1994), pp.55-60.

13. *Tea Tree Oil Answer to Staph.* The Sunday Mail, January 29 1995, p.91.

14. Penoel, D., *The Immune System of Mankind.* AROMA '93 Conference Proceedings, Aromatherapy Publications, UK, (1994), pp.111-9.

15. Hobbs, C., *The Echinacea Handbook.* Eclectic Medical Publications, Portland, (1989).

16. Bauer, R., and Wagner, H., *Echinacea species as potential immunostimulating drugs.* Econ Med Plant Res, Vol. 5, (1991), pp.253-321.

17. Mose, J., *Effect of echinacea on phagocytosis and natural killer cells.* Med Welt, Vol. 34, (1983), pp.1463-7.

18. Schnaubelt, K., *Potential Application of Essential Oils in Viral Diseases.* IJA. Vol. 1, No. 4., (1989), pp.32-5.

19. *Ibid.*

20. *Ibid.*

21. *Ibid.*

22. *Ibid.*

23. Mills, S., *Out of the Earth.* Viking Arkana, England, (1991).

24. Carle, R., and Gomaa, K., *The Medicinal use of Matricaria Flos.* Br J Phytother 2 (4), (1992), pp.147-157.

25. Isaac, O., *Pharmacological investigations with compounds of chamomile.* Planta Med, 35, (1979), pp.118-124.

26. Wagner, H., et al, *In vitro inhibition of prostaglandin biosynthesis by essential oils and phenolic compounds.* Planta Med, June Vol. 3, (1986), pp.184-187.

27. Osieki, H., *The Physician's Handbook of Clinical Nutrition.* Bioconcepts Publishing, Brisbane, (1990).

28. Mills, S., *Out of the Earth.* Viking Arkana, England, (1991).

29. McCarthy, P., et al, *Temperature greater than or equal to 40°C in children less than 24 months of age: A Prospective Study.* Pediatrics, Vol. 59, (1977), pp.663-8.

30. Pizzorno, J., et al, *A Textbook of Natural Medicine.* John Bastyr College Publications, USA, 1993.

31. *Ibid.*

32. Holmes, P., *The Energetics of Western Herbs: Vol. I.* Artemis Press, USA, (1989).

33. *Ibid.*

34. Davies, S., and Stewart, A., *Nutritional Medicine.* Pan Books, UK, (1987)

35. Greene, C., *Overcoming Allergies.* Transworld Publishers, Australia, (1993).

36. Pizzorno, J., et al, *A Textbook of Natural Medicine.* John Bastyr College Publications, USA, 1993.

37. Kroker, G.F., *Chronic candidiasis and allergy.* Food Allergy and Intolerance, WB Saunders, USA (1987), pp.850-72.

38. Leung, A.Y., *Encyclopedia of Common Natural Ingredients Used in Food, Drugs and Cosmetics.* John Wiley & Sons, New York, (1980).

39. Carson, C.F., et al, *The antimicrobial activity of tea tree oil.* Medical Journal of Australia, Vol. 160, (1994), p.236.

40. Belaiche, P., *Treatment of vaginal infections of candida albicans with essential oils of Melaleuca alternifolia.* Phytotherapy, Vol. 15, (1985), pp.13-14.

41. Williams, L., et al, *Oils of Melaleuca alternifolia.* IJA, Vol. 2, No. 4, pp.12-13.

42. Larrondo, J.V., et al, *Effects of essential oils on Candida albicans.* Biomed Letters, Vol. 46, (1991), pp.269-272.

43. Hmamouchi, M., et al, *Illustration of antibacterial and antifungal properties of eucalyptus oils.* Plantes Med Phytother, Vol. 24, No. 4, (1990), pp.278-289.

44. Soliman, F.M., *Analysis and biological activity of the essential oil of Rosmarinus officinalis.* Flavour & Fragrances Journal, No. 9, (1994), pp.29-33.

45. Onawumni, G.O., *Evaluation of the antifungal activity of lemongrass.* Int J Crude Drug Res, No. 27, (1989), pp.121-126.

46. Garg, S.C., et al, *Antifungal activity of some essential oil isolates.* Pharmazie, Vol. 47, (1992), pp.467-468.

47. Worwood, V., *The Fragrant Pharmacy.* MacMillan, UK, (1990).

48. Tisserand, R., *Myalgic Encephalomyelitis.* IJA. Vol. 2, No. 2., (1989), pp.14-6.

49. Pizzorno, J., et al, *A Textbook of Natural Medicine*. John Bastyr College Publications, USA, 1993.

50. Hoffman, R., *Tired All The Time*. Poseidon Press, New York, 1993.

51. *Ibid.*

52. Wilkinson, S., *ME and You*. Wellingborough, UK, (1988).

Chapter 28 Digestive System

1. Somerville, K. W., et al, *Delayed release peppermint oil capsules for spastic colon syndrome: a pharmokinetic study*. Br J. Clinical Pharmacology. Oct; 18(4), pp.638-40.

2. Rees, W. D., et al, *Treating irritable bowel syndrome with peppermint oil*. British Medical Journal Oct 6; 2(6194), pp.835-6.

3. Rangelov, A., *An experimental characterisation of cholagogic and cholesteric activity of a group of essential oils*. Folia Med (Plovdiv), 31(I), pp.46-53.

4. Mills, S., *Out of The Earth: The Essential Book of Herbal Medicine*. Penguin Group, England, (1991), p.52.

5. Harrison, J., *Love Your Disease: It's Keeping You Healthy*. Angus & Robertson Publishers, Australia, (1984), p.40.

6. Hay, L., *You Can Heal Your Life*. Specialist Publications, Australia, (1987), p.161.

7. Krupp, M.A., et al, *Current Medical Diagnosis and Treatment*. Lange Medical Publications, USA, (1980).

Chapter 29 Aromatherapy Skin Care

1. Maury, M., *Marguerite Maury's Guide to Aromatherapy: The Secret of Life and Youth*. First published in French as 'Le Capital Jeunesse' in 1961. English version published by C.W.Daniel, UK, 1964.

2. Tortora, G.J., *Principles of Anatomy and Physiology*. 4th Ed., Harper & Row (1984).

3. Begoun, P., *Blue Eyeshadow Should Still be Illegal*. Beginning Press, USA. (1988).

4. *Ibid.*

Bibliography

A Safety Guide on The Use of Essential Oils. Compiled by the International School of Aromatherapy. Published by Nature by Nature Oils Ltd, London (1993).

Arcier, M., *Aromatherapy*. Hamlyn Publishing Group. London. (1990).

Balch, J., *Prescription for Nutritional Healing*. Avery Publishing Group, USA, (1990).

Berkow, R., *The Merck Manual*. Merck Sharp & Dome Research Laboratories, USA, (1982).

Bettelheim, F. A., *Introduction to general, organic and biochemistry*. Saunders Golden Sunburst Series, USA, (1984).

Bowles, J., *The basic chemistry of aromatherapeutic essential oils*. Australia, (1991).

Campbell, N., *Biology*. The Benjamin/Cummings Publishing Company, USA, (1987).

Chaitow, L., *Soft-Tissue Manipulation*. Thorsons Publishing Group, Great Britain, (1988).

Davies, S., *Nutritional Medicine*. Pan Books, Great Britain, (1987).

De Haas, C., *Natural Skin Care*. Nature & Health, Australia, (1986)

Ebner, M., *Connective Tissue Manipulations*. Robert E. Krieger Publishing Co. USA, (1985).

Facetti, A., *Natural Beauty*. Ebury Press, London, (1991).

Gach, M., *Acupressure's Potent Points*. Bantam Books, USA, (1990).

Harrison, J., *Love your Disease: It's Keeping you Healthy*. Angus & Robertson Publishers, Australia, (1984).

Hay, L., *You Can Heal Your Life*. Specialist Publications, Australia, (1987).

Jackson, J., *Scentual Touch*. Henry Holt and Co., USA, (1986).

Juhan, D., *Job's Body: A Handbook for Bodywork*. Station Hill Press, USA, (1987).

Kaptchuk, T., *Chinese Medicine: The Web That Has No Weaver*. Hutchinson Publishing Group, UK, (1983).

Kenyon, J., *Acupressure Techniques*. Thorsons Publishing Group, UK, (1987).

Kushi, M., *How to See Your Health: Book of Oriental Diagnosis*. Japan Publications, Tokyo, (1980).

Lavabre, M., *Aromatherapy Workbook,* Healing Art Press, (1990).

Lawless, J., *The Encyclopedia of Essential Oils*. Element, Great Britain, (1992).

Little, K., *Kitty Little's Book of Herbal Beauty*. Penguin Books, UK, (1981).

Montagu, A., *Touching: The Significance of the Skin.* Harper & Row Publishers, USA, (1986).

Nice, J., *Looking Good Naturally.* Doubleday, Australia, (1986).

Osiecki, H., *The Physician's Handbook of Clinical Nutrition.* Bioconcepts Publishing, Brisbane, (1990).

Pizzorno, J., *A Textbook of Natural Medicine. Vol. I & II.* Bastyr College Publications, USA, (1993).

Professor Song Tian Bin, *Atlas of the Tongue and Lingual Coatings in Chinese Medicine.* Publication of People's Medical Publishing House, Beijing, (1981).

Theiss, B., and P., *The Family Herbal.* Healing Arts Press, Vermont, USA, 1993.

Thie, J., *Touch for Health.* Second Back Row Press Pty Ltd, NSW, (1979).

Tisserand, R., *The Art of Aromatherapy.* Destiny Books, USA, (1977).

Tisserand, R., *The Essential Oil Safety Data Manual.* Tisserand Aromatherapy Institute, Brighton, England, (1988).

Williams, D., *Aromatic Chemicals.* Perfumery Education Centre, Great Britain, (1980).

Williams, D., *Aromatic Materials from Natural Sources.* The Perfumery Education Centre, (1980).

Worwood, V., *The Fragrant Pharmacy.* MacMillan, London, (1990).

Botanical Index

A

Abies alba 164
Achillea millefolium 206
Acorus calamus 233
Agothosma betulina 233
Amyris balsamifera 47, 199
Andropogon citratus 175
Andropogon flexuosus 175
Andropogon martinii 187
Andropogon muricatus 205
Andropogon nardus 155
Angelica archangelica 140
Aniba rosaeodora 197
Anisum officinalis 141
Anthemis nobilis 42, 152
Arnica montana 228
Artemisia absinthium 242
Artemisia vulgaris 237

B

Bacopa monniera 367
Balsamodendrom myrrha 182
Boswellia carteri 165
Brassica nigra 237

C

Calendula officinalis 228
Cananga odorata 207
Candida albicans 93
Cedrus atlantica 43, 149
Cedrus deodorata 43
Chamaemelum nobile 152
Chamomile recutita 27
Chenopodium anthelminticum 242
Cinnamomum cassia 235
Cinnamomum zeylanicum 154, 235
Cinnamomun camphora 234
Cistus ladaniferus 192
Citrus aurantium 145, 184, 190
Citrus cinensis 187
Citrus limon 174
Citrus medica 176
Citrus nobilis 177
Citrus paradisi 167

(continued)

Citrus racemosa 167
Citrus reticulata 177
Citrus reticulata blanco 201
Cochlearia armoracia 236
Commiphora myrrha 182
Cupressus sempervirens 158
Cymbopogon citratus 175
Cymbopogon martinii 187
Cymbopogon nardus 155

D

Daucus carota 148, 229

E

Elettaria cardamomum 148
Eucalyptus citriodora 159
Eucalyptus dives 159
Eucalyptus globulus 159
Eucalyptus polybractea 159
Eucalyptus radiata 159
Eucalyptus smithii 159
Eugenia aromatica 157
Eugenia caryophyllata 157, 235

F

Foeniculum vulgaris 163

G

Gaultheria procumbens 242

H

Helichrysum angustifolium 162
Helichrysum italicum 82
Hypericum perforatum 229
Hyssopus officinalis 168

I

Illicium verum 141
Inula helenium 236

J

Jasminum grandiflorum 169
Jasminum officinalis 169
Juniperus communis 44, 170
Juniperus oxycedrus 44
Juniperus sabina 44, 240
Juniperus virginiana 44, 150

L

Laurus nobilis 144
Lavendula angustifolia 44, 171
Lavendula fragrans 44
Lavendula latifolia 173
Lavendula officinalis 44
Lavendula spica 44, 173
Litsea cubeba 180

M

Marjorana hortensis 45, 178
Matricaria chamomilla 42, 151
Matricaria recutita 151
Melaleuca alternifolia 202
Melaleuca cajuputi 147
Melaleuca leucadendron 147
Melaleuca quinquenervia 147
Melaleuca viridiflora 185
Melissa officinalis 180
Mentha arvensis 189
Mentha piperita 189
Mentha pulegium 238
Mentha spicata 200
Mentha viridis 200
Myristica aromata 185
Myristica fragrans 185
Myrtus communis 183

O

Ocimum basilicum 27, 142
Origanum marjorana 178
Origanum vulgare 238
Ormensis mixta 42

P

Panax ginseng 367
Pelargonium graveolens 27, 56, 166
Peumus boldus 233
Pimento racemosa 144
Pimpinella anisum 141
Pinus mugo 46
Pinus mugo var. *pumilio* 191
Pinus palustris 46, 191
Pinus strobus 191
Pinus sylvestris 46, 191
Piper nigrum 146
Pogostemon patchouli 188
Prunus amygdalus 232

R

Rosa centifolia 193
Rosa damascena 193
Rosmarinus officinalis 28, 195
Ruta graveolens 239

S

Salvia lavendulaefolia 46, 198
Salvia officinalis 27, 46, 197
Salvia sclarea 155
Santalum album 47, 199
Santalum spicatum 47
Sassafras albidum 240
Satureia hortensis 240
Saussurea lappa 236
Syzygium aromaticum 157

T

Tanacetum vulgare 241
Thuja occidentalis 44, 241
Thymus mastichina 46, 179
Thymus serpyllum 49, 203
Thymus vulgaris 28, 49, 203
Thymus zygis 203
Trachyspermum copticum 232

U

Unona odorantissimum 207

V

Vetiveria zizanoides 205

Z

Zingiber officinalis 167

General Index

A

abortifacients 133
absinthe 131
absolute 37
acne 93, 348
adulteration 55, 122
ajowan 232
alcohols 79
   monoterpene 79
   sesquiterpene 80
aldehydes 81
allergic reaction 128
allergies 398
almond oil, bitter 232
almond oil, sweet 220
alterative 90, 377
amenorrhoea 337
analgesic 314
angelica root 140
aniseed 141
ankle sprain 324
anti-inflammatory 91, 314, 346, 422
anti-microbial 346
anti-rheumatic 314
antibacterial 91, 303
antidepressant 358
antifungal 91, 377
antimicrobial 328
antiphlogistic 314
antiseptic 303, 421
antispasmodic 98, 303, 329, 358, 405
antiviral 377
anxiety 362
apricot kernel oil 220
Arcier, Micheline 21
arnica 84, 228
aromatherapist
   counselling skills 249
   personal hygiene and health 250
   professional ethics 249
   professionalism 248
   role of 248
aromatherapy

definition 4
   holistic 4, 89
   medical 10, 89
aromatherapy clinic
   equipment and products 251
   setting up 250
aromatherapy massage 282
   contra-indications 280
   guidelines 280
aromatherapy treatment
   dosage 266
   duration 266
arthritis 315
   osteo- 317
   rheumatoid 315
asthma 304
   atopic 304
   intrinsic 304
astringent 93, 293
atherosclerosis 215
autonomic nervous system 357
Avicenna 17
avocado oil 221

B

Bach, Dr 9, 263
backache 319
bacteria 386
bactericidal 377
barberry 401
base notes 269
base oils 113
basil 50, 142
   eugenol 50
   exotic 50
   methyl cinnamate 50
   sweet 50
bay 144
bergamot 145
bergaptene 84
black pepper 146
blending 268
blood sugar 366
blood-brain barrier 117

boils 347
boldo 233
bronchitis 307
   acute 307
   chronic 307
bruises 320, 325
buchu 233
bunions 321
bursitis 321

C

cade 44
cajeput 147
calamus 233
calendula 96, 228
camphor 234
cancer 130
candida 341, 400
canola oil 221
carbuncle 347
carcinogenesis 129
cardamom 148
carminative 94, 405
carpal tunnel syndrome 325
carrier oils 110
carrot infused oil 229
carrot seed 148
cassia 235
castor oil 215
catarrh 308
cedarwood 43
   Atlas 43, 149
   Himalayan 43
   Virginian 44, 150
cellulite 378
chamomile 42
   German 43, 151, 396
   Moroccan 43
   Roman 43, 152
chemotype 28
chilblains 294
Chinese medicine 422
cholesterol 215
chologague 406
chronic fatigue syndrome 401
cicatrisant 346
cinnamon 49, 154
   bark 49

leaf 49
cinnamon bark 235
circulatory stimulant 377
cistus 192
citronella 155
clary sage 155
cleansing 424
clinical research 62
clinical trial 63
   ethical considerations 67
   experimental research 67
   patient evaluation 65
   patient selection 64
   pharmacokinetic research 66
   pharmacological research 66
   problems with 65
   randomised 64
   single case studies 65
   types of 63
clove 49, 235
   bud 49, 157
   leaf 49
   stem 49
cohobation 33
cold pressed oils 219
colitis 406
concrete 36
constipation 407
contamination 122
contraindications
   dermal irritation 136
   epilepsy 136
   high blood pressure 136
   not to be used at all 136
   not to be used on skin 136
   pregnancy 136
costus 236
cotton seed oil 214
coughs 309
coumarins 84
cramps 322
cyanide 232
cypress 158
cystitis 342

D

degradation 122
depression 363

depurative 314, 377
dermatitis 349
dermis 112, 416
detoxifier 314, 377
diaphoretic 90, 94
diarrhoea 409
diet 292, 405
digestive system 404
Dioscorides 15
distillation 32
    cohobation 33
    fractional 34
    hydro-diffusion 35
    rectification 34
    steam 33
    water 32
    water and steam 34
diuretic 90, 94, 376
dosages 134
douche 401
dysmenorrhoea 337
dyspepsia 410

E

ebola virus 384
eczema 113, 349
EEG 106, 358
elbow sprain 325
elbow tendonitis 325
elecampane 236
elemicin 186
emmenagogue 90, 95, 329
emotions . . . . 103 - 104, 422
endometriosis 339
enfleurage 37
epidermis 112, 416
epilepsy 370
essential fatty acids
    linoleic acid 212
    linolenic acid 213
essential oil testing 52
    gas chromatography 54
    mass spectrometry 54
    odour evaluation 53
    optical rotation 54
    refractive index 54
    specific gravity 53
essential oils

adulteration 55
character of 265
definition 24
glands 24
hazards 125
natural versus synthetic 57
esters 83
ethers 84
eucalyptus 34, 42, 159
    blue gum 159
    blue mallee 159
    broad-leaved peppermint 159
    gully gum 159
    lemon scented 159, 162
    narrow-leaved peppermint 159
evening primrose oil 221
everlasting 82
excretion 119
exercise 292, 367
expectorant 90, 95, 304
expeller pressing 217
extraction processes
    distillation 32
    expression 30
    solvent extraction 36
    summary 40

F

fatty acids 210
    essential 212
    saturated 211
    toxic 214
    unsaturated 211
fennel 163
fever 375, 396
feverfew 370
finger sprain 325
fir needle 164
flatulence 412
floral waters 425
food flavouring 42
frankincense 165
functional groups 77
fungi 387
fungicide 347

G

galactagogue 329
garlic 296
gas chromatography 54
Gattefosse 5, 20
geranium 56, 166
German chamomile 151
ginger 167, 317
gotu kola 367
gout 322
granulation stimulation 96
grapefruit 167

H

hawthorn berries 296
hayfever 309
headaches 368
healing 62
helichrysum 162
hepatic 90, 406
hepatotoxicity 132
herbalism 10
herpes simplex 350
hip strain 325
Hippocrates 15
history
    China 15
    Egypt 14
    Greece 14
    India 15
    Middle Ages 17
    Middle East 15
hormones 132
horseradish 236
hybridisation 27
hydrogenation 216
hypercritical carbon dioxide extraction . . . 38
hypericin 229
hypericum 229
hypertension 294
hypertensives 293
hypodermis 418
hypotensives 293
hypothalamus 102
hyssop 168

I

immortelle 162
immune system
    non specific resistance 389
    specific resistance 389
immune-stimulant 304
incense 103
indigestion 410
infection 393
inhalation 116
insomnia 365
internal ingestion 10
intuition 265
irritable bowel syndrome 406
isomers 71
    cis-trans 72
    functional group 71
    optical 72
    positional 71
    structural 71
isoprene 73
italidone 162

J

jasmine 37, 169
jojoba oil 224
juniper 44, 75, 170

K

ketones 82, 124
Kirlian photography 58
knee synovitis 326
kyphi 14, 103

L

labdanum 192
lactones 84
lavandin 44
lavender . . . . 19 - 20, 44, 97, 171
    extraction of 51
    spike 44, 173
    true 44
laxative 90
leg sprain 326
lemon 174
lemongrass 81, 175
lethal dose 126
leucocytosis 377
liquorice root 306

life force 57
limbic system 102, 104
lime 49, 176
   cold pressed 49
   distilled 49
linoleic acid 212, 296
linolenic acid 213
linseed oil 224
liver 118, 376
lungs 302
lymph nodes 375
lymphatic 90
lymphatic massage 377
lymphatic stimulants 422
lymphoedema 381

M

macadamia oil 225
macerated oils 228
mandarin 177
marjoram 45
   Spanish 46, 179
   sweet 45, 178
massage
   acupressure 279
   autonomic nervous system 280
   benefits 8
   lymphatic 279
   neuromuscular 278
   polarity therapy 279
   reflexology 279
   shiatsu 279
   Swedish 278
Maury, Marguerite 21, 416
may chang 180, 293
meditation 358, 367
melissa 180
memory association 263
menopause 338
menstrual problems 334
mental fatigue 366
metabolism 118
method of administration
   bath 273
   compress 274
   creams and lotions 275
   dermal 110
   douche 275

ingestion 276
inhalation 116, 272
   massage 272
   ointment 275
   oral 116
   rectal 116
middle notes 269
migraines 369
moisturising 425
monoterpene hydrocarbons 74
mucociliary escalator 302
mugwort 133, 237
mustard 237
myalgic encephalomyelitis 401
myristicin 186
myrrh 182
myrtle 183

N

nausea 413
neroli 184, 293
nervine 97
nervines 293, 358
neurotoxicity 130
   convulsant 131
   psychotropic 131
niaouli 185
nutmeg 185, 293

O

oedema 296
olfaction 9, 100
olfactory bulb 101
olibanum 165
olive oil 225
oral ingestion 116
orange
   bitter 49
   sweet 187
organic chemistry 70
organoleptic testing 53
origanum 238
oxidation 75, 122
oxides 85

P

packaging and labelling 123
palmarosa 187
palpitations 297

Paracelsus 19
parasites 388
parsley seed 133
parturient 329
patchouli 56, 188
pennyroyal 133, 238
peppermint 98, 189
petitgrain 190
phagocytosis 389
pharmacology 7
phenols 78, 124
phenyl ethyl alcohol 34
Photosynthesis 25
pine 46, 191
    dwarf 46, 191
    long leaf 191
    longleaf 46
    Scotch 46, 191
pituitary gland 102
placebo effect 9
plague 19
post-natal care 334
post-natal depression 334
poultice 347
pre-menstrual syndrome 335
pregnancy 329
    varicose veins 331
    backache 330
    constipation 330
    exhaustion 332
    flatulence 331
    fluid retention 331
    haemorrhoids 331
    heartburn 332
    labour 333
    leg cramps 332
    miscarriage 333
    morning sickness 329
    safety 132
    skin problems 332
    stretch marks 332
prostaglandins 221
psoriasis 351
psycho-aromatherapy 103
pumpkin seed oil 226
purines 323

Q
Qi 58
quality control 41-57

R
rape seed oil 214
rectification 34, 42
remedy absorption 110
Rescue Remedy 333
resinoid 36
Rideal-Walker test 92
rock rose 192
rose 33, 193
rosehip oil 226
rosemary . . . . 19 - 20, 51, 195
rosewood 197
rubefacient 97, 293, 315, 422
rue 133, 239

S
safflower oil 226
sage 46, 133, 197
    clary 155
    Dalmatian 46
    Spanish 46, 198
sandalwood 20, 46, 199
    Australian 47
    Indian 47
    West Indian 47
sassafras 133, 240
savin 44, 133, 240
savory 240
sciatica 323
sebaceous glands 112, 418
sebum 422
sedative 97
sesame seed oil 226
sesquiterpenes 76
shingles 372
shoulder strain 326
Siberian ginseng 367
sinusitis 310
sitz bath 274
skin
    functions 110, 418
    hydration 113
    occlusions 113
    permeability of 112

physiology of 114
structure 110
structure of 416
types 418
skin reactions 127
  idiosyncratic sensitisation 129
  irritation 127
  photosensitisation 128
  sensitisation 128
skin types
  combination 420
  dry 419
  mature 421
  normal 420
  oily 419
  sensitive 420
slipped disc 325
smoking 293
solvent extraction
  different solvents used 37
  enfleurage 37
  hypercritical carbon dioxide 38
  of essential oils . . . . 35 - 36
  of vegetable oils 219
soporifics 359
soyabean oil 227
spagyric preparation 30
spasmolytic 97
spearmint 200
specific gravity 53
sports injuries 324
St John's wort 229
stimulant 98
stratum corneum . . . . 112 - 113
stress 293, 357, 359
stress management 107
sunburn 353
sunflower oil 227
suppository 116
surfactants . . . . 113 - 114
sweat glands 418
synthetic oils 57

T

T cell
  delayed hypersensitivy 390
  helper 390
  killer 390

suppressor 390
tangerine 201
tansy 134, 241
tea tree 202
tendonitis 324
teratogenesis 133
throat infections 311
thrush 341
thuja 44, 133, 241
thyme 48, 203
  red 49
  wild 49
tissue inflammation 395
tonic 98
toning 425
tonsillitis 312
top notes 269
toxicity
  acute 125
  chronic 125
  dermal 125
  hepatotoxicity 132
  oral 125
tryptophan 366
turpentine 191

U

ulcerative colitis 406
uterine tonic 329

V

Valnet, Dr Jean 20
varicose veins 297
vetiver 205, 266
viruses 384
vomiting 413

W

wheatgerm oil 227
wintergreen 11, 242
wormseed 242
wormwood 134, 242
wrist sprain 326

Y

yarrow 206
ylang-ylang 34, 207, 265
  extraction of 52